Child Abuse

Medical Diagnosis and Management

Child Abuse

Medical Diagnosis and Management

Second Edition

Editors

Robert M. Reece, M.D.

Clinical Professor
Department of Pediatrics
Tufts University School of Medicine
Director
Child Protection Program
Department of Pediatrics
The Floating Hospital for Children at New England Medical Center
Director
Institute for Professional Education
Massachusetts Society for the Prevention of Cruelty to Children
Boston, Massachusetts

Stephen Ludwig, M.D.

Professor
Department of Pediatrics
University of Pennsylvania School of Medicine
Associate Physician-in-Chief
The Children's Hospital of Philadelphia
Philadelphia, Pennsylvania

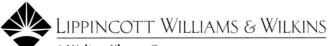

LIPPINCOTT WILLIAMS & WILKINS
A **Wolters Kluwer** Company
Philadelphia • Baltimore • New York • London
Buenos Aires • Hong Kong • Sydney • Tokyo

Acquisitions Editor: Timothy Y. Hiscock
Developmental Editor: Pamela Sutton
Production Editor: Donna Carty
Manufacturing Manager: Ben Rivera
Cover Designer: Mark Lerner
Compositor: Lippincott Williams & Wilkins Desktop Division

© 2001 by **LIPPINCOTT WILLIAMS & WILKINS**
227 East Washington Square
Philadelphia, PA 19106-3780 USA
LWW.com

Printed in China

Library of Congress Cataloging-in-Publication Data

Child abuse : medical diagnosis and management / editors, Robert M. Reece, Stephen Ludwig.--2nd ed.
  p. ; cm.
  Includes bibliographical references and index.
  ISBN 0-7817-2444-9
  1. Abused children. 2. Battered child syndrome. 3. Child abuse. I. Reece, Robert M. II Ludwig, Stephen, 1945–
  [DNLM: 1. Child Abuse. WA 320 C534202 2000]
  RJ375 .C48 2000
  617.1′0083--dc21

                                                                00-065521

Care has been taken to confirm the accuracy of the information presented and to describe generally accepted practices. However, the authors, editors, and publisher are not responsible for errors or omissions or for any consequences from application of the information in this book and make no warranty, expressed or implied, with respect to the currency, completeness, or accuracy of the contents of the publication. Application of this information in a particular situation remains the professional responsibility of the practitioner.

The authors, editors, and publisher have exerted every effort to ensure that drug selection and dosage set forth in this text are in accordance with current recommendations and practice at the time of publication. However, in view of ongoing research, changes in government regulations, and the constant flow of information relating to drug therapy and drug reactions, the reader is urged to check the package insert for each drug for any change in indications and dosage and for added warnings and precautions. This is particularly important when the recommended agent is a new or infrequently employed drug.

Some drugs and medical devices presented in this publication have Food and Drug Administration (FDA) clearance for limited use in restricted research settings. It is the responsibility of the health care provider to ascertain the FDA status of each drug or device planned for use in their clinical practice.

10 9 8 7 6 5 4 3 2 1

To my family.

RMR

To my family
Zella, Susannah and Mike, Elisa, and Aubrey for their love and support.

SL

Contents

Contributing Authors

Randell C. Alexander, M.D.   *Director, Center for Child Abuse, Morehead School of Medicine, Atlanta, Georgia*

Jan Bays, M D.   *Child Abuse Response and Evaluation Services, Emanuel Children's Hospital and Healthcare Center; and Clinical Assistant Professor, Department of Pediatrics, Oregon Health Sciences University, Portland, Oregon*

Maureen Black, Ph.D.   *Professor, Department of Pediatrics, University of Maryland School of Medicine; and Director, Growth and Nutrition, University of Maryland Medical System, Baltimore, Maryland*

Jennifer S. Bleiker, B.A.   *Research Assistant, The Growth Clinic, Department of Pediatrics, Boston Medical Center, Boston Massachusetts*

Cindy W. Christian, M.D.   *Assistant Professor, Department of Pediatrics, University of Pennsylvania School of Medicine; and Director, Child Abuse Services, The Children's Hospital of Philadelphia, Philadelphia, Pennsylvania*

John T. Cook, Ph.D.   *Assistant Professor, Department of Pediatrics, Boston University School of Medicine, Boston, Massachusetts*

Daniel R. Cooperman, M.D.   *Attending Physician, Department of Orthopedic Surgery, University Hospitals of Cleveland; and Associate Professor, Department of Orthopedic Surgery, Case Western Reserve University, Cleveland, Ohio*

Allan R. DeJong, M.D.   *Pediatric Sexual Abuse Program, Thomas Jefferson University Hospital, Philadelphia, Pennsylvania*

Dennis Drotar, Ph.D.   *Chief of Behavioral and Pediatric Psychology, Department of Pediatrics, Rainbow Babies' and Children's Hospital; and Professor, Department of Pediatrics, Case Western Reserve University School of Medicine, Cleveland, Ohio*

Howard Dubowitz, M.D.   *Professor, Department of Pediatrics, University of Maryland School of Medicine; and Chief, Division of Child Protection, University of Maryland Hospital, Baltimore, Maryland*

Kenneth W. Feldman, M. D.   *Clinical Professor, Department of Pediatrics, University of Washington School of Medicine; Pediatrician, Child Protection Team, Children's Hospital and Regional Medical Center; and Odessa Brown Children's Clinic, Seattle, Washington*

Martin A. Finkel, D.O.   *Medical Director, Center for Children's Support, and Associate Professor, Department of Pediatrics, University of Medicine and Dentistry of New Jersey School of Osteopathic Medicine, Stratford, New Jersey*

Deborah A. Frank, M.D.   *Director, Growth Clinic, Department of Pediatrics, Boston Medical Center; and Associate Professor, Department of Pediatrics, Boston University School of Medicine, Boston, Massachusetts*

Kent P. Hymel, M.D., F.A.A.P.   *Medical Director, Pediatric Forensic Assessment and Consultation Team (FACT), Department of Pediatrics, INOVA Fairfax Hospital for Children, Falls Church, Virginia; and Associate Professor of Clinical Pediatrics, Department of Pediatrics, University of Virginia Health System, Charlottesville, Virginia*

Carole Jenny, M.D.   *Director, Child Protection Program, Hasbro Children's Hospital; and Professor, Department of Pediatrics, Brown University School of Medicine, Providence, Rhode Island*

Dorothy Kasper, R.N.   *Nurse, Ready Set Grow Program, Department of Pediatrics, Rainbow Babies' and Children's Hospital, Cleveland, Ohio*

Robert H. Kirschner, M.D.   *Clinical Associate, Departments of Pathology and Pediatrics, University of Chicago; and University of Chicago Hospitals, Chicago, Illinois*

Henry F. Krous, M.D.   *Director, Department of Pathology, Children's Hospital-SanDiego, San Diego, California; and Adjunct Professor, Departments of Pathology and Pediatrics, University of California at San Diego, LaJolla, California*

Alex V. Levin, M.D., F.A.A.P, F.A.A.O., F.R.C.S.C.   *Staff Opthalmologist, Department of Opthalmology, The Hospital for Sick Children; and Associate Professor, Departments of Pediatrics, Genetics, and Opthalmology, University of Toronto, Toronto, Ontario, Canada*

Carolyn J. Levitt, M.D.   *Midwest Children's Resource Center, Department of Pediatrics, University of Minnesota, Saint Paul, Minnesota*

Stephen Ludwig, M.D.   *Professor, Department of Pediatrics, University of Pennsylvania School of Medicine; and Associate Physician-in-Chief, The Children's Hospital of Philadelphia, Philadelphia, Pennsylvania*

David F. Merten, M.D.   *Department of Radiology, University of North Carolina School of Medicine, Chapel Hill, North Carolina*

Lynn Douglas Mouden, D.D.S., M.P.H., F.I.C.D., F.A.C.D.   *Associate Clinical Professor, University of Missouri Kansas City School of Dentistry; Assistant Professor, University of Tennessee College of Dentistry; and Director, Office of Oral Health, Arkansas Department of Health, Little Rock, Arkansas*

John E. B. Myers, J.D.   *Professor of Law, McGeorge School of Law, University of the Pacific, Sacramento, California*

Robert M. Reece, M.D.   *Clinical Professor, Department of Pediatrics, Tufts University School of Medicine; Director, Child Protection Program, Department of Pediatrics, The Floating Hospital for Children at New England Medical Center; and Director, Insitute for Professional Education, Massachusetts Society for the Prevention of Cruelty to Children, Boston, Massachusetts*

Lawrence R. Ricci, M.D.   *Director, Spurwick Child Abuse Program, Portland, Maine; Clinical Assistant Professor, Department of Pediatrics, University of New England College of Osteopathic Medicine, Biddeford, Maine; and Clinical Assistant Professor, Department of Pediatrics, University of Vermont College of Medicne, Burlington, Vermont*

Donna Andrea Rosenberg, M.D.   *Department of Pediatrics, University of Colorado Medical Center, Denver, Colorado*

Desmond K. Runyan, M.D., Dr.P.H.   *Professor and Chair, Department of Social Medicine, University of North Carolina School of Medicine at Chapel Hill; and Attending Physician, Department of Pediatrics, North Carolina Children's Hospital, Chapel Hill, North Carolina*

Wilber L. Smith, M.D.   *Radiologist, Imaging Department, Children's Hospital of Michigan; and Professor, Department of Radiology, Wayne State University School of Medicine, Detroit, Michigan*

Rebecca R. S. Socolar, M.D., M.P.H.   *Clinical Associate Professor, Departments of Pediatrics and Social Medicine, University of North Carolina School of Medicine at Chapel Hill; and Attending Staff, University of North Carolina Hospitals, Chapel Hill, North Carolina*

Betty S. Spivack, M.D.   *Pediatric Forensic Consultant to the Medical Examiner Division of the Kentucky Justice Cabinet, Office of the Chief Medical Examiner, Louisville, Kentucky*

Harry Wilson, M.D.   *Staff Physician, Department of Pathology, Providence Memorial Hospital, El Paso, Texas*

Robert A. Zimmerman, M.D.   *Chief, Department of Neuroradiology and Vice-Chairman, Department of Radiology, The Children's Hospital of Philadelphia; and Professor, Department of Radiology, University of Pennsylvania, Philadelphia, Pennsylvania*

Preface

Since the publication of the first edition of this book, there have been over four hundred peer-reviewed articles appearing in the world's English-language medical literature about child maltreatment or related conditions. Some of these articles have been significant enough to alter our concepts about the medical aspects of child maltreatment. Some have added persuasive information to bolster past concepts. Others have described new manifestations or presented clinical cases to clarify our thinking. These contributions have been found in a broad range of publications encompassing the field of pediatrics and the pediatric subspecialties in radiology, neurosurgery, orthopedics, infectious disease, surgery, gynecology, dermatology, and psychiatry. There have also been important contributions to the fields of pathology, forensic pathology, and the law.

All professionals working in the evaluation and treatment of abused or neglected children need a single resource incorporating information appearing in the diverse range of clinical and research journals. While the information contained in this book is written from a medical perspective, it is, by virtue of the clarity of writing, accessible to all professionals who seek to understand the signs, symptoms, and injuries of the abused child. The first edition is used extensively by social workers, law enforcement, lawyers, judges, physicians and nurses, and mental health professionals. The book is designed to provide a guide through the medical, surgical, radiographic, and laboratory terrain of child abuse and neglect. For the medical practitioner, the book advises about the best diagnostic and therapeutic approaches to diagnose and treat victims of child abuse. For nonmedical professionals, it provides authoritative information about current medical knowledge. For those who must present their findings and opinions in court, it offers the collective knowledge and experience of the contributing authors, all experts in the field of child maltreatment.

In this second edition, there are completely new chapters covering advances in the field. A chapter on biomechanics analyzes the types and amounts of forces required to produce particular injuries. New imaging modalities in pediatric neuroradiology are described in another chapter. A chapter about unusual manifestations of child maltreatment has also been added. In addition, all the chapters from the first edition have been extensively revised in light of new information.

Robert M. Reece, M.D.
Stephen Ludwig, M.D.

Acknowledgments

Our thanks go to all the contributing authors who gave of their time and talent. Thanks also to Timothy Y. Hiscock and Pam Sutton at Lippincott Williams and Wilkins for their patience and hard work in bringing this book to fruition. Finally, we thank our families who gave us the time and encouragement to complete the task.

Child Abuse

Medical Diagnosis and Management

1

The Biomechanics of Physical Injury

Kent P. Hymel and *Betty S. Spivack

*Pediatric Forensic Assessment and Consultation Team (FACT), Department of Pediatrics, INOVA Fairfax Hospital for Children, Falls Church, Virginia; and Department of Pediatrics, University of Virginia Health System, Charlottesville, Virginia; *Medical Examiner Division, Kentucky Justice Cabinet, Office of the Chief Medical Examiner, Louisville, Kentucky*

Nature and nature's law lay hid in night
God said, "Let Newton be," and all was light
Alexander Pope,
"Epitaph for Sir Isaac Newton"

The human, financial, emotional, and societal costs of traumatic injury in the United States are staggering. To prevent accidental traumatic injury first requires an understanding of its pathogenesis. This, in turn, requires an understanding of the basic principles of mechanics and an appreciation of the special properties of biologic tissues. *Biomechanics* is the study of the effects of mechanical forces on living tissues and organisms. An understanding of the biomechanics of physical injury also can assist physicians in answering the central questions in cases of suspected inflicted trauma or child abuse: "How did it happen? Does this story make sense?"

Our objectives for this discussion of the biomechanics of physical injury are (a) to define and describe basic principles of mechanics, and (b) to apply these principles to understand the pathogenesis of traumatic fractures and head injuries.

BASIC MECHANICS

The Physics of Linear Motion

Newton's first law of motion states: *In the absence of forces acting upon it, an object will move with constant linear velocity.* Mass (m) is a measure of an object's resistance to change in its motion. In the M-K-S or scientific system, mass is measured in kilograms (kg). Mass is an inherent property of matter (40,42).

The first law of motion implies that *acceleration* (a) of an object, or the rate of change of its *velocity* (v) over time, occurs only as the result of *forces* (F) acting on the object. In the M-K-S system, *time* (t) is measured in seconds (sec), *distance* (d) is measured in meters (m), velocity is measured in m/sec, and acceleration is measured in m/sec². Newton's second law states: *The force needed to cause a given amount of acceleration is proportional to the acceleration and to the mass of the object.* This is expressed by the formula $F = ma$. Force is measured in newtons (N), equivalent to kg/m/sec².

Gravity also is an inherent property of matter and describes the attractive interaction between two objects. Matter generates a gravitational field that causes the uniform acceleration of any other object within that field. On or near the surface of the Earth, the strength of its gravitational field causes any object to accelerate toward the Earth's center at 9.8 m/sec² (g).

Weight is the downward force associated with a mass under the acceleration of a gravitational field. Because it is a force, in the M-K-S system, it is measured in newtons. It is incorrect to say that a kilogram (a unit of mass) equals 2.2 pounds (a unit of weight). On Earth, an object with a mass of 1 kg has a weight of 9.8 N, equivalent to 2.2 pounds. On the moon, that same object would still have a mass of 1 kg, but its weight would be much reduced because of the moon's smaller mass and gravitational field.

Work (W) is force exerted over a distance (d), and it is measured in joules (J), equivalent to N/m or kg/m^2/sec^2. It is described by the equation $W = Fd$. *Energy* (E) is the capacity to do work and also is measured in joules. The rate of use of energy to perform work is *power,* which is measured in watts (J/sec). One hundred joules of energy is sufficient to light a 100-watt bulb for 1 second, or a 50-watt bulb for 2 seconds.

Energy can be described as *kinetic* (associated with a moving object) or *potential* (associated with the position of the object). The total energy (kinetic plus potential) of a system is constant, but the potential energy can be converted into kinetic energy, and vice versa. The amount of kinetic energy associated with an object is described by the equation $E = 1/2mv^2$. The potential energy of an object in the gravitational field of the Earth is described by $E = mgh$, where h is the height above the nearest surface. As an object falls and is accelerated by gravity, its potential energy is progressively changed to kinetic energy. At the instant just before impact, all of the potential energy has been converted to kinetic energy. If the object bounces, some portion of the kinetic energy is again converted to potential energy. Alternatively, some or all of the kinetic energy may be expended in doing destructive work on the surface it falls upon (or on the falling object itself). In the context of trauma, the degree of injury is the work resulting from the application of the traumatic force. For this reason, the amount of available energy is as important as the magnitude of the traumatic force.

> Example 1: A 5-kg bowling ball sits at rest on the floor. It has no kinetic energy because its velocity is 0 m/sec. It has no potential energy because its height above the floor is 0 m. In a zero-energy state, we do not regard the bowling ball as intrinsically dangerous, but only as a potential obstacle.

> Example 2: If the bowling ball is placed on a shelf 2 m above the floor, our perception of it changes. It is now a potentially dangerous object. Sitting 2 m above the floor, it has a potential energy of 98 joules (5 kg × 9.8 m/sec^2 × 2 m). Its kinetic energy is still 0 because it is at rest. If the bowling ball is dislodged from the shelf, it will fall toward the floor under the acceleration of gravity, and the potential energy will be progressively changed to kinetic energy. Just before it strikes the floor, potential energy will be 0, and the kinetic energy will be 98 joules, as total energy will remain unchanged. The bowling ball will have fallen to the floor in approximately 0.64 seconds and will be moving at approximately 6.3 m/sec on impact. [In this example, time is calculated by solving for time (t) in the equation: $d = 1/2 \, at^2$, where distance (d) is 2 m and acceleration (a) is 9.8 m/sec^2. The velocity at impact (v impact) can be calculated from the equation: $v_{impact} = v_{initial} + at$; where initial velocity ($v_{initial}$) is 0 m/sec, acceleration (a) is 9.8 m/sec^2, and time (t) is 0.64 seconds. At the moment before impact, the bowling ball's kinetic energy (E) is 98 joules (i.e., the same as its initial potential energy), calculated as $E = 1/2mv^2$, where mass (m) = 5 kg and the impact velocity (v_{impact}) is 6.3 m/sec].

As the ball strikes the floor, some of the energy may be used in doing destructive work on the floor, depending on the intrinsic strength of the floor. If the floor has some elastic properties, the ball may bounce to a greater or lesser degree, temporarily converting a portion of the kinetic energy back to potential energy, before the ball again strikes the floor, with considerably less kinetic energy than previously.

The force with which the bowling ball strikes the floor is dependent on the rate of deceleration from its terminal velocity of 6.3 m/sec. The bowling ball is rigid and does not deform easily. If the floor is made of a very rigid substance, such as concrete, the stopping distance will be extremely minimal, and the stopping time may be as little as 1 msec (0.001 sec). The deceleration will be rapid, 6,300 m/sec^2 ($a = v/t$), and the force associated with this acceleration also will be high, 31,500 N ($F = ma$). If the floor is constructed from a more yielding substance, such as a soft foam mat, the stopping distance will be much greater, and the stopping time may exceed 0.1 seconds. This would lead to a much smaller deceleration, less than 63 m/sec^2, and a force of less than 315 N. It is for this reason that foam mats are piled near places of expected falls from a height, such as in a high-jump or pole-vault landing pit, or alongside gymnastic equipment.

Both energy and *momentum* (M) are conserved during any interaction between two or more objects. Momentum is described by the equation $M = mv$. Because both energy and momentum are conserved, a two-object interaction leads to two equations in two unknowns (the velocities of the objects after the interaction) and therefore to a unique solution. The presence of three or more objects increases the complexity of the situation and is less predictable.

The Physics of Rotational Motion

Newton's first law implies that any object that does not experience a force acting on it will continue with constant linear motion. Rotational motion requires the application of a force acting in a direction different from the initial motion of the object. *Rotational inertia* is the equivalent of mass in equations describing rotational motion. It represents the resistance of an object to initiation or change of rotatory motion, and it is a function of both the mass of the object and the distance over which the force is exercised. Therefore it is harder to swing an object on a long string than on a short one.

Torque is the rotational equivalent of force, a measure of the rotational impact of the exerted force. It is equal to the force exerted multiplied by the *lever arm* (i.e., the perpendicular distance between the pivot point and the line of application of that force; Fig. 1.1).

> Example 3: If we are using a wrench to turn (tighten or loosen) a bolt, the wrench is positioned horizontally while the force is directed downward, which maximizes the torque exerted on the bolt. Once the wrench has rotated to reach the bottom of its arc, reducing its torque to zero, it is repositioned.

Rotational velocity and *acceleration* are described in terms of radians or degrees per unit of time (rotational velocity), or per unit of time squared (rotational acceleration). A rotating object has both rotational velocity and acceleration and an instantaneous linear velocity. If the force causing the rotation is discontinued, the object will fly off in a

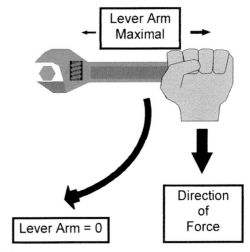

FIG. 1.1. Torque is the rotational equivalent of force, a measure of the rotational impact of the exerted force. It is equal to the force exerted multiplied by the lever arm.

straight line tangent to the arc through which it had been rotating (e.g., if the string to which a twirling object is attached breaks, its velocity will be equal to its linear velocity at the time the string snapped). During rotation, there is conservation of *angular momentum,* which is the product of rotational inertia and rotational velocity.

> Example 4: A figure skater is executing a spin and slows when the arms are extended. The rotational inertia of the body has increased because more of the mass is farther from the axis of rotation, and rotational velocity decreases to preserve angular momentum. The opposite effect is seen when the arms are brought in toward the body.

The Effect of Mechanical Loading

Loading (Fig. 1.2) is the application of a force to an object. Loads may be *tensile* (acts to stretch the material), *compressive* (acts to compress the material), or *shearing* (acts to change the angular relations of portions of the material). Loads may exist in combination. *Bending* (Fig. 1.3) causes tensile forces on the far side of the neutral axis and compressive

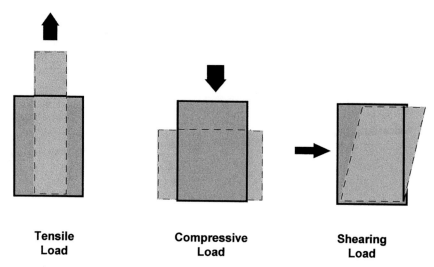

Tensile Load   **Compressive Load**   **Shearing Load**

FIG. 1.2. Loading is the application of a force to an object. Loads may be tensile, compressive, or shearing.

forces on the near side. *Torsion* (Fig. 1.4) causes tension and compression at 45-degree angles to the axis of rotation and maximal shearing effects at maximal distances from the axis of rotation.

Stress (equivalent to pressure) is a measure of force or load applied per unit area of application. It is measured in pascals, equivalent to newtons per square meter or $kg/m/sec^2$. The *ultimate strength* of a material is the maximal stress that it can experience without rupture. If a given stress is tolerable, Newton's third law of motion expresses the reciprocal nature of force: *Every action has an equal and opposite reaction.* If the stress exceeds the ultimate

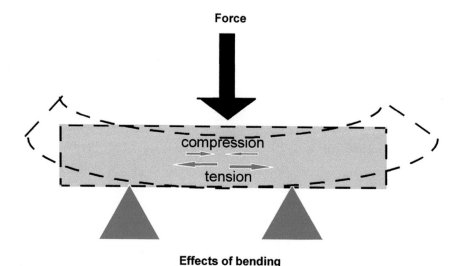

Effects of bending

FIG. 1.3. Loads may exist in combination: bending causes tensile forces on the far side of the neutral axis and compressive forces on the near side.

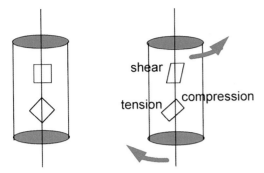

FIG. 1.4. Torsion causes tension and compression at 45-degree angles to the axis of rotation and maximal shearing effects at maximal distances from the axis of rotation.

strength and the recipient object cannot push back with equal force, it will rupture.

> Example 5: A 1-kg book, with surface area 0.1 m, rests upon a large wooden table. The book pushes down with a force equivalent to its weight, 9.8 N, and exerts a stress on the table of 98 pascals (9.8 N/0.1 m^2). This does not exceed the ultimate strength of the table, and it pushes back on the book with an equivalent stress of 98 pascals.

> Example 6: The same 1-kg book is resting on a long, unsupported sheet of thin paper. The ultimate strength of the paper is far less than 98 pascals, and the paper will tear, allowing the book to fall to the floor.

Strain is the ratio of linear or angular deformation induced by the application of a force to the original length or angle of the object. Because it is a ratio, it is dimensionless and has no unit of measure. Materials (and tissues) have different deformational responses to the stresses and strains induced by loading forces.

Elastic Deformation

Some strain may be temporary, lasting only as long as the force is applied. Such a strain is called *elastic*. An example of elastic strain is the stretching of a rubber band, which returns to its original length when the stretching ceases. If the strain is excessive, the object may rupture. In this case, the strain has exceeded the breaking strain of the material.

In an elastic deformation (Fig. 1.5), the amount of deformation is proportional to the applied load. The energy used in causing the deformation is stored in the material and is fully released after elastic recovery. Because the energy is stored, it is available to do other work. In a fully elastic collision, kinetic energy is completely converted back into potential energy (i.e., the object will bounce back to its original height). In a purely elastic deformation or collision, no work is done, as no energy is expended; the situation at the end of the application of the force is exactly as it was before the force was applied. In the real world, there are no purely elastic deformations or collisions. Some energy is always lost either in work due to friction or because of nonelastic properties of the material.

> Example 7: A slingshot elastic band is stretched backward, causing considerable elastic strain, storing a significant amount of energy. A marble is inserted in the slingshot, and the elastic band is released, propelling the marble a considerable distance. The stored energy has been released, and the elastic band returns to its initial conformation. If the wielder of the slingshot is overzealous and pulls back on the elastic, causing a deformation in excess of the breaking strain, the elastic band will rupture.

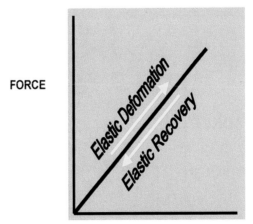

FIG. 1.5. In an elastic deformation, the amount of deformation is proportional to the applied load.

Plastic Deformation

Materials may be permanently deformed without rupture; such a property is called *plasticity.* A good example of plastic deformation is the mark left by pushing one's thumb into wet clay or Silly Putty; the material is not torn, but a permanent deformation has occurred. In a plastic deformation (Fig. 1.6), no deformity occurs until the *yield point* is reached; thereafter, the amount of deformation is dependent on the length of time in which the force is operating. Pure plasticity is uncommon in biologic materials, but many materials exhibit *elastoplastic* behavior (Fig. 1.7). Elastoplastic materials behave elastically, with recoverable deformation, until the yield point of the material is reached, at which point, permanent plastic deformation occurs proportional to the length of time the force operates. In such a situation, some of the deformation (and associated energy) may be recoverable, whereas the remainder has led to permanent deformation (and expenditure of energy). Many biologic materials demonstrate elastoplastic properties.

Viscous Deformation

Some materials are highly responsive to the rate at which a force is applied. Such deformations are described as viscous (Fig. 1.8). Viscous substances are stiff when a force is

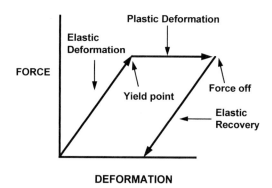

FIG. 1.7. Elastoplastic materials behave elastically, with recoverable deformation, until the yield point of the material is reached.

applied rapidly, but yield readily when a force is slowly and steadily applied. Biologic materials are unlikely to be "purely" viscous, although liquids such as blood have more viscous properties than plastic or elastic properties. Most soft body tissues can be described as *viscoelastic* (Fig. 1.9). Their susceptibility to injury is dependent on the rate of force application.

Example 8: Silly Putty is highly plastic under slow rates of force application. It may be shaped rather like clay, without rupture of the material. However, if it is shaped into a ball

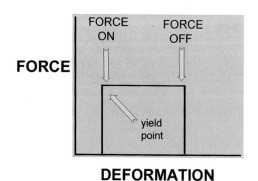

FIG. 1.6. In plastic deformation, no deformity occurs until the yield point is reached. The amount of deformation depends on the length of time in which the force is operating.

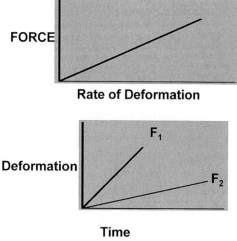

FIG. 1.8. Viscous deformation.

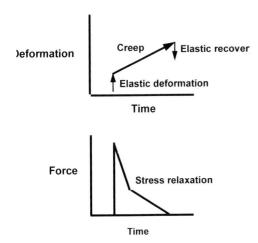

FIG. 1.9. Most soft body tissues can be described as viscoelastic.

and thrown at the floor with considerable force, it exhibits a strong viscoelastic nature. Instead of deforming and sticking to the floor as clay would, it bounces like an elastic object, with little or no deformation. In other words, it strongly resists deformation under conditions of sudden application of force and stress.

Scaling

To understand and predict injury thresholds, we must consider the concept of *scaling*. Some body dimensions increase linearly (e.g., proportional to length), and others increase in a squared (e.g., proportional to surface area) or cubed (e.g., proportional to volume, mass, or weight) manner. This has importance for both body structure and response to injury. In compression, the strength of a support structure (e.g., a leg bone) is dependent on the cross-sectional area of the bone. However, the compressive load it must bear is dependent on the weight of the individual. Weight increases as the cube of length, whereas cross-sectional area increases as the square (i.e., less quickly). Therefore as mass increases, the compressive load-bearing capacity of the leg bone (i.e., its strength) may be less able to "keep up" with its weight-bearing requirements. Whenever ultimate strength (and therefore susceptibility to injury) is dependent on the surface area of a body part, but its

load is described in terms of volume, mass, or weight, then the exponent of increase is likely to be 2:3 (i.e., the ratio of the power of growth in surface area to the power of growth in volume). Scaling is an important consideration when comparing the relative injurious effects of falling in infants, children, and adults.

> Example 9: If the mass of a squirrel (0.2 kg) were increased to that of an elephant (5,400 kg), its mass would grow by a factor of 27,000. If its body proportions were preserved, limb and body length would increase by a factor of 30, and the cross-sectional surface area of the supporting limb bones would increase by a factor of 900. The stress on the supporting limb bones would increase by 30 times, leading to a high risk of compressive fracture. For this reason, large animals such as elephants have different body proportions than those of small animals such as mice and squirrels. The limb bones of the elephant are thicker, which reduces but does not eliminate the stress caused by the disproportionate increase in mass, length, and surface area. Not only is the elephant stouter than the squirrel, but it is not so nimble and must place its limbs more carefully to avoid injury.

BIOMECHANICAL ASPECTS OF SPECIFIC PEDIATRIC INJURIES

Fractures

To understand the mechanism of injury of fractures (87), we must first consider the structure and mechanical properties of bone. The special characteristics of growing bone lead to different patterns of response to loading forces during early life. For this reason, the pattern of bony injury in young infants is very different from that seen in older children and adults.

Bone Anatomy

Bone is constructed from several constituent parts. *Cortical* or *compact* bone is a dense material that is usually well mineralized. It is the major support structure of the body. When it is mature, it is composed of secondary osteons with a central haversian canal containing a neurovascular bundle, and surrounded by concentric lamellae of bone tissue. The lamellae are separated by lacunae, which are connected to each other and to the central haversian canal by canaliculi.

However, these anatomic features are not seen in fetal and infantile bone. Cortical bone develops in two ways depending on whether it is membranous or endochondral in origin. The earliest phase of true compact bone is the primary spongiosa, in which there is no lamellation, and the collagen fibers are randomly arranged. The next phase of development is the production of primary osteons or atypical haversian systems. These are roughly concentric, nonlamellar bone deposited in parallel fibers along the walls of the vascular spaces in the bone. Early in life, this represents a large proportion of cortical bone. As the ossification process continues, the primary osteons and intervening interstitial bone are increasingly incorporated into mature, secondary osteons.

Trabecular or *cancellous* bone, by contrast, consists of a meshwork of calcified strands within which are easily visible spaces. The open meshwork is laid down in a manner determined by loading patterns of the bone. Although this pattern has been noted for more than 100 years, the mechanism by which osteocytes recognize strain patterns and lay down calcium to maximize support while minimizing skeletal weight is just starting to be elucidated (30,49,118,120).

Disuse leads to a marked decrease in bone mass and a higher susceptibility to fracture. This process is seen in spinal cord injury, immobilization of an extremity, bed rest, cerebral palsy, and in astronauts who have spent long periods in a weightless environment. Patients with spinal cord injury display very rapid and severe bone loss from disuse, with most of their bone loss occurring in the first 4 months after injury (34).

Long bones generally have a thick cylinder of cortical bone forming the shaft. The middle of the shaft has a few spicules of trabecular bone but is occupied chiefly by the marrow cavity. This cavity extends in both directions outward during bone development,

and in maturity, extends almost to the epiphyseal fusion line. Trabecular bone is found under synovial joints, where forces are diffused over large areas.

Long bones are formed from cartilage, followed by chondrocyte death and secondary ossification. This process occurs in fetal life at the primary ossification centers in the diaphysis or shaft, and throughout childhood in the secondary ossification centers, usually located at each end in the epiphyses. In childhood, the diaphysis and epiphysis are separated by the metaphyseal regions, where columns of chondrocytes are mineralized in the zone of provisional calcification.

Mechanical Properties of Adult and Pediatric Bone

The mechanical properties of specific bones differ, depending on several variables. In particular, properties of both compact and trabecular bone are dependent on the density and mineral content of the bone (60,127), as well as on the nature of the loading force. The properties of compact bone also are dependent on the proportion of secondary and primary osteons. Ox femora consisting only of secondary osteons were 35% weaker than primary bone (100). This observation may partially explain the greater resistance of pediatric bone to fracture. Secondary osteons have been hypothesized to develop because their structure is more resistant to fatigue-induced microfractures (78).

Compact bone is stiffer than trabecular bone. It withstands greater stress but less strain before failure. Because of its open network of support strands, trabecular bone is highly elastic, with great ability to store and release energy. Trabecular bone may develop up to 75% strain before fracture. Comparable ultimate strain limits for cortical bone are 2% change in initial dimensions (15). Small differences in bone mineralization may make large differences in the strength of both types of bone.

Bone is also a viscoelastic substance (23,72,107). At high loading rates, it is stiffer, sustains a higher load before failure, and stores more energy before fracture (even though maximal strain is unchanged). When the bone fractures, the stored energy is released, doing destructive work. For this reason, higher energy fractures are associated with increased splintering (e.g., *greenstick fracture, comminuted fracture*) and increased displacement of the fracture segments.

Adult cortical bone is strongest in compression (ultimate strength, 193 MPa), weaker in tension (133 MPa), and weakest in shear loading (68 MPa) (100). The mechanical properties of infant bone are less well studied than are those of adults, but the increased energy storage capacity and increased plasticity of juvenile bone is a well-known phenomenon. Adult bone has little or no capacity to store energy after fracture has begun. The persistent ability of pediatric bone to store energy under these conditions results in the preponderance of greenstick fractures in children, as opposed to transverse or oblique fractures under similar bending circumstances.

A current area of research in adult bone biomechanics relates the mechanical properties of the bone to noninvasive determinations of bone density (21,82,102), high-resolution digital radiography (82), or computed tomographic anatomy (102,112,119). This approach holds a great deal of potential for determination of fracture thresholds in a particular patient, but no similar pediatric research has yet been published.

Initial studies now under way shed some light on the biomechanical characteristics of the infant skeletal system. Morild et al. (84) performed three-point bending tests on the fibulae of 24 infants, aged 31 to 381 days, who had died suddenly. After autopsy and investigation, the causes of death were recorded as sudden infant death syndrome (SIDS; n = 21), homicide (n = 1), motor vehicle accident (n = 1), and meningitis (n = 1). Bending progressed until the development of greenstick fracture. The mean ultimate load to fracture in this study was 90.286 ± 36.539 N. Biomechanical properties were strongly correlated to age,

height, weight, bone length, anterior–posterior diameter, m–l diameter, and square area of the fibula cross section. Similar studies are needed on the other components of the infant skeletal system to establish the numeric ranges for pediatric fracture thresholds. In life, however, the fibula is fastened in strut fashion to the tibia, which provides the bulk of support for the lower limb. Therefore one would not expect fibular fracture to occur with such minimal forces in a living child. Similarly, skeletal elements do not exist in isolation. The ability of the skeletal musculature to contract provides a balancing force to tensile stresses incurred during bending, reducing the probability of fracture. Decreases in muscle mass and function may contribute to the increased fracture rate in children with cerebral palsy or spinal cord injury.

Geometric Properties of Bone That Affect Fracture Mechanics

The geometry of a loaded object will affect its ability to support a load. In bending, the distribution of material around the neutral axis and the cross-sectional area are important for stress distribution. The measure of these parameters is the *moment of inertia,* and developed stress is proportional to its square root. The moment of inertia is proportional to the width of the object (length perpendicular to the neutral axis) and the cube of the height (length parallel to the neutral axis). In contrast, the length perpendicular to the bending contributes to the *bending moment,* which represents the amount of work done at any distance from the application of the force. Stress magnitude is proportional to the bending moment.

To minimize the stress and reduce the risk of fracture, bones of the appendicular skeleton are long in the direction of supportive compression and relatively narrow perpendicular to that same axis. This maximizes the moment of inertia and minimizes bending moment during walking. The *rotational* or *polar moment of inertia* plays a similar role in protection from torsional forces. The higher the rotational moment of inertia, the stronger and stiffer the object is while undergoing torsion.

> Example 10: The width of the proximal tibia is greater than that of the distal tibia in humans, but the thickness of the cortex is decreased, with a slightly smaller cross-sectional area. The rotational moment of inertia of the proximal segment is much higher than that of the distal segment because more of the bone mass is farther from the axis of rotation. The distal section, despite its increased cross section, is subjected to higher shear stress during torsion (approximately double) because much of the bone is distributed close to the neutral axis. For this reason, most accidentally incurred spiral fractures of the tibia, such as the toddler's fracture, occur in the distal third of the tibia. Spiral fractures of the upper tibia require higher forces and energies and imply stabilization (e.g., by hand gripping) of the more susceptible lower portion of the bone.

Scaling properties are important to consider in the pathogenesis of pediatric fractures. As we noted before, as size increases, mass (a function of the cube of length) grows

more rapidly than the cross-sectional area of the supports, causing increased stress and increasing the risk of fracture. Although adult cortical bone is denser than juvenile bone, this only partly compensates for the increased stress experienced by the adult skeleton. As a result, children are less susceptible to compressive fractures than are adults.

Diaphyseal Fractures

Various fracture patterns (87) are seen in long bones, arising from the different load patterns acting on the bone (see Fig. 1.10). Increased strain rate and increased available energy will tend to increase comminution and separation of fracture fragments in any pattern of distribution.

Tensile forces cause separation of individual osteons at the cement line, leading to a *transverse fracture,* perpendicular to the axis of force. Compressive loads cause failure because of shear stresses angulated relative to

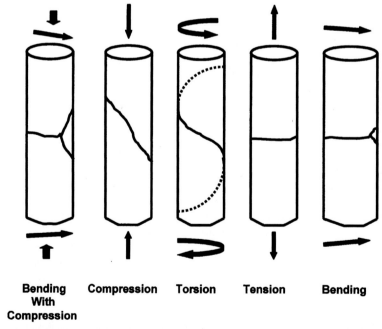

Bending With Compression   Compression   Torsion   Tension   Bending

FIG. 1.10. Various fracture patterns are seen in long bones, arising from the different load patterns acting on the bone. (From Carter D. The biomechanics of bone. In: Nahun AM, Melvin J, eds. *The Biomechanics of Trauma.* Stamford, Connecticut: Appleton and Lange, 1984: 1590, with the permission of the McGraw-Hill Companies.)

the axis of compression; this results in a complex of modestly angled *oblique fractures.* Distal radius fractures are a special case of compressive fracture occurring when a child or adult falls with full force on a single outstretched hand. In adults and older children, this produces a *Colles' fracture.* Infants and toddlers, with a better ratio of mass to bone surface area, and a higher proportion of primary osteons, are more likely to sustain a *partial buckle* or *torus fracture.* Bending leads to transverse fracture on the side of tension, with a butterfly fragment on the side of compression.

Torsional fractures begin with shear failure parallel to the main axis of rotation, and then propagate at a 30- to 45-degree angle, generating an oblique–spiral fracture with a splintered end. Accidental spiral fractures in areas with low polar moment of inertia (e.g., the distal tibia) may occur with relatively little force, especially when the lever arm is long (e.g., a spiral fracture of the distal tibia resulting from the muscular contraction of the strong upper thigh musculature). This common *toddler's fracture* typically occurs with no displacement along the fracture line. Spiral fractures occurring in areas of higher polar moment of inertia (e.g., the femur or proximal tibia) result from higher force and higher energy events, such as motor vehicle accidents or inflicted trauma.

Metaphyseal Fractures

Classic *metaphyseal fractures* have long been recognized as highly specific for inflicted injury (14,62). Caffey (14) proposed that these fractures, described previously as "corner" and "bucket handle" lesions, were the result of pulling, with tension on the periosteum. This explanation was accepted until the late 1980s, when the meticulous radiographic, pathologic, and histologic work performed by Kleinman et al. (63) demonstrated that the corner and bucket-handle lesions were different radiologic appearances of the same lesion, distinguished by the orientation of the x-ray beam relative to the fracture segment.

The principal lesion that they identified was a shearing fracture across the calcified chondrocyte columns of the metaphysis and the underlying, uncalcified chondrocyte columns of the epiphysis.

The fundamental shearing nature of this injury, especially in its most common location in the distal femur, proximal tibia, and distal tibia, clarifies its frequent coexistence with posterior rib fractures and abusive head trauma. Flailing of the limbs during violent shaking may lead to anteroposterior shearing forces in these bony locations acting on the chondrocyte columns perpendicular to their direction of support. Essentially identical fracture patterns have been produced experimentally (125) by shearing forces. In this model, shearing strength was increased when the tissues were undergoing simultaneous compression. During shaking, the bone is not compressed at all, because it is not supporting weight against gravity. Broom et al. (11) demonstrated that the osteochondral junction has a 1.5 times greater fracture toughness in the mature individual than in immature bone.

Posterior Rib Fractures

Rib fractures, especially posterior rib fractures, are uncommon injuries in childhood, with a high degree of specificity for inflicted injury (62). Once again, meticulous radiologic, histopathologic, and experimental work by Kleinman et al. (61,64,65) has clarified the mechanism of injury seen almost exclusively in abused children. The site of the posterior rib fracture, especially at the neck of the rib at the costovertebral junction, always included the ventral surface, and less frequently included the dorsal surface of the bone. Kleinman et al. concluded that such fractures were the result of levering of the rib end against the transverse processes of the vertebral body, with initial failure in tension on the ventral surface of the rib.

Such a mechanism requires an unsupported back, allowing the rib to move behind the vertebral process. Cardiopulmonary resuscitation (CPR) in adults is a frequent cause of rib fracture; the opposite is true of infants (8,33,113). The increased elasticity of the infant rib and the decreased depth of compression, even when performed by lay rescuers, provides a setting in which the transmitted energy is easily stored and released by the infant rib.

Kleinman's proposed mechanism of posterior rib fracture is consistent with forceful grasping and squeezing of the chest during a shaking episode. Experimental reproduction of shaking/squeezing and CPR in rabbits (65) demonstrated posterior rib fractures resulting from manual thoracic compression with an unsupported back, but no fractures from external cardiac massage with the rabbit lying on a firm surface. The fractures produced by squeezing were identical radiographically and pathologically with the posterior fractures seen in abused infants.

Cranial Injuries

Primary traumatic cranial injuries begin at the moment of injury and result from one of two possible mechanisms: contact or noncontact. *Contact injuries* require that the head strike or be struck by an object, regardless of whether the collision initiates cranial acceleration. Contact injuries can be viewed as the deformation injuries that occur if the head is prevented from moving. *Noncontact injuries* result from whole head cranial acceleration, irrespective of whether this cranial acceleration was the result of a cranial collision.

Contact or noncontact primary injury mechanisms may result in compressive, tensile, and/or shearing tissue strains (i.e., deformations). Primary traumatic cranial injuries result when these strains exceed injury thresholds and tissues do not return to their original conformation. Contact forces primarily cause focal strains, particularly at the impact site. Intracranial hemorrhage and/or brain parenchymal injuries resulting from contact forces may cause coma or death, if sufficiently large to cause brain shifts, herniation, or brainstem compression (35). Noncontact forces may cause injury by one of two mechanisms: (a)

Whole brain movement or deformation relative to the rigid skull and dura may produce rupture of bridging veins; and (b) Cranial acceleration may produce strains within the brain itself.

Assuming that impact force and energy are sufficient, the biomechanical circumstances of cranial impact that favor cranial contact injuries include restriction of cranial motion (i.e., *fixity*) and a small surface area of contact (i.e., *nondistributed loading*). Conversely, the biomechanical circumstances of cranial impact that favor whole head cranial acceleration (i.e., noncontact) injuries are cranial freedom to move and a relatively large surface area of contact (i.e., *distributed loading*).

Severe or fatal primary traumatic cranial injuries in humans are most often the result of whole head cranial acceleration, not contact strains (37,38). Because cranial impact may induce severe cranial acceleration, contact and noncontact cranial injuries frequently coexist. The absence of external contact injuries or skull fracture does not exclude cranial impact as a cause of severe acceleration injury (29).

Soft Tissue Injuries

External soft tissue injuries of the head and face are contact injuries. Although cranial impact resulting in soft tissue cranial or facial injury may result in secondary noncontact injuries, soft tissue injuries themselves do not require cranial acceleration. Infants who do not cruise rarely bruise (115). Facial or scalp soft tissue injuries in very young children have been linked to subtle intracranial injuries (43,44,57). Unlike other soft tissue injuries, the location of subgaleal hematoma may not always reflect the site of cranial impact (6). Scalp, hair, and padding afford considerable protection from skull fracture (31,46).

Skull Fracture

Skull fracture is a contact injury. Cranial impact may produce skull fracture even when secondary cranial acceleration is restricted. Conversely, if the cranium is free to move, cranial impacts of sufficient energy and force magnitude to produce skull fracture may precipitate associated noncontact injuries.

Cranial impact over a small surface area of contact (i.e., nondistributed loading) may result in *depressed skull fracture* or even skull perforation (e.g., bullet wound). The increased plasticity of pediatric bone is reflected in the occurrence of *ping-pong skull deformation* rather than depressed skull fracture occurring after moderate focal injury in young children.

In contrast, *linear skull fractures* require impact over a large surface area of contact (i.e., distributed loading) (46). For example, linear skull fractures have been reported in 1% to 3% of witnessed indoor accidental falls to the floor by young children (50,66,76,86,124). Bilateral, prolonged, distributed cranial loading (i.e., crushing injuries) may produce complex "mirror image" skull fracture patterns (51). In patients who survive crushing cranial injury, the absence (or slight degree) of associated concussion and other noncontact injuries is a striking clinical feature (28,105).

The viscoelastic properties of the adult human skull play a significant role in fracture pathogenesis. Using fresh cadaver heads, Yoganandan et al. (128) demonstrated a nonlinear response dependent on the rate of impact and the loading site. Quasistatic (i.e., slow) loading resulted in fractures with markedly lower force (mean, $6,399 \pm 1,134$ N) than dynamic (i.e., rapid) loading ($11,938 \pm 885$ N). Similar degrees of difference were seen in stiffness (812 N/mm ± 139 vs. $4,023 \pm 541$ N/mm) and deflection (12.0 ± 1.6 mm vs. 5.8 ± 1.0 mm).

Cranial impacts to specified locations of the adult cranium produce predictable fracture patterns if injury thresholds are exceeded (46). Similar research has not been reported in young children. The location of linear skull fracture may not reflect the specific location of skull impact with inbending (6,128). Instead, linear skull fractures begin on the outer surface of the skull in a region of skull outbending and tension somewhere around the impact site (25,46). More distant linear skull fractures show greater diastasis of edges, reflective of the lever action with increased bending moment. A unilateral, linear parietal skull fracture is the most common inflicted pediatric skull fracture. It is also the most common accidental skull fracture in children. Therefore linear skull fracture(s) should not be considered specific for inflicted head trauma. At least two very different mechanisms for *basilar skull fracture* have been described in adults: temporomandibular loading in conjunction with neck tension (79) and occipital impact (46).

Epidural Hemorrhage

Epidural hemorrhage is a contact injury. It may occur as an unfortunate complication of cranial impact, even when cranial motion is restricted. Epidural hemorrhage occurs below a cranial impact site or skull fracture when local strains exceed tolerances of underlying blood vessels. An expanding epidural hemorrhage may precipitate delayed clinical deterioration and/or death as a complication of an apparently benign fall onto a rigid surface (101,103,126). Epidural hemorrhage is not considered a specific indicator of inflicted cranial trauma (110).

Subdural Hemorrhage

Subdural hemorrhage can occur as a contact injury. Even if the head is fixed, localized subdural bleeding may result from focal contact strains underlying skull impact or fracture. In this regard, subdural and epidural hemorrhages may represent analogous contact injuries complicating cranial impact or fracture. Small subdural collections can disappear rapidly on neuroimaging (27). If impact loading of sufficient force and energy is widely distributed (e.g., crush injury), larger underlying subdural hemorrhage may occur as a contact injury (54).

Subdural hemorrhage also can occur as a noncontact injury. Whole head cranial acceleration induced by impact or impulsively (i.e., by nonimpact) may rupture parasagittal bridging veins, frequently leading to large, bilateral, and/or interhemispheric subdural collections not limited to the impact or fracture site. More specifically, subdural hematoma as a noncontact injury results from superficial tensile and/or shearing strains to vascular tissues caused by the differential acceleration of the skull and brain, resulting from anteroposterior cranial acceleration of relatively short duration and high magnitude (38). The absence of external cranial soft tissue injuries or skull fracture does not exclude cranial impact (or confirm shaking) as the cause of noncontact subdural hemorrhage (29). Subdural hemorrhage is a frequent finding in pediatric abusive head trauma (4,5,13,22,26,32,47,55,56, 75,80,81,108,117).

Brain Contusions

Bruises of the brain can occur as a contact injury. Contusions occurring beneath the site of cranial impact are called coup contusions. Cranial inbending from impact may cause direct compressive injury to the brain and its surface blood vessels. Alternately, high negative pressures that develop when an area of inbent skull snaps back into place may precipitate underlying brain contusion. Brain laceration underlying an impact site may occur as an extension of these same processes.

In more elastic (i.e., younger) skulls, impact onto thicker regions of the skull anteriorly or posteriorly may precipitate global changes in skull shape and sudden fluctuations in intracranial volume. These changes may precipitate remote contusions underlying regions of skull outbending, herniation of intracranial contents through various foramina (particularly the foramen magnum), and periventricular petechial hemorrhages (36).

Whatever the site of cranial impact, the majority of brain contusions in adults are clustered in the frontal and temporal lobes and the region of the sylvian fissure (45,94,97). In adults, these brain regions are most vulnerable to shearing injury because of their relatively greater restraint by the sphenoidal

ridges and other irregularities of the frontotemporal fossa (94).

In contrast to the contusions seen in the mature brain, very young victims of fatal blunt head trauma younger than 5 months more frequently reveal grossly visible tears in the cerebral white matter and microscopic tears in the outermost cortical layers (73). Lindenberg and Freytag (73) hypothesized that these infantile tear lesions were related to the soft consistency of the unmyelinated brain, the smoothness of the intracranial fossa, the pliancy of the skull, and the shallowness of the subarachnoid space in this age group.

Brain contusions also can occur as an isolated noncontact injury. Ommaya et al. (91) induced brain contusions, subdural hemorrhage, and experimental concussion in monkeys by inducing whiplash without cranial impact. The distribution and severity of brain contusions observed in these animals differed somewhat from those created by the combination of cranial rotation and skull distortion from impact (94).

Diffuse Brain Injuries

Diffuse brain injuries are noncontact injuries. More specifically, these injuries result from diffuse strains throughout the brain caused by coronal (i.e., lateral) cranial acceleration of relatively long duration and low magnitude (39). Functional impairments or structural injury may result. Examples of diffuse brain injury include concussion, diffuse axonal injury (i.e., widespread, traumatically induced axonal injury), prolonged traumatic coma, and tissue-tear hemorrhages (i.e., deep petechial hemorrhages).

Concussion is the beginning of the clinically apparent continuum of primary diffuse brain injury. If the head is fixed at the moment of cranial impact, and cranial acceleration is prevented, there will be no concussion (24,52). More specifically, concussion requires *rotational* cranial acceleration (i.e., rotation of the head about the brain's center of gravity) as opposed to *translational* (i.e., straight line) cranial acceleration (1,93).

However, cranial rotational acceleration alone is insufficient to explain fully the pathogenesis of traumatic cerebral concussion. Minimizing the contribution of contact strains, Holbourn (52) predicted in 1943 that primary diffuse brain injuries (including concussion) result from shearing strains created by cranial acceleration alone. Decades later, Ommaya et al. (90,92,95) tested Holbourn's theory experimentally using primates. They reasoned that, if Holbourn was correct, cerebral concussion should be produced at identical levels of rotational velocity of the head whether cranial rotation was initiated by impact or nonimpact. Their experiments disproved Holbourn's theory regarding the primacy of acceleration-induced shearing strains in the pathogenesis of concussion. As compared with experimental whiplash (i.e., nonimpact), direct head impact produced similar grades of cerebral concussion in primates at about half the amplitude of rotational velocity. Although concussion requires cranial rotational acceleration (24,93,105), contact strains clearly play a more significant role in the pathogenesis of traumatic cerebral concussion and diffuse primary brain injury than originally theorized by Holbourn (52).

More recently, Duhaime et al. (29) reached similar conclusions using infant models. In this experiment, adults vigorously shook and/or impacted infant models with implanted cranial accelerometers. Vigorous shaking alone did not achieve sufficient rotational velocity or acceleration magnitudes to exceed extrapolated injury thresholds for concussion, subdural hemorrhage, or diffuse axonal injury (even using three variations of neck structure in the infant models). Conversely, even "soft" cranial impacts created rotational velocity and acceleration measurements above these extrapolated injury thresholds. Taken together, these works of Ommaya et al. (90,92,95) and Duhaime et al. (29) demonstrated that contact and noncontact strains are additive.

Brain and other viscoelastic tissues behave more stiffly when a mechanical load is applied suddenly or briefly, a protective property that lessens vulnerability to deeper tissue strains and injury. Conversely, tissues behave less stiffly (and are more vulnerable to deeper and diffuse strains and injury) when a mechanical load is applied slowly. It follows logically that concussion and other deeper and diffuse brain injuries are facilitated when the duration of cranial acceleration is prolonged.

Ommaya et al. (91) verified the importance of prolonged load duration in the pathogenesis of diffuse brain injury by inducing experimental concussion in primates using whiplash (i.e., without cranial impact). As load duration was prolonged, the magnitude of cranial acceleration required to produce experimental concussion was lowered. With shorter load duration, greater cranial acceleration magnitude was required to produce loss of consciousness.

More severe primary diffuse brain injury may manifest clinically as immediate loss of consciousness with prolonged traumatic coma and without mass lesions. Frequently this clinical constellation is associated with widespread traumatic axonal injury (i.e., *diffuse axonal injury*). Histopathologic evidence of diffuse axonal injury includes axonal swelling and axonal retraction balls (2,98,99,114). Demonstration of diffuse axonal injury in very young victims of head trauma may require older silver staining (9,121) or newer immunohistochemical techniques (41). Macroscopically, diffuse axonal injury has been linked to petechial tissue-tear hemorrhages in the corpus callosum, the rostral brainstem, and other central portions of the mature brain (36,83,114,123,129). In very young victims of diffuse axonal injury, younger than 5 months, petechial tissue-tear hemorrhages are less common. Instead, macroscopic *parenchymal contusional tears* may be a marker for underlying diffuse axonal injury in this age group (73,121). In pediatric victims of inflicted traumatic brain injury, diffuse axonal injury is found frequently to coexist with subdural hemorrhage and other indicators of cranial acceleration injury (41). Because the specific biomechanical circumstances of cranial rotational acceleration pathogenic for diffuse axonal injury (39) and noncontact subdural hemorrhage (38) differ substantially, their frequent coexistence in young victims of inflicted head trauma may imply multiple injury events and mechanisms (54,121) and portend a more severe clinical outcome (32).

The Centripetal Theory

What principles underlie the distribution of focal and diffuse strains in neural tissues found in cerebral concussion? Correlating clinical, experimental, and pathological observations, in 1974 Ommaya and Gennarelli (93) proposed a unifying *centripetal theory* for traumatic cerebral concussion. They began by observing the following:

1. Both impact and nonimpact can injure the brain by the stresses and strains of inertial (i.e., acceleration or noncontact) loading.
2. Impact adds the effect of contact phenomenon.
3. Because nonimpact inertial loading can produce traumatic unconsciousness, it is reasonable to assume that inertial loading is the major cause of brain damage in blunt head injuries.
4. At equivalent levels of input acceleration, rotation of the head appears to be necessary for loss of consciousness.
5. The distribution of damaging strains induced by inertial loading decreases in magnitude from the surface to the center of the approximately spheroidal brain mass.

To explain these observations, Ommaya and Gennarelli (93) concluded that traumatic cerebral concussion represents "... a graded set of clinical syndromes following head injury wherein increasing severity of disturbance in level and content of consciousness is caused by mechanically induced strains affecting the brain in a centripetal sequence of disruptive effect on function and structure." In other words, increasing severity of primary brain injury (i.e., strains) causes more extensive disconnections between the cortex and the mesencephalic–diencephalic "core" of the brain. Outcome is dependent . . .

on the mechanical properties of various cranial tissues, as well as the location of bony protrusions, dural partitions, vascular anatomy, and other sources of tissue interfaces with different densities. . . .It would follow that those parts of the cortex covered by smooth surfaces (e.g., the occipital lobes) should suffer the least damage, whereas those portions covered by rough surfaces (e.g., the temporal lobes, frontal poles, and orbital cortex) would suffer the most.

This paradigm has been validated in adult and in pediatric populations (70,71).

Applying a Biomechanics-Based Approach to Case Analysis

Does the caretaker's history of accidental cranial impact explain your patient's constellation of primary traumatic cranial injuries? If not, child abuse must be considered. The analysis of primary cranial injuries may seem highly complicated. However, the task can be simplified if approached logically. Hymel et al. (54) proposed a biomechanics-based paradigm for the analysis of primary traumatic cranial injuries. Using a logical series of questions, this paradigm guides injury analysis backwards from injury to history:

1. What are the specific cranial injuries?
2. How can these specific cranial injuries be classified?
3. Was cranial contact or noncontact (i.e., acceleration) required to produce each specific primary cranial injury?
4. What biomechanical circumstances of cranial impact were necessary to create these required contact and/or noncontact primary injury mechanisms?
5. Are these specific required biomechanical circumstances evident in the history provided? If not, child abuse must be considered.

To evaluate the validity of a caretaker's report of accidental cranial impact, we must define the specific biomechanical circumstances of a single cranial-impact event necessary to produce the observed cranial injuries. When a child's head strikes or is struck by an object with sufficient force and impact energy, only three combinations of primary cranial injury are possible. The child may sustain isolated contact injuries, isolated noncontact injuries, or a combination of both contact and noncontact injuries. There are no other possibilities.

Analyzing Cases of Isolated Primary Contact Injuries

Cranial impact occurred. This impact was sufficient to cause one or more contact injuries, but insufficient to cause clinically significant secondary whole-head cranial acceleration. If the head was struck by a moving impactor, the absence of associated noncontact injuries implies (a) high cranial fixity, (b) isolated static cranial loading (e.g., crushing), (c) nondistributed loading, and/or (d) insufficient impactor force and energy. Conversely, if the moving head struck a fixed surface, the absence of associated noncontact injuries implies that impact force and energy of the decelerating cranium were insufficient (e.g., a fall from an indoor height and/or cranial impact onto a deformable surface).

Analyzing Cases of Isolated Primary Noncontact Injuries

Clinically significant whole-head cranial acceleration occurred. This may have been the result of impact or nonimpact cranial loading (e.g., violent shaking). Even in the absence of external soft tissue injuries or skull fracture, impact cannot be excluded (29). If noncontact injuries resulted because the head was struck by a moving impactor, then (a) cranial motion was unrestricted, (b) isolated static cranial loading (e.g., slow crushing) did not occur, (c) cranial loading was more likely distributed, and (d) sufficient impactor force and energy were available. Conversely, if noncontact injuries occurred because the moving head struck a fixed surface, then the impact force and energy of the decelerating cranium were sufficient (e.g., a fall from a outdoor height and/or onto a rigid surface). In either example

of cranial impact, the absence of associated contact injuries implies (a) distributed loading, and/or (b) high deformability of the impactor or impacted surface.

Analyzing Cases of Combined Primary Contact and Noncontact Injuries

Contact injuries confirm that cranial impact occurred. Assuming a single contact event, impact was sufficient to cause both contact injuries and clinically significant whole-head cranial acceleration. If the head was struck by a moving impactor, then (a) cranial motion was unrestricted; (b) isolated static cranial loading did not occur; (c) cranial loading was more likely distributed; and (d) impactor force and energy were sufficient. Conversely, if the moving head struck a fixed surface, then the impact force and energy of the decelerating cranium were sufficient (e.g., a fall from an outdoor height and/or cranial impact onto a rigid surface). In either example of cranial impact, the presence of associated contact injuries implies (a) less well-distributed loading, and/or (b) low deformability of the impactor or impacted surface.

The Timing of Cranial Injuries

Because *immediate* loss of consciousness is an overt clinical manifestation occurring at the moment of primary diffuse brain injury (39), objective evidence of this specific injury classification (41) may allow accurate determination of the timing of cranial injury. In the presence of diffuse primary brain injury (e.g., diffuse axonal injury), the caretaker who witnessed onset of loss of consciousness was present at the moment of injury (54). Biomechanical conditions favoring diffuse axonal injury (DAI) include distributed loading, "soft" impact (i.e., longer duration), cranial motion favoring rotation over translation, coronal direction of cranial rotation, and negligible contact phenomenon (39,88,89).

In the absence of diffuse primary brain injury (e.g., crush injuries with cranial fixation), immediate loss of consciousness is unlikely unless vital deep brain structures are injured primarily (28,54). Biomechanical conditions favoring "non-DAI" primary injuries include focused loading, "hard" impact (i.e., shorter duration), cranial motion favoring translation over rotation, anteroposterior direction of cranial rotation, and more prominent contact phenomenon (38,88,89).

Occasionally, "non-DAI" cases are complicated by *delayed* loss of consciousness occurring as a manifestation of secondary brain injury (12,74,77,101,103,111). *Secondary* brain injuries, mediated primarily by hypoxia and/or ischemia, may be due to apnea (59), altered autoregulation of cerebral blood flow, venous vasospasm (96), space-occupying intracranial hemorrhage (101,103,126), seizures (101,103, 111), acquired coagulopathy (53), hypovolemic shock (69), and/or brain swelling (3,12,69).

Compared with adults, young children appear to be uniquely vulnerable to severe brain swelling after cranial trauma (3,12).

Falls

Cranial acceleration and deceleration are analogous events, differing only in direction. Cranial deceleration on impact with the ground or floor may cause clinically significant noncontact injuries if impact velocity and energy are very high (e.g., an outdoor fall from a significant height) and impact duration is brief (e.g., a fall onto a rigid, nondeformable surface such as concrete). These same biomechanical circumstances increase the risk of resultant contact injuries, as does nondistributed loading (e.g., cranial impact onto a small, rigid object resting on the floor).

Compared with that of an adult, the cranium of an infant or young child represents a larger percentage of the total body mass, so cranial impact is a frequent consequence of accidental pediatric falls. In specific circumstances, accidental pediatric falls may cause severe cranial injury (albeit rarely). These potentially dangerous circumstances include stairway falls in an infant walker, stairway falls in the arms of an adult, or falls from an elevated bunk bed (19,20,58,109).

Nevertheless, an extensive body of medical literature confirms the following:

1. The vast majority of indoor pediatric falls do not result in severe injury (50,76, 86,116,124);
2. Children frequently survive falls from significant heights (7,16,48,85,124); and
3. Serious pediatric injuries are rare in day care centers (10,17,18,67,68,104,106).

Taken together, these reports provide compelling evidence that the vast majority of accidental pediatric falls are benign events. To date, only a single descriptive biomechanical study (122) stands in apparent contrast to this general conclusion.

Anatomic, biomechanical, and developmental factors combine to protect infants and young children from injury when their heads strike the ground as the result of an accidental fall from a standing height. Younger skulls are more elastic. In addition, the nonrigid conformation of the unfused, younger skull further increases its elasticity and resistance to fracture. The surface area of the young skull is large relative to the mass of the body. The scalar features of mass and surface area decrease the compressive stress of cranial impact after a fall and decrease skull-fracture susceptibility during childhood.

Cranial impact onto a rigid surface (i.e., a brief stopping time) will increase the magnitude of cranial deceleration ($a = v/t$) and the resultant impact force ($F = ma$). Nevertheless, even these brief deceleration events rarely cause severe cranial injury in young children. Young children are short and small (i.e., lower mass). They are protected because their indoor falls from a standing height translate into minimal impact velocity [thereby lessening deceleration ($a = v/t$), force ($F = ma$), and impact kinetic energy ($E = 1/2\ mv^2$)]. Finally, parachute and protective reflexes (i.e., the reflex actions to reorient your body while falling and to break your fall with outstretched hands) typically develop before the ability to cruise and/or walk.

CONCLUSION

Social service, investigative, and legal authorities look to child abuse medical specialists to differentiate between accidental and inflicted pediatric trauma. In the absence of a witnessed injury event or a confession of inflicted trauma, these determinations can be very difficult. Biomechanics-based research linking witnessed abusive actions to specific inflicted physical injuries is virtually nonexistent.

Increasingly, child abuse medical specialists seek improved objectivity in their case analyses. Indeed, many courtrooms and even the media are demanding it! A biomechanics-based approach to the analysis of pediatric traumatic injury offers substantial hope of improved objectivity. What caused this injury? Does the history make sense? If not, child abuse must be considered.

REFERENCES

1. Adams JH, Gennarelli TA, Graham DI. Brain damage in non-missile head injury: observations in man and in subhuman primates. In: Smith R, Cavanaugh J, eds. *Recent advances in neuropathology.* Livingston: London, 1982:165–190.
2. Adams JH, Mitchell DE, Graham DI, et al. Diffuse brain damage of intermediate type: its relationship to "primary brain stem damage" in head injury. *Brain* 1977;100:489–502.
3. Adelson PD, Clyde B, Kochanek PM, et al. Cerebrovascular response in infants and young children following severe traumatic brain injury: a preliminary report. *Pediatr Neurosurg* 1997;26:200–207.
4. Alexander RC, Schor DP, Smith WL. Magnetic resonance imaging of intracranial injuries from child abuse. *J Pediatr* 1986;146:97–102.
5. Aoki N, Masuzawa H. Subdural hematomas in abused children: report of six cases from Japan. *Neurosurgery* 1986;18:475–477.
6. Arnholz D, Hymel KP, Hay TC, et al. Bilateral pediatric skull fractures: accident or abuse? *J Trauma Injury Infect Crit Care* 1998;45:172–174.
7. Barlow B, Niemirska M, Gandhi RP, et al. Ten years of experience of falls from a height in children. *J Pediatr Surg* 1983;18:509–511.
8. Betz P, Liebhardt E. Rib fractures in children: resuscitation or child abuse? *Int J Legal Med* 1994;106:215–218.
9. Blumbergs PC, Jones NR, North JB. Diffuse axonal injury in head trauma. *J Neurol Neurosurg Psychiatry* 1996;52:839–841.
10. Briss PA, Sacks JJ, Addiss DG, et al. A nationwide study of the risk of injury associated with day care attendance. *Pediatrics* 1994;93:364–368.
11. Broom ND, Oloyede A, Flachsmann R, et al. Dynamic fracture characteristics of the osteochondral junction undergoing shear deformation. *Med Eng Phys* 1996;18:396–404.
12. Bruce DA, Alavi A, Bilaniuk L, et al. Diffuse cerebral swelling following head injuries in children: the syndrome of "malignant brain edema." *J Neurosurg* 1981;54:170–178.
13. Bruce DA, Zimmerman RA. Shaken impact syndrome. *Pediatr Ann* 1989;18:482–494.
14. Caffey J. Some traumatic lesions in growing bones other than fractures and dislocations: clinical and radiological features. *Br J Radiol* 1957;30:225–228.
15. Carter DR, Hayes WC. Bone compressive strength: the influence of density and strain rate. *Science* 1976;194:1174–1176.
16. Chadwick DL, Chin S, Salerno C, et al. Deaths from falls in children: how far is fatal? *J Trauma Injury Infect Crit Care* 1991;31:1353–1355.
17. Chadwick DL, Salerno JJ. The rarity of serious head injury in day care centers [Letter]. *J Trauma Injury Infect Crit Care* 1993;35:968.
18. Chang A, Lugg MM, Nebedum A. Injuries among preschool children enrolled in day-care centers. *Pediatrics* 1989;83:272–277.
19. Chiavello CT, Christoph RA, Bond GR. Infant walker-related injuries: a prospective study of severity and incidence. *Pediatrics* 1994;93:974–976.
20. Chiavello CT, Christoph RA, Bond GR. Stairway-related injuries in children. *Pediatrics* 1994;94:679–681.
21. Cody DD, McCubbrey DA, Divine GW, et al. Predictive value of proximal femoral bone densitometry in determining local orthogonal material properties. *J Biomech* 1996;29:753–761.
22. Cohen RA, Kaufman RA, Myers PA, et al. Cranial computed tomography in the abused child with head injury. *AJR Am J Roentgenol* 1986;146:97–102.
23. Currey JD. Strain rate and mineral content in fracture models of bone. *J Orthop Res* 1988;6:32–38.
24. Denny-Brown, Russell WR. Experimental cerebral concussion. *Brain* 1941;64:93–164.
25. DiMaio DJ, DiMaio VJM. Trauma to the skull and brain: craniocerebral injuries. In: DiMaio DJ, DiMaio VJM, eds. *Forensic pathology.* New York: Elsevier, 1989:139–169.
26. Duhaime AC, Alario AJ, Lewander WJ, et al. Head injury in very young children: mechanisms, injury types, and ophthalmologic findings in 100 hospitalized patients younger than 2 years of age. *Pediatrics* 1992;90:179–185.
27. Duhaime AC, Christian CW, Armonda R, et al. Disappearing subdural hematomas in children. *Pediatr Neurosurg* 1996;25:116–122.
28. Duhaime AC, Eppley M, Margulies S, et al. Crush injuries to the head in children. *Neurosurgery* 1995;37:401–406.
29. Duhaime AC, Gennarelli TA, Thibault LE, et al. The shaken baby syndrome. *J Neurosurg* 1987;66:409–415.
30. Duncan RL, Turner CH. Mechanotransduction and the functional response of bone to mechanical strain. *Calcif Tissue Int* 1995;57:344–358.
31. Evans FG, Lissner HR, Lebow M. The relation of energy, velocity, and acceleration to skull deformation and fracture. *Surg Gynecol Obstet* 1958;107:593–601.
32. Ewing-Cobbs L, Kramer L, Prasad M, et al. Neuroimaging, physical, and developmental findings after

inflicted and noninflicted traumatic brain injury in young children. *Pediatrics* 1998;102:300–307.

33. Feldman KW, Brewer DK. Child abuse, cardiopulmonary resuscitation and rib fractures. *Pediatrics* 1984;73:339–342.

34. Garland DE, Stewart CA, Adkins RH, et al. Osteoporosis after spinal cord injury. *J Orthop Res* 1992; 10:371–378.

35. Gennarelli TA. Clinical and experimental head injury. In: Aldman B, Chapon A, eds. *The biomechanics of impact trauma.* Amsterdam: Elsevier Science, 1984:103–115.

36. Gennarelli TA, Meany DF. Mechanism of primary brain injury. In: Wilkins R, Rengachery S, eds. *Neurosurgery.* New York: McGraw-Hill, 1996:2611–2621.

37. Gennarelli TA, Spielman GM, Langfitt TW. Influence of the type of intracranial lesion on outcome from severe head injury. *J Neurosurg* 1982;56:26–32.

38. Gennarelli TA, Thibault LE. Biomechanics of acute subdural hematoma. *J Trauma Injury Infect Crit Care* 1982;22:680–686.

39. Gennarelli TA, Thibault LE, Adams JH, et al. Diffuse axonal injury and traumatic coma in the primate. *Ann Neurol* 1982;12:564–574.

40. Gibbs K. *Advanced physics.* 2nd ed. Worcester, U.K.: Cambridge University Press, 1990.

41. Gleckman AM, Bell MD, Evans RJ, et al. Diffuse axonal injury by β-amyloid precursor protein immunohistochemical staining. *Arch Pathol Lab Med* 1999; 123:146–151.

42. Gonick L, Huffman A. *The cartoon guide to physics.* New York: Harper Perennial, 1990.

43. Greenes DS, Schutzman SA. Occult intracranial injury in infants. *Ann Emerg Med* 1998;32:680–686.

44. Gruskin KD, Schutzman SA. Head trauma in children younger than 2 years: are there predictors for complications? *Arch Pediatr Adolesc Med* 1999;153:15–20.

45. Gurdjian ES, Lissner HR, Hodgson VR. Mechanisms of head injury. *Clin Neurosurg* 1966;12:112–128.

46. Gurdjian ES, Webster JE, Lissner HR. The mechanism of skull fracture. *Radiology* 1950;54:313–338.

47. Guthkelch AN. Infantile subdural haematoma and its relationship to whiplash injuries. *Br Med J* 1971;2: 430–431.

48. Hajivassiliou CA, Azmy A. Physical parameters of free fall in a child. *Injury* 1996;27:739–741.

49. Harrigan TP, Hamilton JJ. Bone strain sensation via transmembrane potential changes in surface osteoblasts: loading rate and microstructural implications. *J Biomech* 1993;26:183–200.

50. Helfer RE, Slovis TL, Black M. Injuries resulting when small children fall out of bed. *Pediatrics* 1977; 60:533–535.

51. Hiss J, Kahana T. The medicolegal implications of bilateral cranial fractures in infants. *J Trauma Injury Infect Crit Care* 1995;38:32–34.

52. Holbourn AHS. Mechanics of head injuries. *Lancet* 1943;2:438–441.

53. Hymel KP, Abshire TC, Luckey DW, et al. Coagulopathy in pediatric abusive head trauma. *Pediatrics* 1997; 99:371–375.

54. Hymel KP, Bandak FA, Partington MD, et al. Abusive head trauma? A biomechanics-based approach. *Child Maltreat* 1998;3:116–128.

55. Hymel KP, Rumack CM, Hay TC, et al. Comparison of intracranial computed tomographic (CT) findings in pediatric abusive and accidental head trauma. *Pediatr Radiol* 1997;27:743–747.

56. Jayawant S, Rawlinson A, Gibbon F, et al. Subdural haematomas in infants: population based study. *Br Med J* 1998;317:1558–1561.

57. Jenny C, Hymel KP, Ritzen A, et al. Analysis of missed cases of abusive head trauma. *JAMA* 1999;281: 621–626.

58. Joffe M, Ludwig S. Stairway injuries in children. *Pediatrics* 1988;82:457–461.

59. Johnson DL, Boal D, Baule R. Role of apnea in nonaccidental head injury. *Pediatr Neurosurg* 1995;23: 305–310.

60. Keller TS. Predicting the compressive mechanical behavior of bone. *J Biomech* 1994;27:1159–1168.

61. Kleinman PK. Radiologic and histopathologic correlates of posterior rib fractures in abused infants: an alternate mechanism of injury. *Pediatr Radiol* 1987;17: 83–91.

62. Kleinman PK. Skeletal trauma: general considerations. In: Kleinman PK, ed. *Diagnostic imaging of child abuse.* 2nd ed. St. Louis: Mosby, 1998:8–25.

63. Kleinman PK, Marks SC Jr, Blackbourne BD. The metaphyseal lesion in abused infants: a radiologic-histopathologic study. *AJR Am J Roentgenol* 1986;146: 895–905.

64. Kleinman PK, Marks SC Jr, Nimkin K, et al. Rib fractures in 31 abused infants: postmortem radiologic-histopathologic study. *Radiology* 1996;200:807–810.

65. Kleinman PK, Schlesinger AE. Mechanical factors associated with posterior rib fractures: laboratory and case studies. *Pediatr Radiol* 1997;27:87–91.

66. Kravitz H, Driessen G, Gomberg R, et al. Accidental falls from elevated surfaces in infants from birth to one year of age. *Pediatrics* 1969;44(suppl):869–876.

67. Landman PF, Landman GB. Accidental injuries in day care centers. *Am J Dis Child* 1987;141:292–293.

68. Leland NL, Garrard J, Smith DK. Injuries to preschool-age children in day care centers. *Am J Dis Child* 1993;147:826–831.

69. Levin HS, Aldrich EF, Saydjari C, et al. Severe head injury in children: experience of the traumatic coma data bank. *Neurosurgery* 1992;31:435–444.

70. Levin HS, Mendelsohn D, Lilly MA, et al. Magnetic resonance imaging in relation to functional outcome of pediatric closed head injury: a test of the Ommaya-Gennarelli model. *Neurosurgery* 1997;40:432–441.

71. Levin HS, Williams D, Crofford MJ, et al. Relationship of depth of brain lesions to consciousness and outcome after closed head injury. *J Neurosurg* 1988;69:861–866.

72. Linde F, Norgaard P, Hvid I, et al. Mechanical properties of trabecular bone: dependency on strain rate. *J Biomech* 1991;24:803–809.

73. Lindenberg R, Freytag E. Morphology of brain lesions from blunt trauma in early infancy. *Arch Pathol* 1969; 87:298–305.

74. Lobato RD, Rivas JJ, Gomez PA, et al. Head-injured patients who talk and deteriorate into coma. *J Neurosurg* 1991;75:256–261.

75. Ludwig S. Shaken baby syndrome: a review of 20 cases. *Ann Emerg Med* 1984;13:104–107.

76. Lyons TJ, Oates RK. Falling out of bed, a relatively benign occurrence. *Pediatrics* 1993;92:125–127.

77. Marshall LF, Toole BM, Bowers SA. The National

Traumatic Coma Data Bank (Part 2): patients who talk and deteriorate: implications for treatment. *J Neurosurg* 1983;59:285–288.

78. Martin RB, Burr DB. *The structure, function and adaptation of compact bone.* New York: Raven Press, 1990.

79. McElhany JH, Hopper RH, Nightingale RW, et al. Mechanisms of basilar skull fracture. *J Neurotrauma* 1995;12:669–678.

80. Merten DF, Carpenter BLM. Radiologic imaging of abusive injury in the child abuse syndrome. *Pediatr Clin North Am* 1990;37:815–837.

81. Merten DF, Osborne DRS, Radowski MA, et al. Craniocerebral trauma in the child abuse syndrome: radiological observation. *Pediatr Radiol* 1984;14:272–277.

82. Millard J, Augat P, Link TM, et al. Power spectral analysis of vertebral trabecular bone structure from radiographs: orientation dependence and correlation with bone mineral density and mechanical properties. *Calcif Tissue Int* 1998;63:482–489.

83. Mittle RL, Grossman RI, Hiehle JF, et al. Prevalence of MR evidence of diffuse axonal injury in patients with mild head injury and normal CT findings. *AJNR Am J Neuroradiol* 1994;15:1583–1589.

84. Morild I, Gjerdet NR, Giertsen JC. Bone strength in infants. *Forens Sci Int* 1993;60:111–119.

85. Musemeche CA, Barthel M, Cosentino C, et al. Pediatric falls from heights. *J Trauma Injury* 1991;31:1347–1349.

86. Nimityongskul P, Anderson L. The likelihood of injuries when children fall out of bed. *J Pediatr Orthop* 1987;7:184–186.

87. Carter D. The biomechanics of bone. In: Nahun AM, Melvin J, eds. *The biomechanics of trauma.* Stamford, Connecticut: Appleton and Lange, 1984:159.

88. Ommaya AK. Head injury mechanisms and the concept of preventive management: a review and critical synthesis. In: Bandak FA, Eppinger RH, Ommaya AK, eds. *Traumatic brain injury bioscience and mechanics.* Larchmont, NY: Mary Ann Liebert, Inc. 1996:19–38.

89. Ommaya AK. The head: kinematics and brain injury mechanisms. In: Aldman B, Chapon A, eds. *The biomechanics of impact trauma.* Amsterdam: Elsevier, 1984:117–125.

90. Ommaya AK, Corrao P. Pathogenic biomechanics of central nervous system injury in head impact and whiplash trauma. In: Brinkhouse KM, ed. *Accident pathology.* Washington, DC: U.S. Government Printing Office, 1969.

91. Ommaya AK, Faas F, Yarnell P. Whiplash injury and brain damage. *JAMA* 1968;204:285–289.

92. Ommaya AK, Flamm ES, Mahone RM. Cerebral concussion in the monkey: an experimental model. *Science* 1996;153:211–212.

93. Ommaya AK, Gennarelli TA. Cerebral concussion and traumatic unconsciousness. *Brain* 1974;97:633–654.

94. Ommaya AK, Grubb RL, Nauman RA. Coup and contre-coup injury: observations on the mechanics of visible brain injuries in rhesus monkey. *J Neurosurg* 1971;35:503–516.

95. Ommaya AK, Hirsch AE. Tolerances for cerebral concussion from head impact and whiplash in primates. *Brain* 1971;4:13–20.

96. Ommaya AK, Thibault LE, Boock RI, et al. Head injured patients who talk before deterioration and death: the TADD syndrome. In: Hoerner EF, eds. *Proceedings of the ASTM, International Symposium on Head and Neck Injuries in Sports.* Philadelphia: American Society for Testing Materials, 1993.

97. Pilz P. Axonal injury in head injury. *Acta Neurochir* 1993;32:119–123.

98. Povlishock JT. Traumatically induced axonal injury: pathogenesis and pathobiological implications. *Brain Pathol* 1992;2:1–12.

99. Povlishock JT, Christman CW. The pathobiology of traumatically induced axonal injury in animals and humans: a review of current thoughts. In: Bandak FA, Eppinger RH, Ommaya AK, eds. *Traumatic brain injury bioscience and mechanics.* Larchmont, NY: Mary Ann Liebert, 1996:51–60.

100. Reilly DT, Burstein AH. The elastic and ultimate properties of compact bone tissue. *J Biomech* 1975;8:393–405.

101. Reilly PL, Graham DI, Adams JH, et al. Patients with head injury who talk and die. *Lancet* 1975;2:375–377.

102. Rho JY, Hobatho MC, Ashman RB. Relations of mechanical properties to density and CT numbers in human bone. *Med Eng Phys* 1995;17:347–355.

103. Rose J, Valtonen S, Jennett B. Avoidable factors contributing to death after head injury. *Br Med J* 1977; 2:615–618.

104. Rivara FP, DiGuiseppi C, Thompson RS, et al. Risk of injury to children less than 5 years of age in day care versus home settings. *Pediatrics* 1989;84:1011–1016.

105. Russell WR, Schiller F. Crushing injuries to the skull: clinical and experimental observations. *J Neurol Neurosurg Psychiatry* 1949;12:52–60.

106. Sacks JJ, Smith JD, Kaplan KM, et al. The epidemiology of injuries in Atlanta day-care centers. *JAMA* 1989;262:1651–1655.

107. Sammarco GJ, Burstein AN, Davis WL, et al. The biomechanics of torsional fractures: the effect of loading on ultimate properties. *J Biomech* 1971;4:113–117.

108. Sato Y, Yuh WTC, Smith WL, et al. Head injury in child abuse: evaluation with MR imaging. *Radiology* 1989;173:653–657.

109. Selbst SM, Baker MD, Shames M. Bunk bed injuries. *Am J Dis Child* 1990;144:721–723.

110. Shugerman RP, Paez A, Grossman DC, et al. Epidural hemorrhage: is it abuse? *Pediatrics* 1996;97:664–668.

111. Snoek JW, Minderhoud JM, Wilmink JT. Delayed deterioration following mild head injury in children. *Brain* 1984;107:15–36.

112. Snyder SM, Schneider E. Estimation of mechanical properties of cortical bone by computed tomography. *J Orthop Res* 1991;9:422–431.

113. Spevak MR, Kleinman PK, Belanger PL, et al. Cardiopulmonary resuscitation and rib fractures in infants: a postmortem radiologic-pathologic study. *JAMA* 1994;272:617–618.

114. Strich SJ. Diffuse degeneration of the cerebral white matter in severe dementia following head injury. *J Neurol Neurosurg Psychiatry* 1956;19:163–185.

115. Sugar NF, Taylor JA, Feldman KW, et al. Bruises in infants and toddlers. *Arch Pediatr Adolesc Med* 1999; 153:399–403.

116. Tarantino CA, Dowd MD, Murdock TC. Short vertical falls in infants. *Pediatr Emerg Care* 1999;15:5–8.

117. Tsai FY, Zee CS, Apthorp JS, et al. Computed tomography in child abuse head trauma. *J Comput Tomogr* 1984;4:277–286.

118. Turner CH. On Wolff's law of trabecular architecture. *J Biomech* 1995;25:1–9.

119. Ulrich D, van Rietbergen B, Weinans H, et al. Finite element analysis of trabecular bone structure: a comparison of image-based meshing techniques. *J Biomech* 1998;31:1187–1192.

120. Van der Meulen MCH, Carter DR. Developmental mechanics determine long bone allometry. *J Theoret Biol* 1995;172:323–327.

121. Vowles GH, Scholtz CL, Cameron JM. Diffuse axonal injury in early infancy. *J Clin Pathol* 1987;40: 185–189.

122. Weber W. Biomechanical fragility of skull fracture in infants. *Z Rechtsmed* 1984;92:87–92.

123. Wilberger JE, Rothfus WE, Tabas J, et al. Acute tissue tear hemorrhages of the brain: computed tomography and clinical pathological correlations. *Neurosurgery* 1990;27:208–213.

124. Williams RA. Injuries in infants and small children resulting from witnessed and corroborated free falls. *J Trauma Injury* 1991;31:1350–1352.

125. Williams JL, Vani JN, Eick JD, et al. Shear strength of the physis varies with anatomic location and is a function of modulus, inclination and thickness. *J Orthop Res* 1999;17:214–222.

126. Wilman KY, Bank DE, Senac M, et al. Restricting the time of injury in fatal inflicted head injuries. *Child Abuse Neglect* 1997;21:929–940.

127. Yeni YN, Brown CU, Norman TL. Influence of bone composition and apparent density on fracture toughness of the human femur and tibia. *Bone* 1998;22: 79–84.

128. Yoganandan N, Pintar FA, Sances A Jr, et al. Biomechanics of skull fracture. *J Neurotrauma* 1995;12: 659–668.

129. Zimmerman RA, Bilaniuk LT, Gennarelli TA. Computed tomography of shearing injuries of the cerebral white matter. *Radiology* 1978;127:393–396.

2

Cutaneous Manifestations of Child Abuse

Carole Jenny

Child Protection Program, Hasbro Children's Hospital; and Department of Pediatrics,
Brown University School of Medicine, Providence, Rhode Island

SKIN: AN OVERVIEW

Human skin is an extraordinary organ, accounting for 16% of the weight of the human body (135). It serves many important functions, including control of thermoregulation, regulation of blood pressure, protection from microorganisms and toxins, and maintenance of hydration. Normal skin is supple, allowing facial expressions and joint mobility. The skin interfaces with the environment, providing many of our sensory experiences as well as the unique visage with which we interact with our environment (116).

Skin varies in thickness, depending on the location of the body. On the eyelid, it is 0.5 mm thick. On the soles of the feet, it can be up to 4 mm thick and can tolerate constant abrasion (135). Skin consists of two basic layers.

The Epidermis

The epidermis is the outer protective layer. It is made up of five cellular layers, all of which gradually migrate to the surface from the most basilar layer impinging on the basement membrane. In addition to epithelial cells and their main product, keratin, the epidermis contains melanocytes, providing melanin to protect and color the skin. Keratin constitutes 85% of the mass of the epidermis. The epidermis is replaced every 2 to 4 weeks (38).

The Dermis

The underlying dermis provides the skin's elasticity and strength. The dermis itself is composed of two layers, containing the proteins collagen, elastin, and reticulin, permeated by a mucopolysaccharide ground substance. Blood vessels, lymph vessels, and nerve fibers traverse the dermis. Fibroblasts, macrophages, and mast cells reside in the dermis. Hair follicles, sweat glands, and sebaceous glands protrude from the dermis to the epidermis and skin surface, providing regenerative potential after loss of the epidermis through illness or injury. Below the dermis, a subcutaneous layer attaches to fascia. This layer contains immune cells, blood and lymph vessels, nerves, and fatty tissue, and also provides protection to the body.

PROPERTIES OF SKIN

Skin has biomechanical properties that affect its function and healing. It has a distinctly nonlinear deformation response to loading. Small loads produce great deformation, but as the load increases, skin becomes progressively stiffer. Within limits, it also is elastic, and ideally reverts to its original state when loads are removed. Skin is viscoelastic and capable of both deformation and flow with load. If held in a stretched position, the tension on the skin decreases with time. Thus it exhibits a time-dependent response to load. Temperature, humidity, and pH affect the biomechanical properties of skin. Skin is thinner but more dense on the extremities. It increases in stiffness from the head to the foot (107).

Human skin is constantly under tension in most areas of the body. If a portion of skin is

23

removed from the body, the wound edges retract, and the excised skin shrinks. The lines of tension on the human body were first described by Langer in 1861. Langer noticed that if round pieces of skin were removed from cadavers, the wound contracted into a slit-shaped opening along the long axis of the elastic tension on the skin. "Langer's lines" are often used to guide the choice of sites and directions for surgical incisions, to minimize scarring and stretch on the wound. If healed by secondary intention, a circular or elliptical excision will form a linear scar. If a square of skin is removed, the resulting scar will take on the shape of a four-pointed star (10).

Dermal fibers in children are tortuous, unbranched, and loosely arranged. The lack of connection among fibers gives young skin greater mobility and elastic properties. When skin is strained, dermal fibers reorient to the direction of the load, becoming straightened and compact to minimize strain. With excess stress, the fibers fail and rupture, causing tissue failure. Young skin is less protected against large strains than is older skin. It is more viscous and less elastic (28).

The upper layers of the bloodless epidermis are relatively colorless. Skin coloration comes from the melanin (brown pigment) in the basilar layers of the epithelium, as well as from chemicals in the dermal tissues, including oxygenated hemoglobin (red), deoxygenated hemoglobin (blue), and bilirubin (yellow) (70). Normal skin can appear erythematous because of either increased blood flow through capillaries or increased number of capillaries.

THE WOUNDING OF SKIN

When sufficient force is delivered to skin, deformation and injury result. The injury experienced depends on the nature of the insult, the amount of force or energy applied, and the extent of surface area experiencing the force (26). Injuries are categorized into four types by the nature of disruption to the tissues.

1. Abrasions: Abrasions result from friction removing superficial layers of skin. They are also called scrapes. "Skinned knees" are a typical example of abrasions (30).
2. Contusions: Contusions cause discoloration of the skin because of hemorrhage into the skin after blunt trauma. Contusions can be diffuse (bruise) or focal (hematoma).
3. Lacerations: Lacerations are tears into the skin caused by shearing or crushing forces. Sharp or blunt objects can lacerate the skin, depending on the amount of force applied.
4. Burns: A burn is destruction of tissue by a physical agent applied to skin. Burns can result from the application of heat, chemical agents, or electromagnetic radiation. Although burn injuries caused by different types of agents can appear similar, their basic pathophysiology at the cellular level is quite different. This is described in more detail in a later section.

THE HEALING OF WOUNDED SKIN

Once skin is wounded, the complex process of wound healing begins. Wound healing is a dynamic process involving soluble mediators, blood cells, extracellular material, and parenchymal cells (114). A procession of overlapping steps occurs in wound healing, including formation of a blood clot; infiltration of the site with neutrophils, macrophages, and monocytes; progressive migration of epithelial cells over the wound; wound contraction; fibrinolysis of the original clot; formation of granulation tissue; and neovascularization of the healing wound.

Clot formation and inflammation begin almost immediately to preserve the integrity of the body after the skin is wounded. Within hours after injury, epidermal cells from the skin appendages begin to remove blood clot and damaged tissues. Epithelial cells at the wound edges dissolve their bonds to each other, and by 1 to 2 days after injury begin proliferating. Granulation tissue begins to invade the wound space approximately 4 days after injury. The fibroblast-rich granulation tissue establishes the matrix to support the migration of epithelial cells across the scar (114). Angiogenesis begins within 2 to 3 days. During the second week of healing, fibroblasts are transformed into myofibroblasts that aid in the contraction of the wound.

Wounds gain 20% of their strength in the first 3 weeks. As time goes on, the tensile strength of a wound increases slowly as collagen accumulates and remodels. A fully healed wound, however, is only 70% as strong as uninjured skin (10).

Many factors can slow the rate of wound healing, including hypoxia, ischemia, chronic shear forces, hyperthermia, infection, foreign bodies in the wound, use of antiinflammatory medications, tobacco use, poor nutrition (including deficiencies of vitamins A, B, C, and E, zinc, copper, calcium, methionine, proteins, and essential fatty acids), and metabolic diseases (such as diabetes), and other systemic disease (122). Wound desiccation and eschar formation also are detrimental to healing.

The central nervous system and the cutaneous sensory nerves play a role in wound healing. Wound pain provides protection for the healing wound. In addition, cutaneous sensory neurons secrete neuropeptides that actually modulate the wound-healing process. Denervated tissue heals more slowly than enervated tissue (4). Wounds on areas of the body that have better blood supply heal faster. The mouth, anus, and genitals heal most quickly, followed by the head and trunk. Healing of the extremities is slowest (106). Rewounding an injury causes acceleration of the healing process (18).

Wound healing is faster in children than in adults. Human fetal tissue in the first 6 months of pregnancy heals perfectly, without scar formation (82). Larger wounds require longer to heal than smaller, less deep wounds, and crush injuries cause more devitalization of tissue than do shear injuries, thus delaying healing (58). The compressive force of crush injuries delivers more energy to larger amounts of tissue, causing more tissue disruption and greater risk of infection (16). A scar (cicatrix) results from the deposition of fibrous tissue in the healed wound. A hyper-

trophic scar is limited to the original wound margin. A keloid, conversely, results from collagen deposited beyond the margins of the original wound. Keloids form when fibroblasts are less responsive to tissue-modulating agents, resulting in excess collagen formation during the remodeling phase (18). Keloids are more likely to form on darkly pigmented children, and on certain areas of the body, including the earlobes, sternum, back, shoulder, and upper arm (74).

THE HEALING OF BRUISES

Bruises differ from other wounds because the skin itself remains intact. With bruises, blood vessels are ruptured, and blood seeps into interstitial spaces. In addition, local inflammation and capillary dilation may add to the bright red color of a fresh bruise. As the blood cells and hemoglobin break down, the bruise exhibits a succession of colors, including red, violet, black, blue, yellow, green, and/or brown. There does not seem to be a predictable order or chronology of color progression (109). One study of visible bruises concluded that a bruise with any yellow coloration must be older that 18 hours; the colors red, blue, purple, or black may appear in the bruise at any time from 1 hour of injury to resolution of the bruise; red can appear in the bruise at any time and does not predict age; and bruises of identical age and cause on the same person may not appear the same and may change colors at different rates (72).

Many factors affect the rate of bruise resolution, including the amount of blood extravasated after the injury, the distance of the leakage of the blood from the skin surface, the amount of force applied and the amount of tissue damage incurred, the vascularity of the underlying tissue, the age of the person injured, and the underlying color of the injured person's skin (124). Bruises are often less obviously noted on the skin of more darkly pigmented children (126). The location of the bruise also can be a factor. Loosely attached skin, such as the skin around the eyes or gen-

TABLE 2.1. *Studies of skin trauma in normal children by age*

Location	Study	Population	Lesions studied	Age	% with lesions
Health clinics (U.K.)	Roberton et al. (1982) (104)	Normal children (N = 400)	Bruises and abrasions	2 wk–2 mo 3–9 mo 18 mo–11 yr	3.3 0.1 50–65
Health clinics (U.K.)	Mortimer et al. (1983) (87) N = 620	Normal children	Bruises	<1 y	0.9
Physician offices (U.S.A.)	Sugar et al. (1999) (126) N = 930	Well-child visits	Bruises	0–2 mo 3–5 mo 6–8 mo 9–11 mo 12–14 mo 15–17 mo 18–23 mo 24–35 mo	0.04 0.7 5.6 19.3 22.6 42.8 49.4 60.9

itals, will bruise more readily than skin that is under more tension. Drugs, (e.g., corticosteroids) can alter the rate of bruise dispersion. Aspirin or other antiinflammatory drugs can increase susceptibility to bruising by platelet inhibition, and the bruised person's underlying clotting mechanisms can increase or decrease the size of the initial bruise that must be cleared (124).

Given the many variables involved, the aging of bruises is an inexact process requiring judicious caution and healthy skepticism.

SKIN AND SOFT TISSUE INJURIES IN ABUSED AND NONABUSED CHILDREN

Bruises, lacerations, abrasions, and soft tissue swelling are commonly found in abused children. Table 2.1 summarizes several studies of skin injuries in *nonabused*

children. The studies show that soft tissue injury is extremely uncommon in children younger than 6 months and increases in frequency as children become older and more adventurous. Bruising in normal children also relates to developmental stage (Table 2.2) Infants who do not pull to standing are highly unlikely to suffer bruises. Two studies have shown that infants who do not yet "cruise" holding onto furniture are unlikely to be bruised (126,132). Both found that the amount of bruising in toddlers increased as their motor skill increased.

The distribution on the body also differs by age and developmental stage, and abusive bruises have been found to be located on parts of the body where bruises are not normally found. Roberton et al. (104) found injuries on the lower legs to be uncommon in children younger than 18 months. Head and face injuries were more common in 10- to 18-month-olds, and uncommon in children

TABLE 2.2. *Studies of skin trauma in normal children by developmental stage*

Location	Study	Population	Lesions studied	Motor development	% with lesions
Hospital (U.K.)	Wedgwood (1990) (132) N = 24	Hospitalized children, not suspected of being abused	Bruises	Precruisers Walk up stairs	0 100
Physician offices (U.S.A.)	Sugar et al. (1999) (126) N = 930	Well-child visits	Bruises	Precruisers Cruisers Walkers	2.2 17.8 51.9

TABLE 2.3. *Studies of location of skin trauma in normal children by developmental stage or age*

Location	Study	Population	Location of injury	Age or stage of motor development	% with lesions
Health clinics (U.K.)	Roberton et al. (1982) (104)	Normal children N = 400	Lower leg	18 mo–3 yr	>40.0
				3–11 yr	34.3
			Thigh and buttocks	<18 mo	2.4
				>18 mo	17.0
			Arms	<18 mo	2.4
				>18 mo	15.4
			Face and head	18 mo–3 yr	16.6
				>3 yr	<5.0
Health clinics (U.K.)	Mortimer et al. (1983) (87) N = 620	Normal children	Face	<1 yr	0.6
Physician offices (U.S.A.)	Sugar et al. (1999) (126) N = 930	Well-child visits	Lower leg	Precruiser	0.6
				Cruiser	11.9
				Walker	44.7
			Forehead	Precruiser	0.6
				Cruiser	3.0
				Walker	5.7
			Scalp	Precruiser	0.6
				Cruiser	5.0
				Walker	0.6
			Upper leg	Precruiser	0.2
				Cruiser	1.0
				Walker	4.4

older than 4 years. Whereas fewer than 1% of children younger than 3 years had lumbar bruises, the lumbar areas of 14% of school-aged children were bruised (Table 2.3). Sugar et al. (126) also found lower leg bruising to be common in children who could pull to standing or walk (Table 2.3). They found bruising to be rare in normal children on the hands, buttocks, cheek, nose, forearms, or chest.

Whereas facial injury has been shown to be uncommon in normal children, it is a frequent finding in abused children. McMahon et al. (83) found facial bruises to be common in abused children. Roberton et al. (104) found bruising to be much more common in abused children compared with normal children, in every body location except the lower legs.

In summary, accidental bruises and other soft tissue injuries are very unlikely to occur in children who are not pulling to standing. As children get older and become more developmentally advanced, they are more likely to get accidental bruises. The distribution of these bruises, however, tends to be different than that in abused children, with bruises to "exploratory surfaces" such as the lower legs being common, and bruises to the trunk less common (29).

VARIATIONS OF BRUISES AND SOFT TISSUE INJURIES IN ABUSED CHILDREN

Although many nonabused children will manifest injuries, certain patterns of injury have been recognized to be frequently caused by the abuse of children.

Pattern Marks

Injury inflicted with an object will often leave marks that reflect the outline of that object. The hand itself can leave a negative imprint, particularly on the face, when capillaries break between the fingers as blood is pushed away from the point of impact (101) (Fig. 2.1). Cords, ropes, shoes, kitchen implements, and belt buckles can leave notable out-

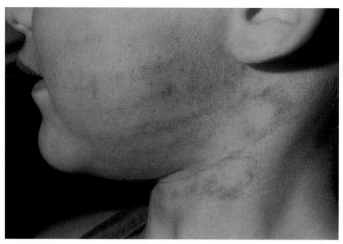

FIG. 2.1. Inflicted hand print on the face of a child, leaving an outline of the fingers.

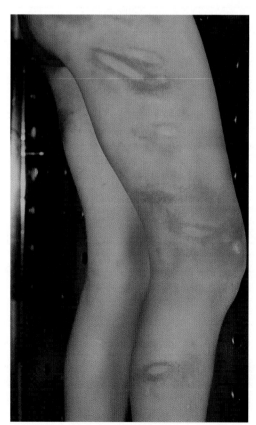

FIG. 2.2. Inflicted pattern mark on a child's body.

lines on the skin (112,117) (Fig. 2.2) Loop marks are generally worse at their extreme ends because the far end of the flexible cord travels at a faster rate of speed around the hand of the batterer.

Subgaleal Hematomas

Violently pulling on a child's hair can cause subgaleal hematomas (hemorrhage under the scalp) (50). The scalp is lifted off the calvarium at the aponeurotic junction. In addition to scalp swelling, traumatic alopecia (traumatic hair loss) can occur (134). The hair loss is usually seen on the top of the head and is patchy. The underlying scalp can appear normal, or petechial bruising can be seen (Fig. 2.3).

Petechiae on the Face and Neck Resulting from Strangulation

Conjunctival hemorrhages and facial and neck petechiae (masque ecchymotique) can result from compression of the chest and neck, causing increased venous pressure (Fig. 2.4). In one case, the petechial eruption resulted from folding the child in half at the waist by

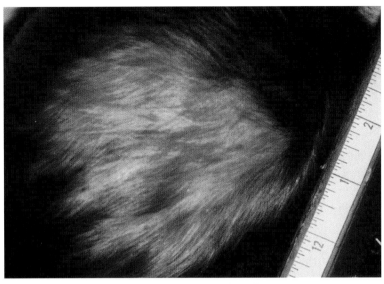

FIG. 2.3. Traumatic alopecia.

applying pressure to the neck and buttocks (96). Strangulation or suffocation by occlusion of the airway can cause similar lesions.

Bite Marks

Human bite marks are sometimes an abusive injury. They appear most frequently on the upper extremities (128). The incisal edges of the mandibular teeth will be more clearly delineated than those of the maxillary teeth because as the upper and lower incisors meet through the tissues, the skin is often impacted by the lower incisor edges against the lingular surface of the upper teeth (119). Bite marks should be carefully photographed with and

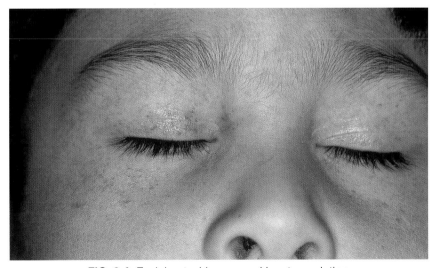

FIG. 2.4. Facial petechiae caused by strangulation.

without a size standard, and swabbed with sterile water or saline to recover genetic markers left behind from saliva.

Purpura of the External Ear

Blows to the side of the head can cause purpuric or petechial hemorrhages to occur on the external ear, often in the interior folds of the ears (52). Pulling or pinching the top of the ear leaves bruises on the helix or behind the pinna. If a blow sharply folds and crimps the pinna at the apex of the helix, petechiae can result (33).

Vertical Bruises of the Gluteal Cleft

Blows to the buttocks can leave vertical marks at the junction where the buttocks curve into the gluteal cleft (33).

Subungual Hematomas

Abusive biting of a child's fingers can cause chronic subungual hematomas. Leukonychia and swelling of the hands and feet also can be seen (41). Hitting a child's fingers with an object might leave subungual hemorrhages as well.

Tattooing

Purposely disfiguring a child's skin by tattooing the skin with an ink-filled needle has been reported (65).

Factitious Dermatitis (Dermatitis Artefactia)

Many different types of skin injuries can be purposefully inflicted on children by their caretakers to gain medical attention (67,123). This factitious disorder by proxy often presents with chronic dermatitis or skin ulcers that heal poorly. They are more likely found on the face, chest, anterior surfaces of the legs, and dorsal surfaces of the arms. The condition goes away when the child is removed from the abuser.

Children who have been victims of abuse (especially sexual abuse) are more likely to "self-inflict" injuries on themselves, cutting or burning themselves to distract themselves from emotional pain (49).

Air Rifles or Pellet Guns

These weapons are unregulated and readily available. They propel pellets at adequate velocities to penetrate human skin. A pellet-gun pellet has been reported to traverse the skin and lodge in the sagittal sinus in a purposefully inflicted injury to an infant (15).

SKIN CONDITIONS CONFUSED WITH ABUSIVE INJURIES TO SKIN AND SOFT TISSUES

Many different pathologic conditions have been described as lesions confused with inflicted injury. Table 2.4 lists these lesions by type of wound. The more common conditions are described.

Dermal Melanosis (Mongolian Spots)

These slate-blue or blue-green patches with indistinct borders are commonly seen in newborns. From 80% to 90% of African-American infants, 75% of Asian infants, and 10% of white infants have dermal melanosis. They are most often found on the lumbosacral region, but can occur anywhere on the body. Most fade by age 5 years (21). These common lesions can be confused with inflicted bruises. The lack of an inflammatory, reddened appearance can help differentiate dermal melanocytosis from bruising (Fig. 2.5). Whereas bruises fade over a few weeks, mongoloid spots remain unchanged during that time period.

Chilblain (Pernio)

Chilblain occurs when tissues are exposed to wet, cold weather (43). Bluish discoloration, erythema, and swelling occur, espe-

TABLE 2.4. *Skin lesions confused with inflicted injuries*

Injury	Other lesions confused with type of injury	Reference
Bruises, ecchymoses, and petechiae	Dermal melanosis (mongolian spots)	21
	Chilblain (pernio)	43
	Bleeding disorders (leukemia, von Willebrand disease, idiopathic thrombocytopenic purpura, hemophilia)	31,63,92
	Henoch–Schönlein purpura	11,73
	Phytophotodermatitis	45,56
	Hemangiomas	79
	Maculae ceruleae (secondary to pediculosis)	100
	Cao gio (coin rolling)	34,125
	Cupping	34,125
	Quat sha (spooning)	125
	Erythema nodosum	71
	Ink, paint, or dye to the body	133
	Hypersensitivity vasculitis	131
	Cystic lymphangiomas	
	Osteoma cutis (Albright hereditary osteodystrophy)	68
	Urticaria pigmentosa	44
	Popsicle panniculitis	23
	EMLA cream application	13
	Epidermal nevi	110
	Prominent facial veins	133
	Subconjunctival hemorrhages from pertussis	133
	Facial bruising from dental treatment	133
	Disseminated intravascular coagulation	131
	Meningococcemia	131
	Congenital indifference to pain	118
Contusions, hematomas, and ulcerated lesions	Erythema multiforme	1
	Erythema nodosum	71
	Angioedema	127
	Loxosceles reclusa (brown recluse spider) bite	88
	Calcium chloride necrosis	140
	Eczema	133
	Hemangiomas	79
	Hypersensitivity vasculitis	131
	Phytophotodermatitis	45,56
	Streptococcal toxic shock syndrome	89
	Chilblain (pernio)	43
	Postmortem insect bites	24
	Congenital indifference to pain	118
	Osteoma cutis (Albright hereditary osteodystrophy)	68
	Urticaria pigmentosa	44
Abusive scarring and lacerations	Striae	19
	Ehlers–Danlos syndrome	94
	Self-injurious behavior	49
	Epidermolysis bullosa	136
Traumatic alopecia	Loose anagen syndrome	134
	Trichotillomania	5
	Alopecia areata	133
Bite marks	Defibrillator injuries	47
Abusive tattoos	Religious tattoos associated with Afro-Caribbean religions such as Santeria and Palo Mayombe; cultural body ornamentation (Maori culture)	65 91
Intentional banding	Accidental banding of digits	
	Ainhum (dactylosis spontanea)	64
Sexual abuse	Perianal streptococcal cellulitis and vaginal streptococcal infections	27
	Lichen sclerosis	62
	Hemangiomas	79
	Lymphangioma circumscriptum	22
	Chronic bullous disease of childhood	20
	Perianal Langerhans cell histiocytosis	95
	Crohn's disease	95
	Lichen planus	95
	Hemolytic uremic syndrome	95
	Bullous pemphigoid	80

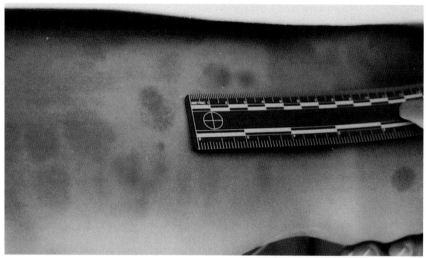

FIG. 2.5. Child with extensive, dark mongoloid spots (dermal melanosis) and many red, inflamed, inflicted bruises on her back.

cially on the hands, feet, and face. Blistering or ulceration also can develop. Vasospasm induced by the cold leads to hypoxemia and localized inflammation of the tissues.

Bleeding Disorders

One study found that 16% of children evaluated for child abuse because of excessive bruising had a bleeding disorder (92). The most common inherited bleeding disorder is von Willebrand disease, affecting about 1% of the population (31). It is caused by a deficiency of the protein, von Willebrand factor, and a variable deficiency of factor VIII:C. In some cases, impaired platelet adhesiveness occurs. The severity of symptoms in patients with von Willebrand disease varies. Some patients are completely asymptomatic, whereas others experience epistaxis, gingival bleeding, severe postoperative bleeding, menorrhagia, and easy bruisability. Idiopathic thrombocytopenia purpura and the hemophilias also have been confused with child abuse (63).

When extensive unexplained bruising occurs, particularly in the absence of associated injuries, bleeding disorders should be considered. A complete blood count with platelet count, an activated partial thromboplastin time, a prothrombin time, a bleeding time (in children older than 1 year), and levels of von Willibrand factor antigen and ristocetin cofactor are useful in screening for unrecognized bleeding disorders. In some cases, a fibrinogen level, thrombin time, clotting factor levels, and platelet kinetic studies may be helpful. Of note, patients with bleeding disorders should exhibit ongoing problems with bruising, rather than an isolated episode, although the severity of von Willebrand disease is known to wax and wane over time.

Henoch–Schönlein Purpura

Henoch–Schönlein purpura causes a nonthrombocytopenic purpuric rash that can be complicated by abdominal pain and bleeding, nephritis, and/or arthritis that can be confused with abusive injury (11). The symmetrical rash tends to be more common over the buttocks and lower extremities, but can be found in other places as well, including the face or ears. The lesions can look like multiple bruises, especially early in the course of the disease. Patients often have a thrombocytosis and an elevated erythrocyte sedimentation rate. Lesions occur in crops over a period of time (73).

Phytophotodermatitis

Phytophotodermatitis is an acute photo-toxic skin eruption occurring after contact with certain fruits or plants, followed by sun exposure. The lesions often have bizarre configurations, making them appear to be inflicted burns or contusions (45) (Fig. 2.6) As the lesions heal, they often become hyperpigmented and can mimic bruises. Citrus fruits and fruit juices, bergamot oil, figs, angelica, cow parsley, scurf pea, celery, wild parsnips, and rue are among the plants that can "photosensitize" the skin. Furocoumarins (psoralens) are the agents in the plants causing the reaction (56).

Hemangiomas

Hemangiomas can look like bruises and also can ulcerate. They are not always obvious at birth, and can become obvious later in infancy. On the genitals, they can mimic sexual abuse–related trauma (79).

Maculae Ceruleae

Flat, purpuric macules can be associated with pediculosis. They occur distant from the actual site of the lice infestation. The exact cause of the lesions is unknown. Although maculae ceruleae are more commonly seen on the body as a complication of pubic crab lice, they have been associated with head lice as well (100).

Folk Remedies

Cao gio (coin rolling) is a Southeast Asian remedy for fever, chills, and headache. The back or chest is massaged with mentholated oil and then vigorously rubbed with the edge of a coin until petechiae or purpura appear (34). *Cupping* (glass leach) is used by Mexican and Eastern European immigrants to treat a variety of ailments. Alcohol is ignited in a cup. The cup is then placed on the skin. As it cools, a round vacuum forms in the cup, causing an ecchymotic lesion to develop at the site. Spooning (*quat sha*) is a Chinese remedy used to relieve pain and headaches. Skin is scratched with a porcelain spoon until ecchymotic lesions appear (125).

Erythema Multiforme

Erythema multiforme often presents with red skin blotches that then darken. The lesions resemble traumatic contusions and bruises. The lesions evolve into the classic "target lesions" with central clearing associated with the disease (1).

Erythema Nodosum

Erythema nodosum presents as tender erythematous nodules that can evolve to bruise-like marks. It occurs most commonly on the lower limbs, and lesions can mimic trauma (71).

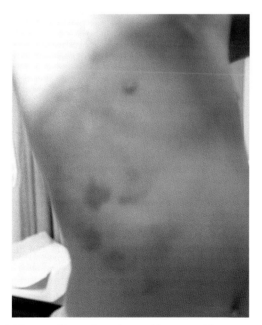

FIG. 2.6. Phytophotodermatitis caused by exposure to lemon juice, mimicking inflicted injury.

Angioedema

Thakur et al. (127) described in an infant a case of recurrent angioedema limited to the scalp and face. The diagnosis of trauma to the head and face was initially considered.

Loxosceles (Brown Recluse Spider) Bites

Loxosceles reclusa (brown recluse spiders) are widespread in the United States (88). They commonly live in homes, barns, and garages, where they come in contact with humans. The bite itself is often painless, and the biting spider is rarely captured or identified. The bite becomes extremely painful and pruritic over 6 to 12 hours. The lesion enlarges and can develop into a significant necrotic ulcer. By day 6 or 7, an eschar develops over the lesion. Because the lesion is so dramatic and usually unexplained, it could be confused with an inflicted injury.

Calcium Chloride Necrosis

Exposure to calcium chloride can cause progressive, necrotic skin ulcers. A case was reported of a child who contacted calcium chloride used to melt ice on sidewalks, causing an initially unexplained necrotic ulcer (140).

Striae

Physiologic striae ("stretch marks") are common and are sometimes found in adolescents who are growing rapidly. Striae in the lumbar area can occur horizontally across the back and hips, appearing to be linear inflicted pattern marks (19). Over time, they fade and take on a sclerotic appearance.

Ehlers–Danlos Syndrome

Ehlers–Danlos syndrome is an inherited disease caused by the production of defective collagen. Various types of the disease have been described, ranging from dramatic to subtle skin findings (94). The defective collagen causes skin to be soft, friable, and easily traumatized. Injured skin heals with wide scars, appearing to have healed by secondary intention. Scars are thin and shiny ("cigarette paper scars"). Other findings include hyperextensible joints, history of premature rupture of membranes at birth, and ocular fragility. Late complications include heart valve defects, ruptured bowel, or aortic aneurysms. Ehlers–Danlos syndrome also has been reported to cause subdural bleeding (8).

Loose Anagen Syndrome

Loose anagen syndrome is a genetic disease frequently causing abrupt, patchy hair loss (134). There is a lack of cohesion between the hair root sheaths and the cuticle during the growth phase of the hair-growth cycle (anagen). Anagen hairs can be pulled out easily and painlessly. The affected hair has a characteristic microscopic appearance, with dystrophic roots, longitudinal groove, lack of root sheaths, and a ruffled cuticle. It is more commonly seen in young, fair-haired children (5).

Ainhum (Dactylosis Spontanea)

This disease of tropical countries causes fibrous bands of tissue to encircle the toes and fingers, leading to autoamputation of the digit. It can be confused with intentional banding (64).

Skin Conditions Confused with Sexual Abuse

Streptococcus pyogenes infections can cause erythema of the anus and vagina, as well as vaginal and anal discharge, anal fissuring, pain on defecation, and blood-streaked stools, simulating sexual abuse injuries (27). Lichen sclerosis, a skin disease, causes subepidermal bleeding around the genitals and anus that can be confused with genital and anal bruising (62). Perianal lymphangioma circumscriptum (dilated lymph channels formed from maldeveloped, sequestered lymphatic sacs) are difficult to distinguish from perianal condylomata (22).

Other conditions confused with child abuse–related skin diseases are listed in Table 2.4.

THE BURNING OF SKIN

The term "burn" is used to describe a variety of physical and chemical insults to tissue, including thermal, electrical, chemical, and radiation. Although the injuries caused by these insults can appear quite similar, their molecular basis and biologic consequences are quite different. In common, they all can lead to tissue inflammation.

Thermal burns cause damage by coagulating tissue proteins. As temperature rises, the number of molecular collisions and the transferred molecular momentum increase in tissues. The transmitted energy deforms proteins and other macromolecules, causing denaturation and structural breakdown. The cell membrane is the most vulnerable component of the cell to heat damage (77).

Damage from electrical burns is not actually mediated by the heat generated by supraphysiologic electrical currents alone. Whereas the passage of electrical current produces damage by the generation of Joule heating effects, additional damage results from the direct action of electrical forces on electrically charged or polarized molecules in tissues. Both mechanisms lead to alteration of molecular conformation and disruption of macromolecular structures. Although thermal forces are random in direction, electric forces produce vectorial electrical coupling in tissues. These vectorial forces can cause changes in protein conformation (76).

Electrical burns cause damage to tissues above the macromolecular level. The bilayer cell membrane acts as an insulating shell for the intracellular contents. As electrical field strengths outside the cell increase, the cell membrane can no longer maintain its integrity, and "electroporation" occurs. Structural defects, or "pores," are formed in the membrane, which causes it to be permeable to ions and molecules, leading to cellular breakdown. In thermal injury, all components of cells are damaged, whereas in electrical injuries, only the cell membrane is damaged (76).

Radiation injuries also are called "burns," but heating has no role in the tissue damage caused by ionizing radiation (76). Ionizing particle beams and electromagnetic irradiation alter atomic structures, which mediate damaging chemical reactions in tissues. The most common radiation burn is caused by excessive ultraviolet light exposure (sunburn). Ionizing UV light penetrates only the most superficial layers of the epidermis. High-frequency ionizing radiation (x-rays or gamma rays) can penetrate the entire body. High-energy irradiation causes damage to proteins, polysaccharides, nucleic acids, and lipids.

Chemicals (acids and alkalis) can cause direct tissue damage by chemically altering the extracellular matrix, cellular membranes, and intracellular structures and molecules. In addition, chemical reactions are exothermic or endothermic and can result in damaging changes in tissue temperature.

All of these mechanisms (thermal burns, electrical burns, radiation injury, and chemical burns) have in common the disruption of cell membranes and the loss of their barrier functions. In addition, cold injury and barotrauma disrupt cell membrane integrity (77). Whereas the biochemical denaturation caused by heat and chemical burns is usually obvious to the observer, the physicochemical effects of ionizing radiation and electricity may not be observable, even though tissue damage has occurred (76).

EVALUATING THERMAL BURNS

The severity of a thermal burn depends on many factors, including the thickness of the skin, the temperature of the burning agent, the length of time the agent contacted the skin, and the heat-dissipating capacity of the burned tissue (the tissue blood flow). Skin thickness varies with the age and sex of the individual, as well as by the location of the tissue on the body. A scald burn in an infant will be more severe than the identical burn inflicted on an adult (120). Infant skin in many parts of the body is less than half as thick as adult skin (54). Skin thickness reaches adult levels by age 5 years. The dermis is thickest on the palms and soles, whereas that of the eyelids and genitals is the thinnest.

Heat is most effectively removed from tissues by vascular perfusion. If the burn wound is poorly perfused, the heat affects the tissues for a longer period. In addition, if shock and hypotension occur after a burn, potentially viable tissue may die. Infection is more likely to become established, and the burn depth increases. In abusive burns, a delay in seeking care can turn a more superficial burn into a deeper, more serious burn, by delaying fluid resuscitation and pain and infection control. Tissue burns are dynamic, and a burn that appears shallow initially can worsen with time, and later appear to be a deep burn.

Early experimental work determined burn tolerances in adult tissues (86). At 44°C (111.2°F), 6 hours is required to cause a superficial epidermal burn. For each degree centigrade above 44°C, and up to 51°C (123.8°F), the time required to produce a burn of given depth decreases by approximately one half. Infants and young children can sustain partial- and full-thickness burns after 10 seconds of exposure at 54.4°C (130°F), 4 seconds at 57°C (135°F), 1 second at 60°C (140°F), and 0.5 seconds at 64.9°C (149°F) (103). Thus very transient exposures to high temperatures can cause serious burns.

Superficial epidermal burns cause redness of tissues without blister formation. They heal quickly and spontaneously. Superficial dermal burns include only the upper layers of the papillary dermis. They often form blisters at the interface of the dermis and epidermis. The wound is pink and hypersensitive once blisters are removed. These burns heal completely within a few weeks. Charred, full-thickness burns are leathery, firm, and insensitive to touch. They often appear white and dry. Noncharred full-thickness burns are more difficult to evaluate. They may be modeled and dry, and sometimes clotted vessels are visible. Full-thickness scald burns may be red in appearance, and can be confused with partial-thickness burns, although capillary refill is not demonstrated (54).

When deaths occur from flame burns, several mechanisms may be at work. Often the death itself is caused by the inhalation of soot or poisonous gases or from heat exposure, and actual tissue burns occur after death. Physical injuries can occur when buildings collapse on the victims before or after death. Burns occurring after death will not show vital reaction. Skin and soft tissues can contract and split, causing lesions that resemble incised wounds. Muscle proteins contract and coagulate, causing rigid flexion of the extremities (a "pugilistic attitude") resembling attempts at self-protection. Spontaneous bony fractures can occur in desiccated bones, including skull fractures. Extradural hemorrhage can occur as brain tissue contracts from the heat, causing hemorrhage that resembles traumatic injury (75).

THE HEALING OF BURNS

Burns that heal within 3 weeks generally leave no scars or functional impairment. More serious burns require early excision and grafting (54). Many of the physiologic, immunologic, and biochemical processes involved in healing burns are the same as those found in other skin injuries, with some essential differences. First, a full-thickness burn actually forms an eschar of coagulated tissue rather than a scab or crust of clotted blood. Surrounding this zone of necrosis is a zone of stasis, where impaired blood supply is caused by leukocytes sticking to damaged capillary endothelium. Around this zone is a zone of increased blood flow (hyperemia). Important in burn healing, if deep skin structures are preserved (glands and hair follicles), epithelial migration can occur from these structures as well as from the wound edges (46).

Systemic responses to serious burns include diffuse tissue edema (probably caused by cytokines and growth factors spilling over into the circulatory system) and a generalized, hypermetabolic inflammatory response causing fever and hyperdynamic circulation. If large areas of skin are burned, severe fluid and electrolyte disturbances can occur from dehydration and protein loss. After extensive burns, the body's immune system also is impaired, increasing the risk of serious infection (48). Not only is the body's skin barrier to microbial invaders broken down, but actual immune suppression occurs, decreasing the body's ability to fight infection (53).

THE EPIDEMIOLOGY OF INFLICTED BURNS IN CHILDREN

Reported proportions of inflicted burns in all children with burns vary greatly, depending on the study sample and diagnostic criteria used for abuse. Table 2.5 reviews several studies determining the proportion of abusive or neglectful burns in children. Abusive burns have been found to be more common in younger children (9,55,60,85,98,105) and in children from single-parent families (9,60,85,101,105). Abuse-related burns are generally more serious and more likely to require excision and grafting and to be full-thickness burns (35,85,98), and have longer hospital stays than accidental burns (60). Parents of abused burned children are more likely to be poor and unemployed than are parents of nonabused children with burns

(9,60). Two studies found that children who were small for their ages using standardized growth charts were at increased risk of abusive burns (7,102).

Ninety-five percent of tap-water scalds occur in the home (6). In the U.S., burns from tap water are the most common form of abusive burns (85,98), and the most common form of all burns (115), whereas in Africa, flame burns and burns with hot objects are the most common forms of abusive burns (36).

Children who sustain abusive burns are at risk for long-term emotional problems (137,138). Some researchers have hypothesized that families with severe emotional problems are more likely to have a child sustain a serious burn than are other families (81,129). The preexisting and complicating emotional problems of abusively burned children complicate their management in the burn unit and in long-term rehabilitation (39,59). Abusive burns and genital and buttocks burns in children are more likely to be complicated by depression than are other types of burns (14).

Certain characteristics are considered to be more likely to indicate an abusive burn rather than an accidental burn. Table 2.6 reviews the common patterns thought to be associated with abusive burns. In some of these studies, abusive burns were diagnosed based on the presence of these factors.

TABLE 2.5. *Proportion of burns caused by abuse or neglect*

Location	Population	Burns caused by abuse and/or neglect	Reference
Detroit, MI	431 emergency department patients	19.5% abuse or neglect	105
San Francisco, CA	60 inpatients	25% abuse or neglect	85
Cincinnati, OH	1,203 inpatients	4.3% abuse	60
Chicago, IL	321 inpatients	24.6% abuse or neglect	9
Dallas, TX	678 inpatients	10.5% abuse	98
Plymouth, U.K.	269 inpatients	<1% abuse	57
Seattle, WA	56 inpatients admitted for tap-water scalds	28.6% abuse	35
Columbus, OH	872 inpatients	16% abuse	55
Columbus, OH	139 inpatients and outpatients	10% abuse	113
Sydney, Australia	507 inpatients	8% abuse or neglect	3
Miami, FL	47 inpatients	12% abuse	51

TABLE 2.6. *Case characteristics attributed to burns caused by abuse*

Characteristic	References
Historic factors	
Discrepant history	3,17,51,55,105
Burn incompatible with developmental age of child	3,17,51,55,57,105
Vague, inconsistent history	3,17,51,55,57,105
Unwitnessed burn	55,105
Denial that lesion is a burn	105
Speculative account of what occurred	57,105
Burn attributed to sibling or babysitter not present at time of presentation	3,17,51,55,57,105
Child contradicts history	3,105
Burn patterns	
Cigarette burn	105
Iron or radiator grill	105
Stocking- or glove-pattern burn	3,105
Mirror-image burns of the extremities	17,51,55,105
Symmetric burns on buttocks	105
Sparing of flexor creases	105
Burns of posterior head, chest, neck, or extremities	105
Burns localized to perineum, genitalia, or buttocks	3,51,55,57,85,98,105
Absence of splash marks in immersion burn	3,105
Crisp margins of burned surface	3,105
Central sparing on buttocks and perineum (doughnut appearance)	3,98,105
Deep scald with running water appearance	105
Multiple burn sites	105
Other factors	
Unexplained delay in seeking care	3,35,51,55,57,85,105
Associated or previous injuries	3,17,51,55,57,105
Previous burns or evidence of previous abuse or neglect	105
Inappropriate level of concern by (affect of) caretakers	3,17,51,55,105
Child excessively withdrawn, submissive, or fearful	3,51,55,57,105
Malnourished child	3,105
Child left with inappropriately young caretaker	105
Unkempt, dirty child	3,105
Inappropriate behavior of caretaker (drunk, impaired, euphoric, depressed)	57,105
Parents do not accompany child to hospital	3,35,51,55,57
Patient is male	35
Adult in the room when victim is scalded	35

VARIATIONS OF BURN INJURIES IN ABUSED CHILDREN

Similar to lacerations and abrasions, some patterns of burns are highly correlated with abuse. This section reviews burns more commonly seen as "abusive" rather than accidental.

Scald Burns

Scald burns are the most common inflicted burns. The burns usually involve the lower trunk, buttocks, perineum, and legs. They can also appear as "stocking" or "glove" burns involving the feet and hands. Abusive burns are more likely to have a clear demarcation between burned and normal skin and to have an absence of splash marks (102,103) (Fig. 2.7). Sometimes sparing of the buttocks and soles of the feet is seen if the child's body is pushed down against the cooler surface of the tub or sink. The flexor creases also may be spared, reflecting the body's flexed position in the hot water (78).

In accidental scald burns, the child is less likely to have a clear "tide mark" at the top of the burn. Accidental scald burns are rarely full-thickness burns (55). The burn margins are more likely to be irregular and asymmetric (139).

Cigarette Burns

Inflicted cigarette burns are circular, uniform-sized, deep burns ranging from 0.75 to

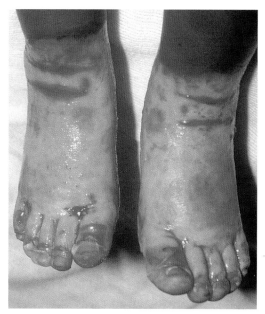

FIG. 2.7. Immersion burn of the extremities.

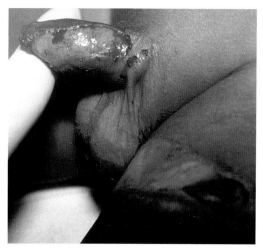

FIG. 2.8. Burn inflicted with a curling iron.

1.0 cm in diameter. They are often grouped, and often found on the hands and feet (37). Accidental contact with cigarettes usually causes "brushed lesions," which appear ovoid, and causes superficial burns instead of deep burns.

Hair Dryer Burns and Other Appliance Burns

Hair dryers can reach very high temperatures in a short time. In one study, the metal grids of hair dyers remained at temperatures above 68°C for up to 2 minutes after the dryers were turned off (97). In normal use, a hair dryer is in constant motion to avoid "hot spots." When a hair dryer or other appliance is held on the skin, deep pattern burns can result in just a few seconds (Fig. 2.8).

Stun Gun Injuries

Stun guns administer an electric shock with a high-voltage, low-amperage impulse, causing the victim to experience muscular tetany, numbness, confusion, and loss of balance. With a longer administration of current, the victim can be paralyzed for up to 15 minutes (12). The characteristic lesion resulting from a stun gun injury is a pair of superficial, symmetrical, circular burns about 0.5 cm in diameter, located about 5 cm apart. Two additional marks may be seen between the round lesions if the recessed spark-gap pins contact the skin (37).

Microwave Oven Burns

Inflicted microwave oven burns to young infants have been reported (2). Microwave radiation spans the electromagnetic spectrum between radiofrequencies and infrared light. Microwaves cause tissue destruction by dielectric heating of tissues. Water molecules act as dipoles and oscillate rapidly in a microwave field, causing heat by molecular agitation (76). Tissues with high water content will be more affected by microwave heating than will those with low water content. Microwave burns typically show damage to skin and muscle layers, sparing the fatty tissue layers.

VARIATION OF BURN INJURIES IN NEGLECTED CHILDREN

Neglecting the supervision or safety of children can cause severe burns. Although these burns result from an act of "omission" rather than an act of "commission," the result for the child can be quite devastating.

House Fires

Many house-fire burns are associated with a lack of adequate smoke detectors. Children and the elderly are particularly vulnerable in house fires. Children can die in house fires resulting from their own unsupervised play, in fires purposefully set by adults, and in fires caused by negligence because of drug or alcohol use by an adult (121). Smoking-related fires are often linked to alcohol use by the smoker.

Walker-Related Burns

Infants in walkers are upright and have increased access to surfaces. Burns have been reported from infants pulling down hot liquids or objects onto themselves when they are in walkers. These burns often resemble hot liquid splash burns (66).

Accidental Scald Burns

Children who accidentally pull hot liquids down onto themselves will usually scald the anterior face and head, neck, palmar surfaces of the hand, arms, and anterior shoulder and chest. The burns generally become less intense as the liquid runs down the body and dissipates heat (98,103). Oily or viscous substances can cause full-thickness burns because they stick to the body and hold heat for longer periods.

The fragile skin of infants and young children can be accidentally burned by bathing the child in hot water. Mirowski et al. (84) reported a case of a newborn bathed in a hospital nursery where the hot water temperature from the nursery faucet was between 56°C (132.8°F) and 59°C (138.2°F). The newborn sustained superficial partial-thickness burns. As part of the case report, they asked nursery nurses to estimate appropriate water temperature for bathing babies using an ungloved hand or brief immersion of the elbow. On days when the water temperature in the nursery was higher, the nurses' estimates of correct temperature for bathing babies was also higher. The authors speculated that because of repeated hand washing, the nurses became accustomed to higher temperatures. Higher estimates also were associated with nurses who held their hand or elbow in the bath for less than 10 seconds. The authors recommended that a thermometer be used to measure water temperature before babies are bathed. The correct temperature for infant bath water is between 36°C (96.8°F) and 39°C (102.2°F).

THE SPECIAL CASE OF ELECTRICAL BURNS AND ELECTROCUTION

Electrical burns and electrocution injuries have not been described in the literature as a mechanism of child abuse. However, when unexplained death or loss of consciousness occurs, electrocution should be considered as a possible cause of injury. Signs of electrocution and electrical burns may be quite subtle. Skin lesions can be inconspicuous or completely absent. The hands are the most common sites of lesions. A thermal blister can be present if the hand actually touched the current source. With intermittent contact or if an arc forms between the hand and current source, a "spark burn" will occur, with a central core of coagulated keratin surrounded by a blanched halo. With high-voltage burns, multiple spark lesions can be seen, causing "crocodile skin" (69). Exit wounds can be seen on the foot. Death occurs secondary to thermal injury to organs, electrical shock to the heart or brain, or paralysis of the respiratory muscles, depending on the nature of the current and location of contact (76).

SKIN CONDITIONS CONFUSED WITH ABUSIVE BURNS

Many different pathologic conditions have been described as lesions confused with inflicted burns. Table 2.7 lists these lesions by

TABLE 2.7. *Skin lesions confused with inflicted burns*

Type of burn	Other lesions confused with type of burn	Reference
Circular		
or patterned burns	Enuresis blanket burn	25
	Moxibustion	34,125
	Maquas	125
	Garlic burns	40
	Therapeutic burns for convulsions by African healers	36,93
	Accidental contact burns	37
	Dermatitis herpetiformis	136
	Impetigo and bullous impetigo	42,91,133
	Phytophotodermatitis	56
	Fixed drug eruption	133
	Varicella	37
	Guttate psoriasis	37
	Pityriasis lichenoides	37
Other burns	Congenital indifference to pain	118
	Epidermolysis bullosa	136
	Staphylococcal scalded-skin syndrome	42
	Allergic contact lesions	61
	Innocent pressure injuries	32
	Car-seat burns	108
	Chemical burns from home remedies	90
	Dishwasher effluent burns	111
	Accidental scald burns	35
	Chilblain	43,133
	Sunburn	130

type of burn. The more common conditions are described.

Accidental Contact Burns

Accidental contact with hot objects can leave burns on children. These burns usually have indistinct margins and do not occur in multiples. They are unlikely to occur on parts of the body that are normally clothed.

Accidental home radiator burns also have been found to be more frequent in houses served by steam radiators versus hot water radiators (99). Steam radiators operate at 82°C (179.6°F) to 109°C (228.2°F), whereas hot-water radiators operate at about 49°C (120.2°F). The difference in temperature means that very brief contact with steam radiators can cause serious burns.

Innocent Pressure Injuries

Pressure injuries to infant skin can be confused with dry contact burns. Feldman (32) described four cases in which patterned lesions in parallel lines with sharply demarcated edges were caused by ischemia from pressure of objects on the skin. These lesions resembled burns.

Staphylococcal Toxin Syndromes

Infections with *Staphylococcus aureus* can release toxins that affect the desmosomes holding epidermal cells together, causing bullous lesions or areas of red, denuded skin (staphylococcal scalded skin syndrome and bullous impetigo). These lesions can be confused with burns (42,91) (Fig. 2.9).

Car Seat Burns

Car seats left in hot cars can reach high temperatures on warm days. When infants' and toddlers' skin contacts the hot upholstery or buckles, pattern marks can result (108) (Fig. 2.10).

Enuresis Blanket Marks

Circular scars from enuresis blankets have been reported. The marks are linear and 0.4 to

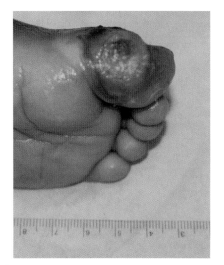

FIG. 2.9. Bullous impetigo, resembling a burn.

cense, or even with a cigarette, to draw out illness (34). The burns appear as circular full- or partial-thickness burns. Bedouins, Arabs, Druses, Russians, and Oriental Jews use the folk remedy *Maquas,* deep burns caused by hot metal spits, to cure illness (125). The belief is that when pus oozes from the burn, the disease drains out. Garlic is sometimes used as a remedy for infections. Garty (40) reported an infant with partial-thickness chemical burns of the wrist caused by the caustic effect of garlic taped to the wrist to treat fever. Other home remedies can cause chemical burns, such as topical methyl salicylate for sprains (90). In some African countries, burning of the skin is an accepted treatment for convulsions (36,93).

0.6 cm in diameter. They occur on the same side of the body (25).

Folk Remedies

Moxibustion is a variant of acupuncture. The moxa herb (*Artemesia vulgaris*) is burned on the skin with a piece of yarn, in-

Postmortem Insect Bites

Insect bites can be confused with burns or abrasions. Cockroaches (*Dictyoptera blattaria*) are notorious for scavenging bodies, particularly after death. They bite hands, toes, eyelashes, and areas of the skin with thin epidermis such as the face and ears. The bites are small and well circumscribed, but

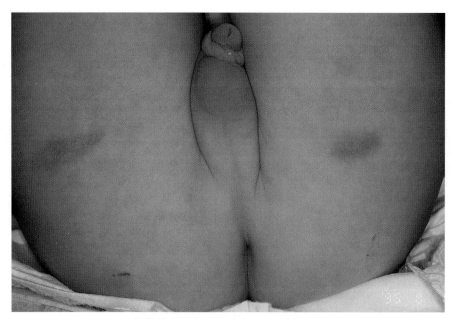

FIG. 2.10. Accidental car seat burn.

irregular. They can sometimes be inflicted in a row. Smaller bites can coalesce into larger lesions (24).

CONCLUSION

The cutaneous manifestations of abuse are varied and often nonspecific. Careful consideration by the practitioner, including the medical history, the physical examination, and the psychosocial context, is necessary to diagnose child abuse accurately.

REFERENCES

1. Adler R, Kane-Nussen B. Erythema multiforme: confusion with child battering syndrome. *Pediatrics* 1983; 72:718–720.
2. Alexander RC, Surrell JA, Cohle SD. Microwave oven burns to children: an unusual manifestation of child abuse. *Pediatrics* 1987;79:255–260.
3. Andronicus M, Oates RK, Peat J, et al. Non-accidental burns in children. *Burns* 1998;24:552–558.
4. Ansel JC, Kaynard AH, Armstrong CA, et al. Skin-nervous system interactions. *J Invest Dermatol* 1996; 106:198–204.
5. Baden HP, Kvedar JC, Magro CM. Loose anagen hair as a cause of hereditary hair loss in children. *Arch Dermatol* 1992;128:1349–1353.
6. Baptiste MS, Feck G. Preventing tap water burns. *Am J Public Health* 1980;70:727–729.
7. Barillo DJ, Burge TS, Harrington DT. Body habitus as a predictor of burn risk in children: do fat boys still get burned? *Burns* 1998;24:725–727.
8. Beighton P, Horan F. Orthopaedic aspects of the Ehlers-Danlos syndrome. *J Bone Joint Surg* 1969;51: 444–453.
9. Bennett B, Gamelli R. Profile of an abused burned child. *J Burn Care Rehabil* 1998;19:88–94.
10. Bernstein G. Healing by secondary intention. *Dermatol Clin* 1989;7:645–660.
11. Brown J, Melinkovich P. Schönlein-Henoch purpura misdiagnosed as suspected child abuse. *Am J Dis Child* 1986;256:617–618.
12. Burdette-Smith P. Stun gun injury. *J Accid Emerg Med* 1997;14:402–404.
13. Calobrisi SD, Drolet BA, Esterly NB. Petechial eruption after the application of EMLA cream. *Pediatrics* 1998;101:471–473.
14. Campbell JL, LaClave LJ, Brack G. Clinical depression in burn cases. *Burns* 1987;13:213–217.
15. Campbell-Hewson GL, D'Amore A, Busuttil A. Non-accidental injury inflicted on a child with an air weapon. *Med Sci Law* 1998;38:173–176.
16. Cardany CR, Rodeheaver G, Taacker J, et al. The crush injury: a high risk wound. *J Am Coll Emerg Physicians* 1976;5:965–970.
17. Clark KD, Tepper D, Jenny C. Effect of a screening profile on the diagnosis of nonaccidental burns in children. *Pediatr Emerg Care* 1997;13:259–261.
18. Cohen BH, Lewis LA, Resnik SS. Would healing: a brief review. *Int J Dermatol* 1975;14:722–726.
19. Cohen HA, Matalon A, Mezger A, et al. Striae in adolescents mistaken for physical abuse. *J Fam Pract* 1997;45:84–85.
20. Coleman H, Shrubb VA. Chronic bullous disease of childhood: another cause for potential misdiagnosis of sexual abuse? *Br J Gen Pract* 1997;47:507–508.
21. Cordova A. The mongolian spot. *Clin Pediatr* 1981; 20:714–722.
22. Darmstadt GL. Perianal lymphangioma circumscriptum mistaken for genital warts. *Pediatrics* 1996;98: 461–463.
23. Day S, Klein BL. Popsicle panniculitis. *Pediatr Emerg Care* 1992;8:91–93.
24. Denic N, Huyer DW, Sinal SH, et al. Cockroach: the omnivorous scavenger: potential misinterpretation of postmortem injuries. *Am J Forensic Med Pathol* 1997; 18:177–180.
25. Diez F, Berger TG. Scarring due to an enuresis blanket. *Pediatr Dermatol* 1988;5:58–60.
26. DiMaio DJ, DiMaio VJ. *Forensic pathology.* New York: Elsevier, 1989:87–88.
27. Duhra P, Ilchyshyn A. Perianal streptococcal cellulitis with penile involvement. *Br J Dermatol* 1990;123: 793–796.
28. Edward C, Marks R. Evaluation of biomechanical properties of human skin. *Clin Dermatol* 1995;13: 375–380.
29. Ellerstein NS. The cutaneous manifestations of child abuse and neglect. *Am J Dis Child* 1979;133:906–909.
30. Evans RC, Jones NL. The management of abrasions and bruises. *J Wound Care* 1996;5:465–468.
31. Falaki NN. Case 3 presentation of facial bruises. *Pediatr Rev* 1998;19:247–248.
32. Feldman KW. Confusion of innocent pressure injuries with inflicted dry contact burns. *Clin Pediatr* 1995;34: 114–115.
33. Feldman KW. Patterned abusive bruises of the buttocks and pinnae. *Pediatrics* 1992;90:633–636.
34. Feldman KW. Pseudoabusive burns in Asian refugees. *Am J Dis Child* 1984;138:768–769.
35. Feldman KW, Schaller RT, Feldman JA, et al. Tap water scald burns in children. *Pediatrics* 1978;62:1–7.
36. Forjuoh SN. Pattern of intentional burns to children in Ghana. *Child Abuse Negl* 1995;19:837–841.
37. Frechette A, Rimsza ME. Stun gun injury: a new presentation of the battered child syndrome. *Pediatrics* 1992;89:898–901.
38. Fuchs E. Keratins and the skin. *Annu Rev Cell Dev Biol* 1995;11:123–153.
39. Galdston R. The burning and the healing of children. *Psychiatry* 1972;35:57–66.
40. Garty BZ. Garlic burns. *Pediatrics* 1993;91:658–659.
41. Gavin LA, Lanz MJ, Leung DY, et al. Chronic subungual hematomas: a presumed immunologic puzzle resolved with a diagnosis of child abuse. *Arch Pediatr Adolesc Med* 1997;151:103–105.
42. Ginsburg CM. Staphylococcal toxin syndrome. *Pediatr Infect Dis J* 1991;10:319–321.
43. Giusti R, Tunnessen WW. Picture of the month. *Arch Pediatr Adolesc Med* 1997;151:1055–1056.
44. Gordon EM, Bernat JR Jr, Ramos-Caro FA. Urticaria pigmentosa mistaken for child abuse [Letter]. *Pediatr Dermatol* 1998;15:484–485.

45. Goskowicz MO, Friendlander SF, Eichenfield LF. Endemic "lime" disease: phytophotodermatitis in San Diego County. *Pediatrics* 1994;93:828–830.

46. Greenhalgh DG. The healing of burn wounds. *Dermatol Nurs* 1996;8:13–23.

47. Grey TC. Defibrillator injury suggesting bite mark. *Am J Forensic Med Pathol* 1989;10:144–145.

48. Griswold JA. White blood cell response to burn injury. *Semin Nephrol* 1993;13:409–415.

49. Gupta MA, Gupta AK. Dermatitis artefacta and sexual abuse. *Int J Dermatol* 1993;32:825–826.

50. Hamlin H. Subgaleal hematoma caused by hair-pull. *JAMA* 1968;204:129.

51. Hammond J, Perez-Stable A, Ward CG. Predictive value of historical and physical characteristics for the diagnosis of child abuse. *South Med J* 1991;84:166–168.

52. Hanigan WC, Peterson RA, Njus G. Tin ear syndrome: rotational acceleration in pediatric head injuries. *Pediatrics* 1987;80:618–622.

53. Heideman M, Bengtsson A. The immunologic response to thermal injury. *World J Surg* 1992;16:53–56.

54. Heimbach D, Engrav L, Grube B, et al. Burn depth: a review. *World J Surg* 1992;16:10–15.

55. Hight DW, Bakalar HR, Lloyd JR. Inflicted burns in children: recognition and treatment. *JAMA* 1979;242:517–520.

56. Hill PF, Pickford M, Parkhouse N. Phytophotodermatitis mimicking child abuse. *J R Soc Med* 1997;90:560–561.

57. Hobson MI, Evans J, Stewart IP. An audit of non-accidental injury in burned children. *Burns* 1994;20:442–445.

58. Hollander JE, Singer AJ. Laceration management. *Ann Emerg Med* 1999;34:356–367.

59. Holter JC, Friedman SB. Etiology and management of severely burned children: psychosocial considerations. *Am J Dis Child* 1969;118:680–686.

60. Hummel RP III, Greenhalgh DG, Barthel PP, et al. Outcome and socioeconomic aspects of suspected child abuse scald burns. *J Burn Care Rehabil* 1993;14:121–126.

61. Inman JK. Cetrimide allergy presenting as suspected child abuse. *Br Med J* 1982;284:385.

62. Jenny C, Kirby P, Fuquay D. Genital lichen sclerosis mistaken for child sexual abuse. *Pediatrics* 1989;83:597–599.

63. Johnson CF. Bruising or hemophilia: accident or abuse? *Child Abuse Negl* 1988;12:409–415.

64. Johnson CF. Constricting bands: manifestations of possible child abuse: case reports and a review. *Clin Pediatr* 1988;27:439–444.

65. Johnson CF. Symbolic scarring and tattooing. *Clin Pediatr* 1994;33:46–49.

66. Johnson CF, Ericson AK, Caniano D. Walker-related burns in infants and toddlers. *Pediatr Emerg Care* 1990;6:58–61.

67. Jones DP. Dermatitis artefactia in mother and baby as child abuse. *Br J Psychiatry* 1983;143:199–200.

68. Kappy M, Kummer M, Tyson RW, et al. Pathological case of the month. *Arch Pediatr Adolesc Med* 1999;153:427–428.

69. Knight B. Forensic problems in practice: XI. Injury from physical agents. *Practitioner* 1976;217:813–818.

70. Kollias N. The physical basis of skin color and its evaluation. *Clin Dermatol* 1995;13:361–367.

71. Labbe L, Perel Y, Maleville J, et al. Erythema nodosum in children: a study of 27 patients. *Pediatr Dermatol* 1996;13:447–450.

72. Langois NEI, Bresham GA. The aging of bruises: a review and study of the color changes with time. *Forensic Sci Int* 1991;50:227–238.

73. Lanzkowsky S, Lanzkowsky L, Lanzkowsky P. Henoch-Schoenlein purpura. *Pediatr Rev* 1992;13:130–137.

74. Laude TA. Approach to dermatologic disorders in black children. *Semin Dermatol* 1995;14:15–20.

75. Lawler W. Bodies associated with fires. *J Clin Pathol* 1993;46:886–889.

76. Lee RC. Injury by electrical forces: pathophysiology, manifestations, and therapy. *Curr Probl Surg* 1997;34:677–764.

77. Lee RC, Astumian RD. The physicochemical basis for thermal and non-thermal burn injuries. *Burns* 1996;22:509–519.

78. Lenoski EF, Hunter KA. Specific patterns of inflicted burn injuries. *J Trauma* 1977;17:842–846.

79. Levin AV, Selbst SM. Vulvar hemangioma simulating child abuse. *Clin Pediatr* 1988;27:213–215.

80. Levine V, Sanchez M, Nestor M. Localized vulvar pemphigoid in a child misdiagnosed as sexual abuse. *Arch Dermatol* 1992;128:804–846.

81. Long RT, Cope O. Emotional problems of burned children. *N Engl J Med* 1961;264:1121–1127.

82. Martin P. Wound healing—aiming for perfect skin regeneration. *Science* 1997;276:75–81.

83. McMahon P, Grossman W, Gaffney M, et al. Soft-tissue injury as an indication of child abuse. *J Bone Joint Surg Am* 1995;77:1179–1183.

84. Mirowski GW, Frieden IJ, Miller C. Iatrogenic scald burn: a consequence of institutional infection control measures. *Pediatrics* 1996;98:963–965.

85. Montrey JS, Barcia PJ. Nonaccidental burns in child abuse. *South Med J* 1985;78:1324–1326.

86. Moritz AR, Henriques FC. Studies of thermal injury: the relative importance of time and surface temperature in the causation of cutaneous burns. *Am J Pathol* 1947;23:695–720.

87. Mortimer PE, Friedrich M. Are facial bruises in babies ever accidental? *Arch Dis Child* 1983;58:75–76.

88. Newcomer VD, Young EM Jr. Unique wounds and wound emergencies. *Dermatol Clin* 1993;11:715–727.

89. Nields H, Kessler SC, Boisot S, et al. Streptococcal toxic shock syndrome presenting as suspected child abuse. *Am J Forensic Med Pathol* 1998;19:93–97.

90. Nunez AE, Taft ML. A chemical burn simulating child abuse. *Am J Forensic Med Pathol* 1985;6:181–183.

91. Oates RK. Overturning the diagnosis of child abuse. *Arch Dis Child* 1984;59:665–666.

92. O'Hare AE, Eden OB. Bleeding disorders and non-accidental injury. *Arch Dis Child* 1984;50:860–864.

93. Oluwasanmi JO. Burns in Western Nigeria. *Br J Plast Surg* 1973;3:146–148.

94. Owens SM, Durst RD. Ehlers-Danlos syndrome simulating child abuse. *Arch Dermatol* 1984;120:97–101.

95. Papa CA, Pride HB, Tyler WB, et al. Langerhans cell histiocytosis mimicking child abuse. *J Am Acad Dermatol* 1997;37:1002–1004.

96. Perrot J. Masque ecchymotique: specific or nonspecific indicator for abuse. *Am J Forensic Med Pathol* 1989;10:95–97.

97. Prescott PR. Hair dryer burns in children. *Pediatrics* 1990;86:692–697.

98. Purdue GF, Hunt JL, Prescott PR. Child abuse by burning: an index of suspicion. *J Trauma Injury Infect Crit Care* 1988;28:221–224.

99. Quinlan KP. Injury control in practice: home radiator burns in inner-city children. *Arch Pediatr Adolesc Med* 1996;150:954–957.

100. Ragosta K. Pediculosis masquerades as child abuse. *Pediatr Emerg Care* 1989;5:253–254.

101. Raimer BG, Raimer SS, Hebeler JR. Cutaneous signs of child abuse. *J Am Acad Dermatol* 1981;5:203–214.

102. Renz BM, Sherman R. Abusive scald burns in infants and children: a prospective study. *Am Surg* 1993;59:329–334.

103. Renz BM, Sherman R. Child abuse by scalding. *J Med Assoc Ga* 1992;81:574–578.

104. Roberton DM, Barbor P, Hull D. Unusual injury? Recent injury in normal children and children with suspected non-accidental injury. *Br Med J* 1982;285:1399–1401.

105. Rosenberg NM, Marino D. Frequency of suspected abuse/neglect in burn patients. *Pediatr Emerg Care* 1989;5:219–221.

106. Rowell LB. Reflex control of the cutaneous vasculature. *J Invest Dermatol* 1977;69:154–166.

107. Ryan TJ. Mechanical resilience of skin: a function of blood supply and lymphatic drainage. *Clin Dermatol* 1995;13:429–432.

108. Schmitt BD, Gray JD, Britton HL. Car seat burns in infants: avoiding confusion with inflicted burns. *Pediatrics* 1978;62:607–608.

109. Schwartz AJ, Ricci LR. How accurately can bruises be aged in abused children? Literature review and synthesis. *Pediatrics* 1996;97:254–257.

110. Sekula SA, Tschen JA, Duffy JO. Epidermal nevus misinterpreted as child abuse. *Cutis* 1986;37:276–278.

111. Sheridan RL, Sheridan M, Tompkins RG. Dishwasher effluent burns in infants. *Pediatrics* 1993;91:142–144.

112. Showers J, Bandman RL. Scarring for life: abuse with electric cords. *Child Abuse Negl* 1986;10:25–31.

113. Showers J, Garrison KM. Burn abuse: a four-year study. *J Trauma Injury Infect Crit Care* 1988;28:1581–1583.

114. Singer AJ, Clark RAF. Mechanism of disease: cutaneous wound healing. *N Engl J Med* 1999;341:738–746.

115. Smith EI. The epidemiology of burns: the cause and control of burns in children. *Pediatrics* 1969;44:S821–S827.

116. Smith KL, Dean SJ. Tissue repair of the epidermis and dermis. *J Hand Ther* 1998;11:95–104.

117. Solomon BA, Laude TA. A peculiar annular eruption in a child with AIDS. *J Am Acad Dermatol* 1995;33:513–514.

118. Spencer JA, Grieve DK. Congenital indifference to pain mistaken for non-accidental injury. *Br J Radiol* 1990;63:308–310.

119. Sperber ND. Bite marks, oral and facial injuries: harbingers of severe child abuse? *Pediatrician* 1989;16:207–211.

120. Spillert CR, Vernese NA, Suval WD, et al. The effect of age on severity of murine burns. *Am Surg* 1984;50:660–662.

121. Squires T, Busuttil A. Child fatalities in Scottish house fires 1980-1990: a case of child neglect? *Child Abuse Negl* 1995;19:865–873.

122. Stadelmann WK, Digenis AG, Tobin GR. Impediments to would healing. *Am J Surg* 1998;176(2A suppl):39S–47S.

123. Stankler L. Factitious skin lesions in a mother and two sons. *Br J Dermatol* 1977;97:217–219.

124. Stephenson T. Aging of bruising in children. *J R Soc Med* 1997;90:312–314.

125. Stewart GM, Rosenberg NM. Conditions mistaken for child abuse: Part II. *Pediatr Emerg Care* 1996;12:217–221.

126. Sugar NF, Taylor JA, Feldman KW. Bruises in infants and toddlers. *Arch Pediatr Adolesc Med* 1999;153:399–403.

127. Thakur BK, Kaplan AP. Recurrent "unexplained" scalp swelling in an eighteen-month-old child: an atypical presentation of angioedema causing confusion with child abuse. *J Pediatr* 1996;129:163–165.

128. Vale GL, Noguchi TT. Anatomical distribution of human bite marks in a series of 67 cases. *J Forensic Sci* 1983;28:61–69.

129. Vigliano A, Hart LW, Singer F. Psychiatric sequelae of old burns in children and their parents. *Am J Orthopsychiatry* 1964;34:753–761.

130. Wardinsky T, Vizcarrondo F. The mistaken diagnosis of child abuse: a three-year USAF Medical Center analysis and literature review. *Milit Med* 1995;160:15–20.

131. Waskerwitz S, Christoffel KK, Hauger S. Hypersensitivity vasculitis presenting as suspected child abuse: case report and literature review. *Pediatrics* 1981;67:283–284.

132. Wedgwood J. Childhood bruising. *Practitioner* 1990;8:598–601.

133. Wheeler DM, Hobbs CJ. Mistakes in diagnosing non-accidental injury: 10 years' experience. *Br Med J Clin Res Ed* 1988;296:1233–1236.

134. Whiting DA. Traumatic alopecia. *Int J Dermatol* 1999;38(suppl 1):34–44.

135. Wilkes GL, Brown IA, Wildnauer RH. The biomechanical properties of skin. *CRC Crit Rev Bioeng* 1973;1:453–495.

136. Winship IM, Winship WS. Epidermolysis bullosa misdiagnosed as child abuse: a report of 3 cases. *S Afr Med J* 1988;73:369–370.

137. Woodward JM. Emotional disturbances of burned children. *Br Med J* 1959;5128:1009–1013.

138. Woodward JM, Jackson DM. Emotional reactions in burned children and their mothers. *Br J Plast Surg* 1961;13:316–324.

139. Yeoh C, Nixon JW, Dickson W, et al. Patterns of scald injuries. *Arch Dis Child* 1994;71:156–158.

140. Zurbuchen P, LeCoultre C, Calza AM, et al. Calcium necrosis after contact with calcium chloride: a mistaken diagnosis of child abuse. *Pediatrics* 1996;97:257–258.

3

Abusive Head Trauma

Randell C. Alexander, *Carolyn J. Levitt, and †Wilbur L. Smith

*Center for Child Abuse, Morehouse School of Medicine, Atlanta, Georgia; *Midwest Children's
Resource Center, Department of Pediatrics, University of Minnesota, Saint Paul, Minnesota; †Imaging
Department, Children's Hospital of Michigan, and †Department of Radiology, Wayne State University
School of Medicine, Detroit, Michigan*

Abusive head trauma is the most common cause of death from child abuse and is the leading cause in all trauma-related deaths among children. Lesser degrees of injury result in brain damage, psychological dysfunction, and physical impairments. Other consequences of child abuse (e.g., a fracture that heals) also are unacceptable, but they are not usually of the magnitude of severe head injuries.

The concept that the head is vulnerable is confirmed by studies of accidental pediatric trauma. Physical abuse statistics parallel those of "accidental" trauma, in that the leading cause of death is head injuries (126). Abusive head trauma occurs not only when direct forces are applied to the brain, but also when neglect places brain function at risk owing to such diverse etiologies as malnutrition or psychological deprivation. Abusive head injuries often lead to brain damage, manifest as a wide range of deficits affecting personality, learning, or functional skills (25). Thus head injuries can cause many types of physiologic and psychological trauma of varying severity.

Head trauma was recognized as a form of child abuse early in the evaluation of this field of pediatric practice (143). In 1946, Caffey (27) described the relationship between intracranial hemorrhage, long-bone fractures, and trauma. Although researchers subsequently identified child abuse as a source of head trauma (134,152), the description of the "battered child syndrome" in 1962 popularized the concept of

inflicted nonaccidental injury to children and included inflicted head injury (79).

In 1971, the scope of abusive brain injuries expanded with a conceptual breakthrough by Guthkelch (59), who first linked whiplash shaking forces to subdural hematomas. Thereafter, Caffey elaborated on the mechanism whereby shearing forces from shaking cause intracranial injuries and retinal hemorrhages (26). His initial description of the whiplash shaken infant syndrome included children with intracranial and intraocular hemorrhages but without evidence of external head trauma or skull fractures. He postulated that shaking alone was sufficient to cause the intracranial injuries, and popularized the widespread awareness of the dangers involved in this practice. More recent studies documented that shaking injuries often are accompanied by evidence of direct impact, especially when substantial efforts are made to identify less apparent injuries that are evident only when the scalp is reflected during autopsy or on cross-sectional imaging (3,46).

The rapid growth in the development of noninvasive brain imaging techniques expanded the understanding of intracranial injury. The use of computed tomography (CT) of the brain became widespread in the late 1970s (48), and more recently, magnetic resonance imaging (MRI) has assumed a key role in documenting the occurrence and severity of head injuries owing to abuse (5,125). Better clinical appreciation of the natural history and symptoms of head injuries has been achieved by the study of analogous accidental injuries (16,33,68). All of these advances have expanded and refined what is recognized as the spectrum of abusive head injuries, and allowed the clinician to better describe the sequence of events causing the injury.

The focus of this chapter is on physically abusive head injuries, especially intracranial injuries from shaken baby syndrome. Such a distinction should not diminish an appreciation of the frequent association between head injuries and injuries to other body parts or neglect. Although the most serious outcomes of head injury are in the context of intracranial trauma, other forms of cranial injury also occur.

EXTRACRANIAL INJURIES

Trauma to the Scalp

In addition to intracranial injuries alone, many studies have found signs of impact as demonstrated by skull fractures, subgaleal hematomas, swelling or edema of the scalp, or bruises of the scalp, which are often obscured by hair (3,46,52,55,63). For example, in a study of 12 children with cervical cord injuries associated with inflicted head injury, Feldman et al. (52) found that eight children had scalp or calvarium surface bruises, and three had swelling of the scalp. Five of the 12 children died, three of whom had bruises under the scalp surface found at autopsy. Additionally, two children had skull fractures, and two had intraoral trauma. The presence of facial or scalp injuries associated with abusive head trauma makes the abuse more quickly apparent (76). In a review of missed cases of abusive head trauma, Jenny et al. (76) found that 20 (37%) of 54 missed cases had facial and/or scalp injuries compared with 78 (65.5%) of 119 cases in which abuse was recognized at first presentation. In the latter group, abusive head injuries may have been suspected because of the more obvious injuries in these visible areas. More recent studies that looked at predictors of occult intracranial injuries found that lo-

cal scalp findings are present in nearly all infants with skull fractures and/or intracranial injuries (36,57,81). If there is no soft tissue swelling, and accidental impact is the purported history, the history becomes suspect.

External signs of abusive head trauma may be minimal, even in life-threatening and fatal head injuries. Therefore normal measurements of extracranial soft tissue thickness on postmortem skull radiographs are needed for comparison. Strouse et al. (143) measured the soft tissue thickness at five standardized locations on postmortem skull radiographs of 18 infants who had no evidence of trauma on subsequent autopsy and compared them with soft tissue thickness on skull films of 100 living children, all younger than 3 years with no history of trauma. The authors demonstrated that minimal extracranial soft tissue swelling is a normal finding on postmortem skull radiograph. However, the presence of greater amount or any asymmetric soft tissue swelling raises suspicions of impact injury.

Subgaleal hematoma is a common finding in accidental trauma that is generally associated with, but not limited to, impact injuries causing skull fractures. It most often occurs over the temporoparietal area but may be frontal, causing the appearance of "raccoon eyes" from the blood seeping into the soft tissue spaces around the eyes. The apparent bruising caused by the subgaleal hematoma tends to be of uniform color and appearance, reflecting a large collection of blood under the surface that forms recognizable patterns around the eyes, ears, and back of the neck. These may become more noticeable 1 to 2 days after the injury and take several weeks to months to resolve. Subgaleal hematomas also can be caused by extremely forceful hair pulling, which also results in areas of alopecia in young children. Extreme traction forces on the scalp vessels cause them to break and form subgaleal hemorrhages, which feel cystic in structure because of the amount of blood contained within the fascial planes. Forensic pathologists have recognized subgaleal hematoma from hair pulling in homicide cases, but this finding has not been given much attention in the pediatric child abuse literature.

Spinal Cord Injuries

In the past, injuries to the cervical spine due to child abuse have been described as part of skeletal trauma or associated with abusive head trauma (52,63,83). Spinal cord injuries among infants and young children most commonly are "spinal cord injury without radiographic abnormality" (SCIWORA), first described by Pang and Wilberger in 1982 (115). The malleability (mechanical tolerances) of the spinal ligaments and dura is greater than that of the spinal cord (115), allowing spinal cord injury in this young age group without signs of fractured vertebrae or ruptured ligaments (52) (Fig. 3.1). Consequently, spine ra-

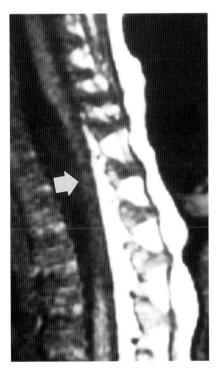

FIG. 3.1. Severe spinal cord atrophy after trauma is documented by the extreme thinning of the cord from C4 through T1 (*arrow*). Cord injury such as this results either from direct trauma due to whiplash with hyperextension or from injury to the anterior spinal artery. No spine fracture was documented.

diographs and CT are not helpful in diagnosis. Subtle findings of the cervical cord, such as edema causing fusiform swelling and hemorrhage into the cord (hematomyelia), are demonstrated only by MRI (115).

Piatt and Steinberg (117) recently reported an abusive cervical spinal cord injury in a 15-month-old child with sudden onset of quadriplegia. The mother's boyfriend had left the child on a couch watching television while he prepared supper in the kitchen. By report, she initially was trying to crawl, but fell onto her back and was unable to move. Of particular note were linear bruises in front of the right ear and jaw and showers of petechial hemorrhages on the left side of the neck, just below the mandible, over both ears, on the right side of the jaw, and on the upper chest. Fusiform swelling of the midcervical cord and hematomyelia were seen on MRI acutely; 2 months later MRI documented atrophy of the cervical cord in this area. Parrish (116) has reported a 2-month-old infant with contusion of the upper cervical cord and lower medulla with associated eye findings including bilateral anterior chamber bleeding, dislocated lens on the left side, and vitreous hemorrhage, suggesting direct compression of the eyes. It was postulated that the infant was picked up by the head with the thumbs positioned over the eyes and that the body was violently shaken while the head was held stable. Case (32) has described two infants in the same family, both at age 3 months, one who was found dead, and the other who survived with a cervical cord injury (central cord syndrome). The father in this case admitted to many abusive acts perpetrated on the deceased child in response to the child's crying, including shaking and bending the child's head to one side. Autopsy demonstrated hematomyelia of the upper cervical cord and conjunctival petechial hemorrhages of the right eye. The father admitted to grasping the second infant by her head with his hands and shaking her body. Levitt reviewed a similar case of a 2-year-old with sudden onset of quadriplegia apparently occurring when his stepfather was alone with him putting him to bed. Autopsy demonstrated severe distraction injury resulting in hemorrhage around the vertebral arteries.

INTRACRANIAL INJURIES

Etiology and Pathogenesis

For the purposes of this discussion, a simple classification system for the mechanisms of head injury follows (4): direct impact; penetration; asphyxiation/hypoxia; ischemia; shaking; neglect; and dermal injuries to the scalp.

Impact

In most instances, direct-impact injuries occur when high-speed objects hit a relatively stationary head. This type of injury is probably the most common form of abusive head trauma. Examples include slapping, hitting with an object, punching, or hitting the head with a thrown object. Facial, eye, ear, nose, oral, brain, scalp, and skull injuries may result. Neglectful as well as overtly abusive practices may result in direct-impact head trauma, probably the most common being failure to use proper automobile safety restraints for children.

Direct-impact injuries also occur when the child's head is propelled against a stationary object. Most accidental injuries occur when the child is moving and the head impacts against an object in the environment (e.g., the floor, a table, a toy, a doorframe) (120). Medically, it may be difficult to distinguish whether it was the object, the head, or both that were moving. If a high-speed impact leaves a specific pattern on the skin (e.g., if a slap mark is identified), it is safe to assume that it was the hand, not the skull, that was moving.

An important exception to the principle that abusive impact trauma is usually caused by the object moving, not the head, is that small children may be swung into hard objects, sometimes as part of the overall pattern described as shaken baby syndrome. Children who also are victims of shaken baby syndrome often have skull fractures, subgaleal hemorrhages, or subtle external bruising, in-

dicating that an impact occurred (46). Although this type of injury may have happened by punching or from the impact mechanisms mentioned previously, it is also common that part of the shaking sequence is to slam the head into a wall or other hard object, or to throw the child against a hard surface. In these instances, the child was moving, not the object, but the physiologic effect is the same as regards the impact-injury component. The tremendous discrepancy in mass between the child and the adult perpetrator facilitates this type of injury. Dropping a child from a great height, either as physical abuse or occurring from neglect, is another method whereby it is the motion of the child and not the object that contributes to the injury. The frequency of this particular injury is unknown.

Penetrating Injuries

Either neglectful or willful practices with firearms are responsible for a number of deaths or serious brain injuries to children (7,9). Bullet impact to the brain causes substantial injury beyond that of the direct penetration. In this sense, it is useful to consider a comparison: a bullet may cause substantial tissue damage along its track, but neurosurgical operations actually remove more tissue, and the patient survives. This apparent discrepancy occurs because, unlike surgery, the high speed of a bullet causes sudden tissue damage, a pressure wave that disrupts neurons beyond the bullet track, and rapid intracranial pressure changes for which the brain has no time to compensate (Fig. 3.2). Pellet or BB guns may achieve a high muzzle velocity but have less range and vary more in their effect once their load impacts (86).

Low-speed penetrating injuries disrupt the skin or scalp, and may fracture bone or cause brain or sensory organ damage. In many instances, an overlap exists between penetrating injuries and direct impact injuries. If a child is hit with an object, the object not only causes direct impact damage, but also, if it is irregular and hard enough, it may penetrate. More specific penetrating injuries result from

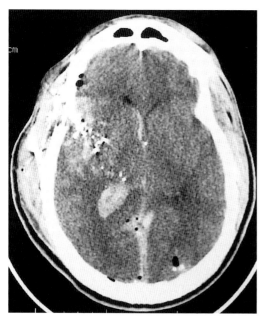

FIG. 3.2. Computed tomography of a teenager obtained 2 hours after a gunshot wound to the right frontal area of the head demonstrates multiple metallic fragments, pneumocephalus, and hemorrhage. These findings were generated by the extreme energy of the bullet as it tracked through the brain tissue. Note that the right lateral ventricle is filled with blood. The internal structures of the brain are unrecognizable owing to the severe brain edema.

knives, glass (often thrown at the child), or objects shaped like spears. Unlike direct-impact injuries, which transmit crushing or pressure forces, penetrating injuries directly interact with underlying tissues. In general, the lower the velocity of penetration, the easier it is to assess what tissues are involved in the injury.

Asphyxia, Hypoxia, and Ischemia

Asphyxiation causes cellular hypoxia, which may be acute or chronic. Choking at the neck, prolonged squeezing forces to the chest, or gagging of the mouth often are discovered as an acute problem but may in fact be part of an ongoing pattern of abusive behaviors. In cases of Munchausen syndrome by proxy, for example, parents have repetitively put their hands over a child's mouth to induce

apneic symptoms (123). In one case, the mother had often "saved" her child by suffocating the child to the point of apnea and then performing mouth-to-mouth resuscitation as medical personnel arrived (6). The child's significant brain atrophy and neurologic damage resulted from these many episodes. Anoxia or repetitive hypoxia lead to cerebral atrophy with ventricular enlargement and cortical brain tissue changes, with the potential for causing microcephaly, cognitive limitations, and other neurologic problems (Fig. 3.3). A previously described practice of placing children in gas ovens to "quiet them down" resulted in multiple episodes of sublethal hypoxia and subsequent brain injury.

In the acute situation, both hypoxia and compromise of circulation to the brain often

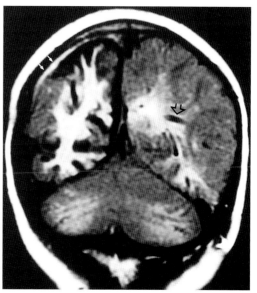

FIG. 3.3. A 3-year-old child who was severely shaken at age 8 months with resultant symptoms of seizures, delayed motor development, and cognitive retardation. The child has a ventriculostomy shunt to control hydrocephalus. The coronal fluid-attenuated inversion recovery (FLAIR) images show a shrunken right (*R*) cerebral hemisphere due to atrophy and extensive gliosis (*white signal*) of the white-matter tracts. The small right-sided subdural fluid collection (*small arrows*) is owing to recent shunt-revision surgery. The ventriculostomy tube (*arrow*) treating hydrocephalus is in the left lateral ventricle.

occur together, from direct trauma such as choking at the neck, as a consequence of shaking, or from cardiovascular instability resultant from acute hypoxia with secondary compromise of circulation to the brain. Injuries owing to suffocation are particularly difficult to document. Obstruction of the carotid arteries leads to unconsciousness and eventually death, if prolonged. Characteristic findings from major vessel occlusion in the neck may be evident on CT scans and with angiography in these instances (17).

In both hypoxia and ischemia, neurologic damage at the cellular level is related to decreased oxygen availability, thereby impairing the ability of mitochondria to continue the metabolic activity of molecular respiration. Owing to the similarities in the clinical presentation, the results of brain imaging, and the mechanisms causing the injuries, it is often not possible to differentiate the two conditions, and the victims are described as sustaining hypoxic–ischemic injury. The swelling of the brain caused by shaking, direct impact, penetration, or other mechanisms may lead to vasospasm of the cerebral vasculature, further compromising blood flow and oxygen delivery to the tissues (24). Although documenting the nature of injury is important, the final pathways of many mechanisms of abusive brain injury overlap.

Shaking

Shaking represents a unique and prevalent form of intracranial injury that can directly cause intracranial, cervical spinal cord, and intraocular injuries (3,27) or may act in combination with impact injuries. In describing the latter instance, some authorities have suggested using the terms "shake/slam" syndrome or shaken/impact syndrome (3,23,46). Although most victims of either type of injury are younger than 1 year, abusive shaking has been reported to occur in children as old as 5 years (4). Thus the term "shaken baby" is not fully descriptive of the population involved.

In instances of abusive shaking, the perpetrator often holds the child by the chest so that they face each other, compressing the chest while violently shaking the infant to and fro. The shaking usually does not cause bruising of the chest or the arms (if they are included in the grip); however, fractures of the humeri or rib fractures may occur. Gripping the child from behind should cause similar intracranial injuries and retinal hemorrhages, but this mechanism has not been described. Infants are usually held off the floor and shaken back and forth at full arm extension, but a toddler may be too heavy to lift. In these instances, the adult may straddle the recumbent child and shake it, gripping primarily the upper torso. In this instance, the child's skull frequently impacts against the floor as the shaking proceeds. Alternative grips occasionally are encountered, including holding the child by combinations of the arms or legs. This grip is rarely used to shake, but it is used to seize the infant preparatory for the chest grip.

No firm answer exists as to the exact number of shakes necessary to create the clinical picture or for how long a person might typically shake a child in abusive circumstances. Because retinal hemorrhages are rarely seen with accidental injuries, such as automobile accidents (1,16,121), the inference is that more than one or two oscillations must be necessary. Four or five shakes would take about 2 seconds if done with extreme force. Anyone who has worked with 8- to 10-pound weights held at arm's length realizes that exhaustion quickly occurs. Shaking probably lasts a maximum of 20 seconds, with up to 40 to 50 shakes. In most cases, the time period of shaking is probably 5 to 10 seconds (10 to 30 shakes). To cause brain damage sufficient to allow clinical detection of the syndrome, severe forces must be used. On mechanical/physiologic grounds and by experience with perpetrators who have been convicted or confessed to the shaking, it is clear that to lift an infant and shake requires an adult or adult-sized person.

The precise manner whereby the brain is injured appears to depend, in part, on repetitive oscillations. Using doll models and published estimates of the force needed to cause brain damage, Duhaime et al. (46) demonstrated that it was difficult or impossible to achieve sufficient peak accelerations from shaking alone to account for the observed injuries. These data suggested that impact with an object (sudden deceleration) is necessary. One of the major difficulties with this concept is that although the pure deceleration model is duplicated in automobile accidents, retinal hemorrhages are very rare. The same observation is true with falls from great heights. Several theoretic explanations exist to reconcile this discrepancy. As the head is shaken through space, it experiences angular accelerations in addition to accelerations along the to-and-fro axis. May et al. (98) have shown that woodpeckers, who experience thousands of strikes a day, use a somewhat awkward thrust of their head to ensure that all accelerations remain in a simple linear direction. If the woodpecker's head rotated about the neck, a different centripetal (angular) force would be exerted at each moment, and the woodpecker would experience brain damage. Instead, the woodpecker only needs to withstand acceleration forces acting in the anteroposterior direction. When an infant is shaken, the head moves in a complex pattern of peak accelerations and perhaps more dangerous angular accelerations; these repetitive oscillations probably contribute to the damage. Ellerstein (47) described the brain and skull as having different densities, and as oscillation proceeds, the brain may be moving in one direction while the skull is moving in the opposite. Compression of the brain against the skull, and stretching, and finally snapping of the bridging veins between the two cause cerebral contusions and intracranial bleeding. Because white and gray neuronal matter have different densities, it is no surprise that the shearing often occurs at the junction between the two. Thus a complex interplay between various accelerations and repetitive movements may determine the pattern and severity of brain injury. Quantification of the forces, concomitant conditions, and billions of cell elements necessary to construct a representation of this complex interplay is not currently possible nor is it clear that by itself, it would be instructive.

The force needed to cause shaking injuries, even in infants, is intense. Severe injuries require severe forces. The general public often does not readily appreciate this fact, and either a doll demonstration or other visual imagery is needed to convey the violence of the shaking. In court, such demonstrations have been accepted as illustrative, by contributing to a better understanding than can verbal descriptions alone (45). Casual "shaking" (i.e. jostling, jiggling) does not cause shaken baby syndrome. Although not condoned, activities such as tossing a child into the air, bouncing on a knee, and jogging with a young child in a backpack represent forces that are orders of magnitude less than necessary to cause shaken baby syndrome injuries.

A unique variation that combines shaken baby syndrome and direct impact is the tin ear syndrome (65). Unilateral ear bruising, ipsilateral cerebral edema, ipsilateral subdural hemorrhage, and retinal hemorrhages are the main findings. The mechanism of injury is a blow to the side of the head, causing the head to spin along the long axis of the neck. Presumably, the head rotates after the blow, compounding the direct impact with angular momentum. The blow is so forceful that a single impact causes severe intracranial injuries, but minimal external bruising. The intracranial bleeding and retinal hemorrhages are theorized to occur from severe angular accelerations. Thus this mechanism of injury consists of a direct impact, but the results are similar to those of a shaken child.

When determining the proximate cause of injury or death in shaken/impact syndrome cases, the answer often is a combination of head injuries. Frequently it is not possible to say that either the impact alone or the shaking alone caused injury; rather, both contributed to the intracranial injuries. Although a distinction is not medically possible, the fact remains that it was head trauma that caused the injuries. Often a legal distinction may be attempted in an effort to diminish or confuse the issue, making possible histories of accidental impact the focus of the inquiry.

Neglect

The mechanisms of head injury mentioned thus far consist of overt trauma. The head can be damaged, however, in other ways. Neglect of medical care for the ears, eyes, or mouth can cause serious injury under certain situations. Failure to thrive has been associated with a higher incidence of microcephaly, as has neglect in general (R. Alexander, unpublished data). Neurologic impairments affecting language development, motor functioning, and cognition can be caused by extreme environmental deprivation.

Incidence

The incidence of shaken baby syndrome is still unknown and will likely remain obscured for some time. The national mortality reporting system, based on county and state health department birth and death certificates, records codes for the underlying and contributing causes of death as well as an external cause of injury code (E-code) and diagnosis code. The E-code specifies both the mechanism and the intent (unintentional, suicide, homicide, or undetermined). The diagnosis code includes the anatomic site and nature of the injury. Specific causes of nonfatal injuries are not readily available because documentation of the injury in the hospital record is most often incomplete or absent (8). The American Academy of Pediatrics Committee on Injury and Poison Prevention (8) called for pediatricians and other providers treating injured children to obtain and document a thorough history, including the who, what, when, where, why, and how of each injury and that each injury-related hospital admission and emergency department visit must include an E-code. In addition, the Committee calls for pediatricians to support legislation mandating the use of E-codes and diagnostic codes and to support training and dissemination of this information.

Currently, an accurate description of the incidence of abusive head injuries in children necessitates considerable analysis and extrapolation. The many studies available report ei-

ther prevalence data within a defined population or frequency data regarding a specific type of injury occurring within a named time period. Neither of these study designs allows direct comparison or compilation; therefore one must sift through studies and extrapolate from large populations to approximate incidence. This imprecision in overall incidence data makes it difficult to measure the effectiveness of preventive actions. Despite these difficulties, some estimates of the incidence of abusive head trauma can be made.

Homicide continues to be the leading cause of death related to injury in the first year of life, making up one third of the infant injury mortality in 1996 (114). Eighty percent of these homicides are fatal child abuse, and strong evidence indicates that homicide and fatal child abuse cases are undercounted when based on death certificates. Death certificates reveal very little about the actual circumstances of the death (114) and are often completed incorrectly, even when the cause of death is known. Consequently, the cause of death is often not captured accurately by the final International Classification of Diseases, Edition 9 coding (40). Based on national linked birth/infant death data sets for 9 years from 1983 to 1991, Brenner et al. (21) found that the infant mortality rate from homicide was 6.72 per 100,000 live births. In comparison, infant mortality from SIDS has been reported as low as or 20 per 100,000 live births in Norway (136). In the Brenner study, homicide accounted for 22.6% of injury-related infant deaths, mechanical suffocation accounted for 17.7%, and motor vehicle incidents accounted for 15.2%. Scholer et al. (128) recently reported that infant deaths due to intentional injuries were second to those due to suffocation.

Data from several states, including those with Child Mortality Review Teams, support these findings. For example, in Washington state, Cummings et al. (40) found intentional injury to be the leading cause of death in children younger than 1 year, with an incidence of 9.1 per 100,000 live births. In contrast, Scholer (128), focusing on injury deaths in children up to age 5 years in Tennessee, found a total injury death rate of 23.5 per 100,000 children; 10.5% of these deaths were due to inflicted injury (2.5 per 100,000 child years). In this study, motor vehicle trauma was the leading cause of injury-related death (28.4% or 6.7 per 100,000 child years), clearly reflecting the decreasing risk of dying of an inflicted injury and the increasing risk of dying of a motor vehicle–related injury as the child grows older.

Other studies have reported head trauma in particular accounts for 45% to 58% of infant homicides (22,29,39). In South Carolina, for example, 27 (45%) of 60 deaths due to homicide in children younger than 5 years over a 10-year period were due to head injuries (39). These results are similar to a report of 40 cases of infanticide occurring over a 7-year period in the United States Air Force, in which 23 (58%) deaths were attributed to head trauma (22). The most accurate estimate of the incidence of fatal abusive head trauma comes from a recent Oklahoma study (29). Over a 5-year period, 30 (46%) of 65 homicide deaths in children younger than 3 years were due to head injuries.

The first population-based study of abusive head trauma focused on the incidence of subdural hematomas in children younger than 2 years known to all the neurosurgical services in three cities in south Wales and southwest England over a 3-year period (75). This 3-year retrospective study identified 27 (82%) of 33 cases definitely due to abuse, an incidence of 12.8 per 100,000 children younger than 2 years and 21 per 100,000 in children younger than 1 year. One additional case was very suggestive of abuse, four were unexplained, and only one was due to a traffic accident.

Perhaps more relevant to the physician caring for children is the number of abused children with life-threatening injuries admitted to pediatric hospitals each year. Although definitive figures are not available and there is much variation due to referral patterns, studies published before 1992 reported prevalences of new cases ranging from four to nine cases annually per hospital (3,65). More re-

cent studies list prevalence ranges from 5.6 per year to 28.8 per year (34,41,71,75,76,78, 87,140). It is difficult to determine whether this is due to a true increase in the number of children being injured each year or to improved recognition of abusive head trauma (71). Another major factor leading to this apparent increase in prevalence is a broader, more inclusive diagnosis of abusive head trauma in some series rather than the more restrictive criteria of life-threatening brain injury due to shaken baby syndrome.

Predisposing Factors

Many factors, some easily quantified and others elusive, place a child at greatest risk for abusive head injury. The child's age, physiologic factors, and the particular type of injury sustained are relatively concrete. Less easily calculated are the factors of caretaker stress and the available capability to manage that stress.

As noted in the discussion of incidence, clearest of the predisposing factors is the young age of the injured child. The mean age of children with abusive head injury is 5 to 9 months (22,41,71,145). with the majority being younger than 9 months. The high susceptibility of the infant brain and cerebral vessels to injury relates to many factors, including the disproportionately large size of the infant's head, relatively weak neck muscles, the pliability of the infant's skull, open sutures (and a large fontanel), the large subarachnoid space, and the high water content of the infantile brain. The vessels involved in subdural and subarachnoid hemorrhages bridging the space between the meninges and the skull are delicate and less tightly bound (132). These factors particularly dispose an infant to serious injury when grabbed by the trunk or shoulders and shaken (25,59).

Injury in young children is also facilitated by the physical helplessness of the infant and the disparity in size between infants and their caretakers. Simply stated, it is quite easy for an adult to shake or to throw an infant. When these violent acts occur, disproportionate weight and size between the victim and the perpetrator facilitates severe injury. Older children are less likely to be shaken or thrown, and if they are shaken, they are less susceptible to severe injuries. This is not to imply that older children cannot suffer abusive head injuries; indeed, severe intracranial injuries to children ages 1 to 4 years do occur with all the spectrum of injuries seen with abusive head injury in younger children. More often, these injuries in older children are associated with other signs of trauma, such as skull or long-bone fractures, abdominal trauma, or extensive bruising (80,98). The young infant is also more likely to have the diagnosis of abusive head trauma missed at first presentation and be susceptible to subsequent abuse unless there are other signs such as facial or scalp injuries, seizures, or abnormal respiratory status (or the infant's parents are not living together) (76).

Social conditions of varying kinds are predisposing factors for abuse that are more difficult to quantify. Poverty and lack of nurturing spousal relationships are risk factors documented to predispose to abusive head injury. Having a child at an early age (younger than 15 years) is strongly associated with infant homicide (114,132), particularly if the mother has previously given birth. Homicide rates are greatest in infants born to mothers who receive late or no prenatal care, are single, black, or Native American and in infants with birth weights less than 2,500 g (16,127). Siegel et al. (133) also found that intentional injury death rates in Colorado were highest for infants of teenage mothers, peaking at 10.5 per 10,000 live births for mothers age 16 years. In Washington state, Cummings (40) also found late prenatal care and low income were associated with intentional infant deaths.

Five percent of infant homicides occur during the first day of life, and half occur by age 4 months (116). The mother is the most likely perpetrator of homicides during the first week of life; after that time, the father, stepfather, or another male is more commonly the perpetrator. In contrast, persons unrelated to the child commit the majority of homicides involving children older than 3 years.

In general, male caretakers are at greatest risk to inflict abusive head trauma to infants (22,87,140). However, babysitters of both sexes are also a concerning risk group (140). Starling et al. (140) reported that fathers, stepfathers, and mother's boyfriends were responsible for 60% of the incidents of abusive head trauma in infants. Female babysitters accounted for 17.3% of cases, and mothers accounted for 12.6%. In the study of infanticide in the United States Air Force (22) in which 58% of victims died of abusive head injury, 84% of the perpetrators were male, 77% were biological fathers, and 54% were first-time parents. When considering all infant homicides in South Carolina, 45% of assailants were men (39). In contrast, when the specific cause of death was asphyxiation, 87% of the assailants were women.

The birth of twins has been shown to increase family stress due to the prenatal complications of twinning, parental lack of sleep and financial pressures (66). There is an increased incidence of abuse in families after the birth of twins both in one or both of the twins and in the siblings of the twins (66). In one report (13), five of eight infants from four sets of twins were seen at one hospital within 11 months for severe injuries due to shaken baby syndrome; two of the infants died from their injuries. It is very clear that the other twin and siblings deserve a complete skeletal survey, MRI, and retinal examination by an ophthalmologist whenever one twin is identified with abusive injuries.

Whether shaped by a cultural force, impulsive response to anger and aggression, and/or other factors, the stimulus to abusive injury is often attributed to the irritation caused by a crying child. The normal infant spends 2 to 3 hours each day crying, and 20% to 30% of infants exceed that amount of time, sometimes substantially (19). Infants often cry on an apparently irrational basis, and may not respond to a parent's initial attempts to comfort them (30). Crying becomes particularly problematic during the 6-week to 4-month age bracket, an age period that coincides with the peak incidence of shaken baby syndrome. In the study of infanticide in the United States Air Force (22), the mean age of the infant victim was 4.9 months. Medical records noted a history of colic in 35% of victims. The infant was reported to have been crying at the time of the incident in 58% of the cases and was alone with the caretaker/perpetrator in 86% of the cases. Forty-seven percent of the incidents occurred during the weekend.

Ironically, the abusive shaking behavior may be self-reinforcing, because the infant who is shaken or otherwise brain injured may cease to cry because of injury inflicted by the shaking. The caretaker may associate such cessation with a gratifying response, in that the infant ceases crying, and the abuser therefore repeats the behavior. Thus an initial action, impulsive and triggered by stress, may have immediate positive results for the caretaker who simply wishes the crying to cease. The quiet, drowsy baby displays the desired behavior and may not exhibit severe symptoms after the first shaking; possibly leading the caretaker to conclude that shaking obtains an appropriate response to irritation or upset (33). In one case cared for at the University of Iowa Hospitals and Clinics, both parents were deaf. Nevertheless, the father admitted shaking the child in response to the visual stimulus of crying.

Diagnosis

Clinical

The presenting complaints of patients with abusive head injury can run a gamut from asymptomatic swelling or bruising of the head to death. Often, the initial symptoms are clouded because of a delay in seeking medical attention. The common clinical symptoms of serious head injury usually involve some combination of loss or alteration of consciousness, vomiting, seizures, and apnea. As a rule, the severity of these symptoms intensifies as the severity of the head injury increases, so that a child presenting with prolonged unconsciousness, apnea, or seizures generally has a severe injury at the time of presentation.

The clinical symptoms correlate roughly with the type of injury in that trauma producing either contusion or diffuse axonal injury generally produces more rapid onset of symptoms of loss of consciousness (124). Conversely, the insidious onset of vomiting and variable diminution of the level of consciousness usually portends cerebral edema. Milder, sublethal cerebral edema maximizes over a 48- to 72-hour period. Therefore, early symptoms of vomiting in a child abuse victim may be the prelude to more severe symptoms that will manifest over the course of the next few hours or days (124). The degree of cerebral edema is related to the severity of the insult, and severe cerebral edema presents clinically in a rapid fashion. Other injuries, such as small subdural hematomas or subarachnoid hemorrhage, may manifest as irritability or may be relatively asymptomatic.

A comprehensive and accurate history elicited from the child's caretakers is paramount in making the correct diagnosis; however, the history is often misleading. In 1973, O'Neill et al. (115) reported, "It is invariably not possible to obtain an accurate history," and documented that the history was inaccurate or deliberately evasive in 95 of 100 cases of child abuse in their series. This duplicity makes it necessary for the physician to depend heavily on objective clinical findings and to document discrepancies between severity of physical injuries and historical explanations. Too often, when faced with a critically ill child, the history is underdocumented and hastily performed by personnel without the specific training and orientation toward meticulous documentation of the potential inaccuracies presented by the historian. The medical personnel should observe and record the history, possibly even on audiotape, with particular attention to details that are inconsistent or change over the course of several interviews. Disparities in history provided by two or more caretakers merit particular attention, as each of these variances reflects on the veracity of the history.

Clinical diagnosis, after obtaining a careful history, begins with a thorough and competent physical examination conducted by a physician familiar with the injuries associated with child abuse. The physician should pay particular attention to cutaneous injuries, particularly bruises in various stages of healing, marks of blunt trauma, or burns. Injuries should be documented by photographs for permanent record and future reference. Such an examination should be conducted daily for several days to assess for other injuries or bruises that had not been noted on the initial examination and to monitor the resolution of the injuries.

External injuries are occasionally subtle and not easily appreciated in child abuse cases. In younger children, bulging of the fontanel or splitting of the cranial sutures may be the only outwardly appreciable sign of trauma. In our experience, local swelling is the most commonly noted sign of external injury, followed by bruising. Bruising is often difficult to document and describe accurately. It is imperative to examine the scalp carefully for bruising, with special attention to those areas covered by hair. In a series of children with abusive head injury, clinically unappreciated signs of external impact were present in a substantial number of patients, as documented by either autopsy or the presence of a subgaleal hematoma during CT imaging (3). Approximately 50% of children with intracranial injury have evidence of impact injury either separately inflicted or inflicted in conjunction with shaking. As previously mentioned, older children are more likely to exhibit external signs of previous injuries to the head and to other parts of the body.

A few specific patterns of external injury may be indicators of specific mechanisms of serious injury.

The tin ear syndrome, due to blows to the head with rotatory force, is characterized by bruising about the pinna of the ear (65). Strangulation may be evident because of a combination of injuries to soft tissues of the neck and evidence of occlusion of one or both carotid arteries with subsequent watershed brain infarcts (17). "Raccoon eyes" indicate bleeding into the subgaleal space with subse-

quent infiltration of the blood into the periorbital space. Patients with this characteristic injury present with darkening of the eyes and forehead some days after the trauma. The darkening is attributable to degradation products of the blood in the scalp that leak ventrally in the upright child into the periorbital space. The initial subgaleal hematoma is often occult because of hair masking the subgaleal swelling.

Photographs of the child should be taken if there are any external signs of abuse.

Ophthalmologic

A careful ophthalmologic evaluation is essential in the diagnosis of suspected abusive head injury (49). The level of expertise available for the examination should be as high as possible, either an ophthalmologist or, ideally, a pediatric ophthalmologist. Dilating the pupils is optimal, but occasionally a compromise has to be struck. Following pupil light reactions is the major clinical criterion in the Glasgow trauma scale, and pharmacologic removal of this criterion by pupil dilation may not be in the overall best interest of the child. Bulging of the optic disk and optic venous hypertension are reliable markers of increased intracranial pressure. Retinal hemorrhages are a hallmark of child abuse; however, other ocular injuries also may be documented (118). Retinal detachment and optic nerve injury have been reported concomitant with severe abusive head injury (85). In the proper clinical setting, it is unusual to find retinal hemorrhages resulting from conditions other than abusive head trauma (1,16,121). Scattered reports document retinal hemorrhage after cardiopulmonary resuscitation (56); however, the paucity of these reports demonstrates the infrequency of this occurrence (111). Retinal hemorrhages may occasionally occur after prolonged increase in intracranial pressure. In the unlikely event this occurs, they should not be numerous, involve the periphery, or be seen in multiple layers. Therefore it is important to document whether these hemorrhages were present on an acute basis or appeared belatedly in the hospital course in a patient with increased intracranial pressure. For this reason, it is imperative that the ophthalmologic examination be done as soon as possible after the child's presentation to the hospital.

A review of the literature suggests that approximately 75% of children with abusive head injury have concomitant retinal hemorrhages (138). The converse figure is not available (i.e., the frequency of retinal hemorrhage in abused children without evidence of intracranial injury). Neonates with birth-related retinal hemorrhages do not have intracranial injuries similar to those of abused children with retinal hemorrhage (139). A child younger than 30 days with intracranial injuries characteristic of child abuse is unlikely to have these injuries as a result of the birth process. The overlap of the finding of retinal hemorrhages in both conditions is merely coincidental.

Imaging

The imaging evaluation of an infant with an acute brain injury depends on the urgency and severity of the clinical situation. A severely injured, apneic, and seizing child should, after a clinical assessment, undergo CT scanning of the brain (102). CT is rapidly available in most trauma centers, and many have life-support systems designed for operation in CT suites. In most instances in which life-saving neurosurgical intervention must be undertaken, CT offers sufficient resolution and detail to allow the surgeon to make the necessary decisions (Fig. 3.4). The initial CT should be obtained without contrast enhancement and at intervals sufficient to cover the brain in a timely fashion but without large interval gaps (Fig. 3.5). For infants younger than 3 months, our standard is to use a 4-mm slice thickness and a 4-mm interslice interval, adjusting these settings to 8 mm and 8 mm for larger children. Rarely is it necessary to use intravenous contrast enhancement in the acute phase. In any case of abusive head trauma, bone windows should be photographed, as well as the standard brain scan.

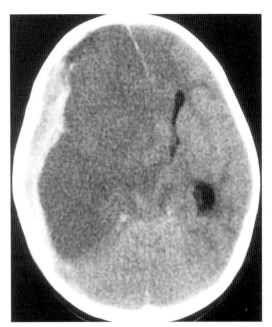

FIG. 3.4. Computed tomography (CT) of the brain of a comatose apneic 22-month-old shaken-impact head injury. CT shows a large hyperacute right subdural hematoma, swelling of the right cerebral hemisphere, and midline shift from right to left. The CT yielded sufficient data to document the need for emergency neurosurgery; the child died despite intervention. Note the blood layering in the subdural area. This was acute blood with no older injury at surgery. The hyperacute layering of blood components in a large, rapidly bleeding subdural hematoma is sometimes confused with an older injury.

MRI gives superior detail for many of the lesions associated with abusive head injury (Figs. 3.4–3.6) (125). Because of the longer scan times and frequent necessity of life-support measures, MRI is often relegated to a confirmatory or supplementary study in patients with abusive head injury; however, with newer scanner and life-support design, this is likely to change, with MR competing with CT as primary imaging. MR scans are often obtained several days to a week after the acute presentation the better to delineate the types of injury and to document extraaxial fluid collections around the brain. More remote to the injury, after 6 to 8 weeks, MRI is useful in showing the changes in brain parenchyma that

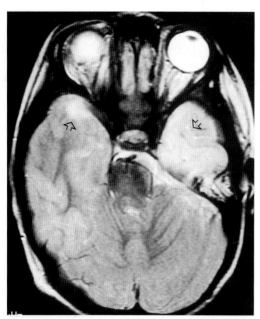

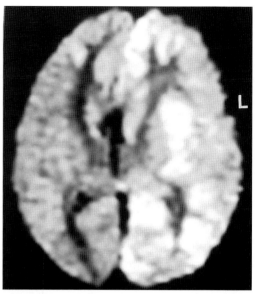

FIG. 3.5. Axial T2-weighted magnetic resonance imaging (MRI) of the brain in a 20-month-
old shaken-impact victim shows high signal
(*white*) in the anterior portions of both temporal
lobes (*arrows*). This is a very typical area for impaction injury of the brain, as rapid deceleration
impacts the temporal lobes against the bony
floor of the middle cranial fossa. The injuries
were not visible on the computed tomography
scan obtained 12 hours earlier.

FIG. 3.6. An echoplanar diffusion image of a
child who has severe symptoms but near-normal
computed tomography (CT) shows a high density of the left (*L*) cerebral hemisphere as well as
some abnormal signal in the right frontal lobe.
The diffusion signal becomes abnormal very
shortly after injury where CT and even conventional MR sequences may not show injury.

take place as a result of the insult. It is not
clear that the MR scan adds much additional
information to CT scanning 6 to 8 weeks after
injury. MR scans typically are obtained using
a spin-echo sequence with T1-weighted views
in the sagittal and coronal planes and T2-
weighted axial and coronal images. Occasionally, proton density imaging may be helpful in
showing smaller foci of bleeding. MR spectroscopy to delineate tissue injury will assume
an increasingly important role.

Table 3.1 indicates our experience with the
relative uses of CT, MR, and plain film imaging of the skull in demonstrating the characteristic lesions of abusive head injury. In general,
parenchymal injuries such as shearing injuries
and diffuse axonal injuries are best seen on
MRI. Small, subdural hematoma or those sub-

dural hematomata that are tangential to the CT
scanning planes are best shown by MRI.
Larger injuries, subarachnoid hemorrhage, and
diffuse hypoxic–ischemic change are often better demonstrated by CT. Most skull fractures
are best shown by skull radiographs.

Accompanying fractures of the skeletal system are identified in up to 50% of cases of abusive head injury. Their presence, if sufficiently
documented, is powerful evidence of an abusive etiology of the injury. Shaking while holding the thorax often causes posterior rib fractures (82). These findings may be occult early
after the injury. It is, therefore, good practice in
suggestive cases to obtain a follow-up radiograph 14 days after the approximate time of
the injury to check for occult rib fractures.
Other authorities have pointed out that bone
scanning is of particular value in identifying
rib fractures, and this method is an alternative,
albeit more expensive, means to document occult rib fractures. False-negative bone scans

Table 3.1. *Imaging techniques used to demonstrate lesions of abusive head injury*

Injury inquiry	Computed tomography	Magnetic resonance imaging	Radiography
Fracture	**	—	***
Subdural hematoma	**	***	—
Epidural hematoma	**	**	—
Subarachnoid hemorrhage	***	*	—
Concussive injury	*	***	—
Shear Injury	*	***	—

Key: *, occasionally useful; **, Moderately useful; ***, very useful; —, not usually of value.

can occur immediately after injury, so a 3-day delay is often helpful. A skeletal survey, which includes detailed views of all extremity long bones, rib detail views, and radiographs of the lateral dorsal lumbar spine, skull, and cervical spine, should be promptly reviewed by the pediatric radiologist who is part of the abuse investigation team.

If the skull is fractured, the cause of the injury may be suggested by the nature of the skull fracture. Hobbs (69) noted that fractures inflicted by abuse are often complex, with involvement of more than one bone, depression of the bone fragments, or wide diastasis of the fracture fragments. The specificity of complex fractures for child abuse is not absolute, although the preponderance of studies supports the concept. In a comparative study, Worlock et al. (153) reported that these fracture patterns did not hold up to statistical scrutiny when used to predict child abuse, a finding also supported by Reece and Sege (119). However, in separate studies, Meservy et al. (103), Billmire and Myers (16), and Leventhal et al. (89) concluded that although not universal, the pattern of complex skull fractures described by Hobbs was more common among their patients who had suffered abuse. In summary, it seems prudent to conclude that a complicated fracture should lead one to suspect child abuse, but a simple fracture should in no way preclude a diagnosis of child abuse.

Laboratory

Laboratory examinations are often of value, principally in excluding other disorders that occasionally superficially mimic abusive head injury. Results of bleeding and clotting studies in patients with head injuries may be abnormal and are correlated with the degree of brain damage (72). However, the "normal" values for prothrombin time (PT) and partial thromboplastin time (PTT) are based on nontraumatized patients and would not be precisely the same in an injured child. In comparing the abnormalities in these clotting functions, they are well short of the abnormalities seen in conditions such as hemophilia. The elevations in PT and PTT, sometimes seen, should be seen as an effect of brain trauma, not as a bleeding disorder (which would not explain the brain injury or pattern of bleeding). They should be documented. In the patient with apnea or hypoxia, blood gas determinations may be vital for management. Lumbar puncture may be helpful but should be undertaken with care in the face of possibly increased intracranial pressure. Some children with shaken baby syndrome have survivable head injuries but actually die of concomitant abdominal injuries. It is important to conduct a full trauma workup for the abused patient, with liver and pancreatic enzymes, and urinalysis as well. Other laboratory examinations should be obtained as required by the clinical condition of the patient.

Differential Diagnosis

Accidental versus Inflicted Injuries

In establishing a diagnosis of abusive head injury, the most troublesome dilemma is sorting out accidental from nonaccidental injury.

The determination is best made by a thorough review and scrutiny of the history including seeking witnesses to the event coupled with assessment of the severity of the injury. Except for cases of clear-cut trauma, such as auto accidents, the literature supports an underlying assumption that the most severe head injuries are those least likely to have been caused by accident (16,45,74,121). Nonabusive injury is the leading cause of morbidity and mortality for children in the United States (61,62,64,92,122,148). Falls are the most frequent cause of injury bringing children to emergency departments and requiring hospital admission (121,141). In one study, falls accounted for one third of pediatric hospital admissions due to trauma (121).

Falls, however, are an infrequent cause of death (121). Differences are substantial between traumatic injuries suffered in falls and other accidents and those inflicted abusively (51). Available studies are disparate, in that each focuses on a separate population and research question. However, each credible study supports the conclusion that severe head injuries purported to be accidental, unless related to a moving vehicle accident, are very likely to be the result of abuse, particularly if injuries are ascribed to falls from short heights. Difficulty remains in sorting out accidental from abusive injury when the head injuries are less severe.

Studies of head injuries in children due to falls are difficult to compare. Some studies are based on all children aged 0 through 18 years in whom a greater proportion of outdoor accidents are represented. Others address a public health threat by focusing on young children who fall down stairways in walkers or from open windows in high-rise buildings. In other studies of falls in children, it is unclear whether cases of abusive injury based on a false history were excluded. It is more likely that errors have been made in other studies by including abusive injuries in the accidental fall category. In addition, the surface on which the child fell is not always clearly defined.

Despite these difficulties, at least 25 studies collectively described injuries of 4,671 children. For comparison, these can best be divided into short falls (n = 1,732), stairway falls (n = 1,037), and falls greater than one story (n = 1,902) (10,35,68,77,84,88,93,107, 110,123,142,150). In the short-fall category, Helfer et al. (68) studied the injuries of 246 children younger than 6 years who had fallen from their beds or sofas. One hundred seventy-six of these falls took place in the children's homes, and 85 occurred in the hospital. The children generally fell from beds or sofas that were elevated 90 cm or less, although several were from heights up to 5 ft. Two of the children sustained linear skull fractures from these accidental falls; however, none of the children had central nervous system damage. Drawing on these findings, Helfer et al. (68) asserted that serious injuries attributed to an accidental fall from a bed or low height should be considered unlikely and, in most instances, the correct diagnosis is child abuse. Nimityongskul and Anderson (111) replicated Helfer's findings, describing 76 children who were injured as the result of a fall while in the hospital. These children experienced minor injuries, and only one patient had a skull fracture. This study also scrutinized the surface onto which the child fell, comparing their data with existing literature on playground safety (67). The authors hypothesized that a carpeted floor or thick rug could cushion falls from high places sufficiently that injury was unlikely, but that a child falling onto a tiled or concrete surface would be more likely to sustain injury.

Other investigators reached similar conclusions after studying the outcomes of accidental head trauma in situations in which the histories were reliable. Focusing only on falls in children younger than 3 years that were witnessed by a person other than the child's caretaker, Williams (150) described 44 children who fell less than 10 feet and 62 who fell 10 feet or more. Those who fell less than 10 feet sustained serious but not life-threatening injuries, including small depressed skull fractures from falling against sharp edges. In contrast, two children died of falls from less than 5 feet among the 53 uncorroborated falls. The only other death was in a child who fell 70 feet. Relying on the accurate history from incident reports in hospital-related falls, Lyons and Oates (93) found no serious, multiple, visceral, or life-threatening injuries in children younger than 6 years, 124 of whom fell from cribs and 83 from beds. Falls from beds ranged from 25 to 41 inches (over the side rails) and up to 54 inches over the top of the crib railing. One 21-month-old child who climbed over the top of the crib rail sustained a fractured clavicle, and one 10-month-old who fell from his crib had a simple linear skull fracture. Studying the safety of bunk beds, Selbst et al. (129) found only six of 68 children who fell from a top bunk required admission to the hospital. Of these, four had concussions, one had a skull fracture with a subdural hematoma, and one had a laceration near the eye.

In a study of injuries of children younger than 18 years at a children's trauma center, Chadwick et al. (35) found one death in 118 children who fell from 10 to 45 feet. No deaths occurred in 65 children who fell from 5 to 9 feet. By contrast, there were seven deaths among 10 children reported to have fallen less than 4 feet. These seven children had subdural hematomas and cerebral edema. Five of the seven deaths alleged to be due to short falls had other injuries to suggest abusive trauma. The authors concluded that the most likely explanation for this exaggerated mortality from shorter distances was that the history provided in these cases was false. To increase the likelihood that histories would be reliable, Chadwick studied serious head injuries occurring at day-care centers. Reviewing 338 records, he found only one child, age 2.5 years, who sustained a somewhat serious head injury at a day-care, falling a distance of 5 feet from a tree onto a concrete walk. The child was temporarily unconscious, a CT of the head was negative, and he recovered completely within a few hours. In a similar study, Levitt and McCormick (unpublished study) reviewed emergency department and hospital records over a 2-year period of 336 infants younger than 2 years who were reported, but

not corroborated, to have fallen from heights less than 8 feet (140). There were nine in this group with subdural hematomas; seven of these nine cases were eventually determined to be due to inflicted injuries. Tarantino et al. (142) limited their study to infants younger than 10 months presenting to the emergency department after falling from distances of up to 4 feet. Twelve of the 167 infants had skull fractures, and seven had long bone fractures. No intracranial hemorrhages were attributed to the short vertical falls. However, two infants with intracranial hemorrhages initially presented with a false history of falling only a short distance. The authors also pointed out that an infant who is dropped appears to be at greater risk for significant injury than one who rolls or falls off a couch or bed. Mayr et al. (97) found no intracranial injuries or neurologic sequelae due to falls from high-chairs in 103 young children whose ages ranged from 7 to 30 months. Almost all of the children were unrestrained, half were trying to stand up when they fell, and 14% tipped the high-chair over as they fell.

Joffe and Ludwig (77) studied 363 stairway falls presenting to their emergency department in children younger than 11 years. Although injuries to the head and neck were the most common, most of the injuries were superficial, and none of the children required intensive care. The authors found that the injuries in the children who fell more than four steps were of no greater severity or number than those who fell less than four steps. Four of 10 infants who fell with their caretakers while being carried on the stairway sustained skull fractures. Infant walkers were involved in 24 of the 40 injuries of children aged 6 to 12 months. Excluding falls down stairs, in walkers, and likely abusive trauma, Chiavello and Bond (37) found that the most serious injuries from falls occurred in infants who were being carried by their caretakers who then fell on the child against the stairs. Of three infants who fell under these circumstances, two sustained skull fractures. One of these two infants also had a subdural hematoma and cerebral contusion as well as a fracture of the second cervical vertebra. Overall, the authors concluded that stairway-related injuries were much less severe than free falls from the same vertical height and that infants who fall in the arms of their caretakers are falling from that height.

Chiavello et al. (38) also studied stairway falls in walkers and found that the majority of these falls result in only minor injuries. However, of 46 stairway walker falls in this study, there was one fatally injured child who had a cervical spine fracture, skull fracture, and subdural hematoma, and four other infants with intracranial hemorrhages. In a current 10-year study of intracranial injuries due to falls involving children younger than 2 years comprising both retrospective and prospective components, Levitt and McCormick (unpublished study) found there were nine of 30 infants with accidental intracranial injuries who sustained these injuries by falls downstairs in infant walkers. This group included three infants with subdural hematomas, three with large parenchymal hematomas, two with small brain contusions, and one with a subarachnoid hemorrhage. Abusive head injuries were excluded from this group by careful scene investigations, corroborating witnesses, and multiple interviews. Smith et al. (137) also reported that intracranial injuries were rare among 260 minor injuries of infants, sustained when they fell downstairs in walkers. This study found that the number of stairs the child fell was significantly associated with the seriousness of the injury. Only 10 patients were admitted to the hospital, all 10 of whom had skull fractures. Three of the skull fractures were depressed, and three had accompanying intracranial hemorrhages. In contrast, Mayr et al. (99), in a study from Austria, found 19 infants had skull fractures, but there were no intracranial injuries among 143 infants falling downstairs in walkers.

Falls from extreme heights are expected to cause serious head injury, but mortality in this group is surprisingly low. Combining the data of eight studies involving 1,962 children younger than 18 years, there were 23 deaths (10,11,35,88,105,121,138,150). Eighteen of these deaths involved falls of greater than three stories (Table 3.2). Most long-fall studies do not describe in detail the morbidity associated with the falls, so correlations between the heights of the falls and the incidence of severe intracranial injuries are not available. One study from Saudi Arabia of 104 children younger than 13 years reported no brain injuries in those children who fell less than 7 m (23 ft.). Fatalities and neurologic morbidity were related to falls from second- and third-floor balconies. Three of 44 children died, two falling from the second floor and one from the third floor. Five other children sustained multiple skull fractures and hemorrhagic cerebral contusions, resulting in moderate neurologic sequelae such as monoparesis, ataxia, or seizures from falls of 7 to 12 m.

As early as 1985, Billmire and Myers (16) provided convincing data that child abuse is the leading cause of serious head injury. In a 2-year study focusing on children up to age 1 year admitted to their intensive care unit, they were able to ascertain that accidental trauma rarely, if ever, caused intracranial injury in infants. They found that 95% of fatal or life-threatening head injuries in children during the first year of life were the result of abuse.

In 1992, Duhaime et al. (45) reported findings of 100 children younger than 2 years who were hospitalized for head injuries. Initial histories attributed injuries in 73 children to household falls. Twenty-four were determined to be abusive head trauma, and 32 others were suggestive of abuse. Epidural hematomas without other intracranial bleeding occurred in three children determined to fall less than 4 feet. Falls greater than 4 feet resulted in focal parenchymal contusions in four children and focal subarachnoid hemorrhages in two others. However, the clinical course for these children was described as benign. In contrast to the accidental injuries, abusive injuries had a disproportionately high incidence of intracranial hemorrhage (13 of 24 children), resulting in the deaths of three children.

In a review of 287 children younger than 6.5 years and who had head injuries, definite

TABLE 3.2. *Summary of published studies regarding pediatric falls: 1969–1994*

Reference	No.	Age	Height/Mechanism	Injuries/Deaths
Short falls				
Helfer et al. (1977)	176	<6 yr	Home: Bed, sofa, etc.	2 skull fxs and 1 humeral fx <6 mo; 3 clavicle fxs >6 mo
Helfer et al. (1977)	85	<6 yr	Hospital: bed, crib	1 skull fx (uncomplicated)
Nimityongskul & Anderson (1987)	76	<16 yr	Hospital: bed, crib	1 skull fx (linear)
Kravitz et al. (1969)	330	<2 yr	Home: changing table	1 skull fx; 1 subdural hematoma
Williams (1991)	44	<3 yr	≤10 feet	3 skull fxs (depressed)
Lyons & Oates (1993)	207	<7 yr	Hospital: bed, crib	1 skull fx (linear); 1 clavicle fx
Selbst et al. (1990)	68	<6 yr	Bunkbeds	6 hospitalized; 7 fxs; 1 skull fx with subdural hematoma
Levitt & McCormick (unpublished)	336	<2 yr	≤8 feet	9 subdural hematomas; 7 with retinal hemorrhage (7 are SBS)
Chadwick et al. (1991)	165	<18 yr	<10 feet	7 deaths; 7 subdural hematomas; 7 with cerebraledema, 5 with retinal hemorrhage; 5 subarachnoid hemorrhage (7 are SBS)
Mayr et al. (1999)	103	<30 mo	Highchairs (some standing up)	No intracranial injuries, 16 had skull fractures
Tarantino et al. (1999)	167	<10 mo	<4 feet	No intracranial hemorrhages, 12 had skull fractures
Gruskin & Schutzman (1999)	72	<12 mo	≤3 feet	4 with intracranial injuries
Total	**1,829**			**8 with nonintentional intracranial injuries**
Stairway falls				
Joffe & Ludwig (1988)	363	<19 yr	24 in walker; 10 carried by adults	No intracranial hemorrhage or cerebral contusions; 22 fxs: 6 skull fxs (<3 yr) and 16 extremity fxs (15 >4 yr)
Chiavello et al. (1994)	69	<5 yr	Excluded walkers; 3 carried by adults	5 skull fxs; 1 small subdural hematoma; 1 cervical spine fx; 2 cerebral contusions
Levitt & McCormick (unpublished)	156	<2 yr	75 in walkers	2 with subdural hematomas & retinal hemorrhage (1 flame)
Total	**588**			**5 with intracranial injuries**
Stairway falls in walkers				
Chiavello et al. (1994)	46	<1 yr	Walker	5 with intracranial hemorrhages (1 death with C-spine fracture, skull fracture and subdural hematoma)
Mayr et al. (1994)	143	7–14 mo	Walker	No intracranial injuries. 19 skull fractures
Smith et al. (1997)	260	Mean, 9.2 mo	Walker	3 depressed skull fractures with intracranial hemorrhage
Total	**449**			**8 with intracranial hemorrhages**
Falls >1 story				
Rivara et al. (1993)	1,371	<10 yr	Specific height not included	1 death, height not known
Williams (1991)	62	<3 yr	≥10 feet	1 death (70 feet)
Barlow et al. (1983)	61	<16 yr	≥1 story	14 deaths (>3 stories)
Smith et al. (1975)	42	<15 yr	≥1 story	2 deaths (4 stories)
Chadwick et al. (1991)	118	<18 yr	≥10 feet	1 death (10–45 feet)
Musemeche et al. (1991)	70	<15 yr	≥10 feet	No deaths
Lehman & Schonfeld (1993)	134	<16 yr	Windows, balconies, rooftops	1 death
Annobil et al. (1995)	44	<13 yr	≥2 stories	2 deaths at 7 m (23 ft) and 1 death at 9 m (29.5 ft); 5 others had cerebral contusions and moderate neurologic sequelae
Total	**1,902**			**23 deaths (18 more than three stories)**

Prepared by Carolyn Levitt, M.D.

abuse accounted for 19% (121). Abused children were younger (0.7 vs. 2.5 years) and had higher incidences of intracranial bleeding. Cutaneous, skeletal, visceral, and retinal injuries were significantly more common in the abuse group.

Recent studies looking at predictors of intracranial injury found that young infants may be asymptomatic and require neuroimaging, either CT or preferably MRI to document intracranial injury (57). In a retrospective study focusing on head injuries in children younger than 2 years who were seen in the emergency department, Gruskin and Schutzman (58) found 12 intracranial injuries in a group of 278 children evaluated over a 1-year period, 236 of whom sustained falls. Specifically these injuries consisted of four epidural hematomas, two subdural hematomas, three cerebral contusions, two cerebral edema, and one subarachnoid hemorrhage. From the data, it is impossible to determine which intracranial injuries come from the 227 falls in which the height of the fall was known. However, they do describe four infants of 72 infants younger than 12 months who had intracranial abnormalities from falls 3 feet or less. If these authors carefully excluded abusive head trauma, it can be concluded that benign intracranial injuries in this age group rarely do occur from short, accidental falls. In another retrospective study from the same tertiary care hospital, Greenes and Schutzman (57) reviewed the charts of children younger than 2 years hospitalized over a 6.5-year period with intracranial hemorrhage, cerebral contusion, or cerebral edema. These authors found that 19 of 101 infants had asymptomatic intracranial injuries, and 14 of these 19 infants sustained their injuries in short falls or downstairs. Based on the physicians' and/or social workers' chart notes, only one infant was thought to be a victim of child abuse. None of the 19 infants were seriously injured, and all were normal at the time of discharge.

The existing studies cited here, taken in totality, support the conclusion that not only are accidental falls from heights of less than several stories unlikely to result in death, but also that severe intracranial injuries ascribed to short falls likely indicate abusive injury. Accidental falls, even down stairways, are not generally the cause of intracranial injuries in infants. Household falls from furniture or down stairs most commonly result in minor trauma, but these falls, particularly when from the arms of a caretaker, may cause skull fractures, some of which may be complex or depressed, epidural hematomas, and at times clinically benign focal subarachnoid hemorrhages or small parenchymal contusions. Falls downstairs in walkers infrequently cause large intraparenchymal hematomas with potential neurologic consequences, but only one death has been reported (38). High-velocity impact injuries, falls from extreme heights, or falls onto extremely hard surfaces provide the opportunities for more severe injury. Rarely do these catastrophic events occur without a corroborated history. If these factors are not present to account for severe head injury, the examining physician must strongly consider abuse.

Other household accidents in young children occur rarely, but have severe neurologic consequences and often death. The most frequently described event causing significant morbidity and mortality is a television set toppling from an unstable location falling and crushing the child. Bernard et al. (15) reported that there were 73 cases of falling television sets reported to the Consumer Products Safety Commission (CPSC) over the 7-year period beginning in January 1990, resulting in 28 deaths. Head injuries were the most common and accounted for 72%. A crushing injury of the head was found in 13 of 14 deaths further investigated by the CPSC. The authors conclude that serious injury and death does occur from children toppling television sets from elevated heights, particularly crushing injuries to the head. The base on which a television is set is of fundamental importance in preventing these types of injuries and may offer a clear explanation for the severe injury or death after a thorough investigation of the injury scene. Duhaime et al. (44) described crush injuries to the head occurring in seven children, four whose heads were run over by a motor vehicle in a driveway or parking lot. In the other three, the children pulled on a heavy object, causing it to fall on their heads. All patients had basilar skull fractures, and calvarial fractures were often multiple and complex and associated with subarachnoid and parenchymal hemorrhages. All surviving children made good cognitive recoveries, suggesting a good long-term prognosis despite their alarming history and initial appearance.

Accidental suffocation has been a leading cause of infant deaths and is a challenge to separate from abusive head trauma or deliberate suffocation, as seen in cases of infanticide or Munchausen syndrome by proxy. Drago and Dannenberg (42) reviewed 2,178 deaths by mechanical suffocation occurring in the U.S. over a 17-year period beginning in 1980 in infants 12 months or younger. They found the most frequent cause of suffocation was being wedged between a bed or mattress and the wall, and the second was oral nasal obstruction by a plastic bag. Astute first responders, crime scene investigators, and death review teams must assess and weigh these cases very carefully.

In our experience, the most frequently offered reason for abusive head injury is accidental trauma; therefore when evaluating the cause of head injury, the care team must consider all potential origins and causes of the findings suggestive of head trauma. Hampered by an inaccurate history that is often intentionally misleading, the physician must weigh each diagnostic possibility, assessing the characteristics of the finding and the statistical likelihood of those findings correlating with the history provided. The other conditions that mimic abusive head injuries include accidental injuries, metabolic disorders, preexisting intracranial vascular abnormalities, and SIDS.

Intracranial Hemorrhages

Many of the lesions described with abusive head injury have intracranial hemorrhage as a prominent feature. Trauma is by far the most common cause of intracranial head injury in young children. In reviewing 2,000 cases of subarachnoid hemorrhage, Matson (95) found only three instances of spontaneous intracranial bleeding occurring in children ages 1 through 5 years. Reviewing additional studies from 1966 to 1973, totaling 10,000 cases, Newton (109) found no instances of spontaneous subarachnoid hemorrhage in children younger than 1 year (109).

Although a common cause of subarachnoid hemorrhage in adults is a ruptured aneurysm, the incidence of cerebral aneurysms in childhood and adolescents is low, increasing with advancing age. Aneurysms occur twice as frequently in male subjects (33,104,111). A review of recent case reports yielded 72 cases of spontaneous rupture of cerebral aneurysms in children younger than 5 years, 66 cases in children younger than 2 years, and 20 cases in infants 1 year or younger (33,104,111).

Infection, especially herpes simplex encephalitis, may be associated with hemorrhage. Infants may present with seizures, bulging fontanel, and fever. Retinal hemorrhages are not present, and radiologic imaging should enable the physician to differentiate this condition from abusive head injury (109).

Spontaneous intracranial bleeding may result from vitamin K deficiency or from clotting abnormalities related to disease processes such as hemophilia. Spontaneous bleeding associated with vitamin K deficiency occurs when vitamin K is not administered prophylactically after birth. In studies of selected newborn populations in Japan and England, the incidence of spontaneous intracranial hemorrhage among those deficient in vitamin K was substantial (81.2%). The disorder is especially prevalent in breast-fed babies, generally occurs between 4 and 8 weeks, and is rapidly corrected by administration of vitamin K (100,106). The issue is moot in most areas in which vitamin K is administered to the newborn as a matter of routine postnatal care. A check of the birth records documents administration of vitamin K.

Intracranial bleeding in neonates attributable to prematurity, mechanical injury from traumatic birth, or the use of forceps occa-

sionally becomes an issue in children with injuries in the first few days of life. Generally,
intracranial bleeding and dural sinus thromboses related to birth trauma are present
within the first 24 hours of life, but recognition may be delayed for up to 4 days, particularly in instances in which there is a small
continuing hemorrhage (101). Occasionally, it
is difficult to ascertain whether subarachnoid
bleeding in the first days of life is due to birth
trauma or to inflicted injury. Frequently in
this dilemma, the birth history, the dynamics
of the caretakers, and review of postnatal care
yield clues.

To keep these data in perspective, intracranial hemorrhage in children from causes other
than trauma is rare. Of the few cases of spontaneous intracranial bleeding in young children, one third result from a ruptured
aneurysm, another one third from congenital
arterial venous malformation, and the final
one third from no recognizable cause (109). It
is best to assume that all unexplained intracranial bleeding in children is due to
trauma. Little harm is done if a nontraumatic
intracranial bleed is discretely approached as
traumatic; however, a traumatic injury incorrectly viewed as spontaneous or accidental results in time and information lost in the
process of identifying circumstances surrounding the injury. Further diagnostic studies, additional historic factors, and characteristics of the hemorrhage usually separate
traumatic from nontraumatic causes.

Sudden Infant Death Syndrome

Possibly the most vexing differential diagnosis in fatal cases of child abuse is sudden
infant death syndrome (SIDS; see also Chapter 20). SIDS is perceived as a condition of
substantial prevalence, and only a minority
of SIDS deaths are the result of child abuse.
SIDS is a diagnosis of exclusion and can be
established reliably only through a careful,
meticulously conducted autopsy by a pathologist familiar with causes of death in childhood, a death-scene evaluation, and a review
of the clinical circumstances. The patholo-

gist must have access to proper imaging results, specialized consultants, and experienced death-scene investigators. In one of
the few studies attempting to analyze the
misdiagnosis of SIDS, Bass et al. (12) found
two definite cases of shaken baby syndrome
and a third probable case among 27 consecutive cases initially labeled as SIDS.

Recent data emphasize the importance of
careful assessment of the spinal cord at the cervical medullary junction in SIDS autopsies.
Towbin (144) described autopsy findings in
four cases of SIDS that included cervical cord
injury with hemorrhage into the epidural
space, meninges, and spinal cord parenchyma.
The author described this injury as resembling
a spinal injury after forceful delivery, and suggested that the flailing head was the source of
such an injury. [Note that Hadley et al. (63)
showed that five of six infants dying of shaken
baby syndrome and undergoing autopsy had
injuries of the spinal cord at the cervical
medullary junction, but others have found such
injuries only rarely].

SIDS is therefore a diagnosis of exclusion.
As the name implies, no available diagnostic
test unequivocally establishes the diagnosis.
The documentation of injuries to the brain,
bones, or other major organs excludes SIDS
as a diagnostic consideration.

Miscellaneous Conditions

Both Menkes' syndrome and osteogenesis
imperfecta are associated with skeletal findings suggestive of child abuse (see also Chapter 7); however, the intracranial imaging findings of these syndromes should not be
confused with the findings of child abuse.
Metabolic disorders and encephalitis are often
mentioned as a possible differential diagnosis
in abusive head trauma. In most instances,
imaging, appropriate screening tests for toxins, and the patient's clinical course can make
these diagnoses clear. Unless the situation is
one of self-limited toxin exposure (e.g., drug
overdose), in general, metabolic conditions
continue to worsen unless identified and
treated, whereas abusive head trauma usually

is at its worst at the time of hospitalization of the child.

Glutaric Aciduria Type I

Glutaric aciduria type I (GA 1) is an autosomal recessive inborn error of metabolism due to a deficiency of glutaryl-CoA dehydrogenase required for lysine and tryptophan metabolism (151). Infants with this rare disorder appear normal at birth and have normal early developmental milestones (151). Macrocephaly may be present at birth, or develops rapidly within the first few weeks of life (54). Ultrasound demonstrates cyst-like dilatation of the sylvian fissures by age 3 weeks (54). Often GA 1 remains undiagnosed, misdiagnosed (54), or the diagnosis is delayed until there is an onset of encephalopathy associated with minor illness or the gradual loss of motor abilities with dystonic or choreoathetotic movements (recognized usually between ages 7 and 18 months) (54,70). Radiologic imaging at the time symptoms appear characteristically shows frontotemporal atrophy as well as diffuse cortical atrophy, changes in basal ganglia, white matter hypodensities, and internal and external hydrocephalus (151). Subdural hematomas, often of different ages, and retinal hemorrhages occur in some cases and in conjunction with the clinical neurologic deterioration raise the suspicion of abusive head trauma (70).

Making the diagnosis of GA 1 by measuring urinary glutaric acid, 3-OH glutaric acid, and glutaconic acid can be confounded because these metabolites are not always present in the urine when the infant is clinically stable and also can be elevated in other conditions (105). Measuring glutaryl-CoA dehydrogenase activity in leukocytes or cultured fibroblasts is the definitive diagnostic test, but because it is expensive and time-consuming, it should be reserved for those infants in whom the diagnosis is clearly suspected, and not for all infants with subdural hematomas. Morris et al. (105) recently reported some guidelines to help sort out GA 1 from abusive head trauma. They remind us that GA 1 is not associated with fractures, and subdural hematomas in GA 1 have not been reported without frontotemporal atrophy or widening of the sylvian fissure. If these characteristic features of GA 1 are present, they further recommend urinary organic acid analysis and blood-spot glutarylcarnitine, combined with total free plasma carnitine concentration. If these results suggest GA 1, or there is low plasma carnitine or equivocal findings, the diagnosis should be determined by measuring glutaryl-CoA dehydrogenase activity. Most important, it should be noted that GA 1 is a potentially treatable condition if diagnosed early when neurodevelopment is still normal, before the metabolic encephalopathy leaves the infant with a severe irreversible dystonic movement disorder (36).

Ehlers–Danlos Syndrome

Connective tissue diseases, particularly those associated with bleeding and coagulation abnormalities, can be difficult to distinguish from abusive head trauma. Nuss and Manco-Johnson described a 3-year-old child with Ehlers–Danlos syndrome who had presented at age 13 weeks with a seizure, chronic and acute subdural hematomas, retinal hemorrhages, and normal coagulation except for a prolonged bleeding time. The infant had been placed in a foster home for 3 months because of the presumptive diagnosis of shaken baby syndrome. To help prevent errors in diagnoses, the authors recommended obtaining a thorough family history and coagulation screening, including a bleeding time. This laboratory screen comprises PT, PTT, TT, fibrinogen, platelet count, fibrin degradation product (FDP), and bleeding time. However, the risk of misdiagnosing abusive head trauma in these rare conditions must be balanced by the high risk of recidivism and the severity of subsequent brain injuries in abused infants. In each case, information from an extensive medical history, family history, thorough child protection and police investigations, assessment for other abusive injuries including a complete bone survey, initially and 2 weeks later, and screening for coagulation abnormalities must be weighed against the specific physical and radiographic findings to minimize errors in diagnosis.

Timing of Injuries

The natural history of head injuries is important not only when planning medical treatment, but also when defining the cause of the injury. In addition to assisting in predicting the child's prognosis, medical data help to identify a time frame during which the injury likely occurred, thereby helping to establish possible perpetrators. Occasionally, information about injury timing establishes a delay in seeking medical treatment.

Three major sources of information are used to establish the timing of intracranial injuries: clinical history, physiologic data, and imaging. These sources work in synergy and, if used separately, may lead to apparent disagreements between experts. In most instances, imaging dating is less precise than physiologic data; clinical history, if reliable, is the most precise.

Imaging-based estimates of the timing of intracranial bleeding principally depend on a recognizable course as the hemoglobin changes into its breakdown components. Standards exist for dating of blood seen on CT or MR scans. Under some circumstances, it may be possible to narrow the time frame for the bleeding to a matter of days. In other instances, it may be possible to document only that several episodes of bleeding occurred (3,4,125). The usual time course for developing acute cortical necrosis and the evolution of encephalomalacia also are known. Cerebral atrophy begins to be evident about 4 weeks after a severe brain insult. The effects, as documented by imaging, of a single episode of brain injury are maximal at about 3 months after injury. Subgaleal hematomas form within minutes of the trauma and are seen in the earliest brain imaging studies, even when they are not apparent clinically. As with other forms of limited internal bleeding (e.g., ankle sprains), they tend to peak in size within 24 to 72 hours, and then they slowly resolve. Skull fractures

and fractures associated with shaking (e.g., ribs) can be categorized by appearance into likely time frames (see Chapter 7).

Physiologic information includes data from various measures, including autopsy, laboratory, and clinical assessments of the child. Using clinical assessment, head injuries can be dated by correlating the extent and type of injury with the child's condition at a particular time. For example, if a child with massive head injuries is brought to an emergency department with agonal respirations and dies soon thereafter, it is possible to predict that such injuries could not have existed for an extended period.

Xanthochromia in the cerebrospinal fluid (CSF) develops within 12 to 24 hours of insult. It is a marker of the age of a particular bleed, or it may confirm that a previous bleed was also present. Consequently, all CSF specimens (usually obtained while ruling out meningitis and before intracranial bleeding is suspected) should be examined for xanthochromia once intracranial bleeding is diagnosed.

Autopsy findings may demonstrate the extent of the injuries, allowing the determination that the more severe the initial damage, the shorter the elapsed time before intensive medical attention is required or death of the child results. Autopsy or neurosurgical interventions may distinguish between old and new blood (e.g., the organization of the clot in old subdural hematomas). Microscopic analysis of brain tissue can distinguish between acute and chronic hypoxia–ischemia. Whereas radiologic dating may encompass a period of days to weeks, physiologic dating may allow a prediction within days to hours.

Clinical dating combines imaging and physiologic data with the history and is often the most precise. The more severe the head injury, the more stereotyped the clinical course should be. At the extreme, massive head injuries should result in immediate death, coma, or severe symptoms that are unmistakably serious, even to the medically uneducated parent. If several observers report that the child was apparently normal, eating, walking, and/

or playing, such histories would be inconsistent with a child already fatally injured. Thus if a fatal injury occurred, it would have had to occur later. Mild head injuries, such as concussions, are easily confused with other medical entities such as gastroenteritis if the proper history is not forthcoming (76). In general, the more severe the trauma, the more precisely it can be dated.

The following cases illustrate the way in which data can be combined to yield accurate estimates of the time of injury.

Case Histories

Case 1

A 4-month-old boy is brought to the emergency department by his parents. They report that he had a 2-minute, left-sided seizure. He now appears healthy, perhaps slightly fussy, but is drinking his formula well. Spinal fluid is obtained and shows xanthochromia. Further physical examination reveals retinal hemorrhages in the right eye. The CT scan is normal, but the MR scan shows a thin subdural hemorrhage over the frontal aspect of the right cerebral hemisphere. By MRI criteria, the blood collection appears subacute (2 days to 2 weeks old). Additional history includes the fact that the child has had five caretakers over the last 2 weeks.

Comment. The clinical symptoms are minimal. Although the child must have been in considerable pain after the shaking, this pain would have diminished over several hours, and it might be difficult for anyone later to know that anything was significantly wrong with the child. Only because of the seizure (which could happen any time after the trauma) was the correct diagnosis suspected. Radiologically, physiologically, and clinically, the injury could have happened any time within several days of the seizure.

Case 2

An 18-month-old girl is seen at 10 a.m. for vomiting and dehydration. Reportedly, the vomiting began about 24 hours ago and has worsened. She was unsteady on her feet yesterday, but refuses to walk now. Physical examination is significant for bilateral retinal hemorrhages, esotropia, 10% dehydration, and stupor. CT scanning reveals acute bilateral subdural hemorrhages over the frontal–parietal areas, cerebral edema, and an interhemispheric subdural hemorrhage. Skeletal survey shows a left 8th rib posterior fracture with beginning callus formation. Her serum sodium level is 166 mEq/L. She is admitted to the intensive care unit and has neurosurgical interventions. Additional history establishes that she was active, eating, and happy during a party at noon yesterday, but was symptomatic with vomiting, esotropia, and an inability to walk when visited by her grandmother at 7 p.m. last night. Only her mother was present between noon and 7 p.m.

Comment. Radiologically, the bleeding must have occurred within several days of the CT study. The rib fracture is 7 to 10 days old, indicating an earlier trauma, probably shaking. Thus it is probable that whoever broke the rib also caused this recent shaking (narrowing the list of possible perpetrators). Physiologically, the dehydration and the hypernatremia require time, often 24 hours or more, and are unlikely to be less than 12 hours. If the vomiting is the result of the shaking, the episode could have happened between noon and 7 p.m. yesterday. If the shaking is because of caretaker stress related to the child's illness, the shaking could have occurred more recently. Her injuries are extensive, and cerebral edema over the first 24 to 48 hours would require medical attention to avert possible death. Clinically, it is clear that she was not injured before noon yesterday. It is probable that the unsteadiness and esotropia observed by the grandmother represent head injuries and not gastroenteritis. Thus the shaking almost certainly occurred between noon and 7 p.m. yesterday. Social or law-enforcement, not medical, investigation will establish whether the mother really was the only caretaker present during this time (and thus is the perpetrator).

Case 3

The mother's boyfriend was watching a 10-month-old boy while she went out shopping for 30 minutes. He was playful, interactive, and crawling when she left. When she returned, the boyfriend reported that 10 minutes ago, the child had fallen down from a sitting position and his eyes rolled back. The mother found the boy gasping, dusky, and unresponsive. Ambulance personnel intubated the boy. Examination in the emergency department showed bilateral retinal hemorrhages and a large right parietal scalp swelling. Emergency CT scans showed massive bilateral subdural hemorrhages over the entire frontal–parietal–temporal areas, several shearing injuries at the gray–white matter junctions within the brain, and numerous areas of intraparenchymal bleeding. A depressed left parietal skull fracture was present. The child died shortly after admission. Autopsy showed free-flowing subdural blood. The postmortem skeletal survey showed the parietal fracture to be 8 cm in length.

Comment. Using only imaging data, this case must be dated within a window of several days. When the physiologic data are added, we get a better perception of these rapidly fatal, extensive injuries. The child could not have lasted more than 1 to 2 hours after the injuries were incurred. That he was still alive when seen in the hospital means that he most likely was injured sometime within the last hour, certainly within the last 2 hours. Clinically, he most likely was rendered unconscious from the trauma, and the onset of symptoms would be immediate. If he had prior injuries of this magnitude, he could not have acted the way the mother described. If her history is true, the shake/slam occurred sometime during the time that the boyfriend had sole access.

MANAGEMENT CONSIDERATIONS

The clinical management of the child with head injuries must focus simultaneously on diagnosis and treatment. No single order of steps is taken, because these rest exclusively on the clinical status of the child. Because the head-injured child is likely to be critically ill at the time of presentation, multiple assessments and interventions are likely to be required, calling for the involvement of numerous specialists with a clear understanding of the forensic and clinical considerations. It is beyond the scope and intent of this chapter to provide a manual of specific treatment for head-injured children; therefore only a brief overview is offered.

A child who is apneic or convulsing or presents with signs of severely increased intracranial pressure requires airway support. Placement of a large-bore intravenous line is necessary for the administration of medications. Careful consideration should be given before performing lumbar puncture because of the theoretic possibility of causing herniation of the cerebellar tonsils. Some authorities recommend imaging of the brain as the diagnostic step of choice, with lumbar puncture held in abeyance of the results of the imaging study. In the face of cerebral edema, fluid restriction, steroids, and osmolar drugs aimed at limiting intracranial pressure may be needed. Once the child's emergency clinical condition is stabilized, an ongoing coordinated forensic and clinical assessment begins. Depending on the complexity of services needed, the clinician may consider transferring the child to a specialized pediatric center.

From the standpoint of both effective clinical intervention and investigative accuracy, the interval during which the child is undergoing initial examination, diagnosis, and treatment is the optimal time for a physician to elicit a thorough history from the caretakers. Each person involved in the caretaker role should be interviewed separately. It is appropriate for the interviewing physician to be supportive and interested, but also to gather historic data rather than to provide information regarding suspicion of abuse until the entire assessment is completed. One should address a parent by noting that he or she may be able to provide information useful in the diagnosis and treatment of the infant, and that separate interviews are conducted because each caretaker may see the child somewhat differently. The interview then proceeds with questions that probe the time the caretaker last saw the child behaving normally. Specific questions regarding feeding difficulties, vomiting, irritability, or other subtle neurologic signs should be carefully elicited.

The child protective services representative and police investigator should be involved immediately when suspicion arises that an injury is nonaccidental. Child abuse injury is often misdiagnosed or incorrectly reported when child protective services or investigative activities, including adequate death-scene investigation, are not implemented promptly (50,149). For these professionals, the lack of certainty as to the child's condition, the early remorse of the caretaker, and the small window of time during which the caretaker may not recognize the potential consequences of the action make critical the earliest possible contact with caretakers, physicians, and child. "Crime scene" information fades rapidly, as does the capacity for police professionals to apply specialized interviewing and investigative techniques aimed at determining veracity and investigative direction. Child-protection assessment must be available immediately to assess the ongoing safety of the injured child as well as the safety of siblings in the home. Subsequently, complete medical examinations performed by physicians understanding the subtle nature of child abuse injuries should be performed on all children who have had contact with the caretakers of the injured child.

OUTCOME AND PROGNOSIS

Mortality from abusive head trauma is high, with figures varying from 12% to 30% (41,75,108,140). Nachelsky and Dix(110) compiled data from the 24 shaken baby syndrome studies published prior to 1993 and found 84 deaths in 278 total shaken baby syndrome cases, for a mortality rate of 30%. Some authorities have estimated that for every child who dies of inflicted cranial cerebral trauma, four are left neurologically handicapped. Although this statement can be con-

strued as speculative, support for it is found in the works of Sinal and Ball (137), Benzel and Hadden (14), Ludwig and Warman (92), and McClelland et al. (99).

In a prospective study comparing 20 children with intentional head injuries with 20 children with nonintentional head injuries, Ewing-Cobbs et al. (51) found intentional injuries to be more devastating. There was short-term good recovery in 55% of the nonintentional head injury group compared with 20% of the intentional head injury group. Moderate disability was present in 65% of the intentional injury group compared with 20% of the nonintentional injury group. Forty-five percent of the victims of intentional head injury scored in the mentally deficient group as compared with only 5% of the nonintentional head injury group. In a study of pediatric intensive care unit (PICU) admissions (67), 15 infants with abusive head injury were compared with 10 age-matched children comprising all children younger than 2 years who were admitted with severe head injury caused by accidental impact trauma. Two of the abused infants died, and 69% of the survivors showed major neurologic handicaps. Of the 10 accidental-impact trauma group, one died, another had severe neurologic damage, and six (67%) of nine were thought to be normal at discharge. Five of these accidental impacts were due to falls, three were due to road traffic accident, one was the result of being kicked by a horse, and one was due to being struck by a hammer.

In the past, outcome studies have been based on the short-term follow-up of infants surviving abusive head trauma. One fourth to one third of abusive head injury victims recover and leave the hospital without apparent neurologic deficit (18). Twenty percent to 50% are symptom-free 1 year after the incident (18). Hampered by difficulties in locating survivors because of family instability and confidentiality restrictions, few studies have documented the long-term effects (43). However, some studies have shown that cognitive, behavioral, and neurologic deficits are common even in those with apparent good early recovery

(18,43,53). These studies, in conjunction with clinical scrutiny of follow-up CT and/or MRI examinations, provide a vivid picture of the devastating long-term effects of cranial cerebral trauma in abused children (18,43,53, 67,73).

Duhaime et al. (43) followed up 14 surviving infants for an average of 9 years after their injuries and found only five with good neurologic outcomes. However, three of these five children had repeated years in school and/or required tutoring or management of behavior problems. Similarly Fischer and Allasio (53) were able to locate 10 long-term survivors of 25 infants with shaken baby syndrome. Three of the 10 infants were normal, and seven were moderately to severely impaired at discharge. Only one of these three "normal" infants remained normal on long-term follow-up. The other two had either clumsiness and poor vision or problems with gait, reclusiveness, and required special education. Bonnier et al. (18), following up 13 infants for a mean of 7 years, found that it took up to 2 years for epilepsy to develop and up to 3 to 6 years for behavioral and neuropsychological abnormalities to be recognized. Six of the 13 infants apparently had recovered fully with normal neurologic, psychomotor, and general examinations 2 months after injury from shaking. However, all but one of these infants demonstrated disabilities between 6 months and 5 years after the injury. Hemiparesis was detected 12 months after the shaking in two cases, and psychomotor retardation, especially problems with language, adaptability, and social behaviors became apparent 24 months after the injury. Mental retardation requiring special education was confirmed in five of the six cases within 5 years, and severe behavioral disorders appeared in three of the six cases. Only one child was clinically normal 5 years after the injury.

Neurologic deficits and diminished productive life potential are correlated with the findings of encephalomalacia, cerebral atrophy, ventriculomegaly, porencephaly, or localized cranial nerve lesions. Many children are left with cortical blindness, seizure disorders, profound mental retardation, spastic diplegia, or quadriplegia. Some continue to live in a persistent vegetative state. Although based on small numbers, the series by Duhaime et al. (43) pointed out some factors noted immediately that predict these severe outcomes. All infants who presented with unresponsiveness and all who had bilateral diffuse hypodensity with loss of gray–white differentiation or unilateral hemispheric hypodensity on CT within the first few days of injury became vegetative or blind, nonverbal, and wheelchair bound. Only two of five with focal areas of hypodensity or contusion were severely disabled. Bonnier et al. (18) found impairment of cranial growth to predict severe neurologic sequelae in one third of infants, all of whom were neurologically impaired at the time of discharge.

In addition to these poor outcomes, the cost of care for these severely injured infants is staggering. Comparing the costs of 13 infants with abusive head trauma among 937 admissions to the PICU, Irazuzta et al. (73) found that infants with abusive head injuries were younger and had a higher severity of illness ranking and greater hospitalization charges averaging $35,641 per case (range, $12,200–$150,600). Yet seven patients died, and four of the six survivors were left with serious enough disabilities to require permanent medical assistance. Financial cost of one child who is ventilator dependent due to a cervical cord injury is estimated at $1,000,000 every 3 years that he survives, with estimated costs in excess of $26,000 per month (Levitt C, personal communication).

Other outcome considerations are the proper societal management of both the other children at risk in the family constellation and the injured child if and when he or she returns home. Given the fact that etiologic factors often do not change and are not easily treated, the likelihood of recidivism or abuse of other siblings is high (2,13,26,76). Protective custody is a serious consideration in circumstances in which available information indicates a nonaccidental injury. No single professional can make this decision as confidently as a team of professionals representing the multiple disciplines called for in a child abuse investigation. Naturally, this task calls for a well-orchestrated team effort with clear role definition, mutual respect, and sound professional thinking. A child abuse team with a history of cooperation and collaboration can develop this type of synergism through ongoing case consultation in a non-crisis setting. Whereas the police and child protection workers develop their own documentation, physicians should not allow medical findings merely to be incorporated into the findings of these professionals, but should ensure that their own findings, judgment, and conclusions lead early discussions and are documented and available as input into these long-term decisions.

Legal sanctions may not be the normal province of the medical professional, but criminal prosecution of the perpetrator may be a strong determinant of long-term outcome for a child. Such a strong systematic response may serve to break through denial on the part of either the offending or nonoffending care-taker and family, resulting in both accurate fact disclosure and possible therapeutic intervention, or at least long-term separation of the perpetrator from the victim and from other potential child victims. The medical care team must, therefore, be prepared to participate within the legal system in the best interest of the child and of justice.

MYTHS

Clinical presentations of shaken baby syndrome tend to be very similar across cases. Likewise the stories told by the perpetrator, and the courtroom arguments that it is something else, form distinct patterns. For example, commonly the constellation of injuries is claimed to have occurred by a fall. Other such myths around shaken baby syndrome include rebleeds, genetic/metabolic diseases, vulnerable physiology of the infant, children being too old for shaken baby syndrome, retinal hemorrhages always mean shaken baby syndrome, and profiling the abuser.

Subdural hemorrhages, like any hemorrhage, may rebleed some time after the original injury. However, this is a rare phenomenon, most likely to occur in conjunction with neurosurgical procedures for other conditions, and does not mimic shaken baby syndrome. As part of the process of healing, subdural hematomas develop new delicate blood vessels within several weeks. Although some trauma is probably necessary to damage these vessels, it may be relatively minor. Typically, subdural rebleeding is contained within the original clot or is adjacent. It is not associated with retinal hemorrhages, or with cerebral edema. The symptoms are slow, with increasing lethargy, diminished appetite, and perhaps some irritability. An expanding head size may be seen if several weeks pass and there is sufficient bleeding to cause a mass effect. Rebleeds should not be sudden or fatal. They represent bleeding, not a brain-injury process like that seen with shaken baby syndrome. Thus the combination of retinal hemorrhages and new subdural hemorrhages, when in the presence of old subdural hemorrhages, represents a new episode of severe shaking and not rebleeding (2).

Sometimes professionals may find it personally difficult to accept the diagnosis of shaken baby syndrome, and may postulate that there must be some sort of obscure medical explanation such as a genetic or metabolic disorder (see Chapter 9). Genetic conditions that have been suggested as possibly mimicking shaken baby syndrome inevitably entail some sort of bleeding disorder (usually involving liver dysfunction). The difficulty with these explanations is that shaken baby syndrome is a brain-damage problem, with the intracranial and retinal bleeding as secondary. Bleeding disorder rationales fail to explain even the pattern of bleeding. Hemophiliacs, individuals who develop disseminated intravascular coagulation (DIC), idiopathic thrombocytopenic purpura (ITP), and others with true bleeding disorders do not present with the pattern of bleeding or brain damage seen with shaken baby syndrome. Thus there is no reasonable metabolic or genetic disorder in the differential diagnosis of shaken baby syndrome.

Since the first descriptions of shaken baby syndrome (26–28), it has been claimed that infants and young children are especially vulnerable to shaking. This claim has been repeated in the medical and child abuse prevention literature, but it never has been experimentally verified. The major reason for children's susceptibility is the difference in size between the child and the perpetrator. However, it was also claimed that their physiology makes them more vulnerable. Although it is true that infants have a somewhat enlarged subarachnoid space, any CT of an infant's brain shows that it occupies virtually all of the intracranial space. It is therefore unlikely that this small difference has any practical significance. It is also claimed that the infant's neck muscles are relatively "weak." An infant's head relative to its body is much larger than an adult's. Were an adult to have a proportionally large head, no doubt it would be difficult to control. There is no evidence that a child's neck muscles are proportionally weaker. No matter how strong children's neck muscles, it is unlikely that they could "tense" them enough to withstand the assault by an adult 10 times their size who is violently shaking them. Thus the claim of special infant vulnerability to shaking has no experimental support and makes no practical medical sense.

A related claim is made by some physician practitioners unfamiliar with shaken baby syndrome. This infrequent assertion is that some children (e.g., 3-year-olds) are too old for shaken baby syndrome. Yet there is no physiologic reason as to why children of any age could not suffer these injuries were they shaken hard enough. Most children who are victims of shaken baby syndrome are younger than 1 year; some are older, and for all practical purposes, children 5 years old or older are not seen (4). In a case of domestic violence, an adult sustained retinal hemorrhages, and subdural hemorrhage (31). Absent extraordinary circumstances, children older than 4 years do not appear to be at risk, simply because of their size.

Another myth is that retinal hemorrhages always mean shaken baby syndrome. Thirty percent of newborns have transient retinal hemorrhages as part of the birth process (139). Rarely there may be other causes of retinal hemorrhages, including children with head injuries in motor vehicle crashes (see Chapters 5, 9). However, the pattern of multilayer, numerous retinal hemorrhages that extend to the periphery of the eye is almost always from shaken baby syndrome, and when coupled with intracranial brain injury and bleeding, it is diagnostic.

Profiles of the abuser are not legally or scientifically sound. Although many of the perpetrators are men (140), this also is true for physical abuse in general (146). Many perpetrators are young adults because they are the ones most likely to have access to young children. Some of the perpetrators abuse drugs or commit other forms of violence. For an individual case, such information is of no value in determining who did it. Such demographic information is only of value in better understanding the general dynamics of child abuse and perhaps fashioning prevention programs (assuming such targeting is of proven value).

Claims of these types do not reflect the medical literature or mainstream medical opinion. Rather they are "courtroom diagnoses," which are not seriously considered in the medical community.

PREVENTION

Considerable effort has gone into specific targeted programs designed to prevent shaken baby syndrome. Such programs attempt to educate young parents and others about the dangers of shaking.

One older study showed that when given verbal questions about whether shaking a baby is dangerous, college students failed to appreciate its hazards (131). Nonverbal assessments as to whether shaking is perceived as dangerous have not been studied. The American Academy of Pediatrics supports the position that any external observer viewing such shaking would know that it was dangerous and life-threatening (in press).

Only one article attempted to study the effects of a shaken baby syndrome program (130). In that study, mothers of newborns were given materials about shaken baby syndrome. The ones who responded felt that this provided information they did not previously have or previously did not fully appreciate. With only an approximate 20% response rate to what essentially was a satisfaction survey, a serious response bias is likely. Furthermore, these results do not address the more important question of whether such information actually prevents anything.

The presumption of current shaken baby syndrome prevention programs is that a knowledge deficit exists and that once taught what forces are involved, a caregiver would refrain from abusing a child. Yet education alone has never been shown to affect the incidence of other forms of physical abuse nor do laws against child abuse ensure that it will not happen. Programs that attempt to change motivation are more likely to prevent abusive head trauma. Child abuse prevention programs such as intensive home visitation are more likely to redirect behavior than is education about dangers, which attempts the difficult task of getting a potential perpetrator to inhibit.

Another problem with specific shaken baby prevention programs is that stopping one form of physical abuse might only result in the substitution of another. This is not the goal of general physical abuse prevention. Strategies to deal with crying (the usual inciting stimulus) and anger management may prove to be more successful. In a review of home visitation programs, Gutterman (60) demonstrated that trying to target specific populations did not work as well as a more universal approach. Whatever approaches are selected to try to prevent physical abuse (and hence abusive head trauma), the programs should be universal and outcome-based.

REFERENCES

1. Alario A, Duhaime T. Do retinal hemorrhages occur with accidental head trauma in young children? *Am J Dis Child* 1990;144:445.
2. Alexander R, Crabbe L, Sato Y, et al. Serial abuse in children who are shaken. *Am J Dis Child* 1990;144: 58–60.
3. Alexander R, Sato Y, Smith W, et al. Incidence of impact trauma with cranial injuries ascribed to shaking. *Am J Dis Child* 1990;144:724–726.
4. Alexander RC, Smith WL, eds. *Abusive head trauma: proceedings of a consensus conference: supported by the Brain Trauma Foundation.* Ames, IA: University of Iowa Press, 1991.
5. Alexander RC, Schor DP, Smith WL. Magnetic resonance imaging of intracranial injuries from child abuse. *J Pediatr* 1986;109:975.
6. Alexander RC, Smith W, Stevenson R. Serial Munchausen syndrome by proxy. *Pediatrics* 1990;86: 581–585.
7. American Academy of Pediatrics, Committee on Adolescence. Firearms and adolescents. *Pediatrics* 1992; 89:784.
8. American Academy of Pediatrics Committee on Injury and Poison Prevention. The hospital record of the injured child and the need for external cause-of-injury codes. *Pediatrics* 1999;103:524–526.
9. American Academy of Pediatrics, Committee on Injury and Poison Prevention. Firearm injuries affecting the pediatric population. *Pediatrics* 1992;89:788.
10. Annobil SH, Binitie OP, Ranganayakulu Y, et al. A hospital-based study of falls from heights in children in southwestern Saudi Arabia. *Saudi Med J* 1995;16: 133–138.
11. Barlow B, Niemirska M, Gandhii RP, et al. Ten years of experience with falls from a height in children. *J Pediatr Surg* 1991;31:1353–1355.
12. Bass M, Kravath RE, Glass L. Death-scene investigation in sudden infant death. *N Engl J Med* 1986;315: 100–105.
13. Becker JC, Liersch R, Tautz C, et al. Shaken baby syndrome: report on four pairs of twins. *Child Abuse Negl* 1998;22:931–937.
14. Benzel EC, Hadden TA. Neurologic manifestations of child abuse. *South Med J* 1989;82:1347.
15. Bernard PA, Johnston C, Curtis SE, et al. Toppled television sets cause significant pediatric morbidity and mortality. *Pediatrics* 1998;102:e32:627.
16. Billmire M, Myers PA. Serious head injury in infants: accident or abuse? *Pediatrics* 1985;75:340–342.
17. Bird CR, McMahon JR, Gilles FH, et al. Strangulation in child abuse: CT diagnosis. *Radiology* 1987;163: 373–375.
18. Bonnier C, Nassagne MC, Evrard P. Outcome and prognosis of whiplash shaken infant syndrome: late consequences after a symptom-free interval. *Dev Med Child Neurol* 1995;37:943–956.
19. Brazelton TB. Crying in infancy. *Pediatrics* 1962;29: 579.
20. Brenner SL, Fischer H, Mann-Gray S. Race and the shaken baby syndrome: experience at one hospital. *J Natl Med Assoc* 1987;81:183.
21. Brenner RA, Overpeck MD, Trumble AC, et al. Deaths attributable to injuries in infants, United States, 1983-1991. *Pediatrics* 1999;103:968–974.
22. Brewster AL, Nelson JP, Hymel KP, et al. Victim, perpetrator, family, and incident characteristics of 32 infant maltreatment deaths in the United States Air Force. *Child Abuse Negl* 1998;22:91–101.

23. Bruce DA, Zimmerman RA. Shaken impact syndrome. *Pediatr Ann* 1989;18:482–494.
24. Bruce DA, Alavi A, Bilaniuk L, et al. Diffuse cerebral swelling following head injuries in children: the syndrome of "malignant brain edema." *J Neurosurg* 1981; 54:170.
25. Caffey J. The whiplash-shaken infant syndrome: manual shaking by the extremities with whiplash-induced intracranial and intraocular bleedings, linked with residual permanent brain damage and mental retardation. *Pediatrics* 1974;54:396.
26. Caffey J. On the theory and practice of shaking infants. *Am J Dis Child* 1972;124:161.
27. Caffey J. Multiple fractures in long bones of infants suffering from chronic subdural hematoma. *Am J Roentgenol* 1946;56:163.
28. Calder IM, Hill I, Scholtz CL. Primary brain trauma in non-accidental injury. *J Clin Pathol* 1984;37:1095.
29. Cannon TC, Jordan FB, Vogel JS, et al. Child homicide in Oklahoma: a continuing public health problem. *J Okl State Med Assoc* 1998;91:449–451.
30. Carey WB. "Colic"—primary excessive crying as an infant-environment interaction. *Pediatr Clin North Am* 1984;31:993.
31. Carrigan TD, Walker E, Barnes S. Domestic violence: the shaken adult syndrome. *J Accid Emerg Med* 2000; 17:138–139.
32. Case M, Graham M, Wood J. Spinal cord injury in child abuse by shaking. Presented at the Second National Conference on Shaken Baby Syndrome, Salt Lake City, Utah, Sept. 1998.
33. Cedzich C, Schramm J, Rockelein G. Multiple middle cerebral artery aneurysms in an infant. *J Neurosurg* 1990;72:806–809.
34. Chabrol B, Decarie JC, Fortin G. The role of cranial MRI in identifying patients suffering from child abuse and presenting with unexplained neurological findings. *Child Abuse Negl* 1999;23:217–228.
35. Chadwick DL, Chin S, Salerno C, et al. Deaths from falls in children: how far is fatal? *J Trauma* 1991;31: 1353.
36. Champion MP, Lee PJ. Abuse or metabolic disorder? [Letter] *Arch Dis Child* 1999;80:100.
37. Chiavello CT, Bond GR. Stairway-related injuries in children. *Pediatrics* 1994;94:679–681.
38. Chiavello CT, Christoph RA, Bond GR. Infant walker-related injuries: a prospective study of severity and incidence. *Pediatrics* 1994;93:974–976.
39. Collins KA, Nichols CA. A decade of pediatric homicide. *Am J Forensic Med Pathol* 1999;20:169–172.
40. Cummings P, Theis MK, Mueller B, et al. Infant injury death in Washington State, 1981 through 1990. *Arch Pediatr Adolesc Med* 1994;148:1021–1026.
41. Dias MS, Backstrom J, Falk M. Serial radiography in the infant shaken impact syndrome. *Pediatr Neurosurg* 1998;29:77–85.
42. Drago DA, Dannenberg AL. Infant mechanical suffocation deaths in the United States, 1980-1997. *Pediatrics* 1999;103:1020.
43. Duhaime AC, Christian C, Moss E, et al. Long-term outcome in infants with shaking-impact syndrome. *Pediatr Neurosurg* 1996;24:292–298.
44. Duhaime AC, Eppley M, Margulies S, et al. Crush injuries to the head in children. *Neurosurgery* 1995;37: 401–407.
45. Duhaime AC, Alario AJ, Lewander WJ, et al. Head injury in very young children: mechanisms, injury types and ophthalmologic findings in 100 hospitalized patients younger than 2 years of age. *Pediatrics* 1992;90: 179–185.
46. Duhaime AC, Gennarelli TA, Thibault LB, et al. The shaken baby syndrome: a clinical, pathological, and biomechanical study. *J Neurosurg* 1987;66:409–415.
47. Ellerstein NS. *Child abuse and neglect: a medical reference.* New York: Wiley Medical Publications, 1981.
48. Ellison PH, Tsai FY, Largent JA. Computed tomography in child abuse and cerebral contusion. *Pediatrics* 1978;62:151–154.
49. Elner SG, Elner VM, Arnall M, et al. Ocular and associated systemic findings in suspected child abuse. *Arch Ophthalmol* 1990;108:1094.
50. Ewigman B, Kivlahan C. Child maltreatment fatalities. *Pediatr Ann* 1989;18:476.
51. Ewing-Cobbs L, Kramer L, Prasad M, et at. Neuroimaging, physical, and developmental findings after inflicted and non-inflicted traumatic brain injury in young children. *Pediatrics* 1998;102:300–307.
52. Feldman KW, Weinberger E, Milstein JM, et al. Cervical spine MRI in abused infants. *Child Abuse Negl* 1997;21:199–205.
53. Fischer H, Allasio D. Permanently damaged: long-term follow-up of shaken babies. *Pediatrics* 1994;33: 696–698.
54. Forstner R, Hoffmann GF, Gassner I, et al. Glutaric aciduria type 1: ultrasonographic demonstration of early signs. *Pediatr Radiol* 1999;23:138–143.
55. Gilliand MCG, Folberg R. Shaken babies: some have no impact injuries. *J Forensic Sci* 1996;41:114–116.
56. Goetting MG, Sowa B. Retinal hemorrhage after cardiopulmonary resuscitation in children: an etiologic re-evaluation. *Pediatrics* 1990;85:585–588.
57. Greenes DS, Schutzman SA. Occult intracranial injury in infants. *Ann Emerg Med* 1988;32:680–686.
58. Gruskin KD, Schutzman SA. Head trauma in children younger than 2 years. *Arch Pediatr Adolesc Med* 1999; 153:15–20.
59. Guthkelch AN. Infantile subdural hematoma and its relationship to whiplash injuries. *Br Med J* 1971;2:430.
60. Gutterman N. Enrollment strategies in early home visitation to prevent physical child abuse and neglect: "universal vs. targeted" debate: a meta-analysis of population-based and screening-based programs. *Int J Child Abuse Negl* 1999;23:863–890.
61. Guyer B, Gallagher SS. An approach to the epidemiology of childhood injuries. *Pediatr Clin North Am* 1985;32:5–15.
62. Guyer B, MacDorman MF, Martin JA, et al. Annual summary of vital statistics-1997. *Pediatrics* 1998;102: 1333–1349.
63. Hadley MN, Sonntag VK, Rekate HL, et al. The infant whiplash-shake injury syndrome: a clinical and pathological study. *Neurosurgery* 1989;24:536–540.
64. Hahn YS, Raimondi AJ, McLone DG, et al. Traumatic mechanisms of head injury in child abuse. *Childs Brain* 1983;10:229–241.
65. Hanigan WC, Peterson RA, Njus G. Tin ear syndrome: rotational acceleration in pediatric head injuries. *Pediatrics* 1987;80:618–622.
66. Hansen KK. Twins and child abuse. *Arch Pediatr Adolesc Med* 1994;148:1345–1346.

67. Haviland J, Russell RIR. Outcome after severe non-accidental head injury. *Arch Dis Child* 1997;77:504–507.

68. Helfer RE, Slovis TL, Black M. Injuries resulting when small children fall out of bed. *Pediatrics* 1977; 60:533–535.

69. Hobbs CJ. Skull fracture and the diagnosis of abuse. *Arch Dis Child* 1984;59:246.

70. Hoffman GF, Naughten ER. Abuse or metabolic disorder? [Letter] *Arch Dis Child* 1998;78:399.

71. Hymel KP, Rumack CM, Hay TC, et al. Comparison of intracranial computed tomographic (CT) findings in pediatric abusive and accidental head trauma. *Pediatr Radiol* 1997;27:743–747.

72. Hymel KP, Abshire TC, Luckey DW, et al. Coagulopathy in pediatric abusive head trauma. *Pediatrics* 1997; 99:371–375.

73. Irazuzta JE, McJunkin JE, Danadian K, et al. Outcome and cost of child abuse. *Child Abuse Negl* 1997;21: 751–757.

74. Jamison DKL, Kay HH. Accidental head injury in childhood. *Arch Dis Child* 1974;49:376–381.

75. Jayawant S, Rawlinson A, Gibbon F, et al. Subdural hemorrhages in infants: population based study. *Br Med J* 1998;317:1558–1561.

76. Jenny C, Hymel KP, Ritzen A. et al. Analysis of missed cases of abusive head trauma. *JAMA* 1999;281:621–626.

77. Joffe M, Ludwig S. Stairway injuries in children. *Pediatrics* 1988;82:457–461.

78. Johnson DL, Braun D, Friendly D. Accidental head trauma and retinal hemorrhage. *Neurosurgery* 1993;33: 231–235.

79. Kempe CH, Silverman FN, Steele BF, et al. The battered child syndrome. *JAMA* 1962;181:17–24.

80. King J, Diefendorf D, Apthorp J, et al. Analysis of 429 fractures in 189 battered children. *J Pediatr Orthop* 1988;8:585–589.

81. Kleinman PK, Spevak MR. Soft tissue swelling and acute skull fractures. *J Pediatr* 1992;121:737–739.

82. Kleinman PK, Mark SC, Adams VI, et al. Factors affecting visualization of posterior rib fractures in abused infants. AJR *Am J Roentgenol* 1988;150:653–638.

83. Kleinman PK. Spinal trauma. In: Kleinman PK, ed. *Diagnostic imaging of child abuse.* St. Louis: Mosby, 1988:91–102.

84. Kravitz H, Criessen C, Gomberg R, et al. Accidental falls from elevated surfaces in infants from birth to one year of age. *Pediatrics* 1969;44:869–876.

85. Lambert SR, Johnson TE, Hyot CS. Optic nerve sheath and retinal hemorrhages associated with shaken baby syndrome. *Arch Ophthalmol* 1986;104:1509–1512.

86. Lawrence HS. Fatal nonpowder firearm wounds: case report and review of the literature. *Pediatrics* 1990;85: 177–181.

87. Lazoritz S, Baldwin S. The whiplash shaken infant syndrome: has Caffey's syndrome changed or have we changed his syndrome? *Child Abuse Negl* 1997;21: 1009–1014.

88. Lehman D, Schonfeld N. Falls from heights: a problem not just in the northeast. *Pediatrics* 1993;92:121–124.

89. Leventhal JM, et al. Skull fractures in young children: do characteristics of the fractures clearly distinguish child abuse from accidental injuries? *Am J Dis Child* 1990;144:429.

90. Levitt C, McCormick D. Head injuries in infants: accidental or inflicted? Presented at the National Conference on Shaken Baby Syndrome, Salt Lake City, Utah, November, 1996.

91. Levitt C, McCormick D. A closer look at intercranial infuries due to falls in infants less than 2 years. Presented at the Second National Conference on Shaken Baby Syndrome, Salt Lake City, Utah, September, 1998.

92. Ludwig S, Warman M. Shaken baby syndrome: a review of 20 cases. *Ann Emerg Med* 1984;13:104–107.

93. Lyons T, Oates RK. Falling out of bed: a relatively benign occurrence. *Pediatrics* 1993;92:125–127.

94. MacKeith R. Speculations on non-accidental injury as a cause of chronic brain disorder. *Dev Med Child Neurol* 1974;16:2116.

95. Matson DD. Intracranial arterial aneurysm in childhood. *J Neurosurg* 1965;23:573.

96. May PR, Fuster JM, Newman P, et al. Woodpeckers and head injury [Letter]. *Lancet* 1976;19:1347–1348.

97. Mayr J, Gaisl M, Purtschher K, et al. Baby walkers: an underestimated hazard for our children? *Eur J Pediatr* 1994;153:531–534.

98. McClelland CO, Heiple KG. Fractures in the first year of life. *Am J Dis Child* 1982;136:26–29.

99. McClelland CO, Rekate H, Kaufman B, et al. Cerebral injury in child abuse: a changing profile. *Childs Brain* 1980;7:225–235.

100. McNinch AW, Orme RL, Tripp JH. Hemorrhagic disease of the newborn returns. *Lancet* 1983;1:1089–1090.

101. Menezes AH, Smith DE, Bell WE. Posterior fossa hemorrhage in the term neonate. *Neurosurgery* 1983; 13:452–456.

102. Merten DF, Osborne DR, Radkowski MA, et al. Craniocerebral trauma in the child abuse syndrome: radiological observations. *Pediatr Radiol* 1984;14:272–274.

103. Meservy CJ, Towbin R, McLaurin RL, et al. Radiographic characteristics of skull fractures resulting from child abuse. *AJR Am J Roentgenol* 1987;149:173–175.

104. Meyer FB, Sundt TM, 'Fode NC, et al. Cerebral aneurysms in childhood and adolescence. *J Neurosurg* 1989;70:420–425.

105. Morris AAM, Hoffmann GF, Naughten ER, et al. Glutaric aciduria and suspected child abuse. *Arch Dis Child* 1999;80:404–405.

106. Motohara K, Matsukura M, Matsuda I, et al. Severe vitamin K deficiency in breast-fed infants. *J Pediatr* 1984;105:943–945.

107. Musemeche C, Barthel M, Cosentino C, et al. Pediatric falls from heights. *J Trauma* 1991;31:1347–1349.

108. Nachelsky MB, Dix JD. The time interval between lethal infant shaking and onset of symptoms. *Am J Forensic Med Pathol* 1995;16:154–157.

109. Newton RW. Intracranial hemorrhage and non-accidental injury. *Arch Dis Child* 1989;64:188–190.

110. Nimityongskul P, Anderson LD. The likelihood of injuries when children fall out of bed. *J Pediatr Orthop* 1987;7:184–186.

111. Nishio A, Sakagunchi M, Mukata K, et al. Anterior communicating artery aneurysm in early childhood. *Surg Neurol* 1991;35:224–229.

112. Odom A, Christ E, Kerr N, et al. Prevalence of retinal hemorrhages in pediatric patients after in-hospital cardiopulmonary resuscitation: a prospective study. *Pediatrics* 1997;99:E3.

113. O'Neill JA, Meacham WF, Griffin JP, et al. Patterns of injury in the battered child syndrome. *J Trauma* 1973; 13:332–329.

114. Overpeck MD, Brenner RA, Trumble AC, et al. Risk factors for infant homicide in the United States. *N Engl J Med* 1998;339:1211–1216.

115. Pang D, Wilberger JE Jr. Spinal cord injury without radiologic abnormalities in children. *J Neurosurg* 1982;57:114–129.

116. Parrish R. Isolated cord injury in child abuse [Letter]. *Pediatr Trauma Forensic Newsl* 1996;Jan:1.

117. Piatt J, Steinberg M. Isolated spinal cord injury as a presentation of child abuse. *Pediatrics* 1995;96:780–782.

118. Rao N, Smith RE, Choi JH, et al. Autopsy findings in the eyes of fourteen fatally abused children. *Forensic Sci Int* 1988;39:293–299.

119. Reece R, Sege R. Childhood head injuries: accidental or inflicted? *Arch Pediatr Adolesc Med* 2000;154:11–15.

120. Reichelderfer TE, Overbach A, Greensher J. Committee on Accident and Poison Prevention: unsafe playgrounds. *Pediatrics* 1979;64:962–963.

121. Rivara FP, Alexander B, Johnston B, et al. Population-based study of fall injuries in children and adolescents resulting in hospitalization or death. *Pediatrics* 1993;92:61–63.

122. Rivara F, Kamitsuka MD, Quan L. Injuries to children younger than 1 year of age. *Pediatrics* 1988;81:93.

123. Rosenberg DA. Web of deceit: a literature review of Munchausen syndrome by proxy. *Child Abuse Negl* 1987;11:547–563.

124. Sato Y, Smith WL. Head injury in child abuse. *Neuroimaging Clin North Am* 1991;1:475.

125. Sato YS, Yuh WT, Smith WL, et al. Head injury in child abuse: evaluation with MR imaging. *Radiology* 1989;173:653–657.

126. Schmitt B. The child with nonaccidental trauma. In: Helfer R, Kemp R, eds. *The battered child*. 4th ed. Chicago: The University of Chicago Press, 1987.

127. Scholer SJ, Mitchel EF Jr, Ray WA. Predictors of injury mortality in early childhood. *Pediatrics* 1997;100:342–345.

128. Scholer SJ, Hickson GB, Ray WA. Sociodemographic factors identify United States infants at high risk of injury mortality. *Pediatrics* 1999;103:1183–1188.

129. Selbst SM, Baker MD, Shames M. Bunk bed injuries. *Am J Dis Child* 1990;144:721–723.

130. Showers J. "Don't shake the baby": the effectiveness of a prevention program. *Child Abuse Negl* 1992;16:11–18.

131. Showers J, Johnson CF. Students' knowledge of child health and development effects on approaches to discipline. *J School Health* 1984;54:122–125.

132. Shugerman RP, Paez A, Grossman DC, et al. Epidural hemorrhage: is it abuse? *Pediatrics* 1996;97:664–668.

133. Siegel CD, Graves P, Maloney K, et al. Mortality from intentional and unintentional injury among infants of young mothers in Colorado 1986-1992. *Arch Pediatr Adolesc Med* 1996;150:1077–1083.

134. Silverman FN. The roentgen manifestations of unrecognized skeletal trauma in infants. *AJR Am J Roentgenol* 1953;69:413–427.

135. Sinal SH, Ball MR. Head trauma due to child abuse: serial computerized tomography in diagnosis and management. *South Med J* 1987;80:1505–1512.

136. Skadberg B, Morild I, Markestad T. Abandoning prone sleep: effect on the risk of sudden infant death syndrome. *J Pediatr* 1998;132:340–343.

137. Smith GA, Bowman MJ, Luria JW, et al. Babywalker-related injuries continue despite warning labels and public education. *Pediatrics* 1997;100:256.

138. Smith MD, Burrington JD, Woolf AD. Injuries in children sustained in free falls: an analysis of 66 cases. *J Trauma* 1975;15:987–981.

139. Smith WL, Alexander RC, Judisch GF, et al. Magnetic resonance imaging evaluation of neonates with retinal hemorrhages. *Pediatrics* 1992;89:332–333.

140. Starling SP, Holden JR, Jenny C. Abusive head trauma: the relationship of perpetrators to their victims. *Pediatrics* 1995;95:259–262.

141. Strouse PJ, Caplan M, Owings CL. Extracranial soft-tissue swelling: a normal postmortem radiographic finding or a sign of trauma? *Pediatr Radiol* 1998;28:594–596.

142. Tarantino CA, Dowd MD, Murdock TC. Short vertical falls in infants. *Pediatr Emerg Care* 1999;15:5–8.

143. Tardieu A. Etude medico-legale sur les sevices et mauvais traitments exerces sur les enfants. *Ann D Hyg Publ Med-Leg* 1860;13:361–398.

144. Towbin A. Sudden infant death (cot and crib death) related to spinal injury. *Lancet* 1967;2:940.

145. Tzioumi D, Oates RK. Subdural hematomas in children under 2 years: accidental or inflicted? A 10-year experience. *Child Abuse Negl* 1998;22:1105–1112.

146. U.S. Advisory Board on Child Abuse and Neglect. *A nation's shame: fatal child abuse and neglect in the United States*. Washington, DC: U.S. Department of Health and Human Services, 1995.

147. United States vs. Winter. U.S. Air Force Court of Military Review. 32 MJ 901 (AFCMR). p. 901, 1991.

148. Waller AE, Baker SP, Szocka A. Childhood injury deaths: national analysis and geographic variations. *Am J Public Health* 1989;79:310–315.

149. Weston JT. The battered child in medicolegal investigation of death. In: Spitz WV, Fisher RS, eds. *Guidelines for the application of pathology in crime investigation*. Springfield, IL: Charles C Thomas, 1980:477.

150. Williams RA. Injuries in infants and small children resulting from witnessed and corroborated free falls. *J Trauma* 1991;28:1350–1352.

151. Woelfle J, Kreft B, Emons D, et al. Subdural hemorrhage as an initial sign of glutaric aciduria type 1: a diagnostic pitfall. *Pediatr Radiol* 1996;26:779–781.

152. Wooley PV Jr, Evans W Jr. Significance of skeletal lesions in infants resembling those of traumatic origin. *JAMA* 1955;158:539–543.

153. Worlock P, Stower M, Barbor P. Patterns of fractures in accidental and nonaccidental injury in children: a comparative study. *Br Med J* 1986;293:100–102.

4

New Directions in Neuroradiology of Child Abuse

Robert A. Zimmerman

Departments of Neuroradiology and Radiology, The Children's Hospital of Philadelphia; and Department of Radiology, University of Pennsylvania, Philadelphia, Pennsylvania

The past decade, the 1990s, saw rapid techno-logical progress in neuroimaging in both computed tomography (CT) and magnetic resonance imaging (MRI). These advances have improved the ability to examine the abused infant for evidence of neurologic in-jury and have also improved the type of infor-mation possible to derive about the nature of the brain injury. This chapter looks at the hardware and software that has led to these improvements, the various technical applica-tions, and how these are clinically applied.

TECHNICAL ADVANCES

Computed Tomography

At the end of the 1980s in the United States, the average CT scanner used for examining the head was capable of rapid speeds, produc-ing images on the order of multiple seconds per image. Scans of the brain were done one slice at a time, with variable slice thickness de-pending on the make and model of the CT scanner, but with capabilities of as thin as 1.5 mm and as thick as a centimeter. Total scan time for the brain was on the order of 5 min-utes or more. Brain imaging in the infant and young child was done with 5-mm sections through the posterior fossa and supratentorial space. Images were displayed in brain, bone, and intermediate windows (subdural win-dows). Depending on the neurologic picture of the patient, motion artifacts were a problem in children who were either not sedated or not comatose. When additional areas were done, such as the cervical spine, these images were acquired in the same fashion, using axial 2-mm-thick sections. If additional portions of the anatomy, such as the chest, abdomen, or pelvis were examined, then scan times would become significantly longer. The capacity of the x-ray tube used in the CT scanners was of-ten adequate to do a single part of the anatomy, but to continue to the other parts required pe-riods of tube cooling before the CT scanner could be used again.

In the early 1990s, the first spiral CT scan-ners became available for clinical use (21). To-day, depending on the manufacturer, these are described as either spiral or helical CTs. The principles for the method of acquiring the in-formation are essentially the same with both. The concept is as follows: The patient is on a table that, during the scan acquisition, contin-ues to move while the x-ray tube spins around the portion of the anatomy being examined. Thus a volume of CT density information is acquired. How that information is handled in the image-reconstruction phase of the study depends on algorithms that are used in the computer reconstruction of the images. Partial volume effect artifacts are a part of the prob-lem seen in spirally acquired images. These are less an issue with conventionally acquired CT slices. The spiral acquisition of CT infor-mation means that information can be acquired extremely quickly. Time for a brain examination may be only a matter of 15 or 20 seconds (Fig. 4.1). The time for the cervical spine examination is frequently less than a minute. Tube heating and cooling issues still remain, but have decreased as the heat capacity of the x-ray tubes has increased. Motion artifacts can still occur, but, because of the rapidity of the acquisition of the scan, are less. The application of spiral CT scanning, while significantly improving the ability to get CT scans done in traumatized infants and children, has, by the same token, led to the greater use of CT scanning by emergency department physicians in children's hospitals. The ease of acquiring the information is now associated with a much greater utilization of the procedure, the indications for the study being looser than before. Very thin sections can be obtained through the skull base, paranasal sinuses, and orbits, when indicated, to assess for fractures at these sites. In the cervical spine, the thinness of the sections permits both sagittal and coronal reconstruction of the images (Fig. 4.2) to demonstrate vertically the alignment of the

vertebral bodies and the presence of fractures seen as a loss in height of the vertebral body.

As we enter the next millennium, the newest advent in CT scanning that will affect the ease of acquisition of the CT data in pediatric trauma patients is the development of multiple-slice spiral CT scanners. The newest ones, as of 1999, allow multiple simultaneous slices to be obtained with each revolution of the x-ray tube. Slice thickness can be as thin as half a millimeter or as thick as a centimeter. Intermediate slice thicknesses are available. Studies of the brain or cervical spine can often be performed in such a short time that sedation issues in noncooperative children may no longer be a problem. Manual restraint by a protected physician or nurse, or parent, may permit an adequate examination. Although scan times can be reduced to a matter of multiple seconds, the fact remains that patient throughput may not be that dramatically affected. The reason for that is that most of the time spent in obtaining the CT is now spent in moving the patient to the CT scanner and onto the table, in moving whatever support equipment is necessary, and in programming the

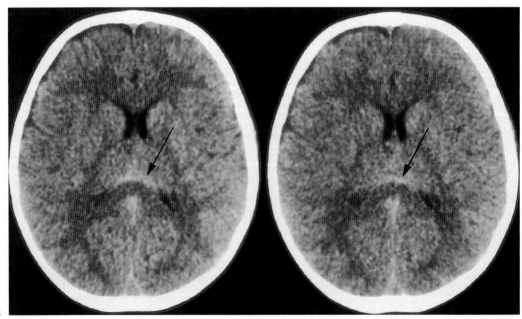

A   B

FIG. 4.1. Conventional computed tomography (CT) versus spiral CT in traumatic brain injury. A 2.5-year-old boy with diffuse axonal injury with tear of fornices in the roof of the third ventricle with bleeding. **A:** Conventional CT shows midline hemorrhage (*arrow*). **B:** Spiral CT examination at the same slice location shows the same information with the same clarity (*arrow*).

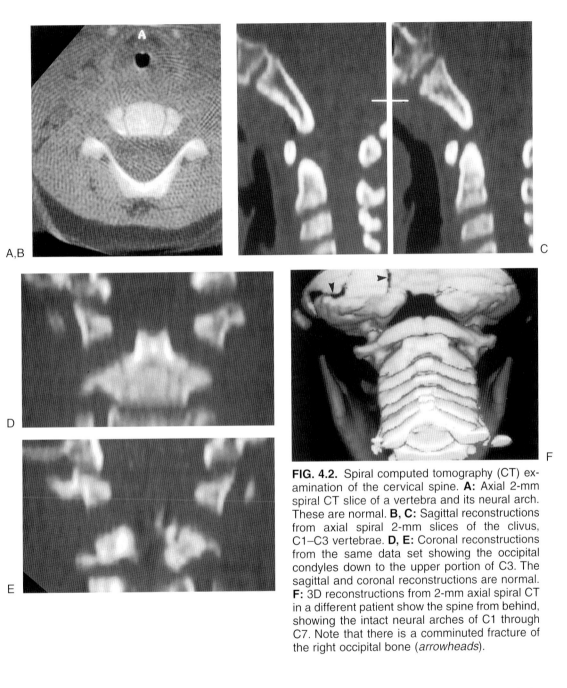

FIG. 4.2. Spiral computed tomography (CT) examination of the cervical spine. **A:** Axial 2-mm spiral CT slice of a vertebra and its neural arch. These are normal. **B, C:** Sagittal reconstructions from axial spiral 2-mm slices of the clivus, C1–C3 vertebrae. **D, E:** Coronal reconstructions from the same data set showing the occipital condyles down to the upper portion of C3. The sagittal and coronal reconstructions are normal. **F:** 3D reconstructions from 2-mm axial spiral CT in a different patient show the spine from behind, showing the intact neural arches of C1 through C7. Note that there is a comminuted fracture of the right occipital bone (*arrowheads*).

scanner. The actual time of the study, that is acquiring the information, becomes an insignificant portion of the total time spent.

Magnetic Resonance Imaging

After the inception of magnetic resonance (MR) scanning as a clinical tool in 1983, most of the early technical advances were made in the realm of software in the form of new pulse sequences. Initially, scanning was with spin echo (SE) techniques, but more recently, multiple echo acquisitions [turbo, spin-echo (TSE) or fast imaging (FSE)] led to T2-weighted images (T2WI) being acquired in 3–4 minutes, whereas conventional SE sequences required

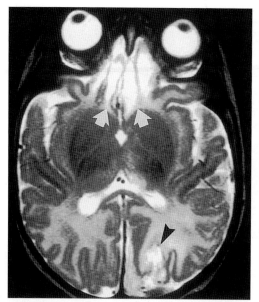
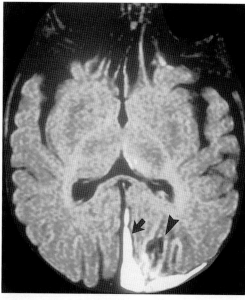

A   B

FIG. 4.3. A 2-month-old boy after whiplash shaken impact injury. **A:** Axial turbo, spin-echo (TSE) 512 × 512 image shows gliding contusions of the inferior frontal lobes (*arrows*) and focal infarction in the left occipital lobe (*arrowhead*) adjacent to a left posterior subdural hematoma. **B:** Axial fluid-attenuated inversion recovery (FLAIR) image shows the subacute subdural hematoma (*arrow*) in the interhemispheric fissure on the left posteriorly, extending around the posterior convexity. There is encephalomalacia at the site of infarction (*arrowhead*) in the left occipital lobe. Note that the gliding contusions in the frontal lobes are predominantly water-filled encephalomalacic spaces, seen as focal linear hypointensities.

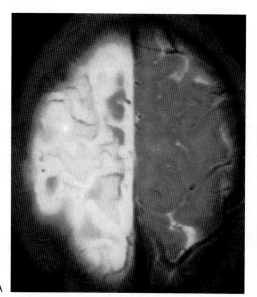
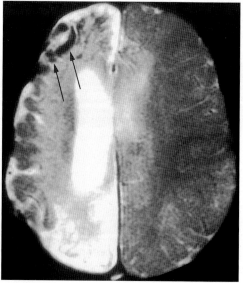

A   B

FIG. 4.4. Chronic posttraumatic cerebral injury in child abuse patient, a 14-month-old girl. **A:** Axial turbo, spin-echo (TSE) 512 × 512 image shows almost complete necrosis of the right cerebral hemisphere. **B:** Axial gradient echo 2D fast low-angle shot (FLASH) susceptibility scan shows evidence of blood products as loss of signal (*arrows*) within the right frontal lobe.

9–12 minutes for the same information (20). These TSE T2WI acquisitions are now standard. More recently, the introduction of higher gradients, phased-array coils, powerful computers, as well as new software, have combined to give the same 1.5-T MR magnet new possibilities, which include not only faster and higher-resolution studies, but the demonstration of cortical activation by functional MR, the decrease in diffusion of water molecules with cytotoxic edema, and the change in brain metabolites with various disease states on proton spectroscopy (2,8,14,22).

Image Resolution

In 1983, most T1- and T2-weighted images were in a matrix size of 128×256. To achieve a 256×256 matrix, with an increase in resolution, the acquisition time had to be doubled. With the development of TSE T2WI, it is now possible to obtain a matrix of 512×512 in scan times that are much shorter than with 256×256 SE T2WI (Figs. 4.3–4.5). With the use of the higher-millitesla gradients, it is now possible also to obtain images with a 1,024 matrix, often 500 or $600 \times 1,024$. This

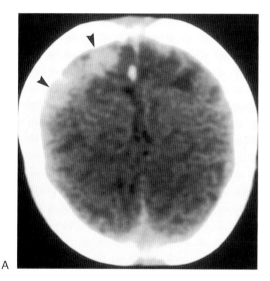

A

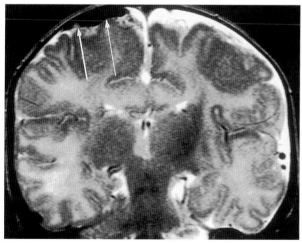

B

FIG. 4.5. Child abuse, shaken impact injury, in a 2-month-old girl. **A:** Axial non–contrast-enhanced computed tomography (CT) shows subdural blood (*arrowheads*) over the right frontal lobe. **B:** Coronal turbo, spin-echo (TSE) 512 × 512 image shows the acute subdural bleeding (*arrows*) as an area of focal hypointense deoxyhemoglobin on top of the right posterior frontal lobe.

further increases the resolution. Increased resolution is translated into better definition, resulting in improved visualization of the cortex and more precise characterization of what is happening within both the brain and the extraaxial spaces.

Fluid-Attenuated Inversion Recovery Imaging

A recently developed pulse sequence that dramatically improves detection of increased water within damaged brain tissue is fluid-attenuated inversion recovery (FLAIR)imaging (25). Signal intensity of cerebrospinal fluid (CSF) within the ventricles or subarachnoid space is nulled and therefore not apparent as an area of increased signal intensity, whereas gliotic brain tissue from previous

damage (Fig. 4.6B) and vasogenic edematous tissue from acute trauma (Fig. 4.6A) are readily demonstrated with an increase in conspicuity relative to conventional SE images or TSE images (1). In this pulse sequence, relaxation goes from negative to positive during longitudinal magnetization, and a point is reached where the longitudinal magnetization is equal to zero. This is the null point, which has been found to be equal to 69% of the T1 value of what is to be nulled. For CSF, the T1 is between 1,900 and 4,300 milliseconds at 1.5 T, so that a null point of 1,728 milliseconds is required. The 90-degree RF pulse is applied at this null point; there is no transverse magnetization from the CSF, because it has been suppressed. However, there is still signal from the abnormal tissue due to increased water in the interstitial space (25).

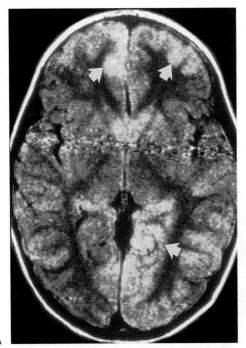
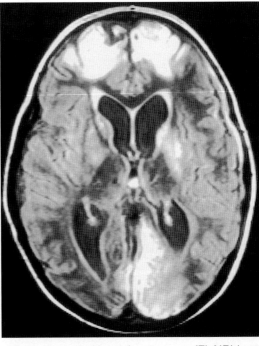

A   B

FIG. 4.6. Child abuse, shaken impact injury, use of fluid-attenuated inversion recovery (FLAIR) imaging. **A:** Axial FLAIR image shows acute cortical brain swelling (*arrows*) in both frontal lobes and in the posterior temporal occipital lobes, predominantly on the left. **B:** Follow-up FLAIR imaging, 2 months after injury, shows atrophy of the brain with enlargement of the lateral ventricles, bifrontal high-signal-intensity encephalomalacia in the frontal lobes, and evidence of cortical injury bilaterally in the posterior temporal occipital lobes, left greater than right, and evidence of injury in the left lenticular nucleus.

Recent software advances have led to fast FLAIR or turbo FLAIR sequences in which the slices are now 5 mm, or thinner, there is no interslice gap, the number of slices is not significantly limited, and the acquisition times are on the order of 2½ minutes for the brain. It is also possible to do EPI FLAIR, but the images have significantly less resolution than those of the turbo FLAIR.

The application of turbo FLAIR in evaluating brain injury has been predominantly in the demonstration of contusions, diffuse axonal injury (DAI), and brain swelling. Infarctions due to vascular events, such as dissections or strangulation, also are well visualized (7). In the fully myelinated brain, past age 2 years, FLAIR appears to be much more sensitive than either the SE T2WI or TSE T2WI. MRI has generally been thought of as not successful at demonstrating subarachnoid hemorrhage (SAH). It is clear that CT is the gold standard for acute SAH. However, a recent publication (15) has demonstrated that subacute and chronic SAH can be shown by FLAIR imaging to a greater extent than with CT or by other MR techniques (Figs. 4.7 and 4.8). Of course, whether FLAIR imaging can compete with CT in acute SAH from the ictus to 3 days, when CT is at its best, remains unknown. The problem in answering that question is in studying acute SAH patients by MR rapidly after the trauma, so that this question is likely to remain unanswered for a while longer. Finally, subacute subdural hematomas are also better demonstrated by FLAIR imaging than by SE T2WI (Figs. 4.3B and 4.8A).

Pitfalls exist with FLAIR imaging, as they do with any technique. The most annoying one is the common flow-related high CSF signal-intensity artifacts that occur when noninverted CSF flows into the slice, such as at the foramen of Monro or the fourth ventricle (25).

Susceptibility Scanning

A T2-weighted two-dimensional gradient-echo FLASH sequence is important in the MRI evaluation of patients with acute or re-

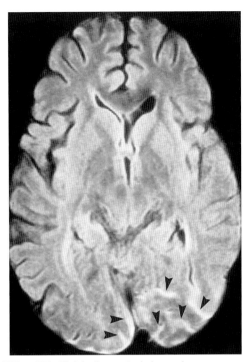

FIG. 4.7. Fluid-attenuated inversion recovery (FLAIR) imaging to demonstrate acute subarachnoid hemorrhage in trauma. Axial FLAIR image shows abnormal increased signal intensity within the subarachnoid space of both occipital lobes (*arrowheads*).

mote history of trauma. Although it is not a new technique, it is one that is often overlooked when MRI is not routinely used in the evaluation of trauma patients. For convenience, this type of sequence is referred to in this chapter as susceptibility scanning. The concept is as follows: The pulse sequence is designed to produce dephasing of protons affected by blood products such as deoxyhemoglobin or hemosiderin. The dephasing is seen on the study as a loss of signal (blackness) at the site of bleeding (Figs. 4.4B and 4.8B). The size of the signal loss is often somewhat larger than the size of the bleed that can be depicted on routine T2 images. It is unknown whether this is due to effects of the blood on protons beyond the bleed site or is due to relatively invisible microscopic blood that extends beyond that which is visible. The im-

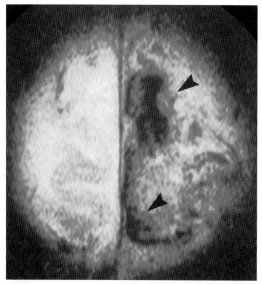
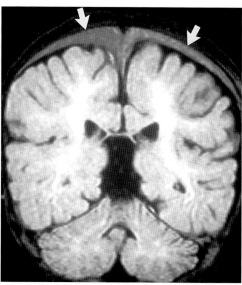

A
B

FIG. 4.8. Acute and subacute subdural bleeding in child abuse. 2-month-old boy. **A:** Axial 2D fast low-angle shot (FLASH) gradient-echo susceptibility scan shows hypointense deoxyhemoglobin (*arrowheads*) in the subdural space over the left hemisphere. **B:** Coronal fluid-attenuated inversion recovery (FLAIR) image shows bilateral parietal chronic subdural hematomas (*arrows*).

portance of this type of scanning is not in demonstrating the obvious but in showing evidence of bleeding that is otherwise invisible on routine MRI and on CT. Small hemorrhages that are acute and those that are weeks, months, or years old (Fig. 4.4B) fall into this category.

Even Faster Imaging

The original T1- and T2-weighted SE images were time consuming, 3–5 minutes for the T1 and 12 minutes for the proton-density and T2WI. The TSE images took less time, gave very attractive T2WI, but had less sensitivity to the depiction of blood products as a susceptibility effect (hypointensity) due to spin dephasing. SE T2WI is highly sensitive to the susceptibility effects of deoxyhemoglobin, methemoglobin, and hemosiderin. Even faster imaging than current TSE techniques have also evolved. Half-Fourier single-shot turbo spin-echo (HASTE) or snapshot imaging can be used, in which each image is a single acquisition, so that motion that occurs

during that slice ruins only that slice, and not the other slices (26). Imaging times are as short as 0.5 seconds per slice. Such imaging times compete with CT for speed. There are, of course, trade-offs in image contrast and overall resolution compared with non–half-Fourier TSE images, in that the HASTE images are less sharp and after infancy have limited gray–white matter contrast. However, in the infant, there is gray–white matter contrast, and infarcts of the cortex are readily demonstrated (Fig. 4.9). The real advantage of the HASTE technique is in the high-risk infant with low oxygen saturation, or the unsuccessfully sedated patients, that can now be more readily studied (26).

The new higher-millitesla gradients allow echo planar imaging (EPI), which produces image acquisition in times that have been previously unprecedented (2). T2-weighted sequences, susceptibility scans, FLAIR, and a wide variety of pulse sequences can now be obtained with acquisitions on the order of 50 msec/section. Typical pulse sequences for encompassing the structures of the brain in the

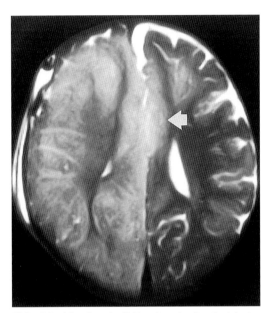

FIG. 4.9. Ultrafast half-Fourier single-shot turbo spin-echo (HASTE) imaging in a child abuse patient with subdural bleeding and acute infarction of the right hemisphere. Axial HASTE image performed in 1 second as part of a series of images, making a total of 13 seconds. This shows the right hemisphere to be diffusely involved in the cortical subcortical white matter, with infarction of the brain. There is involvement of the medial aspect of the left frontal lobe (*arrow*).

axial plane necessitate a total acquisition time of between 2 and 8 seconds. Again, there are trade-offs: image resolution is not so good as that with TSE, and there are problems with artifacts due to susceptibility that occur at the sites of air and bone interfaces at the base of the skull. EPI images are particularly prone to these artifacts. Despite these, hemorrhage within a stroke, as well as a stroke, are demonstrable, and the size of the ventricles is appreciated. EPI acquisitions are now faster than those achievable with conventional CT scanning (26).

Magnetic Resonance Angiography

The demonstration of blood flow within vessels that travel to the brain, and within the intracranial arteries and veins has been achieved with MR by two methods: (a) time-of-flight (TOF) magnetic resonance angiography (MRA), and (b) phase contrast (PC) MRA (23). TOF MRA depends on flow-related enhancement (i.e., production of relatively increased signal intensity within flow coming into a slice plane when the protons in the blood are energized by an RF pulse). To see the flow within the vessel, the background signal of the adjacent stationary brain has to be suppressed by a presaturation RF pulse. Currently, MRA with TOF can produce images with a 512×512 resolution and with multiple submillimeter partitions within a slab that can encompass most of the brain. Artifacts due to flow-related spin dephasing and to saturation effects have, for the most part, been eliminated by using shorter echo times, higher matrices, and by varying the flip angle of each of the slice partitions. In addition, the intravenous injection of gadolinium can improve vascular demonstration by decreasing the relaxation time of blood. For the arterial anatomy of the circle of Willis, a three-dimensional (3D) TOF MRA has become the most used technique. The 2D TOF MRA techniques have proven to be useful for demonstrating the venous anatomy of the brain: dural venous sinuses such as the superior sagittal, both transverse and sigmoid sinuses, and the jugular veins. Phase-contrast MRA depends solely on the motion of the protons in the blood (23). PC techniques have a longer acquisition time and a slightly coarser resolution, but are not affected by high-signal-intensity methemoglobin within clots, as only moving blood is depicted on the images. In 3D and 2D TOF MRA, high-signal-intensity methemoglobin is a problem and is incorporated on the maximum intensity projection (MIP) images of the vessels, producing false information (23). Progress in MRA in the last several years has been the introduction of high-resolution (512 $\times$ 512), thinner sections, faster acquisition times, and techniques that are less affected by spin dephasing and in-plane saturation. With the use of higher-millitesla gradients and newer software, preliminary work has been done with higher-resolution MRA (1,024 $\times$

1,024). Smaller vessels can be seen, but the price paid is the amount of data that must be stored and then handled by the MIP program to produce an image. These are software computer issues that will shortly be resolved.

Turbo MRA techniques that use gadolinium bolus injections have only now become feasible with acquisition times of 3D data sets that take between 2–8 seconds/image and can produce serial sequential images of flow. By timing the contrast injections and the time of image acquisition, it is possible to obtain a serial set of vascular anatomic flow images (e.g., early arterial phase, late arterial phase, and venous phase images). Although this can be used for the intracranial vessels, its use is even more important in the extracranial brachiocephalic vessels of the aortic arch, which are usually not well evaluated by most current 2D and 3D TOF techniques. This is because of swallowing, breathing, and other physiologic causes of motion artifact.

The better the MRA information, the less need for conventional angiography. Relative to the trauma patient and the issues of child abuse, vascular injury can and does occur as dissections, lacerations, and occlusion, transiently or permanently, with strangulation (Fig. 4.10). The venous anatomy becomes of interest in the whiplash shaken impact injury, as disruption of the venous drainage is one of the accepted mechanisms of brain injury.

Diffusion-Weighted Imaging

At both the intra- and extracellular levels, random motion of water molecules occurs within the brain tissue. This random motion is variably restricted by cell membranes and tissue macromolecules. To some extent, characterization of both gross and microscopic structural changes within normal and diseased tissues may be achieved both by making an image of diffusion and by measuring the

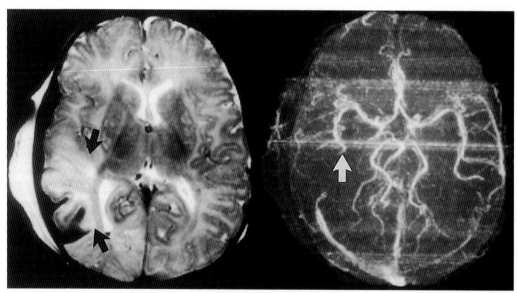

A   B

FIG. 4.10. Child abuse, battering, laceration of right middle cerebral artery with subarachnoid hemorrhage and infarction. **A:** Axial T2WI spin-echo (SE) 256 × 256 image shows swelling of the right scalp, hypointense deoxyhemoglobin filling the subarachnoid space on the right, and hyperintense signal in the white matter and grey matter of the posterior division middle cerebral artery (MCA) vascular territory (*arrowheads*), consistent with infarction (*arrows*). Note a small amount of interventricular blood in the occipital horn of the right lateral ventricle, producing a cerebrospinal fluid blood–fluid level. **B:** Axial magnetic resonance angiography shows absence of the posterior division of the right MCA. Cutoff was demonstrated (*arrow*).

rate at which diffusion occurs. The measurement of the rate of diffusion is known as the apparent diffusion coefficient (ADC) (18). In essence, the ADC is a measurement that contains information regarding both random motion arising from water (proton) diffusion and that from the flow of blood and the protons within the capillary bed, a small but important contribution. Principles of the techniques used to look at diffusion have been known for many years, but unfortunately, the performance of *in vivo* studies has always been hampered by considerable problems. Diffusion-weighted MRI and the quantitative determination of ADC are both very sensitive to movement, both involuntary (head translations and rotations) and physiologic (breathing motion, cardiac driven, brain, and CSF pulsations), on the part of the patient. These motions are indiscriminate, producing large phase shifts in the echo signal intensity from one image to the next. This results in ghosting artifacts and severely compromises voxel registration. Methods developed for overcoming these sources of error generally require extremely rapid imaging acquisition, techniques that have only recently become available in the form of EPI.

Tissue water diffusion is of a complex nature, and its magnitude and direction depend on permeability and the nature of the diffusion barriers as well as the viscosity of the medium and the technical factors related to diffusion measurements. Active tissue water-transport processes and bulk flow of capillary fluid contents contribute to this complex phenomenon. Immobile protons affixed to the brain macromolecules and membranes make no contribution to the diffusion characteristics and have short T2 values. In quantifying the ADC values, the measurements rely on intervoxel alteration and signal intensity as a response to the bipolar gradients that are superimposed. In essence, ADC is measured in any desired direction, usually the x, y, and z axes, by acquiring images in the presence of very large field gradients in each direction. Motion decreases the signal intensity from that expected due to the usual

contrast mechanisms. Regions of tissue with higher ADCs will be less intense on the images, whereas regions with lower ADCs will be brighter.

A relatively new, important concept that must be understood when considering both the diffusion-weighted imaging (DWI) and the ADC values is anisotropy. For axons, the cell wall is thought to restrict the diffusion of water across it, whereas diffusion along the axonal fibers occurs at a normal rate. In the brain, fiber tracts that are perpendicular to the direction at which the images are acquired appear brighter, having less diffusion across those cell membranes. Thus it is expected that during early infancy, the ADC of white matter will change during the months that are associated with the myelination of fiber tracts. As this occurs, the ADC of white matter decreases at the sites where myelin has formed. The ADC changes actually precede the appearance of myelin on T1- and T2-weighted images.

In the normal adult brain, the ADC values fall into three categories: CSF and fluid-filled spaces, gray matter, and white matter. ADC values are often expressed in 10^{-3} mm^2/sec. In these units, typical values are 3.0 for the fluid-filled ventricles, 0.8–1.2 for the gray matter, and 0.4–0.6 for the white matter (9).

The ADC decreases with restriction of the movement of extracellular water into the cell, as occurs with ischemia and infarction (13). With an increase in the interstitial fluid volume, such as occurs in vasogenic edema, the ADC value is increased, and on the diffusion image, the area is darker (11).

This technologic breakthrough has important implications for patient care and evaluation that will lead to the development of practical applications for patient management (24). Animal research work indicates that acute stroke can be recognized approximately 30 minutes after the onset of the injurious process. Application of these techniques to the traumatized infant and child are only now beginning. When cell death occurs, such as is seen in acute contusions and diffuse axonal injuries, the DWI can be contrib-

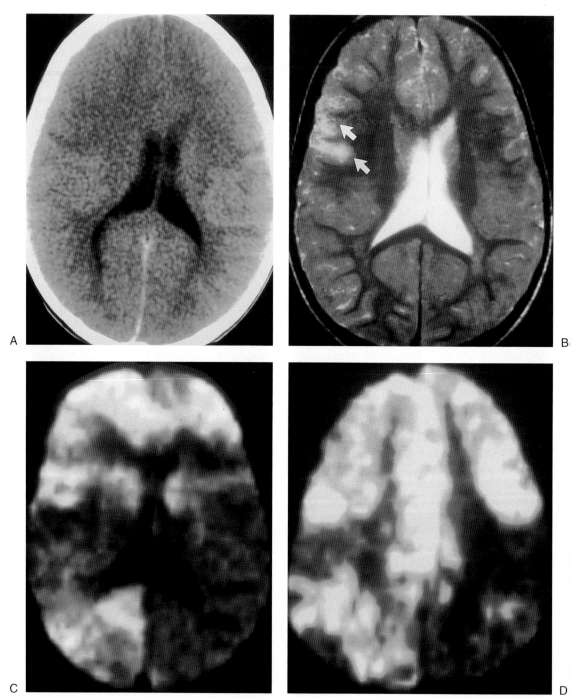

FIG. 4.11. Shaken impact injury, child abuse. **A:** Axial computed tomography shows mass effect. The subdural windows showed a very thin right frontal subdural next to the inner table of the skull. **B:** Axial T2WI spin echo shows cortical swelling involving the posterior right frontal lobe (*arrows*). There is mass effect with displacement of the ventricular system toward the left. **C, D:** Lower and higher axial diffusion-weighted images show abnormal restricted motion of water involving more of the right than the left cerebral hemispheres as high signal intensity.

utory to routine MRI by showing, with great sensitivity, sites of cell death. The major application, however, will be in the demonstration of very early parenchymal brain swelling in patients who have suffered trauma. Particularly, the whiplash shaken impact infant, who presents in the emergency department with only a small smear of a subdural hematoma, can be effectively evaluated by DWI for brain selling that will become more clinically apparent in the near future, as increased intracranial pressure develops (Figs. 4.11 and 4.12). These patients can be demonstrated to have early cytotoxic edema by DWI. This is when even the CT and MRI conventional images are negative. Not only that, but the pattern of early brain swelling is of interest, in that it is not uniform, that there are areas of sparing that become involved subsequently. Early DWI in suspected child abuse patients has potential of providing a tool for assessing the effectiveness of future therapies for controlling brain swelling and preventing cell death.

Proton Magnetic Resonance Spectroscopy

Proton MR spectroscopy (MRS) did not evolve until the signal intensity of water could be suppressed and localization techniques could be developed that would allow determination of where the spectral information was coming from within the brain. In the late 1980s, these techniques became available, and initially, single-voxel proton MRS had been performed (3,5,16). The techniques that have been required have become more user friendly and are gradually coming into wider clinical use (17). The echo times used with proton MRS were initially in the range of 135 to 270 milliseconds. Several important metabolites could be identified with these techniques. These include choline, a cell membrane metabolite; phosphocreatine and creatine, energy metabolites; N-acetyl aspartate (NAA), a metabolite that is thought to be within neurons and perhaps oligodendroglia; and, at these longer TEs, lactate, a by-product of metabolism, primarily of anaerobic metabolism, that

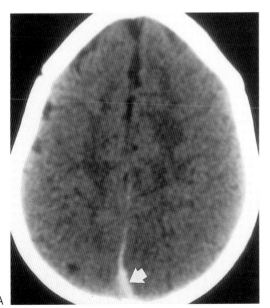 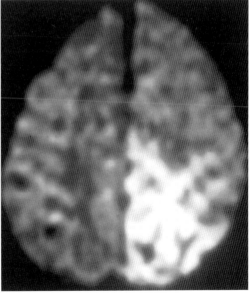

A   B

FIG. 4.12. Child abuse, whiplash shaken impact injury, 2-month-old child. **A:** Axial computed tomography (CT) shows a small amount of subdural blood along the posterior falx (*arrow*). Gray–white matter differentiation appears normal. **B:** Axial diffusion-weighted image at the same level as the CT shown in **A**, shows abnormal restricted water diffusion in the left parietooccipital region, consistent with cytotoxic edema.

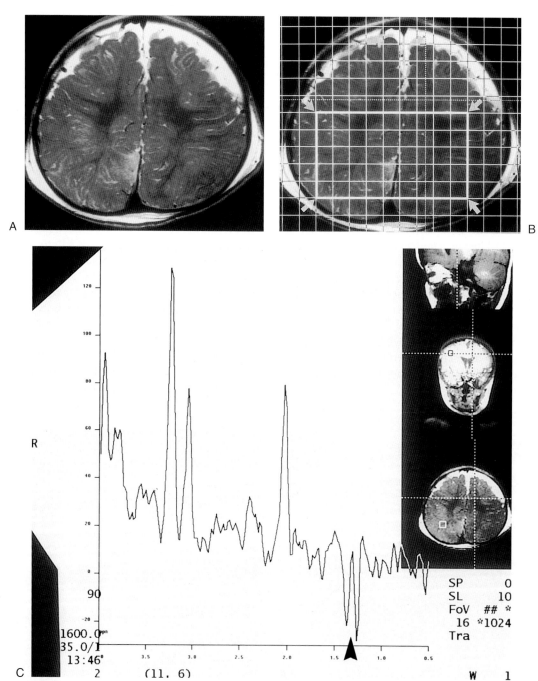

FIG. 4.13. Child abuse, bilateral chronic subdural hemorrhages, with new acute bilateral, right greater than left hemispheric injuries in a 7-month-old boy. **A:** Axial turbo, spin-echo (TSE) 512 × 512 shows anterior bifrontal subdural fluid collections. There is bilateral posterior scalp swelling. Subtle increased signal intensity in the right hemisphere suggests some injury process. **B:** Same axial magnetic resonance imaging as shown in **A**, but with the grid of the 2D chemical shift imaging (CSI) proton spectroscopy superimposed (*arrows*, the margins of the voxel map). **C:** One voxel from the 2D CSI map, taken from the right parietal region, shows markedly elevated lactate at 1.3 ppm (*arrowhead*). The amount of *N*-acetyl aspartate is decreased.

can be seen in very small amounts normally, but increases dramatically in a number of pathologic states such as infarction and in brain swelling, most dramatically with acute cell death. Recently, shorter echo times, down to 5–10 milliseconds, allow the detection of more spectral peaks, representing a larger number of proton-containing compounds within the brain tissue. Among others, these include inositol, glutamate, and glutamine. Inositol is of interest as an osmolite related to intracellular sodium content, the belief being that it is increased with increased osmolality of the brain (10). Glutamate has a role as an excitatory amine that is released with insults to the brain, such as trauma, and leads to further brain injury and brain swelling.

More recently, two-dimensional chemical shift imaging spectroscopy (2D CSI) and 3D CSI spectroscopy have been developed. 2D permits a cross-sectional area of the brain to be studied, containing multiple small voxels, frequently between 20 to 30 (4,12). These may be as small as $1 \times 1 \times 1$-cm voxels. 3D CSI techniques allow four to eight slices to be obtained, when combined with a Hadamard technique, the acquisition time for the multiple voxels (196 in four slices) is on the order of 25 minutes (6). Both 2D and 3D CSI allow regions of the brain to be analyzed metabolically. Differences in regional distribution of metabolites can lead to understanding of the nature of types of brain injury (19). Beyond 2D and 3D CSI lies total brain metabolic quantification. Recent work indicates that total brain metabolites, not regionally localized, quantitatively accurate, can be obtained in relatively short acquisition times of minutes, providing an overall assessment of metabolites. In the posttraumatic patient, the decrease in NAA would be an assessment of the loss of neural mass. In the acute traumatic patient, increase in lactate would be an overall assessment of the degree of brain ischemia/infarction (Fig. 4.13).

REFERENCES

1. Ashikaga R, Araki Y, Ishida O. MRI of head injury using FLAIR. *Neuroradiology* 1997;39:239–242.
2. Bandettini PA, Wong EC, Hinks RS, et al. Time course EPI of human brain function during task activation. *Magn Reson Med* 1992;25:390–397.
3. Bottomley PA. Selective volume method for performing localized NMR spectroscopy. U.S. patent 4 480 2281984.
4. Brown TR, Kincaid BM, Ugurbil K. NMR chemical shift imaging in three dimensions. *Proc Natl Acad Sci U S A* 1982;79:3523–3526.
5. Frahm J, Merboldt KD, Hanicke W. Localized proton spectroscopy using stimulated echoes. *J Magn Reson* 1987;72:502–508.
6. Gonen O, Wang ZJ, Molloy P, et al. Pediatric brain 3D NMR spectroscopy in neurofibromatosis type I disorder. *AJNR Am J Neuroradiol* (in press).
7. Hajnal JV, Bryant DJ, Kasuboski L, et al. Use of fluid attenuated inversion recovery (FLAIR) pulse sequences in MRI of the brain. *J Comput Assist Tomogr* 1992;16: 841–844.
8. Le Bihan D, Turner R, Moonen CTW, et al. Imaging of diffusion and microcirculation with gradient sensitization: design, strategy, and significance. *J Magn Reson Imaging* 1991;1:7–28.
9. Le Bihan D, Turner R, Douek P, et al. Diffusion MR imaging: clinical applications. *AJR Am J Roentgenol* 1992;159:591–599.
10. Lee J, Arcinue E, Ross B. Organic osmolytes in the brain of an infant with hypernatremia. *N Engl J Med* 1994;331:439–442.
11. Matsumoto K, Lo EH, Pierce AR, et al. Role of vasogenic edema and tissue cavitation in ischemic evolution on diffusion-weighted imaging: comparison with multiparameter MR and immunohistochemistry. *AJNR Am J Neuroradiol* 1995;16:1107–1115.
12. Maudsley AA. Spatially resolved high resolution spectroscopy by "four-dimensional" NMR. *J Magn Reson* 1983;51:147–152.
13. Moseley ME, Kucharczyk J, Mintorovitch J, et al. Diffusion-weighted MRI of acute stroke: correlation with T2-weighted and magnetic-susceptibility-enhanced MRI. *AJNR Am J Neuroradiol* 1990;11:423–429.
14. Moseley ME, Glover GH. Functional MR imaging: capabilities and limitations. *Neuroimag Clin North Am* 1995;5:161.
15. Noguchi K, Ogawa T, Seto H, et al. Subacute and chronic subarachnoid hemorrhage: diagnosis with fluid-attenuated inversion-recovery imaging. *Radiology* 1997;203:257–262.
16. Ordidge RJ, Bendall MR, Gordon RE, et al. In: Govil G, Khetrapal CL, Saran A, eds. *Magnetic resonance in biology and medicine.* New Delhi: Tata McGraw-Hill, 1985:387–397.
17. Ross B, Michaelis T. Clinical application of magnetic resonance spectroscopy. *Magn Reson Q* 1994;10: 191–247.
18. Sorensen AG, Buonanno FS, Gonzalez RG, et al. Hyperacute stroke: evaluation with combined multisection diffusion-weighted and hemodynamically weighted echo-planar MR imaging. *Radiology* 1996;199: 391–401.
19. Sutton LN, Wang Z, Duhaime AC, et al. Tissue lactate in pediatric head trauma: a clinical study using 1H NMR spectroscopy. *Pediatr Neurosurg* 1995;22: 81–87.

20. Vinitski S, Mitchell DG, Einstein SG, et al. Conventional and fast spin-echo MR imaging: minimizing echo time. *J Magn Reson Imaging* 1993;3:501–507.
21. Zimmerman RA, Gusnard DA, Bilaniuk LT. Pediatric craniocervical spiral CT. *Neuroradiology* 1992;34: 112–116.
22. Zimmerman RA, Wang Z. Proton spectroscopy of the pediatric brain. *Riv Neuroradiol* 1992;5:5–8.
23. Zimmerman RA, Naidich TP. Magnetic resonance angiography. In: Salcman M, ed. *Current techniques in neurosurgery.* Philadelphia: Current Medicine, 1993.
24. Zimmerman RA. Diffusion-weighted imaging. *Crit Rev Neurosurg* 1997;7:221–227.
25. Zimmerman RA. Recent advances in MR imaging: FLAIR imaging. *Crit Rev Neurosurg* 1998;8:188–192.
26. Zimmerman RA, Haselgrove JC, Wang Z, et al. Advances in pediatric neuroimaging. *Brain Dev* 1998;20: 275–279.

5

Ocular Manifestations of Child Abuse

Alex V. Levin

*Department of Ophthalmology, The Hospital for Sick Children; and Departments of Pediatrics,
Genetics, and Ophthalmology, University of Toronto, Toronto, Ontario, Canada*

Ocular abnormalities may be found in all forms of child abuse. In one study, the eye was the presenting sign for physical child abuse in 4% to 6% of cases (19). Ophthalmology consultations are an important tool in identifying child abuse or differentiating the child who is not abused. This is particularly important in physical abuse, although ocular abnormalities may be found as manifestations in nonorganic failure to thrive, child neglect, sexual abuse, Munchausen syndrome by proxy, and perhaps, emotional abuse. The retinal hemorrhages of the shaken baby syndrome are the most common and familiar ocular sign of child abuse.

SHAKEN BABY SYNDROME

Ocular involvement, in particular retinal hemorrhage, joins skeletal and brain injury as a cardinal manifestation of this disorder. Retinal hemorrhages are seen in approximately 80% of shaken infants, with reports ranging from 30% to 100% depending on the population studied. For example, studies that included abusive nonshaking head trauma are likely to have lower rates, whereas postmortem studies are likely to have higher rates (29). The unique violent shaking that characterizes the shaken baby syndrome results in abnormal shearing forces inside the eye and orbit. Elevation of intracranial pressure, intracranial hemorrhage, damage to the intracranial visual pathways, and increased intrathoracic pressure may also contribute to the ophthalmic abnormalities.

Perhaps the most important aspect of understanding the significance of retinal hemorrhage as a manifestation of shaken baby syndrome is a knowledge of the anatomic correlates used to describe them. The retina lines the inside of the eyeball up to and behind the posterior surface of the iris. It is a vascularized structure made up of multiple layers. It is separated from the sclera (white of the eye) by an interposed vascular layer called the choroid. That area straight back from the pupil and in the center of the visual axis has a specialized anatomy known as the fovea (Fig. 5.1). Just

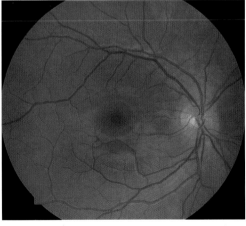

FIG. 5.1. The posterior pole. This area of the retina encompasses the optic nerve and macula as well as the immediately surrounding retina.

nasal to the visual axis, the optic nerve can be seen entering the globe, bringing with it the central retinal artery and vein. These vessels branch out over the superficial retinal layers, starting as four major branches (arcades): two temporal (superior and inferior) and two nasal (superior and inferior) (Fig. 5.1). The area of retina that surrounds the fovea posteriorly, demarcated by the major vessels of the temporal half of the retina (the superior and inferior arcades), is known as the macula (Fig. 5.1). The retina continues to extend along the inner surface of the globe almost up to the back of the iris. The retinal edge is known as the ora serrata and that area of retina leading up to the ora, not easily visible with the direct ophthalmoscope, is known as the peripheral retina.

Hemorrhage may be found lying on the retinal surface (preretinal hemorrhage), underneath the retina (subretinal hemorrhage), or within the retinal tissues proper (intraretinal hemorrhage) (Fig. 5.2). Superficial intraretinal hemorrhage will lie within the nerve fiber layer of the retina, thus causing the blood to stream along the course of the neurons leading to "flame shaped" or "splinter" hemorrhages (Fig. 5.2). Deeper intraretinal

hemorrhage tends to have a round or amorphous geographic appearance (Fig. 5.2), which is arbitrarily referred to as a dot (smaller) or blot (larger) hemorrhage, although there is no specific size cut-off point for the use of one term as opposed to the other. Retinal hemorrhages may have white centers. Although well recognized as a manifestation of endocarditis (Roth spots), this nonspecific sign may be observed in virtually any disorder associated with retinal hemorrhage including shaken baby syndrome (22). Hemorrhage within the gel (vitreous) that fills the back part of the eye (in front of the retina but behind the iris and pupil) is called vitreous hemorrhage and may be mild, moderate, or severe and visually threatening. The ophthalmologist can determine, through the use of indirect ophthalmoscopy, which types of hemorrhages are present. Likewise, the hemorrhages also may be described with regard to the number of hemorrhages observed (by counting or general description: few, moderate, many, or too numerous to count) and the distribution. Hemorrhages may involve the entire retina or one or more specific regions such as the area immediately around the optic

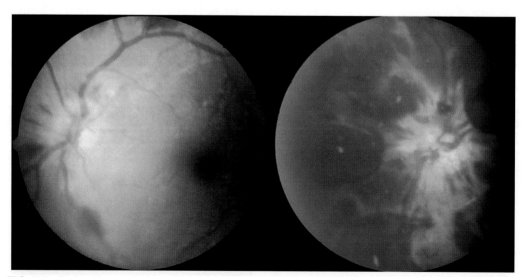

FIG. 5.2. Retinal hemorrhages of various types in the shaken baby syndrome. Note the asymmetry between the two eyes, as may sometimes occur, as well as the variety of hemorrhages. The left eye (on right) demonstrates a severe hemorrhagic retinopathy that is virtually pathognomonic of shaking injury. The right eye (on left) is a more nonspecific retinopathy.

nerve (peripapillary), the area including the macula and peripapillary region (posterior pole), along major branches of the vascular tree (paravascular), the peripheral retina, or the area of retina posterior to the periphery but outside of the macula (midperipheral retina). Retinal hemorrhage due to shaking also may be unilateral or asymmetric between the eyes (10,18,33,37,38,45,47).

Describing the retinal hemorrhages in terms of type, number, and distribution is essential if one is to appreciate the specificity of any particular child's eye examination. A few intraretinal hemorrhages confined to the posterior pole may be very nonspecific and could result from numerous other causes (Fig. 5.2). But the presence of massive retinal hemorrhage throughout the entire retina (subretinal, intraretinal, and preretinal) is virtually diagnostic of shaken baby syndrome, as it is very rare to see such a presentation of any other systemic or ocular disease that would not otherwise be easily distinguished by the presence of other supportive signs (Fig. 5.2). Too often in the medical literature and other settings, comments are made about the specificity or implications of "retinal hemorrhages." The use of this rather generic term is no more helpful in determining a diagnosis of accidental versus nonaccidental injury than is the use of the term "fracture" without describing the involved bone and type of fracture.

The nonophthalmologist is at a distinct disadvantage in achieving an adequate description of intraocular hemorrhage because of lack of routine exposure, failure to dilate the pupil pharmacologically, and the limitations of the direct ophthalmoscope, particularly in the awake and noncooperative infant. False-positive and false-negative examinations may occur; if documented in the medical record, they may lead to confusing evidence in a legal proceeding. It is essential that ophthalmology consultation be obtained in all cases in which shaken baby syndrome is suspected, if not all cases of unexplained sudden infant death. Except in those cases in which a child's pupils may be fixed and dilated because of imminent death, the pupils should always be pharmaco-

logically dilated so that the entire retina may be viewed. If there are concerns about preserving pupillary reactivity for neurologic monitoring, options include the use of short-acting agents (phenylephrine, 2.5%; tropicamide, 1%), which will wear off within 4 to 6 hours, dilating one pupil at a time, or if no other options exist, using small pupil indirect ophthalmoscopy. Ideally, the examination should be conducted within 24 hours of presentation or recognition of the possibility of nonaccidental injury. The ophthalmologist should be encouraged to write a descriptive note and perform retinal photography by using either a standard hand-held fundus camera, video indirect ophthalmoscopy, or the RetCam photographic unit. Such equipment is extremely costly and may not be available at many centers, but detailed drawings and scoring systems also can be useful (29).

One specific retinal abnormality, traumatic retinoschisis (Fig. 5.3), is essential to recognize as it is highly specific for shaken baby syndrome and has never been described in any other condition of infants and young children in the shaken baby age range (17,29). At these ages, the vitreous is quite firmly adherent to the macula and retinal blood vessels, much more so than in the adult (41). As a result, the shaking forces applied indirectly to the vitreous exert shearing tractional forces

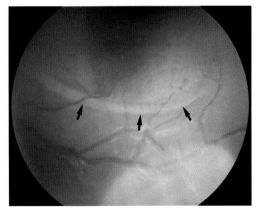

FIG. 5.3. Traumatic retinoschisis. Note the white demarcation line (*arrows*), caused by mechanical disruption of the pigment layer underlying the retina, at the edges of the cystic cavity.

on the retina, in particular the macula, causing it to split its layers, forming a cystic cavity that may be partially or completely filled with blood. It also is important to avoid the common error in identifying these blood collections as "preretinal" or "subhyaloid" (between the vitreous and retina) (48). Recognition of traumatic retinoschisis is aided by the identification of hemorrhagic or hypopigmented circumlinear ridges or lines at the edges of the lesion (Fig. 5.3). These demarcations also have been called paramacular folds. Schisis-like cavities also can form directly over blood vessels (Fig. 5.4), although this is a less specific finding that may be mimicked by virtually any disorder in which a major vessel can have a local bleed (e.g., vasculitis, leukemia). The blood within a retinoschisis cavity may leak into the vitreous, making careful monitoring and follow-up essential (23).

Although the biomechanical mechanism for traumatic retinoschisis is well recognized, the pathophysiology of the other forms of retinal hemorrhage is less certain. Peripapillary flame hemorrhages may be associated with papilledema, a very nonspecific finding, although certainly a marker for increased intracranial pressure or orbital optic nerve com-

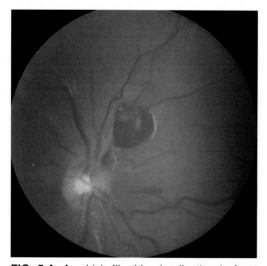

FIG. 5.4. A schisis-like blood collection in front of a blood vessel may be a sign of vessel shearing due to shaking but can be also due to other causes.

pression. Yet many shaken babies do not have papilledema even when increased intracranial pressure is present. A number of theories have been offered to explain hemorrhages not associated with papilledema: increased intracranial pressure, increased intrathoracic pressure, and intracranial hemorrhage are those most commonly offered. Also to be considered are the roles of anoxia, carotid occlusion, and anemia. The reader is referred elsewhere for a more lengthy discussion of the pathogenesis of retinal hemorrhage (29). Some or all of these theories may play a role in the generation of retinal hemorrhages; they are clearly not the major mechanisms.

Retinal hemorrhages are rarely associated with increased intracranial pressure from other causes in young children. When present, they tend to be few in number, intra- or preretinal, and confined to the posterior pole, in particular the peripapillary area. Likewise, intracranial hemorrhage alone, although not uncommonly associated with intraocular hemorrhage in adults (Terson syndrome), occurs in fewer than 5% of children with intracranial bleeding (A.V. Levin, unpublished data) (29). Retinopathy associated with increased intrathoracic pressure (Purtscher retinopathy) might be expected in view of the presence of rib fractures in many shaken babies. Yet Purtscher retinopathy is rarely reported in shaken baby syndrome (44); multiple studies show that retinal hemorrhage is extremely rare and, if possible, confined to a very limited number of retinal hemorrhages after cardiopulmonary resuscitation with chest compression (13,15,21,29), and retinal hemorrhages occur commonly in shaken babies without rib fracture. Anoxia and anemia also are rarely associated with pediatric hemorrhagic retinopathy.

Searching for alternative explanations, one must consider that the shaking itself induces unique shearing forces within the eye that cause intraocular hemorrhage to develop. This concept is additionally supported by the rare occurrence of retinal hemorrhage after accidental head trauma. Retinal hemorrhages are observed in fewer than 3% of such children, and when they occur, the hemorrhages are almost always limited to the posterior pole, predominantly intra- and preretinal, and relatively few in number (4,29). The mechanism for the accidental injury is usually so severe, life-threatening, and obvious (e.g., motor vehicle accident) that child abuse would not even be considered. Yet it is perhaps the severe single acceleration–deceleration of extreme trauma that for a brief moment mimics the severe repetitive shaking of shaken baby syndrome, leading to the comparatively mild retinopathy. Further evidence linking shaking to retinal hemorrhage comes from the studies at our center and others (9), which reveal orbital injury at the optic nerve–scleral junction and the orbital apex: sites of fixation for the optic nerve, orbital vessels, and orbital nerves. The injuries observed to these structures may help to explain not only the retinal hemorrhage, but also the frequent observation of long-term optic atrophy, which is second only to cortical injury as the cause of permanent visual loss or blindness in survivors. Optic nerve sheath hemorrhage is not uncommon in shaken babies (24,29), and although previously attributed to intracranial factors, may also reflect the direct effects of shaking. Optic nerve sheath hemorrhage and damage to vessels or nerves within the orbit may all play a role in generating intraocular bleeding. Postmortem examination of the entire orbital contents, preferably with sections taken after removal *en bloc* by a combined transconjunctival and intracranial route, may have specific utility in identifying pathophysiologic mechanisms that identify the results of shaking.

There are many causes of retinal hemorrhages in children, and these are reviewed at length elsewhere (29). Perhaps the most common cause is normal birth, which can result in an extensive hemorrhagic retinopathy in up to 45% of normal babies at term examined in the first 24 hours of life. Studies in virtually every demographic setting have shown collectively that flame hemorrhages resolve within 7 days after birth, and intraretinal dot/blot hemorrhages are gone usually by 4 weeks. Rarely a large or deep intraretinal hemorrhage may last to 6 weeks (42). Although it may be difficult to distinguish the shaken baby retina from normal before 4 weeks, normal babies do not demonstrate traumatic retinoschisis, and other evidence of shaking injury is absent. In addition, subretinal hemorrhage is much more likely to occur after shaking as opposed to after normal birth. Retinal hemorrhage can occur after any type of delivery but is more common after spontaneous vaginal and vacuum-assisted parturition.

Most important in narrowing the differential is the need to consider a full description of a hemorrhagic retinopathy. Peripapillary hemorrhages due to papilledema or a small number of intraretinal hemorrhages confined to the posterior pole are more nonspecific and can be seen in association with a wide range of disorders. A particular pattern of hemorrhages, such as those that strictly follow blood vessel distributions, may lead to a more specific alternate diagnosis (e.g., vasculitis). A severe hemorrhagic retinopathy, with pre-, intra-, and subretinal bleeding, a large number of hemorrhages with extension out to the ora (3,14,16,24,25), and particularly in the presence of traumatic retinoschisis is virtually pathognomonic for shaken baby syndrome. After the time limitations for resolution of birth hemorrhage have expired, shaking is the most common cause of retinal hemorrhage in children younger than 4 years, with the shaken baby syndrome itself being far more common than many of the disorders listed in the differential diagnosis of retinal hemorrhage in this age group. Nontraumatic causes of vitreous hemorrhage in infants and young children also are quite uncommon (6,29).

Once the diagnosis of shaken baby syndrome has been accepted, there is often a need by criminal investigators to define a window of time within which the shaking may have occurred. Unfortunately, retinal hemorrhages cannot be used in this fashion with acceptable precision. Even though there are some data from adults (36,46) and my own unpublished observations that suggest perhaps a 2- to 3-day delay in the development of vitreous hemorrhage, particularly after traumatic retinoschisis, these data are "soft" and should not be used to rule out the possibility of vitreous hemorrhages occurring at the moment of shaking. This possibility must be true if retinal detachment can rarely be produced by the immediate effects of the shake. The timing of papilledema after increases in intracranial pressure also is not well understood.

Surprisingly, even the severe retinal hemorrhages and traumatic retinoschisis often resolve without long-term visual sequelae (17). More often, long-term visual impairment results from optic atrophy or cortical damage, the latter being from autoinfarction of the occipital cortex, cortical contusion, occipital laceration, or intraparenchymal brain hemorrhage. It also is of note that in the awake and interactive child, not experiencing central nervous system decompensation at the time, no visual impairment may be noted by caretakers despite retinal hemorrhage. This is particularly true if only one eye has sustained the brunt of the ocular injury. Young children will appear to function normally unless both eyes have severe visual damage that is enough to interfere with the relatively few visual demands in their lives. Therefore the history of normal visual function, as observed by caretakers in the home, does not rule out the possibility that hemorrhagic retinopathy has taken place. Our data (unpublished) and those from other centers (34,49) noted a positive correlation between the severity of retinopathy and the severity of intracranial injury. One might thus conclude that the awake visually and neurologically normal child is unlikely to have sustained a severe retinal injury, particularly if the expert pediatric neurosurgeon believes the period of neurologic normality is inconsistent with the degree of brain injury observed at presentation.

Other ocular injuries are less common after shaking and include cataract, hyphema, ptosis, retinal edema, retinal detachment, or total disruption of the ocular contents (29). Some of these injuries may reflect coincident blunt trauma to the eye, either during or in addition to the shaking. Although some authors have suggested that blunt impact is necessary to generate enough acceleration–deceleration to cause severe, and in particular fatal, shaken baby syndrome injury (8), numerous authors have concluded to the contrary that severe injury and death can result from shaking alone (2,29). Not only does this hold true for retinal hemorrhage, but there also is strong empiric and reported evidence that "mild shaking" could result in a lesser hemorrhagic retinopathy that would go undetected because of the absence of a brain injury sufficient to bring the child to medical attention. Retinal hemorrhages due to shaking in the presence of a normal computed tomography (CT) and magnetic resonance imaging (MRI) scan have not been reported. Normal CT scans with abnormal MRI scans (12,31) and CT scans showing edema without hemorrhage have rarely been observed. Yet shaken babies may make their first presentation to the medical system with relatively few or nonspecific symptoms and signs (33), thus underscoring the importance of dilated retinal examination in situations in which a specific diagnosis is unclear, and "covert" shaking is a possibility.

OTHER FORMS OF PHYSICAL ABUSE

Virtually any ocular injury could possibly result from an act of child abuse (26). The face is involved in up to 45% of child abuse cases, with the eyes affected in up to 61% (26). Like all forms of physical injury, a history and complete physical examination, with appropriate diagnostic testing, is essential to elucidate the cause. Yet certain eye injuries are virtually always indicators of trauma, whereas others must at least invoke the consideration of trauma. Table 5.1 offers some diagnostic guidelines for considering a possible traumatic nature of an observed ocular finding, although differentiating accident from abuse would of course require further investigation and evaluation beyond the eye examination. In the absence of intraocular surgery, avulsion of the vitreous base from its attachment to the peripheral retina is virtually diagnostic of trauma. Alternatively, trauma is a less likely cause of unilateral infantile cataract or ectopia lentis than are nontraumatic etiologies.

TABLE 5.1. *Specificity of possibly traumatic ocular abnormalities*

Ocular abnormality	Possible trauma	Traumatic
Periocular ecchymosis	x	
Lid laceration		x
Conjunctival abrasion/ laceration		x
Corneal/scleral laceration		x
Corneal scar	x[a]	
Iritis	x[a]	
Hyphema	x[a]	
Cataract	x[a]	
Ectopia lentis	x[a]	
Retinal detachment	x	
Commotio retinae (Berlin edema retinal bruise)		x
Avulsion of vitreous base		x
Optic atrophy	x	

[a]Less likely to be traumatic when bilateral.

There are many causes of optic atrophy in children, such as optic neuritis and Leber congenital neuropathy, but prior trauma must always be considered a possibility.

It is well beyond the scope of this chapter to discuss every possible physical injury to the eyeball, its diagnosis, and its management. Many general references discuss ocular trauma (28), but particular attention should be paid to the common error of attempting to date periocular hemorrhage in trying to establish a time of injury. The skin of the periorbita is loosely attached to the underlying tissues as compared with other vulnerable body parts. As a result, large quantities of blood can accumulate, thus rendering dating systems (26), which are already subject to inaccuracy, and which were designed with other body parts in mind, largely inaccurate. Periocular ecchymosis will often look darker for its age than subcutaneous accumulations of blood elsewhere on the body. This also will affect resolution time. In addition, the loose skin around the eye allows tracking of blood in the subcutaneous planes both to lower areas on the face and from areas on the forehead or scalp. A single blow to the forehead or anterior scalp can result in tracking of blood to the tissues around both eyes, thus giving the false impression of bilateral injury (Fig. 5.5).

One also may be confronted with a child who has sustained visual loss at some time significantly before the examination and now presents with sequelae that are otherwise of unknown etiology. Although the corneal scar

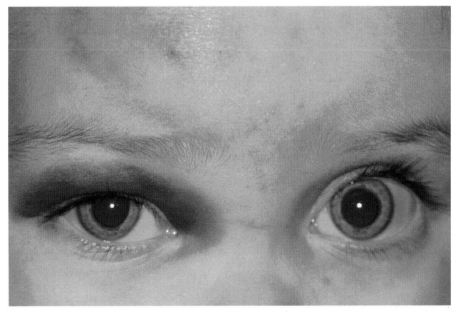

FIG. 5.5. Bilateral periorbital ecchymosis from accidental blunt trauma to the central forehead.

listed in Table 5.1 is an example, as might be an old retinal detachment or vitreous hemorrhage, there may also be situations in which the eye examination is normal, and further investigations, such as neuroimaging, may be required. Old injuries may have particular morphology such as retinal pigmentary clumping, the fixed fold in a retinal detachment, or the whitened residual vitreous collection representing prior hemorrhage. Children also may present with functional visual loss and an otherwise normal eye examination, as a result of unrevealed physical, emotional, or sexual abuse in the home (5). Clearly such causes are far less common than the other stresses and strains of childhood, but it is important to include child abuse in the differential diagnosis.

Munchausen Syndrome by Proxy

Ocular injury may be a primary or secondary manifestation of Munchausen syndrome by proxy (MSP; also referred to as factitious disorder by proxy). This subject is reviewed elsewhere (27). Direct ocular injury from MSP has taken the form of covert instillation of a noxious substance onto the ocular surface, resulting in conjunctivitis or corneal scarring (43), atropine sprayed onto the ocular surface resulting in factitious unilateral pupillary dilation (50), and periorbital/orbital cellulitis due to the injection of noxious substances into the periorbita (11). In the first scenario, that of chronic idiopathic unilateral or bilateral conjunctivitis that is unresponsive to treatment, one might note a predominant involvement of the inferior half of the cornea and conjunctiva. This would result from the upgaze induced by forced opening of a resisting eye (Bell phenomena), thus exposing only these inferior surfaces to the bulk of the noxious agent. Pharmacologic testing is available to help sort out the causes of anisocoria (30). Careful inspection of the involved skin in an area of periorbital cellulitis may reveal needle-puncture marks.

Indirect manifestations may be more difficult to recognize. Subconjunctival hemorrhage or periocular petechiae may result from covert suffocation (35). Although there are other possible causes, such as normal birth and pertussis (which often yields a more severe 360-degree hemorrhage), subconjunctival hemorrhage beyond the neonatal period is actually quite uncommon in the absence of direct blunt trauma to the eye. In any baby or child with sudden explained seizure, altered mental status, or unexplained signs of anoxia, a full eye examination should be requested to rule out not only the retinal hemorrhages of shaken baby syndrome but also the possibility of covert suffocation, as indicated by subconjunctival hemorrhage. This finding may otherwise go unobserved. The ophthalmologist must be alerted to inspect the conjunctiva before proceeding with retinal examination, which itself may induce subconjunctival hemorrhage if instrumentation is used.

Other indirect effects of MSP would include those that result from covert poisoning that has an effect on the central nervous system. The pupils may become bilaterally constricted or enlarged (7,39). Asymmetry of the pupils (anisocoria) may be the result from elevated intracranial pressure. Eye-movement disorders including strabismus (20) and nystagmus (40) can be seen. In addition, the drugged patient may be visually inattentive and appear to be "not focusing."

Neglect

Nonorganic failure to thrive has no specific ocular manifestations, although I have observed bilateral corneal erosions due to exposure in a severely wasted and neglected child who was left listless and unattended for a prolonged period before coming to medical attention. The lids were incompletely closed during this period and the blink rate reduced, thus leaving characteristic exposure desiccation injury involving the lower third of each cornea. More commonly, the ophthalmologist is confronted with issues of less dramatic, chronic, medical neglect and noncompliance. For example, if the caretaker does not adhere to the prescribed regimen of patching to treat amblyopia, the child may be left with a permanently legally blind eye. This is particularly troublesome when one considers that amblyopia is a treatable disorder. Failure to seek prompt medical attention for injury or other obvious ocular disorders also may result in blindness. The subject of child neglect is addressed elsewhere in this book (Chapter 13), but it is essential to note here the importance of consultations and collaboration between ophthalmologist and pediatricians/family physicians in managing such situations.

Sexual Abuse

Although there is one reported case of retinal hemorrhage presumably due to an extreme Valsalva effect in resisting a sexual assault, and I have observed an infant with severe retinal hemorrhages from fatal shaken baby syndrome in which sexual assault also occurred, ocular trauma is an uncommon manifestation of sexual abuse. Also uncommon is the occurrence of ocular involvement from sexually transmitted disease. Syphilis, "the great imitator," can result in a huge variety of ocular manifestations including keratitis, uveitis, retinal abnormalities, and optic nerve changes. It is always transmitted sexually, with the exception of transmission to the fetus or through the birth canal. Congenital syphilis has a different set of ocular manifestations than does acquired infection and should be distinguishable by the ophthalmologist as well as other generalists and specialists. Although nonneonatal transmission of gonorrhea to the urethra, vagina, oropharynx, and rectum occurs exclusively through sexual contact, there is some evidence that the conjunctiva might represent a unique "externalized" mucosal membrane that may make nonsexual transmission by fomites possible (26,32). I am aware of one child who developed mild gonorrheal conjunctivitis after her mother, who had an active vaginal discharge later proven to be from gonorrhea, used a washcloth to clean her own genitals and then directly applied that same washcloth to her child's face during a joint shower. Full sexual

abuse evaluation including examination and culture of other orifices and interview by a trained sexual abuse social worker and physician, as well as a child protective services investigation of the family and home failed to uncover any evidence to support sexual abuse. However, the child was preverbal. Two other similar cases have been reported (32).

If gonorrhea can possibly be transmitted to the conjunctiva in a nonsexual fashion, it raises the possibility that chlamydia conjunctivitis could be initiated in the same way. Human papillomavirus can result in conjunctival lesions, and pubic lice can infest the eyelashes. Cases due to sexual abuse are known, but there are no studies evaluating the possibility of alternate routes of transmission. Human immunodeficiency virus (HIV) can have a wide range of primary and secondary ocular manifestations, but these are less common in infected children as compared with infected adults. Of course, children may acquire HIV through routes other than sexual transmission. Herpes simplex and molluscum contagiosum, although occasionally transmitted by sexual contact, are so much more frequently transmitted by nonsexual routes that the consideration of sexual abuse is usually a low priority in the absence of other risk factors. In light of this information, it seems prudent that, in the absence of neonatal transmission or "consensual" sexual contact in an older adolescent, a full workup for sexual abuse be enacted for the ocular manifestations of syphilis, gonorrhea, chlamydia, human papillomavirus, pubic lice, or, in the absence of other clear risk factors, HIV. At the very least, this intervention may have public health advantages in identifying infected adults in the child's home.

Emotional Abuse

Although perhaps not truly an ophthalmic manifestation of abuse, one must wonder about the psychosocial damage induced by harmful visual experiences in childhood. Children may be subjected to viewing sexual activity or drug-abuse behaviors by their caretakers or other adults. In a study of 1,000 Chicago high school students, 35% had witnessed a stabbing, 39% had witnessed a shooting, and 24% had witnessed a murder (1). There is certain to be an adverse emotional impact of such experiences.

REFERENCES

1. in *Am Med News* AMA 1990: Chicago.
2. Alexander R, Sato Y, Smith W, et al. Incidence of impact trauma with cranial injuries ascribed to shaking. *Am J Dis Child* 1990;144:724–726.
3. Betz P, Püschel K, Miltner E, et al. Morphometrical analysis of retinal hemorrhages in the shaken baby syndrome. *Forensic Sci Int* 1996;78:71–80.
4. Buys Y, Levin A, Enzenauer R, et al. Retinal findings after head trauma in infants and young children. *Ophthalmology* 1992;99:1718–1723.
5. Catalano R, Simon J, Krohel G, et al. Functional visual loss in children. *Ophthalmology* 1986;93:385–390.
6. Dana M, Werner M, Viana M, et al. Spontaneous and traumatic vitreous hemorrhage. *Ophthalmology* 1993; 100:1377–1383.
7. Deonna T, Marcoz J, Meyer H, et al. Epilepsie factice: syndrome de münchausen par procuratio. Une autre facette de l'enfant maltraité: comas à répétition chez un enfant de 4 ans par intoxication non accidentelle. *Rev Med Suisse Romande* 1985;105:995–1002.
8. Duhaime A, Gennarelli T, Thibault L, et al. The shaken baby syndrome: a clinical, pathological, and biomechanical study. *J Neurosurg* 1987;66:409–415.
9. Elner S, Elner V, Arnall M, et al. Ocular and associated systemic findings in suspected child abuse: a necropsy study. *Arch Ophthalmol* 1990;108:1094–1101.
10. Ewing-Cobbs L, Kramer L, Prasad M, et al. Neuroimaging, physical, and developmental findings after inflicted and noninflicted traumatic brain injury in young children. *Pediatrics* 1998;102:300–307.
11. Feenstra J, Merth I, Treffers P. A case of Munchausen syndrome by proxy. *Tijdschr Kindergeneeskd* 1988;56: 148–153.
12. Giangiacomo J, Barkett K. Ophthalmoscopic findings in occult child abuse. *J Pediatr Ophthalmol Strabismus* 1985;22:234–237.
13. Gilliland M, Luckenbach M. Are retinal hemorrhages found after resuscitation attempts? A study of the eyes of 169 children. *Am J Forensic Med Pathol* 1993;14: 187–192.
14. Gilliland M, Luckenbach M, Chenier T. Systemic and ocular findings in 169 prospectively studied child deaths: retinal hemorrhages usually mean child abuse. *Forensic Sci Int* 1994;68:117–132.
15. Goetting M, Sowa B. Retinal haemorrhage after cardiopulmonary resuscitation in children: an etiologic evaluation. *Pediatrics* 1990;85:585–588.
16. Green M, Lieberman G, Milroy C, et al. Ocular and cerebral trauma in non-accidental injury in infancy: underlying mechanisms and implications for paediatric practice. *Br J Ophthalmol* 1996;80:282–287.
17. Greenwald M, Weiss A, Oesterle C, et al. Traumatic retinoschisis in battered babies. *Ophthalmology* 1986; 93:618–625.
18. Harcourt B, Hopkins D. Ophthalmic manifestations of the battered-baby syndrome. *Br Med J* 1971;3:398–401.
19. Jensen A, Smith R, Olson M. Ocular clues to child abuse. *J Pediatr Ophthalmol* 1971;8:270–272.
20. Kahn G, Goldman E. Munchausen syndrome by proxy: mother fabricates infant's hearing impairment. *J Speech Hear Res* 1991;34:957–959.
21. Kanter R. Retinal hemorrhage after cardiopulmonary resuscitation or child abuse. *J Pediatr* 1986;180: 430–432.
22. Kapoor S, Schiffman J, Tang R, et al. The significance of white-centered retinal hemorrhages in the shaken baby syndrome. *Pediatr Emerg Care* 1997;13:183–185.
23. Kuhn F, Morris R, Witherspoon D, et al. Terson syndrome: results of vitrectomy and the significance of vitreous hemorrhage in patients with subarachnoid hemorrhage. *Ophthalmology* 1998;105:472–477.
24. Lambert S, Johnson T, Hoyt C. Optic nerve sheath hemorrhages associated with the shaken baby syndrome. *Arch Ophthalmol* 1986;104:1509–1512.
25. Lancon J, Haines D, Parent A. Anatomy of the shaken baby syndrome. *Anat Rec* 1998;253:13–18.
26. Levin A. Ocular manifestations of child abuse. *Ophthalmol Clin North Am* 1990;3:249–264.
27. Levin A. Ophthalmic manifestations. In: Levin A, Sheridan M, eds. *Munchausen syndrome by proxy: issues in diagnosis and treatment.* New York: Lexington Books, 1995:207–212.
28. Levin A. Eye trauma. In: Fleisher G, Ludwig S, eds. *Textbook of pediatric emergency medicine.* Philadelphia: Williams & Wilkins, 2000:1561–1568.
29. Levin A. Retinal haemorrhage and child abuse. In: David T, ed. *Recent advances in paediatrics.* London: Churchill Livingstone, 2000:151–219.
30. Levin A. Unequal pupils. In: Fleisher G, Ludwig S, eds. *Textbook of pediatric emergency medicine.* Philadelphia: Williams & Wilkins, 2000:237–244.
31. Levin A, Magnusson M, Rafto S, et al. Shaken baby syndrome diagnosed by magnetic resonance imaging. *Pediatr Emerg Care* 1989;5:181–186.
32. Lewis J, Glauser T, Joffe M. Gonococcal conjunctivitis in prepubertal children. *Am J Dis Child* 1990;144: 546–548.
33. Ludwig S, Warman M. Shaken baby syndrome: a review of 20 cases. *Ann Emerg Med* 1984;13:51–54.
34. Matthews G, Das A. Dense vitreous hemorrhages predict poor visual and neurological prognosis in infants with shaken baby syndrome. *J Pediatr Ophthalmol Strabismus* 1996;33:260–265.
35. Meadow R. Suffocation. *Br Med J* 1989;298: 1572–1573.
36. Muller P, Deck J. Intraocular and optic nerve sheath hemorrhage in cases of sudden intracranial hypertension. *J Neurosurg* 1974;41:160–166.
37. Rao N, Smith R, Choi J, et al. Autopsy findings in the eyes of fourteen fatally abused children. *Forensic Sci Int* 1988;39:293–299.
38. Riffenburgh R, Sathyavagiswaran L. Ocular findings at autopsy of child abuse victims. *Ophthalmology* 1991; 98:1519–1524.
39. Rogers D, Tripp J, Bentovim A, et al. Non-accidental poisoning: an extended syndrome of child abuse. *Br Med J* 1976;1:793–796.
40. Rosenberg D. Web of deceit: a literature review of Munchausen syndrome by proxy. *Child Abuse Negl* 1987;11: 547–563.

41. Sebag J. Age-related differences in the human vitreo-retinal interface. *Arch Ophthalmol* 1991;109:966–971.

42. Sezen F. Retinal haemorrhage in newborn infants. *Br J Ophthalmol* 1970;55:248–253.

43. Taylor D, Bentovim A. Recurrent nonaccidentally inflicted chemical eye injuries to siblings. *J Pediatr Ophthalmol* 1976;13:238–242.

44. Tomasi L, Rosman P. Purtscher retinopathy in the battered child syndrome. *Am J Dis Child* 1986;93:1335–1337.

45. Tyagi A, Willshaw H, Ainsworth J. Unilateral retinal hemorrhages in non-accidental injury. *Lancet* 1997; 349:1224.

46. Vanderlinden R, Chisolm L. Vitreous hemorrhages and sudden increased intracranial pressure. *J Neurosurg* 1974;41:167–176.

47. Weinberg H, Tunnessen W. Megacephaly: heeding the head. *Contemp Pediatr* 1996;13:169, 172, 175.

48. Weingeist T, Goldman E, Folk J, et al. Terson's syndrome: clinicopathologic correlations. *Ophthalmology* 1986;93:1435–1442.

49. Wilkinson W, Han D, Rappley M, et al. Retinal hemorrhage predicts neurologic injury in the shaken baby syndrome. *Arch Ophthalmol* 1989;107:1472–1474.

50. Wood P, Fowlkes J, Holden P, et al. Fever of unknown origin for six years: Munchausen syndrome by proxy. *J Fam Pract* 1989;28:391–395.

6

Maxillofacial, Neck, and Dental Manifestations of Child Abuse

Cindy W. Christian and *Lynn Douglas Mouden

*Department of Pediatrics, University of Pennsylvania School of Medicine; and Child Abuse Services, The Children's Hospital of Philadelphia, Philadelphia, Pennsylvania; *University of Missouri Kansas City School of Dentistry; *University of Tennessee College of Dentistry; and *Office of Oral Health, Arkansas Department of Health, Little Rock, Arkansas*

Physical injuries to the structures of the face, mouth, and neck are among the most common seen in abused children. Studies have shown that 65% to 75% of all physical abuse involves injuries to the head, neck, and face, with approximately half involving some form of orofacial injury (8,9,15). For example, Willging (72) reviewed the medical records of 4,340 abused children seen at a large urban hospital over a 5-year period. Injuries to the head and neck were seen in 49% of physically abused children, and of these, the head or neck represented the primary injury in 82% of cases. In another retrospective analysis of hospitalized abused children, Leavitt (36) found the incidence of otolaryngologic findings to be 56%, more than half of which were directly related to physical abuse or neglect.

Abusive injuries to the face and mouth are typically due to blunt trauma by a hand or object, although penetrating trauma to facial cavities is well described. The majority of documented injuries are mild, with ecchymoses, abrasions, and lacerations most common (72). Although many of these injuries are mild, requiring outpatient treatment only, early reports of battering often described extensive facial injuries (66). Orofacial injuries are uncommonly isolated and are often associated with more severe internal injuries. Certain injuries, such as those within the ear, nose, or throat, should arouse suspicion of abuse, especially in infants and young children. When recurrent, these injuries are almost always inflicted (22). Cutaneous injuries are easily recognized, but injuries to the oral cavity may be overlooked by physicians who do not routinely examine the structures within the mouth (15).

FACIAL BRUISING

Contusions are the most common injury seen in abused children and are the most common injury sustained to the head and face (8,15). The specificity of facial bruising for abuse is highest in young children. Facial bruising is notably uncommon during infancy, and is even more atypical in nonambulatory infants (11,43,64). In contrast to accidental injuries, bruises to the head and face are common in abused infants. Identification of such injuries should always elicit concern when identified. McMahon (40) reviewed soft tissue injuries in 341 hospitalized children reported for abuse, and compared patterns of injury by age. Although infants averaged only one soft tissue injury, approximately 50% of these injuries were to the head and face. In contrast, children older than 2 years averaged three soft tissue injuries, of which 25% were to the head and face. Facial bruising in infants may be the only external indication of trauma and is often associated with skeletal or other internal injuries (40).

FACIAL FRACTURES

Facial fractures are uncommon pediatric injuries. Approximately 5% of all facial fractures occur before the age of 12 years, and only 1% occur in the first 5 years of life (59). During adolescence, the frequency of facial fractures increases, and the pattern of fractures begins to resemble that seen in adults. In preadolescent children, fractures to the mid third of the facial skeleton are uncommon, and are extremely rare in infants and preschool children (30,59). Fractures of the zygoma or maxillary fracture of the LeFort type are rare pediatric injuries (70) and have not been reported in abused children. Mandibular fractures are more common. The pediatric mandible, however, is protected from fracture by the elasticity of the developing mandible, the relatively thick soft tissue of the face, and the small size of the mandible compared with the cranium (62). Because of the protection the frontal bone affords the smaller mandible, major head trauma is more likely to be transmitted to the frontal bone than the mandible (59). When mandibular fractures occur, they are likely to be located in the premolar or subcondylar region, and more than one fracture site within the mandible is common throughout childhood (Fig. 6.1) (70).

Mandibular fractures are uncommon but well described in abused children. Siegal (62) reviewed 73 mandibular fractures seen at an urban children's hospital over a 10-year period. Cases were divided by age groups that reflected the developing structure of the mandible and dentition. Mandibular fractures were most common in adolescents and least common in infants and preschoolers. Altercation, with direct blow to the jaw, was the most frequent cause of fracture. Child abuse accounted for 14% of the injuries, with an equal distribution throughout childhood. Surprisingly, although younger children had a higher incidence of extramandibular injuries than did older children, none of the confirmed child abuse cases was associated with extramandibular injuries. The authors concluded that child abuse should be strongly considered when infants present with isolated mandibular fractures.

Clinically, mandibular fractures in the premolar area are not severely painful. Those involving the subcondylar region are associated

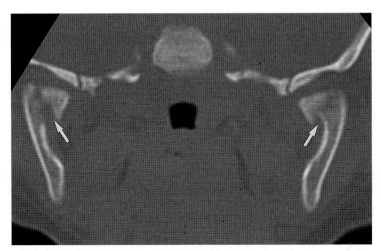

FIG. 6.1. A 3-month-old baby with bilateral, displaced subcondylar fractures of the mandible. The baby had injury to the upper labial frenum, but no other injuries.

with trismus and pain and tenderness in the region of the temporomandibular joint. A contusion in the floor of the mouth may denote a fracture of the mandible. An irregularity in the mandibular arch may be noted, including alteration of the dental occlusion. Treatment varies by age and severity of the fracture (62).

INJURIES TO THE EAR

Injuries to the external and internal structures of the ear are well described in abused children, and may result from either direct or penetrating trauma. Blows to the ear may cause bruising or hematomas of the pinna, abrasions, scarring, or less commonly, meatal wall lacerations, hemotympanum, or perforation of the tympanic membrane (36). Bruises caused by pinching or pulling the ear may reveal a matching bruise on its posterior surface (71). Other unusual injuries include a report of ossicular discontinuity (fractured stapes) from a blow to the ear and simulation of recurrent ear bleeding using beet juice (22). Penetrating trauma with a pointed instrument may result in direct injury to the external meatus, tympanic membrane, and middle or inner ear. Repeated penetrating injuries are rarely accidental, and are described in cases of Munchausen syndrome by proxy (23). Like other orofacial injuries, aural injuries are unlikely to be isolated.

The tin ear syndrome is a pathognomonic triad of abuse consisting of unilateral ear bruising, radiographic evidence of ipsilateral cerebral edema with loss of the basilar cistern, and retinal hemorrhage (26). The ear injuries described in the original report consisted of purpuric hemorrhages in the antitragus, helix, triangular fossa, and in the interior folds of the ear. Internal ear injury was not present. All of the three children described died, and autopsy revealed the presence of an ipsilateral subdural hemorrhage. The mechanism postulated consists of blunt injury to the ear, resulting in rotational acceleration of the head and subsequent brain injury.

INJURIES TO THE NOSE

Abusive trauma to the nose, like other inflicted facial trauma, is often associated with extracranial injury. Blunt trauma to the nose can result in superficial abrasions, bruises, or nasal fractures (72). The development of a hematoma and abscess of the nasal septum (HANS) after direct trauma is a rare complication of abuse. Canty and Berkowitz (10) noted two abused children in their series of septal hematoma and abscess. Unlike the older children who developed HANS after minor, isolated nasal trauma, the abused children were young (younger than 2 years), had severe facial, neck, and nasal injuries, and a history of previous abuse (10).

Collumella destruction and septal perforation, although uncommon, are documented in the abuse literature (53,56). Fischer and Allasio (18) reported 6-month-old twins with traumatic destruction of the nose. One infant had loss of the nasal tip, columella, and distal nasal septum, with collapse of the nares. The other had loss of the alar rim and collapse of the nostril. Further investigation revealed nasal deformities in a 2-year-old sister. The nasal injuries to all three children were isolated and thought to be due to forceful, repeated nasal rubbing.

INJURIES TO THE PHARYNX, LARYNX, AND ESOPHAGUS

Iatrogenic pharyngeal and cervical esophageal perforation in infants is not uncommon and is usually related to instrumentation of the oropharynx. The anatomic weakness of the hypopharyngeal–esophageal junction predisposes this area to perforation (68). Similar perforations due to child abuse are occasionally reported in the literature and are typically caused by penetrating trauma to the child's mouth (21,38,57). Pharyngeal or esophageal lacerations introduce air, oral secretions, and bacteria into the soft tissues of the neck and mediastinum, with potentially life-threatening sequelae (68). Such consequences of injury are well described. In 1971, Morris and Reay (42) described a battered baby with respiratory and feeding difficulties. Investigation revealed pharyngeal atresia, in which the soft palate was fused with the posterior pharyngeal wall. The authors suggested that the atresia was congenital, although considered the (more probable) traumatic etiology. Inflicted tears to the palate, pharynx, tonsillar fossa, and high posterior cervical esophagus have resulted in the development of esophageal abscesses, pneumomediastinum, and a mediastinal pseudocyst (2,35). Bansal and Abramo (7) reported a 2-month-old abused infant with severe subcutaneous emphysema of the scalp, neck, and anterior and posterior chest, with pneumomediastinum and subsequent *Moraxella catarrhalis* sepsis due to traumatic pharyngeal laceration.

Children with perforating injuries may present with fever, drooling, respiratory distress, (erythematous) cervical swelling, dysphagia, dysphonia, subcutaneous emphysema, or pneumomediastinum. Although most traumatic perforations associated with abuse occur in infants, exceptions exist (44). Ablin and Reinhart (1) described a 6-year-old abused child, whose avulsed tooth was impacted in and/or through the esophageal wall, leading to a retropharyngeal and mediastinal abscess. The authors suggested the possibility of sexual assault as the cause of the initial injury.

Oral and esophageal foreign bodies in abused children are well described (22). In a series of abusive ingestions and foreign bodies, Friedman (20) reported a 6-month-old child who was found to have a metallic foreign body in the esophagus and lower gastrointestinal tract, and an 8-year-old boy who drank a glass of lye, causing extensive caustic burns and subsequent esophageal strictures. Foreign bodies being forced into the esophagus as a form of fatal child abuse is rare. Nolte (52) described repeated introduction of coins into the esophagus of a 5-month-old infant who ultimately died with multiple coins found in the esophagus.

Vocal cord paralysis can be a complication of strangulation or abusive head trauma (49). The paralysis is due to either central or peripheral neuropathology. Children with unilateral paralysis may have few acute symp-

toms other than a weak voice or cry, but are at risk for aspiration. Children with bilateral vocal cord paralysis usually have stridor or signs of upper airway obstruction. Bilateral cord paralysis can be an overlooked cause of extubation failure in severely head-injured patients.

INJURIES TO THE NECK

Neck injuries in abused children are less well studied than those of the head, although case reports of inflicted neck injuries are well documented. Cutaneous injuries, usually contusions or abrasions, are reported in series of abused children (29). More unusual injuries have also been documented. Ng et al. (51) reported a 1-year-old who was found to have multiple needles imbedded in her neck. This was discovered after an autopsy of the child's 1-month-old sister revealed multiple needles in the brain and body. The authors speculated that the ethnic and cultural origins of the patients reported (Indian and African) may be relevant in this form of injury (24). Although bruises are familiar injuries, Williams (73) reported a child whose apparent cervical bruising was found to represent a cystic lymphangioma of the neck.

Strangulation is a well-described cause of child homicide (19). The physical examination of a strangled child may reveal linear or circumferential ligature marks. Direct radiologic evidence of strangulation is rare. Carty (13) described the radiologic finding of calcification in the supraclavicular soft tissues of a 3-month-old battered infant. The calcification was thought to be due to fat necrosis from previous strangulation of the baby. Although strangulation or suffocation of a child may cause petechial hemorrhages of the face or neck, this is not a reliable finding. In a series of 14 patients who were intentionally suffocated during covert video surveillance, no child had facial markings that lasted more than 30 to 60 seconds after the attempted suffocation (60). Meadow (41) reviewed the records of 81 children who were smothered to death. Blood in the mouth, nose, or on the face was reported in 39% of the children, and only 10 children had either bruises or petechiae on the face or neck. More than half of the victims had neither bruises, petechiae, nor a history or finding of bleeding.

INJURIES TO THE CERVICAL SPINE

Cervical spine and spinal cord injury are uncommon findings in abused children (55, 63,69). In an early review of spinal and spinal cord injury in battered children, Swischuk (65) reported seven children with spine injury. Most injuries involved the lower spine, but evaluation of a 2-year-old child with neck rigidity, flaccid extremities, and urinary incontinence revealed prevertebral edema and widening at the cervical spine, consistent with trauma. Injuries to the cervical spine and cord may escape detection. Cervical spinal cord injury without radiographic abnormality (SCIWORA) is a well-known phenomenon in young children and is related to the mechanical tolerances of the young spine. Plain radiographs and computed tomography (CT) will fail to detect such cord injuries. Concomitant brain injury in some abused children may obscure signs of cervical cord injury (63). Some injuries to the spine are asymptomatic, identified at the time of a skeletal survey.

In recent years, an association of cervical cord injury and inflicted head injury has been noted, although to date, has not been extensively studied. In 1989, Hadley (25) reported after autopsy subdural or epidural hematomas of the cervical spine with proximal spinal cord contusions in five of six abused infants with shaking injuries. The significance of these findings to the pathophysiology of brain injury or death in abused infants has yet to be delineated. To investigate this relationship further and to determine the utility of screening the cervical spine with magnetic resonance imaging (MRI), Feldman (17) prospectively imaged the cervical spine in head-injured abused infants. In cases of fatal injury, MRI findings

were compared with autopsy data. None of the MRI scans in the 12 patients studied showed evidence of cervical cord injury or extraaxial cord blood. At autopsy, one of five infants who died had a thin subdural hemorrhage at the cervical cord, and three had subarachnoid hemorrhage. No gross or microscopic changes were noted in the spinal cords of the children at autopsy, except for one cord with hypoxic neuronal changes. Although this study confirms the finding of extraaxial hemorrhage in the cervical cord of infants dying of inflicted head injury, MRI was unable to detect these findings.

CERVICAL SPINE FRACTURES

Despite the frequency of abusive head trauma attributed to shaking, fractures to the cervical spine are rare. Cervical spine fractures associated with abuse are reported in infants and have been postulated to be due to forced hyperflexion or hyperextension of the neck during shaking or a direct blow. The actual mechanism of these injuries remains speculative, and concomitant intracranial injury is typically absent (34,58). Cervical spine fractures may present with symptoms related to cord compression, but are often asymptomatic, identified during skeletal survey (58, 67). In almost all case reports, additional skeletal injuries are present. Compression fractures, fracture dislocations, and anterior subluxations all may result from abuse. Hangman's fractures, which result from traumatic spondylolysis of C2, are a rare manifestation of abuse (34,39). Like other cervical fractures, they are thought to be due to severe hyperflexion or hyperextension of the neck. Congenital spondylolysis can be confused with a hangman's fracture, and serial radiographic studies may be needed to distinguish the two (54).

SEXUAL ABUSE

Oral injuries related to child sexual abuse are occasionally seen. Forced fellatio can cause palatal erythema, petechiae, and bruising, and repeated fellatio can cause deep palatal ulcerations (27). Similar injuries can also be seen on the floor of the mouth (28). Sexually transmitted diseases can have variable appearances in the oral cavity, making identification difficult for practitioners (14). For example, oral gonorrhea may present with pharyngitis, exudative tonsillitis, or gingivitis, but is most often asymptomatic in children (16). Condyloma acuminata may be found in the mucosa of the lip, cheek, palate, gingiva, or tongue, but is infrequently considered in the differential diagnosis of oral lesions in children (27).

The primary chancre of syphilis can be located on the lip, although this is rare in children. A careful examination of the oral cavity in sexually abused children is warranted, and on occasion may reveal evidence to substantiate the diagnosis.

DENTAL MANIFESTATIONS OF CHILD ABUSE

Many injuries to facial structures are within the scope of dentistry or easily observed by the dental professional in the course of routine dental treatment. Other types of injuries are pathognomonic for abuse and easily identified by the dentist. Injuries of this type include those that appear simultaneously on multiple body planes (61). Injuries that exhibit patterned marks of implements or the adult's hand or bilateral injuries to the face carry a high index of suspicion of abuse and can occur on easily observable areas of the child's body (47). Various explanations for the mouth as a target of abuse are possible. Injuries to the mouth represent an assault on the communicative "self" of the child and can be a compelling reason behind abuse directed at the mouth. Another factor is the adult's easy access to the head of a child, often well within reach. Any physical injury or emotional trauma also may elicit a cry from the child. Efforts to silence the crying often can result in injuries to the mouth.

Whereas treatment of oral injuries is usually referred to the general dentist, pediatric dentist, or oral surgeon, proper evaluation of the abused child cannot be complete without a thorough visual examination by the primary care provider. Various types of oral injuries may be encountered in any clinical setting. The orofacial injuries that may be encountered in child abuse include trauma to the teeth, trauma to supporting structures, and trauma to surrounding tissues. The principal intraoral injuries of child abuse include missing and fractured teeth, oral contusions, oral lacerations, jaw fractures, and oral burns.

ORAL INJURIES TO INFANTS

Inflicted injuries to oral structures of the infant should be considered separately from those of older children. Infants generally do not have teeth before age 4 to 6 months. The pattern of eruption of primary teeth varies widely and is usually not important in deciding whether or not child abuse has occurred. Delayed eruption of primary teeth may, however, be seen in cases of child neglect resulting from poor nutrition, or may be a result of poor prenatal nutrition during fetal development.

The difficulties and frustrations surrounding an infant's feeding may lead to abuse. Intraoral lacerations have long been recognized as possible indicators of forced feeding and abuse (31). Injury can occur when excessive pressure is used while feeding with a nursing bottle or when a utensil is misdirected during feeding. If the adult feels that the child is uncooperative during bottle-feeding, the adult may use excessive force to introduce the nipple into the child's mouth or press too firmly against oral structures. This can cause mild to severe contusions of the lips and gingivae as well as cause lacerations of the labial frenum (Fig. 6.2) Forced feeding with a utensil can lacerate the tongue, the floor of the mouth, or the lips.

INJURIES TO TEETH

All injuries to teeth and supporting structures should be referred to a dentist as soon as

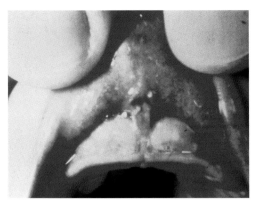

FIG. 6.2. A 2-month-old baby with a laceration of the labial frenum from forced feeding.

possible. The abuse-related injuries to teeth can include movement of the teeth within the socket, fracture, or loss of the tooth. Any trauma to a tooth that does not result in loss of the tooth may, however, move the tooth sufficiently to result in loss of the tooth's vitality. Even relatively minor trauma may disrupt the neurovascular supply through the apex. Evidence of tooth injury may not be evident immediately after the trauma. However, after several weeks or months, nonvital teeth are often characterized by slight to severe color changes of the tooth resulting from the necrotic pulp tissue within. The nonvital tooth appears discolored or markedly darker when compared with the adjacent teeth. Although many etiologies may explain discolored teeth, one or two severely darker teeth in an otherwise normal dentition almost always indicate past trauma.

Displaced or Avulsed Teeth

A tooth that has been moved within its socket often causes tears of the periodontal ligament and may bleed into the tooth's sulcus. Teeth traumatized in this way also may exhibit more mobility than normal. Normal, healthy teeth should move no more than 1 mm within the socket. Palpation to test tooth mobility must be conducted by using two metal instruments or wooden tongue blades. The ex-

aminer should not rely on moving the tooth with fingers to judge the tooth's mobility, because subtle movement of the teeth cannot be felt with the fingertips.

A traumatized tooth can be displaced in any direction. Teeth can be bodily moved anteriorly or posteriorly, intruded into or avulsed from the socket, or moved mesially or distally if adjacent teeth are not in tight contact. This can happen with accidental injuries as well as in abuse. Contact directly on the tooth or from a blow to the face that transfers energy to the teeth can cause the displacement. Either the abuser's hand or an object can deliver sufficient force to displace one or several teeth.

In severe cases, the entire tooth can be forcefully expelled from the alveolar bone (Fig. 6.3). The tendency for a tooth to be avulsed is related to the force and direction of the trauma as well as the anatomy of the tooth. Single-rooted teeth and teeth with conically shaped roots are more easily avulsed without being fractured. Therefore anterior teeth, especially incisors, are most likely to be avulsed, but some premolars (bicuspids) also may have cone-shaped roots. Multirooted, posterior teeth are less likely to be avulsed, both because of their location in the mouth and because of the physics involved in forcing a multirooted tooth bodily out of the alveolar bone. Because root anatomy of a primary

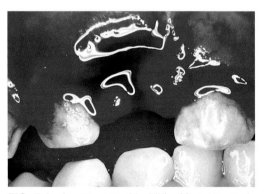

FIG. 6.3. An 11-year-old child with a traumatic avulsion of a permanent central incisor from a beating.

tooth is likely to be less conical in form than its permanent counterpart, avulsion of teeth during physical violence is less common in children with primary dentition. Severe trauma can, of course, remove or shatter any tooth.

At least two cases have been reported of children who were abused by having permanent teeth "extracted" by the parents. In these cases, one adult held the child while another removed the intact teeth without anesthesia (12).

Traumatic tooth avulsion requires immediate dental consultation. The tooth must be kept moist in isotonic saline solution or milk. The chances for successful reimplantation are best if the procedure is accomplished within 30 minutes of the avulsion. No attempt should be made to clean or remove tissue tags from the tooth before the dentist reimplants it. Removing anything from the tooth may result in loss of tissue important for periodontal ligament regeneration. Reimplanted teeth must be stabilized for an absolute minimum of 7 to 10 days with intraoral fixation.

Tooth Fractures

Fractures of teeth can involve the crown, the root, or both. Tooth fractures are sometimes seen in abusive injuries, but they also can be accidental. Fractures occur either when the tooth is struck with a hard object or when the face comes into contact with a hard surface (Fig. 6.4).

Fractures can involve only the enamel, extend into the dentin layer, or involve the tooth's pulp. Teeth may fracture, even bodily through the entire tooth, and still remain held in place by the surrounding bone, periodontal ligament, and gingival tissues. Timely referral to a dentist is mandatory for treatment of tooth fractures. Modern restorative materials and bonding procedures can save teeth with enamel or dentin fractures that only a decade ago would have required full crowns or extraction.

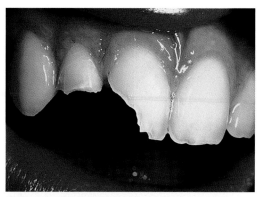

FIG. 6.4. Fractured teeth sustained when a 16-year-old boy hit his mouth against a piece of furniture during a beating.

INJURIES TO ORAL SOFT TISSUES

Gingiva

Trauma that affects teeth also is likely to affect the surrounding gingivae. In addition, trauma from an object striking the child can produce contusions or lacerations of the gingivae without apparent trauma to adjacent teeth. Radiographic examination is necessary in all cases of gingival trauma to diagnose properly any damage to adjacent teeth or alveolar bone (Fig. 6.5)

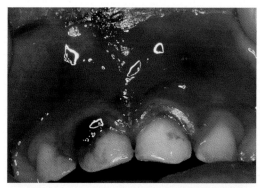

FIG. 6.5. A 10-year-old with multiple oral injuries from an open-handed slap to the face, including laceration of the upper lip, contusions of the vestibule, laceration of the labial frenum, and subluxation of the right central incisor.

Lingual and Labial Frenulae

Inflicted trauma can cause mild to extensive damage of the attachment tissues of the tongue and lips. Along with lacerations cause by forced feeding discussed previously, many forms of abusive trauma can tear these tissues. Blows to the face can displace the lip far enough to stretch the lip's attachment tissue beyond its elastic limit, causing laceration of the frenum itself. Invasive trauma that introduces a hard or sharp object into the mouth also can lacerate these areas. Although accidental frenum tears are common in the 8- to 18-month-old who is learning to walk, similar injuries in young infants (younger than 6 months) and in older, more stable children should raise a suspicion of abuse. Frenum tears will usually heal on their own, although may require sutures if the wound is large, the alveolar bone is exposed, or if the wound separates when the lip is pulled upward (50).

Lips

Any trauma to the mouth can cause contusions and lacerations of the upper or lower lip. Inflicted injuries to the lips are evidenced by marks either from the offending object or from the child's own teeth. When a blow is directed at the face or lips, the oral tissues can come into forceful contact with the child's teeth. The lips may show resulting "bite marks" from the child's own teeth. Bruising or laceration at the corners of the lips also can result from the use of a rope or other material to gag and silence the child. Scarring at the commissures of the lips may result from electrical burns from biting an electrical cord and are more likely to be caused accidentally. In addition, if the child is wearing either fixed or removable orthodontic appliances, these appliances can damage lips during the trauma. The clinician must exercise caution when examining the child's mouth if orthodontic appliances are in place because lips can become trapped in the wires or brackets.

Tongue

Laceration of the tongue can occur from abuse involving a sharp or hard object in the mouth. However, most abusive injuries to the tongue are a result of the child's biting the tongue inadvertently. Any blow to the jaw can trap the tongue between upper and lower teeth. These injuries usually involve the lateral or anterior surfaces of the tongue and resemble jagged indentations seen with any bite mark in soft tissue. If the bite involves posterior areas of the tongue, the marks may appear more like crushed tissue rather than showing definite bite marks.

Bite marks to the tongue inflicted by the child's own teeth are likely to show a curvature consistent with the child's own arch. A bite mark on the tongue from an abuser may show a curve in the direction opposite to the curve of the child's dental arch.

Burns

Burns can affect any oral soft tissue. Abusive burns result from the introduction of a hot object into the mouth, from forced feeding of a food or liquid that is too hot, or from the use of caustic or acidic materials such as drain cleaner.

BITE-MARK ANALYSIS IN SUSPECTED CHILD ABUSE

Bite marks can be important evidence in cases of suspected child abuse. Dentists with experience in forensic odontology are best prepared to evaluate bite marks, but all dental professionals are capable of identifying wound patterns that could be possible bite marks. Health care professionals should seek the advice of a dentist to determine if an investigation should be made into the cause of the mark. The dental professional should be able to recognize the injury as a bite mark, determine and understand the significance, document basic information about the bite mark, and contact the forensic odontologist for the definitive evidence collection and final determination.

Dentists and their staff members can often differentiate between bite marks and other marks caused by different etiologies. If the injury is interpreted as a possible bite mark, the dentist should consider consulting with an experienced forensic dentist as soon as possible for analysis and collection of necessary evidence.

A "typical" bite mark can often be described as a

> circular or oval (doughnut- or ring-shaped) patterned injury consisting of two opposing symmetrical, U-shaped arches separated at their bases by open spaces. Following the periphery of the arches are a series of individual abrasions, contusions, and/or lacerations reflecting the size, shape arrangement and distribution of the class characteristics of the contacting surfaces of the human dentition (4).

Bite marks can be inflicted by an adult, another child, an animal, or by the patient himself. Identification of the perpetrator is determined by size, dentition class characteristics seen in the wound, location of the wound, presence of puncture marks, arch form, and intercanine distance. All of these characteristics may or may not be found in every bite mark.

Bite marks may not only identify the attacker but also may be used to show evidence that the attacker was with the victim at or near the time of the injury, that a violent action was taken, or that the accused is not responsible for the injury (32). Careful analysis may also show that bite marks are in various stages of healing. Repeated similar injuries can be a powerful indicator of continuing abuse. Therefore any bite mark on a child should be immediately and clearly documented for court evidence and to aid child-protective services agencies in determining placement options for the child.

Those attempting to photographically record bite mark evidence should be well trained in forensic photography techniques. Multiple color photos, all including a known color and measurement index and taken perpendicular to each body plane, should be taken by using various exposures to ensure adequate evidence collection. If a standard index, such as the ABFO No. 2 scale is not available, any indexing item of known size and shape, such as a 25-cent piece, can be a suitable index for processing and analysis.

For proper investigation of suspected child abuse, or other forms of family violence, it is imperative that appropriate evidence collection be performed as soon as practical during the examination. Expedited, appropriate evidence collection will help the development of an accurate diagnosis as to the cause of the wound and assist in identification of the perpetrator. Health care professionals who are not forensics experts should seriously consider the assistance of and consultation with a forensic odontologist. Improper or inadequate collection and analysis of information can lead to faulty or misleading conclusions. Improper technique can also lead to exclusion of important evidence in a judicial proceeding. Practitioners are encouraged to contact the American Academy of Forensic Sciences for a list of forensics experts in North America before their services might be needed.

Bite-mark evidence has provided critical information in child abuse cases. However, its usefulness is dependent on early examination, evidence collection, and proper analysis (33). The dental team can provide critical assistance in this process to ensure accurate and complete documentation of the bite mark.

DENTAL IMPLICATIONS OF CHILD NEGLECT

Typically, dental neglect is but one manifestation in the general neglect of a child. It has been defined as lack of care that makes routine eating impossible, causes chronic pain, delays or retards a child's growth, or that makes it difficult or impossible for a child to perform basic daily activities (37). Untreated dental problems are as serious as an untreated wound to any other part of the body because neglected oral health can lead to complications that affect the entire body.

The American Academy of Pediatric Dentistry has defined dental neglect as a willful failure on the part of the child's parent or caregiver to seek and follow through with treatment necessary to ensure a level of oral health essential for adequate function and freedom from pain and infection (3). Previous definitions from the Academy have included the caregiver's failure to seek treatment for a child's untreated rampant caries, untreated pain, infection, bleeding, or trauma. Rampant caries by definition involves gross carious lesions, including the mandibular anterior teeth. These teeth are the least likely to decay and are easily seen by even untrained observers.

Also included in the Academy's definition is the failure to follow through on treatment needs once the caregiver has been informed treatment is needed. Many parents are unaware of conditions in their children's mouths. Often only after the dentist's diagnosis are they aware of even serious problems. However, once they are informed of serious dental conditions and refuse to address these problems according to their personal resources, they have neglected their child. Therefore, parents' failure to follow through with necessary treatment is probably more important in determining reportable dental neglect than is the parents' lack of knowledge. Most practitioners also would agree that no neglect might exist if parents are providing for their children's oral health needs in a manner consistent with their own financial situation or available economic existence. The argument also has been made that, if parents have even taken the child to the dentist who diagnosed a dental problem, the parents are not neglecting the child. However, episodic pain relief is not appropriate dental care when adequate resources exist for more comprehensive care.

The Academy's definitions of dental neglect serve neither as law nor as a standard of practice for reporting suspected cases of child neglect. They are merely a guideline for practitioners evaluating a patient's oral health in light of societal norms and fiscal realities. It is up to the health care professional to weigh the guidelines and legal definitions against such issues as money and access to care.

The most common form of dental neglect is failure to provide treatment for carious teeth. Multiple carious lesions can debilitate an otherwise healthy child, and untreated caries can lead to more serious problems of severe pain, fever, malaise, and lethargy. Pulpal infections can penetrate alveolar bone and exit through the gingiva, usually at or near the tooth's apex, resulting in a parulis or "gum boil." Severe untreated lesions can even lead to facial cellulitis or Ludwig's angina, leading to serious and even fatal consequences.

Baby bottle tooth decay (BBTD), a form of early childhood caries, is a severe form of rampant caries resulting from the habit of putting a child to bed with a nursing bottle or letting the child fall asleep at the breast. The remnants of milk in the child's mouth allow bacterial growth, leading to carious lesions that can amputate teeth at the gingival crest. The clinical pattern of BBTD is typically different from other forms of rampant caries because the most seriously affected teeth are the maxillary anterior teeth. Failure to provide treatment for BBTD severe involvement of a child's teeth can be considered neglect. However, practitioners should keep in mind that BBTD is preventable, and recurrence could be considered a form of physical abuse and reported as such.

Other conditions may constitute dental neglect if left untreated. These include severe malocclusions, abnormal tongue position, cleft lip or palate, missing teeth, or other manifestations that may lead to speech or eating difficulties.

THE ROLE OF DENTISTRY IN PREVENTING ABUSE AND NEGLECT

Dentists and other health care professionals in all 50 states and the District of Columbia are required by statute to report suspected cases of child abuse and neglect (48). A 1995 national study of child-protective services agencies pointed out several facets of dentistry's involvement in the reporting process.

Because only six states currently track the number of dentists making reports, the data on dentists' reporting of child maltreatment must be extrapolated from the small sample. In these six states, from a total of 201,944 reports of child abuse and neglect, only 637 reports came from dentists. This figure represents a reporting rate of 0.32% of all reports (45).

In an effort to change dentists' involvement with child-protective services agencies, the American Dental Association (ADA) added the required recognition and reporting of suspected child abuse to its Principles of Ethics and Code of Professional Conduct in 1993 (5). Official ADA policy states that dentists should become familiar with all physical signs of child abuse that are observable in the course of the normal dental visit (3). In 1999, the ADA further refined its policy to encourage dentists to become better educated about all forms of abuse and neglect and to learn about state-specific legal considerations for reporting suspected victims of abuse and neglect of all ages (6).

In an effort to address prevention issues, the Prevent Abuse and Neglect through Dental Awareness (P.A.N.D.A.) Coalition was established in Missouri. The P.A.N.D.A. Coalition is a public–private partnership between the dental community, public health, social services agencies, and a dental insurance company.

The P.A.N.D.A. message is presented to a vast array of dental audiences, other health care providers, teachers, law enforcement staff, and day care workers. The newest P.A.N.D.A. educational program is targeted for eighth-grade students in a program that not only teaches about the problems of child abuse and neglect but also discusses anger control, conflict resolution, and how to make decisions about proper discipline.

Dentists' increased reporting of suspected cases of child abuse and neglect since the coalition's educational program premiered in 1992 has proven the success of the initiative. Since the inception of the P.A.N.D.A. educa-

tion and awareness programs, the reporting by dentists of suspected child abuse and neglect has increased by 160% (46). P.A.N.D.A. has further proven its success by having Missouri's program replicated in 36 other states; Ontario, Canada; Guam; the states of Timis and Mehedinti, Romania; and Peru. P.A.N.D.A.'s founders are working with individuals in Nigeria, South Africa, the Federated States of Micronesia, Israel, Belgium, and Iceland to replicate the program.

Increased reporting of suspected cases of abuse and neglect encourages the P.A.N.D.A. volunteers around the world. However, true success of the initiative will be proven when the involvement of health care professionals in every discipline results in fewer cases to report and fewer children and adults that suffer from the ravages of family violence.

REFERENCES

1. Ablin DS, Reinhart MA. Esophageal perforation by a tooth in child abuse. *Pediatr Radiol* 1992;22:339–341.
2. Ablin DS, Reinhart MA. Esophageal perforation with mediastinal abscess in child abuse. *Pediatr Radiol* 1990;20:524–525.
3. American Academy of Pediatric Dentistry. *1999-00 American Academy of Pediatric Dentistry reference manual.* Chicago: American Academy of Pediatric Dentistry, 1999.
4. American Board of Forensic Odontology. *Policies, procedures and guidelines.* Colorado Springs, CO: American Academy of Forensic Sciences, 1995.
5. American Dental Association. Minutes of House of Delegates, November 6–10, 1993. In: 1993 transactions, 134th annual session, Chicago: 1994.
6. American Dental Association. Resolution 44-1999, Adopted by the 1999 ADA House of Delegates. Honolulu: October 1999.
7. Bansal BC, Abramo TJ. Subcutaneous emphysema as an uncommon presentation of child abuse. *Am J Emerg Med* 1997;15:573–575.
8. Becker D, Needleman HL, Kotelchuck M. Child abuse and dentistry: orofacial trauma and its recognition by dentists. *J Am Dent Assoc* 1978;97:24–28.
9. Cameron JM, Johnson HRM, Camps FE. The battered child syndrome. *Med Sci Law* 1966;6:1–36.
10. Canty PA, Berkowitz RG. Hematoma and abscess of the nasal septum in children. *Arch Otolaryngol Head Neck Surg* 1996;122:1373–1376.
11. Carpenter RF. The prevalence and distribution of bruising in babies. *Arch Dis Child* 1999;80:363–366.
12. Carrotte PV. An unusual case of child abuse. *Br Dent J* 1990;168:444–445.
13. Carty H. Case report: child abuse-necklace calcifica-

tion: a sign of strangulation. *Br J Radiol* 1993;66: 1186–1188.

14. Casamassimo PS. Child sexual abuse and the pediatric dentist. *Child Abuse Negl* 1986;8:1026.

15. daFonesca MA, Feigal RJ, ten Bensel RW. Dental aspects of 1248 cases of child maltreatment on file at a major county hospital. *Pediatr Dent* 1992;14:152–157.

16. DeJong AR. Sexually transmitted diseases in sexually abused children. *Sex Transm Dis* 1986;13:123–126.

17. Feldman KW, Weinberger E, Milstein JM, et al. Cervical spine MRI in abused infants. *Child Abuse Negl* 1997;21:199–205.

18. Fischer H, Allasio D. Nasal destruction due to child abuse. *Clin Pediatr* 1996;35:165–166.

19. Fornes P, Druilhe L, Lecomte D. Childhood homicide in Paris, 1990-1993: a report of 81 cases. *J Forensic Sci* 1995;40:201–204.

20. Friedman EM. Caustic ingestions and foreign body aspirations: an overlooked form of child abuse. *Ann Otol Rhinol Laryngol* 1987;96:709–712.

21. Golova N. An infant with fever and drooling: infection or trauma? *Pediatr Emerg Care* 1997;13:331–333.

22. Grace A, Grace MA. Child abuse within the ear, nose and throat. *J Otolaryngol* 1987;16:108–111.

23. Grace A, Kalinkiewicz M, Drake-Lee AB. Covert manifestations of child abuse. *BMJ* 1984;289:1041–1042.

24. Hadley GP, Bosenberg AT, Wiersma R, et al. Needle implantation ascribed to "tikoloshe" [Letter]. *Lancet* 1993; 342:1304.

25. Hadley MN, Sonntag VKH, Retake HL, et al. The infant whiplash-shake injury syndrome: a clinical and pathological study. *Neurosurgery* 1989;24:536–540.

26. Hanigan WC, Peterson RA, Njus G. Tin ear syndrome: rotational acceleration in pediatric head injuries. *Pediatrics* 1987;80:618–622.

27. Heitzler GD, Cranin AN, Gallo L. Sexual abuse of the oral cavity in children. *J Mich Dent Assoc* 1994;76:28–30.

28. Jessee SA. Orofacial manifestations of child abuse and neglect. *Am Fam Physician* 1995;52:1829–1834.

29. Jessee SA. Physical manifestations of child abuse to the head, face and mouth: a hospital survey. *ASDC J Dent Child* 1995;62:245–249.

30. Kaban LB, Mulliken JB, Murray JE. Facial fractures in children. *Plast Reconstr Surg* 1977;59:15–20.

31. Kempe CH. Uncommon manifestations of the battered child syndrome. *Am J Dis Child* 1975;129:1265.

32. Kenney JP. Child abuse and neglect. In: Clark DH, ed. *Clark's clinical dentistry.* Philadelphia: Lippincott, 1993:19-1–19-9.

33. Kenney JP, Spencer DE. Child abuse and neglect. In: Bowers CM, Bell G, eds. *Manual of forensic odontology.* 3rd ed. Colorado Springs: American Society of Forensic Odontology, 1996:xx–xx.

34. Kleinman P, Shelton Y. Hangman's fracture in an abused infant: imaging features. *Pediatr Radiol* 1997;27: 776–777.

35. Kleinman PK, Spevak MR, Hansen M. Mediastinal pseudocyst caused by pharyngeal perforation during child abuse. *AJR Am J Roentgenol* 1992;158:1111–1113.

36. Leavitt EB, Pincus RL, Bukachevsky R. Otolaryngologic manifestations of child abuse. *Arch Otolaryngol Head Neck Surg* 1992;118:629–631.

37. Malceez RE. Child abuse: its relationship to pedodontics: a survey. *ASDC J Dent Child* 1979;46:193–194.

38. McDowell HP, Fielding DW. Traumatic perforation of the hypopharynx: an unusual form of child abuse. *Arch Dis Child* 1984;59:888–889.

39. McGrory BE, Fenichel GM. Hangman's fracture subsequent to shaking in an infant. *Ann Neurol* 1977;2:82.

40. McMahon P, Grossman W, Gaffney M, et al. Soft-tissue injury as an indication of child abuse. *J Bone Joint Surg Am* 1995;8:1179–1183.

41. Meadow R. Unnatural sudden infant death. *Arch Dis Child* 1999;80:7–14.

42. Morris TMO, Reay HAJ. A battered baby with pharyngeal atresia. *Laryngol Otol* 1971;85:729–731.

43. Mortimer PE. Are facial bruises in babies ever accidental? *Arch Dis Child* 1983;58:75–80.

44. Morzaria S, Walton JM, MacMillan A. Inflicted esophageal perforation. *J Pediatr Surg* 1998;33:871–873.

45. Mouden LD. A National Survey of Child Protective Services Agencies, 1995; prepared under contract with the Federal MCH Bureau; (unpublished)

46. Mouden LD. Dentistry addressing family violence. *Mo Dent J* 1996;76:21–27.

47. Mouden LD. The role of dental professionals in preventing child abuse and neglect. *Calif Dent Assoc J* 1999;26:737–744.

48. Mouden LD, Bross DC. Legal issues affecting dentistry's role in preventing child abuse and neglect. *J Am Dent Assoc* 1995;126:1173–1180.

49. Myer CM III, Fitton CM. Vocal cord paralysis following child abuse. *Int J Pediatr Otorhinolaryngol* 1988;15: 217–220.

50. Needleman HL. Orofacial trauma in child abuse: types, prevalence, management, and the dental profession's involvement. *Pediatr Dent* 1986;81(1 Spec No):71–80.

51. Ng CS, Hall CM, Shaw DG. The range of visceral manifestations of non-accidental injury. *Arch Dis Child* 1997;77:167–174.

52. Nolte KB. Esophageal foreign bodies as child abuse potential fatal mechanisms. *Am J Forensic Med Pathol* 1993;14:323–326.

53. Orton CI. Loss of columella and septum from an unusual form of child abuse: case report. *Plast Reconstr Surg* 1975;56:345–346.

54. Parisi M, Lieberson R. Shatsky S. Hangman's fracture or primary spondylolysis: a patient and a brief review. *Pediatr Radiol* 1991;21:367–368.

55. Piatt JH, Steinberg M. Isolated spinal cord injury as a presentation of child abuse. *Pediatrics* 1995;96:780–782.

56. Pincus RL, Bukachevsky RP. Medially based horizontal nasolabial flaps for reconstruction of columellar defects. *Otolaryngol Head Neck Surg* 1990;116:973–974.

57. Reece RM, Arnold J, Splain J. Pharyngeal perforation as a manifestation of child abuse. *Child Maltreatment* 1996;1:364–367.

58. Rooks VJ, Sisler C, Burton B. Cervical spine injury in child abuse: report of two cases. *Pediatr Radiol* 1998; 28:193–195.

59. Rowe NL. Fractures of the facial skeleton in children. *J Oral Surg* 1968;26:505–515.

60. Samuels MP, McClaughlin W, Jacobson RR, et al. Fourteen cases of imposed upper airway obstruction. *Arch Dis Child* 1992;67:162–170.

61. Schmitt BD, Kempe CH. The pediatrician's role in child abuse and neglect. *Curr Probl Pediatr* 1973;5:3–47.

62. Siegal MB, Wetmore RF, Potsic WP, et al. Mandibular

fractures in the pediatric patient. *Arch Otolaryngol Head Neck Surg* 1991;117:533–536.

63. Sneed RC, Stover SL. Undiagnosed spinal cord injuries in brain-injured children. *Am J Dis Child* 1988;142:965–967.

64. Sugar NF, Taylor JA, Feldman KW. Bruises in infants and toddlers: those who don't cruise rarely bruise. *Arch Pediatr Adolesc Med* 1999;153:399–403.

65. Swischuk LE. Spine and spinal cord trauma in the battered child syndrome. *Radiology* 1969;92:733–738.

66. Tate FJ. Facial injuries associated with the battered child syndrome. *Br J Oral Surg* 1971;9:41–45.

67. Thomas NH, Robinson L, Evans A, et al. The floppy infant: a new manifestation of nonaccidental injury. *Pediatr Neurosurg* 1995;23:188–191.

68. Tostevin PMJ, Hollis LJ, Bailey CM. Pharyngeal trauma in children: accidental and otherwise. *J Laryngol Otol* 1995;109:1168–1175.

69. Towbin A. Sudden infant death (cot death) related to spinal injury [Letter]. *Lancet* 1967;2:940.

70. Waite DE. Pediatric fractures of jaw and facial bones. *Pediatrics* 1973;51:551–559.

71. Welbury RR, Murphy JM. The dental practitioner's role in protecting children from abuse. 2. The orofacial signs of abuse. *Br Dent J* 1998;184:61–65.

72. Willging JP, Bower CM, Cotton RT. Physical abuse of children: a retrospective review and otolaryngology perspective. *Arch Otolaryngol Head Neck Surg* 1992;118:584–590.

73. Williams CM, Spector R, Braun M. Cervical bruises: a battered child? Cystic lymphangioma. *Arch Dermatol* 1986;122:1066–1070.

7

Skeletal Manifestations of Child Abuse

Daniel R. Cooperman and *David F. Merten

*Department of Orthopaedic Surgery, University Hospitals of Cleveland; and
Department of Orthopaedic Surgery, Case Western Reserve University, Cleveland, Ohio;
*Department of Radiology, University of North Carolina School of Medicine,
Chapel Hill, North Carolina*

GENERAL CONSIDERATIONS

Historical Perspective

The first report of skeletal injury as a manifestation of maltreatment of children was published in Paris in 1860 (130). Ambroise Tardieu, a specialist in pathology, public health, and forensic medicine, described multiple fractures and other injuries in children that were inflicted by parents or others with authority over the victims. This report appears to be the first inclusive concept of the medical, demographic, social, and psychiatric features of child physical abuse that would be defined more than a century later as the battered child syndrome (113). The nidus for current concepts of a "syndrome" of child physical abuse was Caffey's description in 1946 (16) of clinically unsuspected fractures of the long bones associated with subdural hematomas in infants with no history of trauma. His suggestion that the injuries were possibly inflicted by the child's caretaker was confirmed in 1953, when Silverman (115) determined that observed skeletal injuries were the result of repetitive trauma that was unrecognized through unawareness or deliberate denial on the part of the perpetrators. This and later reports led to the formal description and definition of the battered child syndrome by Kempe et al. in 1962 (48).

Incidence and Pathologic Characteristics of Inflicted Skeletal Injuries

The reported frequency of fractures associated with child abuse varies from 11% to 55% (31,41,71,88). Inflicted skeletal trauma may involve virtually any part of the axial and appendicular skeleton. Many injuries (43%) are clinically unsuspected, and multiple fractures are found in over one half of physically abused children (77,88). The true incidence of inflicted skeletal injury is, however, probably greater than these reports would indicate, because radiologic examination is performed inconsistently in suspected cases of abuse, and when performed, it is frequently incomplete or of nondiagnostic quality. Postmortem comparison of high-detail radiographic skeletal surveys, specimen radiography, and histopathologic analysis indicate that the yield of skeletal surveys can be increased from 5% to 92% by specimen radiography (70).

Factors Increasing the Risk of Child Physical Abuse and Skeletal Injury

Age is the single most important risk factor in the incidence of abuse-related skeletal injuries (79), with 55% to 70% of all inflicted skeletal trauma found in infants younger than 1 year (34,77,88). Put another way, 80% of abuse fractures are found in infants younger than 18 months, whereas only 2% of accidental fractures are found in this age group (137). Similarly, occult and multifocal skeletal trauma is in large part limited to the first 2 years of life.

Socioeconomic factors also influence the incidence and severity of physical abuse and skeletal injury. The classic picture of the "battered child" has been that of an infant with multiple skeletal as well as soft tissue and other injuries inflicted over the course of time by a depressed mother. This spectrum of serious physical abuse, resulting in death or requiring hospitalization, appears to be changing, with an increase in the severity of inflicted trauma (i.e., intracranial injuries) and an increasingly prominent role of non-family male friends who are "babysitters" as perpetrators (11). Although overt physical child abuse is more often identified in lower socioeconomic levels, maltreatment of children crosses all social and economic boundaries. Reported statistics should be thought of as delineating the recognition of, rather than the true existence of, child abuse, because better educated and more affluent members of society can more readily disguise physical injury and other forms of abuse (14).

Developmental handicaps and prematurity also increase the risk for child abuse (5,46, 121). Infants and children with cerebral palsy and a variety of developmental disabilities are at increased risk for physical abuse, with the incidence of maltreatment in handicapped children reported in up to 70% of cases (32). Preterm infants are also at increased risk for abuse because of early "bonding failures." Low-birth-weight infants, although accounting for only 10% of the newborn population, constitute approximately 20% to 25% of the physically abused population (121).

Associated Injury

The association of skeletal injuries with head and visceral trauma in the abused child has long been recognized (16), and concur-

rent intracranial injuries and fractures are identified in up to 70% of infants presenting with abuse-related head injury (88). Caffey's original admonition that "the presence of unexplained fractures in the long bone warrants investigation for subdural hematoma" should not go unheeded (16). A screening radiologic skeletal examination should be carried out in all suspected victims of abuse with significant head injuries; conversely, cranial computed tomography (CT) should be performed in any infant with extensive inflicted skeletal injuries, even those without significant neurologic findings (109).

DIAGNOSTIC CONSIDERATIONS

Diagnostic Imaging

Diagnostic imaging plays a fundamental role in the evaluation of suspected child abuse, and judicious application of modern imaging techniques facilitates early and accurate diagnosis in such cases. Diagnostic imaging serves (a) to identify the presence and extent of trauma, and (b) to document, if possible, that observed injuries are the result of abuse (85). In fulfilling this role, the radiologist must determine the location, nature, and extent of skeletal trauma, as well as attempt to determine when and how these injuries occurred. Observed fractures must be assessed in relation to the morphologic response of the skeleton to specific mechanical forces and to established pathologic and radiologic features of accidental versus nonaccidental skeletal injuries. The clinical findings and suspicions must be correlated with the findings of the radiologic evaluation, and the radiologist must be fully informed of the suspicion of abuse before the radiologic examination begins. It is as an integral part of the overall evaluation of suspected child abuse that radiologic imaging has its maximal diagnostic impact.

A complete radiographic skeletal survey (child abuse, Trauma-x, SCAN series) remains the primary imaging study for suspected child abuse (55,86). The routine screening skeletal survey includes 19 separate radiographic exposures tightly collimated to each anatomic region, with axial images viewed in two projections (frontal and lateral), and specific anatomic regions of the extremities viewed in the single projection (frontal) (Table 7.1) (6,55). Additional views including oblique projections may be taken when abnormalities are identified or suspected on the screening survey and/or the clinical findings. A single radiograph of the entire infant ("the babygram") is diagnostically inadequate and must be avoided. When child abuse is strongly suspected clinically and/or radiographically after the initial skeletal survey, a follow-up skeletal survey 2 weeks after the initial examination may facilitate a more accurate assessment of the presence and extent of skeletal injury (68). All studies should be closely monitored by a radiologist for technical and diagnostic adequacy, and because fractures associated with child abuse are often subtle and easily overlooked, and it is essential that skeletal surveys are carried out with a high level of technical excellence.

Because the diagnostic capacity of the skeletal survey depends on the spatial and contrast resolution of the film/screen combination, the radiographic imaging system should have a limiting resolution of at least 10 line pairs per millimeter and a maximal film speed of 200 (6). Although mammographic film/screen systems can provide optimal skeletal detail, newer high-detail double screen/double emulsion film systems appear to produce radiographs of comparable detail with lower radiation doses

TABLE 7.1. *Radiographic skeletal survey for suspected child abuse*[a]

Skull: Frontal and lateral (lateral to include the cervical spine)
Spine: Frontal and lateral thoracolumbar spine
Chest: Frontal and lateral (lateral for sternum)
Extremities
  Upper: Humeri (frontal)
       Forearms (frontal)
       Hands (frontal, oblique as needed)
  Lower: Pelvis (frontal)
       Femora (frontal)
       Tibias (frontal)
       Feet (frontal, oblique as needed)

[a]At least two views of each fracture should be obtained.

(62). Digital ("filmless") radiography has, in recent years, been replacing conventional film/screen radiography, with many departments now using digitally acquired images for skeletal surveys. Clinical experience has shown, however, that currently used digitized radiographic skeletal images may not be adequate for recognition of characteristic metaphyseal lesions associated with abuse because of lower image quality as well as longer interpretation time (138). Careful laboratory study and additional clinical evaluation are necessary before conventional film/screen radiography is replaced by digital skeletal images in the evaluation of suspected child abuse.

Postmortem radiographic skeletal examination also may play an important role in the diagnosis of child abuse (135), and the forensic medical investigator should seek the advice and expertise of a radiologist familiar with the findings of child abuse when this diagnosis is suspected (47).

Skeletal radionuclide scintigraphy (the bone scan) in the evaluation of suspected child abuse is a complementary imaging modality to conventional radiographic examination in the diagnosis and management of child abuse (10,21,28,40,44,125). Scintigraphy is sensitive in defining the extent of skeletal injury and identifying nondisplaced or subtle healing fractures, especially acute rib fractures and periosteal injury inapparent radiographically (21, 117,118,128). At the same time, certain diagnostic considerations limit the use of scintigraphy in the investigation of suspected child abuse including difficulty in the identification of metaphyseal–epiphyseal fractures because of normal uptake of tracer around the physis (growth plate); symmetric fractures; inability to determine the age and type of fracture; and general lack of sensitivity in detecting skull and vertebral body fractures (55). The diagnostic quality of scintigraphic imaging is important, requiring immobilization of the child, correct positioning, magnification techniques in infants, as well as optimized imaging equipment (21,108). As a general rule, skeletal scintigraphy is appropriate as a supplement to the initial skeletal survey when clinical suspicion of abuse is high in the absence of radiographic evidence of skeletal injury.

Occasionally, other imaging methods are needed to evaluate possible inflicted skeletal and soft tissue injury. Ultrasonography may be used to identify nondisplaced fractures before the onset of callus formation and acute subperiosteal hemorrhage in the absence of overt fracture (33,53). In patients with extensive muscle and soft tissue trauma, CT and magnetic resonance imaging (MRI) may further define the type and extent of injury (86,92).

The efficacy of skeletal imaging in the evaluation of child abuse can be increased by clinical criteria based on the age of the child and the type of abuse (55,88). Routine complete skeletal screening for occult fractures is indicated in all infants younger than 2 years with clinical evidence of physical abuse, and in infants younger than 1 year with evidence of significant neglect and deprivation. In older children (age 2 to 5 years), the frequency of occult skeletal injuries decreases, and a selective approach to a complete screening skeleton examination is indicated on the basis of clinical presentation and the results of radiographic examination for clinically evident skeletal injuries. Beyond age 5 years, complete skeletal screening is rarely indicated, because acute occult fractures are rarely present (88). Similarly, victims of isolated sexual abuse and siblings of abused children without clinical evidence of physical abuse do not require routine skeletal surveys.

FRACTURES OF THE APPENDICULAR SKELETON

Fractures of the extremities are the most common skeletal injuries occurring in abused children, and have long been recognized as important indicators of child abuse (16,37,77,79, 113). Fractures may be isolated, involving a single bone, or they may be multifocal; in one study of skeletal trauma in abused children, from one to 15 fractures per child were identified, with an average of 3.6 fractures (5). Long-bone fractures may involve the diaphysis (shaft), as well as the metaphyseal–epiphyseal

complex. Diaphyseal fractures have been reported to be the most common extremity injury in abused children (49,75,88); however, postmortem studies using a combination of high-detail skeletal surveys, specimen radiography, and histopathologic analysis have clearly shown that metaphyseal fractures are identified more frequently than diaphyseal fractures, at least in those fatal cases included in this study (70).

The mechanism of extremity fractures in abused children may be difficult to define in any single case, because the trauma is often unobserved, is inflicted on more than one occasion by a variety of methods, is perpetrated by individuals who are reluctant to confess or discuss the mechanism of injury, and is sustained by children who lack the ability to describe what happened to them. A combination of mechanical forces is probably at play in most cases of abuse-related skeletal injury, reflecting repeated episodes of abuse over time producing more than one fracture in multiple locations and a variety of fracture types in various stages of healing. The broad spectrum of biomechanical forces producing extremity injury results in a variable pattern of fractures, including transverse/greenstick fractures (bending or direct impact from a hand or other blunt object), spiral/oblique fractures and periosteal stripping with subperiosteal hemorrhage (twisting or torsion of the limb), torus/buckle fractures (bending or slamming impact of the limb on a hard surface), and metaphyseal as well as epiphyseal complex fractures (shaking).

Metaphyseal fractures were described as part of the initial definition of the battered child syndrome (48). It was noted that the "classical radiologic features of the battered child syndrome are usually found in the appendicular skeleton" and include "irregularities of mineralization in the metaphysis of the bones of the major tubular bones with slight malalignment of the adjacent epiphyseal ossification centers." Meticulous pathologic–radiographic investigation has now demonstrated that the metaphyseal fracture is not an avulsion at the site of periosteal attachment as was originally thought (17), but rather a planar fracture through the region of the metaphysis abutting the physis (61). Histologic examination reveals a series of subphyseal microfractures through the delicate primary spongiosa and calcified cartilaginous cores traversing this most immature portion of the metaphysis (Fig. 7.1). The result is two contiguous mineralized regions: calcified cartilage in the adjacent subphyseal zone of the metaphysis separated from the calcified cartilage in the physeal–epiphyseal fragment. As the fracture plane extends peripherally to the cortex, it veers away from the growth plate, undercutting a fragment of bone, the subperiosteal collar, producing a disk-like fragment that is thin centrally but has a thicker, mineralized peripheral rim.

Nondisplaced metaphyseal injuries appear radiographically as planar lucencies traversing the subphyseal metaphysis for variable distances (Fig. 7.2A). With a complete fracture,

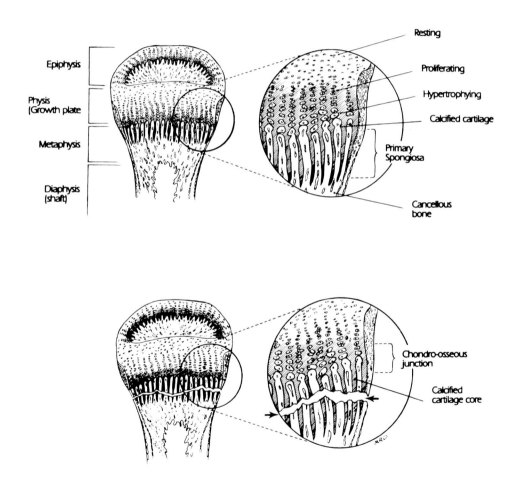

FIG. 7.1. Skeletal manifestations of child abuse. **A:** Normal tubular bone consists of the diaphysis (shaft), metaphysis, physis (growth plate), and epiphysis. Longitudinal growth results from proliferation and calcification of cartilage cells at the chondroosseous junction. The physis is a disk of cartilage extending from the zone of resting cartilage to the zone of calcified cartilage in the metaphysis. In the metaphysis, calcified cartilage is transformed in the bone in the primary spongiosa. **B:** Metaphyseal fracture in the primary spongiosa. The planar fracture separates a disk-like fragment of calcified subphyseal cartilage from the adjacent calcified submetaphysis.

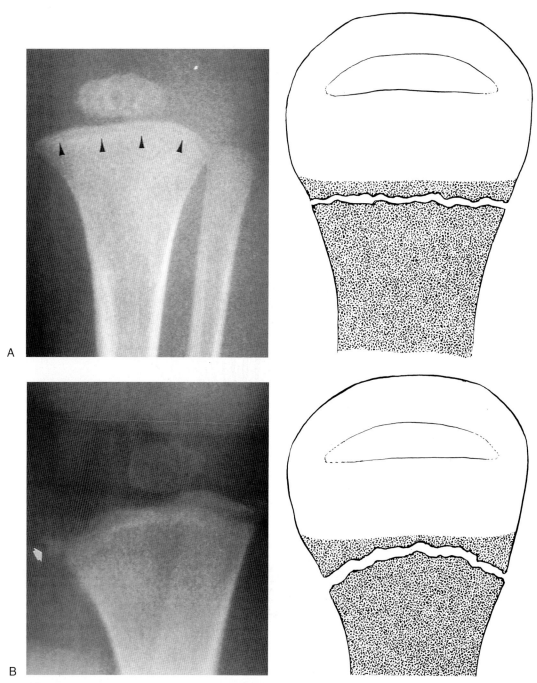

FIG. 7.2. Radiographic appearance of metaphyseal fracture. **A:** Nondisplaced fracture. The fracture line is seen as a subtle linear lucency (*arrows*). **B:** "Corner" fracture. As the fracture is viewed tangentially, the dense peripheral margin of the disk-like metaphyseal fragment may be seen as a discrete bony fragment (*arrow*).

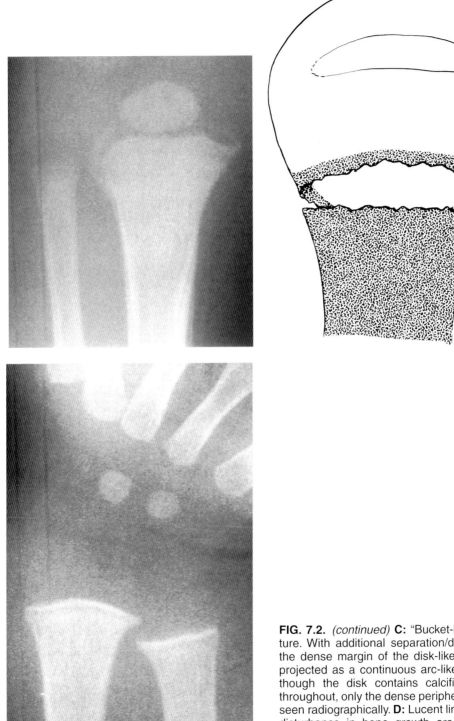

FIG. 7.2. *(continued)* **C:** "Bucket-handle" fracture. With additional separation/displacement, the dense margin of the disk-like fragment is projected as a continuous arc-like density. Although the disk contains calcified cartilage throughout, only the dense peripheral margin is seen radiographically. **D:** Lucent lines reflecting disturbance in bone growth are generalized and symmetric, and traverse the entire metaphysis.

inclusion of the subperiosteal bone collar within the periphery metaphyseal fracture fragment explains the radiographic picture of the "corner" fracture (Fig. 7.2B) or "bucket-handle" pattern (Fig. 7.2C), depending on the degree of displacement and the radiographic projection (73). If no further injury occurs, the fracture will disappear in several weeks. If, however, trauma is continued, with additional trabecular disruption, a wider lucency and metaphyseal irregularity will be seen. The amount of periosteal disruption and subsequent new bone formation depends on the extent of metaphyseal injury and degree of dis-

placement; it is common to see no periosteal reaction with nondisplaced or only slightly displaced metaphyseal fractures. The transmetaphyseal planar lucency of a nondisplaced fracture (Fig. 7.2A) must be differentiated from metaphyseal lucent lines reflecting disturbance in normal bone growth (growth disturbance lines; Fig. 7.2D). Fracture lines are usually asymmetric and often incomplete, whereas the growth-disturbance lines are generalized and symmetric and traverse the entire metaphysis.

Metaphyseal fractures require biomechanical forces that are not produced by the usual accidental trauma of infancy. Rather, rota-

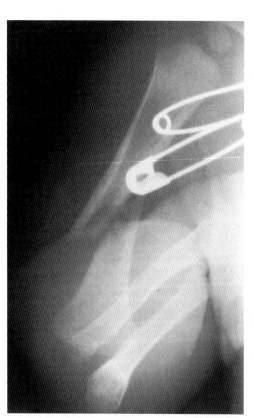 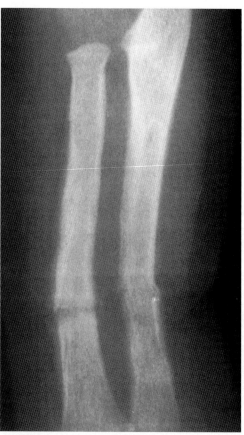

A   B

FIG. 7.3. Diaphyseal fracture. Chest radiograph obtained in a patient with pneumonia identified an unsuspected acute oblique fracture of the right humeral diaphysis **(A)**. A complete skeletal survey revealed older transverse diaphyseal fractures of the left radius and ulna, with evidence of healing **(B)**.

tional forces are generated as the shaken infant is held by the trunk or when the extremities are used as convenient handles for violent shaking (14,52). Rapid acceleration and deceleration delivers planar shearing forces to the metaphysis, resulting in fracture. Cartilaginous epiphyseal fracture with separation occurs when the limb is subjected to massive traction, compression, or rotation. Because of the specificity of metaphyseal fracture in infancy, it has been suggested that resection of "high risk" metaphysis (proximal humeri, knees, distal tibia) followed by high-detail radiography and histologic examination be performed to verify the fracture, on infants for whom cause of death is not determined, and in fatal cases with central nervous injuries or ocular signs of abuse (59,134).

Diaphyseal (shaft) fractures may be transverse or oblique/spiral fractures. Although fractures of the humerus, femur, and tibia are found frequently in abused children, most authors agree that there are no specific types or location of diaphyseal fractures in abused children (7,11,49,97). In contrast to metaphyseal fractures, diaphyseal fractures may result from accidental injury. A careful history and physical examination for other evidence of unexplained injury are necessary, and in cases in which abuse is suspected, a complete skeletal survey must be obtained to search for additional occult injuries (Fig. 7.3). In this context, because extremity injuries are common initial presentations often involving an orthopedic surgeon, it is essential that this physician be familiar with the signs of abuse and make referral to the appropriate child-protection agency (73,116).

Periosteal injury may occur without radiographically evident diaphyseal fracture. The periosteum is most strongly attached to the metaphysis in infants and is loosely attached to the underlying diaphyseal cortex. As a result, twisting or torsion of the limb may result in stripping of the periosteum from the cortex with associated subperiosteal hemorrhage.

These "bone bruises" can be detected radiographically only when periosteal new bone has begun to form 5 to 10 days after injury. Ultrasonographic examination can be used to demonstrate acute periosteal elevation and hemorrhage and, in some cases, the presence of acute nondisplaced incomplete diaphyseal fractures (27,47). On radionuclide scintigrams, tracer activity is increased in the area of acute periosteal stripping and hemorrhage, well before periosteal new bone formation (Fig. 7.4) (21).

Upper Extremities

Clavicular fractures have been reported in 3% to 10% of abused children (5,31,41,49). Because the most common location for both accidental and inflicted clavicular fractures is the middle one third of the shaft, fractures in this location are by themselves of limited diagnostic significance. Clavicular fractures are the most common birth-related skeletal injury, and a healing fracture in the first 7 to 10 days of life must be regarded as accidental; however, any acute clavicular fracture identified after age 10 days without evidence of healing is suggestive of abuse. In older infants, recognition and treatment of both accidental and inflicted fractures of the midshaft may be delayed until abundant callus produces a palpable "lump," and these fractures must be evaluated within the context of the history and other evidence of physical injury and/or abuse. By contrast, accidental fractures in the medial or lateral end of the clavicle are uncommon in children aged 3 years or younger (75). These fractures are adjacent to the sternoclavicular and acromioclavicular articulations and are likely the result of shaking (Fig. 7.5).

Scapular fractures are unusual in abused children (5,31,41,49,75). Fracture or fragmentation of the acromion at the acromioclavicular articulation occurs most commonly and probably results from indirect shearing biomechanical forces generated by shaking or as

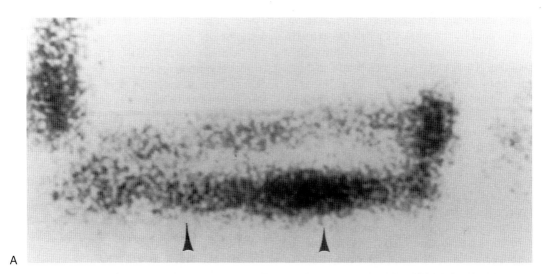

A

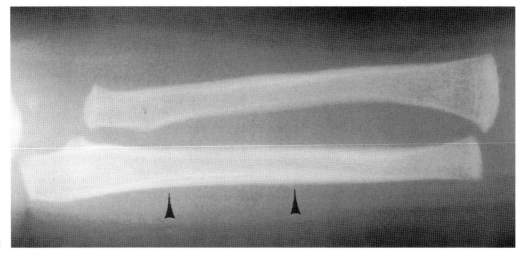

B

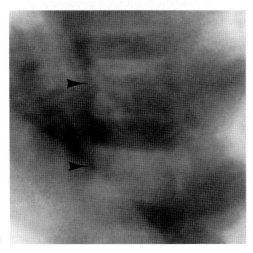

C

FIG. 7.4. A radionuclide bone scan **(A)** reveals increased tracer activity in the right forearm (*arrowheads*), as well as the lower thoracic spine. Radiographic examination of the right forearm **(B)** shows periosteal new bone along the shaft of the ulna (*arrowheads*). A lateral view of the thoracic spine **(C)** shows anterior compression of the T8 and T9 vertebral bodies (*arrows*).

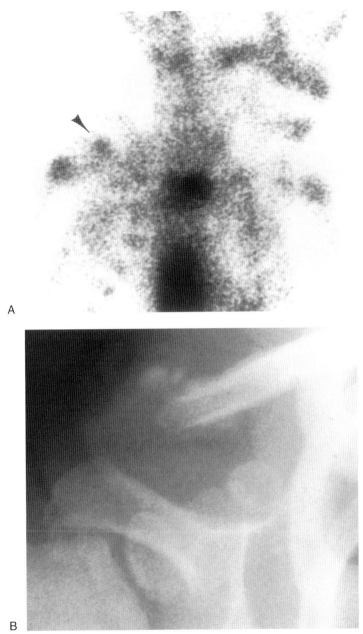

A

B

FIG. 7.5. A radionuclide bone scan **(A)** in a 10-month-old infant with a subdural hematoma reveals an area of tracer uptake in the distal right clavicle (*arrowhead*). A radiograph of the right shoulder **(B)** reveals a healing distal clavicular fracture.

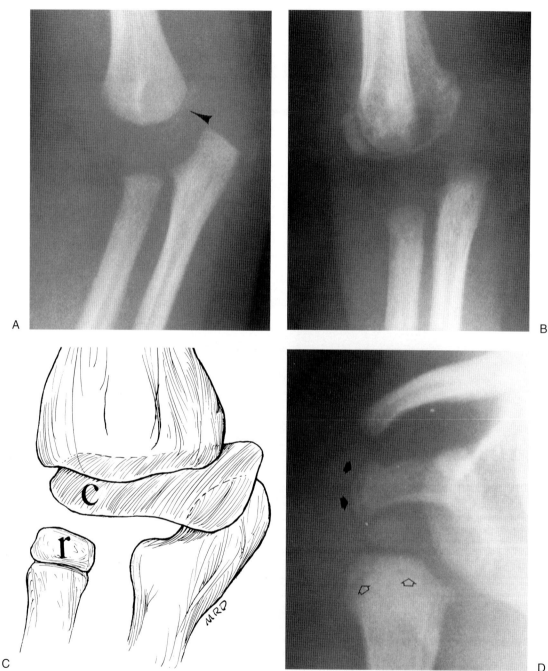

FIG. 7.6. A: Extensive soft-tissue swelling is evident about the right elbow with a subtle curvilinear fragment of bone adjacent to the humeral metaphysis *(arrowhead).* **B:** Five weeks later, abundant callus formation is medially displaced about the distal humeral epiphysis. **C:** The diagram shows separation and displacement of the capitellum *(C).* The radial head *(r)* remains with the capitellum. **D:** A fracture of the right acromion process is shown *(solid arrows),* as well as the adjacent proximal humeral metaphysis *(open arrows).*

traction is applied to the upper extremity (Fig. 7.6D). Rare fractures of the body of the scapula are presumably the result of direct impact. Coracoid fractures are similarly uncommon.

Fractures of the humerus are reported in from 12% to 57% of abused infants and children (5,32,80,112,122,133). The frequency of these fractures in abused children is readily explained: the arms offer a convenient "handle" to the assailant as the infant is pulled, swung, or shaken. Abuse-related transverse or oblique/spiral diaphyseal fractures are found most frequently in the middle or lower one third of the diaphysis. Supracondylar fracture, although a common accidental distal humeral injury in older children, should prompt consideration of possible child abuse when encountered in a child younger than 3 years (53,133). Although less common than diaphyseal fractures of the humerus in abused children, proximal humeral metaphyseal fractures have been demonstrated by postmortem radiologic–histopathologic examination, stressing the need for careful examination of this area in the initial radiographic survey in cases of suspected abuse (67). Inflicted epiphyseal fracture–separation of the proximal and distal epiphyses also may occur, and acute injuries may be difficult to identify radiographically before periosteal new bone and callus formation (Fig. 7.6) (87,111). Ultrasonography and MRI may be useful in establishing the diagnosis of these fractures before epiphyseal ossification and may obviate the need for arthrography (92). Once the capitellum is ossified, the radiographic diagnosis of distal humeral fracture separation should be little trouble, because the radius will remain aligned with the displaced capitellum (24).

Fractures of the radius and ulna are common extremity injuries in abused children (5). As with humeral fractures, their frequency reflects the use of the forearms as handles for shaking. Diaphyseal subperiosteal hemorrhage may be the only sequelae of abuse. Forearm fractures are most frequently paired fractures of the radius and ulna, are found in the distal one third of the shaft, and tend to be transverse (Fig. 7.3). Accidental torus or buckle fractures of the distal radius and ulna are also relatively common in toddlers and small children, and are typically transverse. As in all nonspecific long-bone fractures, the history and age of the child must be used to determine the risk of child abuse in such injuries (80).

Hand fractures have been reported only sporadically in abused children (88). However, these fractures may be subtle, and a study of abused infants revealed both metacarpal and phalangeal fractures that are presumably the result of forced extension (93). Abuse-related hand fractures also may result when older children attempt to shield themselves from a blow (Fig. 7.7). Well-collimated, high-detail initial radiographs with oblique views and follow-up examination may aid in detection of these injuries. Fractures of the hands are often associated with more widespread musculoskeletal and soft tissue injury.

Lower Extremities

Fractures of the pelvis are seldom reported in abused children (5,31,49,88). Fractures of the pubic bones and ischium are reported most frequently and require close radiographic scrutiny for identification (79,86, 102). Radionuclide scintigraphy also may aid in the identification of these fractures (128). Considering the direct force required to produce such injuries, pelvic fractures without a history of vehicular or other severe trauma should be considered nonaccidental injuries.

Femoral fractures are reported in from 12% to 29% of physically abused children (5,38,49). In at least one study, these fractures were the most common long-bone injury identified in abused children (41). Femoral shaft and distal metaphyseal fractures occur most commonly and may result from rotational force applied to the leg during twisting or shaking, torsion when the leg is used as a handle for shaking, or result from a direct blow. Torus/buckle injuries at the end of the diaphysis are impaction fractures that probably occur at the end of a shaking episode as the infant is forcibly brought down against a hard surface (18).

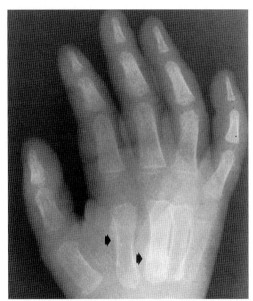

A

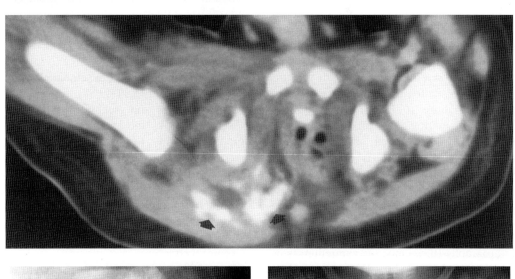

B

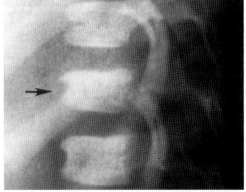

C

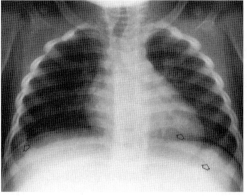

D

FIG. 7.7. A 14-month-old child had multiple bruises and a buttocks mass. **A:** Radiography reveals healing fractures of the second and third metacarpals *(arrows).* Computed tomography of the buttocks mass **(B)** reveals a calcified right gluteal hematoma *(arrows).* An anterior compression fracture of the twelfth thoracic vertebral body **(C)** and multiple healing rib fractures **(D)** also were identified.

Distal metaphyseal fractures initially involve the posteromedial aspect of the femur, with anterior and lateral extension in more extensive lesions (64). Fractures of the proximal femur occur less frequently than distal fractures (7,9). The radiographic diagnosis of the proximal metaphyseal/epiphyseal fractures before ossification of the femoral head is made on a basis of displacement of the femoral shaft relative to the femoral head and acetabulum (Fig. 7.8). Ultrasonography, MRI, and/or arthrography may be necessary to define the fracture further.

With the exception of metaphyseal injuries, femoral fracture patterns cannot be used to rule in or rule out abuse (9). Age is an important consideration in differentiating accidental from nonaccidental femoral fractures (7). In one

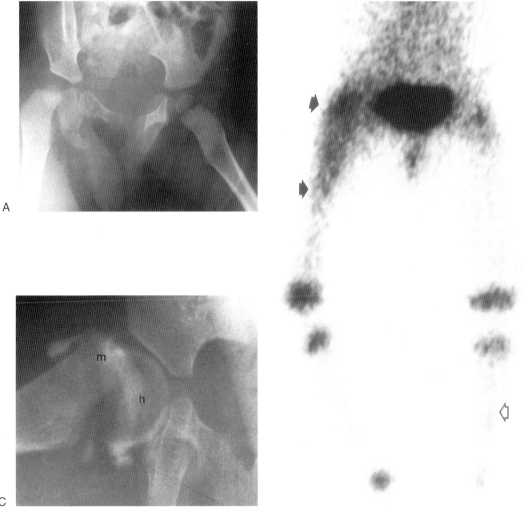

FIG. 7.8. A 10-month-old boy refused to move his right leg. A: The right femoral head is malaligned relative to the adjacent metaphysis when compared with the normal left hip. B: A radionuclide bone scan reveals increased tracer uptake about the right hip, extending to the middle of the femur (*solid arrows*). An area of increased activity in the middle of the left tibial shaft (*open arrow*) was identified later as a healing diaphyseal fracture. C: An arthrogram of the right hip shows complete fracture–separation of the femoral head (*h*) from the metaphysis (*m*).

study, 60% of fractures of the femur occurring in infants aged 1 year or younger were the result of abuse, whereas only 20% of fractures in children aged between 2 and 3 years were determined to be the result of abuse (133). Isolated femoral fractures are not associated with significant accompanying blood loss or shock, and their presence should suggest the possibility of additional visceral injuries (7).

Tibial fractures are the third most common extremity injury in abused children (5,31). By contrast, fractures of the fibula are relatively uncommon as isolated injuries, and most occur in conjunction with a tibial fracture. Most inflicted tibial fractures occur in the distal metaphysis, less frequently in the proximal metaphysis, and only occasionally in the diaphysis (17). Distal tibial metaphyseal fractures are initially seen along the medial aspect of the metaphysis and extend to the lateral metaphysis with more extensive injuries (71). Proximal metaphyseal fractures show a similar pattern of medial involvement and lateral extension (72). Distal fractures show the typical radiographic changes of metaphyseal lucency as well as corner and bucket-handle configurations (Fig. 7.9). Inflicted diaphyseal fractures usually have less obliquity than do accidental spiral tibial fractures, which are relatively common in infants and young children between 9 months to 3 years (toddler fracture) (83,132). These nondisplaced spiral fractures are often the result of trivial or innocuous injuries that are frequently unobserved; soft tissue swelling as well as ecchymoses are unusual, with localized tenderness often being

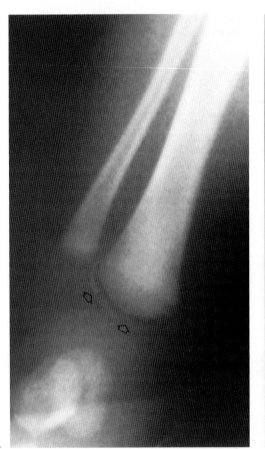
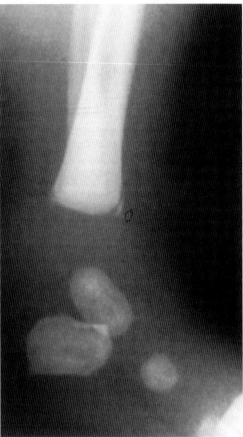

A   B

FIG. 7.9. A 1-month-old infant had a swollen left leg. **A:** Radiography shows a "bucket-handle" fracture *(arrows)* of the distal tibial metaphysis, which, viewed in a lateral projection **(B)**, appears as a "corner" fracture *(arrow)*.

the only physical finding. These children are usually seen because of failure to bear weight, a limp, or the appearance of pain when forced to stand on the involved extremity (99). Radiographic evidence of a toddler fracture is subtle and requires at least two (anteroposterior and lateral) and possibly three (oblique–internal/external rotation) views for diagnosis. Skeletal scintigraphy (bone scan) may be helpful in identifying these subtle fractures when radiographic findings are negative (117). If fracture is suspected but not visualized, immobilization is indicated. Repeated radiographs obtained 7 to 10 days later usually show subperiosteal new bone formation (132).

Fractures of the feet are unusual injuries in abused children (5,31,49). The mechanism is thought to be forced hyperextension with a tendency to involve the first metatarsals and phalanges with few clinical signs of injury (93). Radiographic diagnosis requires careful, focused examination of the feet in at least two projections including oblique views.

Long-Term Sequelae of Long-Bone Fractures

In general, the outcome of a fracture is related to the position of the bone ends after the bone has healed. Three factors correlate with prognosis: (a) maintenance of length, (b) proper rotational alignment, and (c) angulation. If fractures are not displaced or are minimally displaced, the bone will usually be normal after healing, provided the physis (growth plate) has not been damaged. If the fracture alignment is nonanatomic at presentation, the goal of treatment is to align the bones appropriately with respect to length, angulation, and rotation. If children present with nonanatomic alignment but the bones are healed, remodeling can occur to a certain extent, depending on the location and plane of angular deformity. As a general rule, a child can remodel 3 to 4 degrees of flexion deformity at the distal femur with each year of remaining growth. Therefore, if a 3-year-old child's femur heals in 30 degrees of flexion just above the knee, this angulation will be completely remodeled, and the bone will be straight by the time the child has finished growth.

Length also is a plastic property in children. Increased nutrition delivered to the area of injury to aid in healing also stimulates the physes both proximally and distally, resulting in an increased rate of growth in the fractured bone. For example, overgrowth in a femur can range from a few millimeters to 4 cm in children aged 10 years and younger. Consequently, even fractures that heal with considerable shortening may normalize in length. Unfortunately, there is no good prognostic indicator in any individual case to predict the amount of overgrowth the patient will experience. The majority of overgrowth occurs within the first 2 years after injury. If a child has a functionally short limb 2 years after injury, further significant spontaneous correction should not be expected. If limb-length inequalities cause problems, further treatment is required.

Rotational malalignment has less potential for remodeling. No good data exist on what can be reasonably expected in terms of rotational correction after fracture in children. Two mechanisms account for remodeling of bone: epiphyseal, relating to the longitudinal growth of the bone at the growth plate; and diaphyseal, related to the forces acting on the shaft of the bone. In child abuse, the diaphyseal mechanism is rarely disrupted. By contrast, the epiphyseal mechanism may be disrupted, with severe metaphyseal–epiphyseal fractures that damage the physis (96). As a consequence, growth may cease altogether or may become asymmetric, producing an angular deformity. Damage to the physis resulting from child abuse has been described with shortening and deformity of the injured limb, flaring of the metaphysis, and blurring of the growth plate (15). All children with fractures in the epiphyseal region must be followed up carefully for 6 to 12 months to determine if the physis will grow normally.

A rarely encountered but devastating sequela to inflicted proximal femoral fracture is avascular necrosis of the proximal femoral epiphysis (head). If the epiphysis is displaced with respect to the femoral neck or the femoral neck is displaced with respect to the shaft of the femur, the blood vessels nourishing the femoral head can be damaged. If avascular necrosis occurs, the entire proximal femoral epiphysis may collapse, leading to flattening of the proximal femur and loss of longitudinal growth in the proximal femoral growth plate.

Management of Long-Bone Fractures

The management of abuse-related skeletal injury differs little from treatment of accidental fractures. Simple immobilization in a cast is usually sufficient because the children are young, and most inflicted fractures are not displaced or are minimally displaced. Closed reduction and cast immobilization are required for displaced fractures to restore length as well as rotational and angular alignment. Operative management, either open reduction with internal fixation or closed reduction with percutaneous internal fixation, is rarely necessary, except in supracondylar elbow fractures and epiphyseal fracture–separation.

FRACTURES
OF THE AXIAL SKELETON

Thoracic Cage

Rib fractures constitute between 5% and 27% of all skeletal injuries occurring in abused children (53), with almost 90% seen in infants younger than 2 years (88). Most fractures (80%) are located posteriorly near the costovertebral articulation (Fig. 7.10) (88). In contrast to extremity fractures, most rib fractures in abused children are clinically unsuspected. Rib fractures are rarely if ever the result of minor accidental trauma in otherwise healthy infants and children, because the compliance and mobility of the thoracic cage in childhood normally prevent rib fracture in situations other than massive vehicular or other major accidental trauma (17,28). Rib fractures have not been found after cardiopulmonary resuscitation in children, and only rarely from over-enthusiastic physiotherapy (18,29).

Most rib fractures are thought to result from violent shaking (52) rather than from direct impact (118) or lateral compression of the chest (17). As the infant is grasped, the assailant's palms are usually situated laterally, with the thumbs positioned anteriorly and the fingers

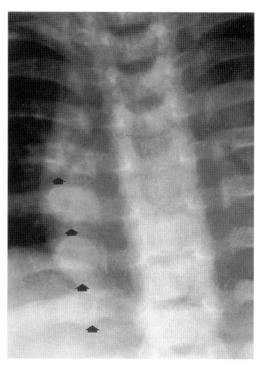

FIG. 7.10. Multiple healing fractures of the right fourth through seventh ribs (*arrows*) at the costovertebral junction, adjacent to the tip of the transverse processes.

placed posteriorly (Fig. 7.11). Compression of the chest is from front to back, with levering of the proximal rib over the fulcrum of the transverse process. Animal studies confirm that these fractures require excessive levering associated with massive forces that entail violent anteroposterior compression, as with child abuse or deceleration associated with automobile accidents (66). Posterior fractures are seen initially at the costovertebral junction and subsequently tend to occur laterally along the posterior arc of the rib as compressive force increases. Because these compressive forces are distributed more or less equally over the thoracic cage during shaking, rib fractures often are multiple and bilateral. Although anterior and costochondral junction fractures are identified less frequently (88), these injuries are likely more common than reported because they are often difficult to detect (60). Lateral and anterior arc fractures tend to occur along the inner cortex of the rib. Costochondral junc-

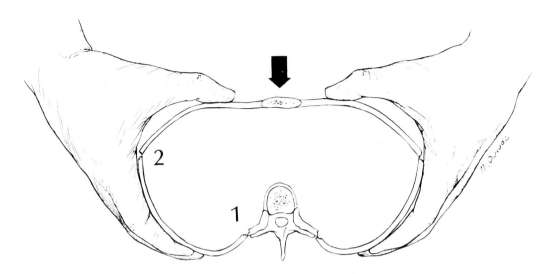

FIG. 7.11. With anteroposterior compression of the chest, rib fractures occur initially in the proximal rib over the transverse process of the adjacent vertebrae (*1*) and more laterally along the posterior arc of the rib to the midaxillary line (*2*).

tion fractures are usually bilateral and symmetric and tend to involve the sixth through ninth ribs (90). Costochondral junction fractures impact along the inner aspect of the osteochondral interface with an osseous fragment analogous to metaphyseal corner and bucket-handle fractures (69). These fractures are almost always associated with major intraabdominal injuries. Fracture of the first rib is less commonly seen in abused infants and may be due to impact force or acute axial load (slamming), producing an indirect fracture (123).

Whereas rib fractures are readily detected radiographically with healing and callus formation, acute nondisplaced rib fractures are difficult to identify (69). Costovertebral fractures may be subtle, appearing only as slight expansion of the head and neck of the rib (60). Asymmetry in the appearance of the ribs at the costovertebral junction may be the only radiographic evidence of fracture. In addition to the routine frontal and lateral thoracic views, in the skeletal survey, right and left posterior oblique views should be obtained to define further rib fractures identified on initial examination. Skeletal scintigraphy may contribute

to the detection of acute and healing rib fractures in abused children (21,45,118).

Fractures of the sternum are infrequently reported in abused infants and children (37,75). These injuries result from direct blows or violent compression of the thorax with sternal displacement at the sternomanubrial articulation or along the cartilaginous margins of the sternal ossification centers. When present, fractures of the sternum are pathognomonic of abuse (53). Detection requires careful inspection of the chest in the lateral projection.

Spine

Vertebral fractures are reportedly uncommon skeletal injuries with child abuse (4,31, 79,88). Personal experience and postmortem study of abused infants, however, suggest that these fractures are more common than reported previously (54). In most cases, vertebral fractures are asymptomatic and may go unrecognized without careful radiographic screening and scrutiny of the spine in lateral projection. Radionuclide scintigraphy can demonstrate fractures of the trans-

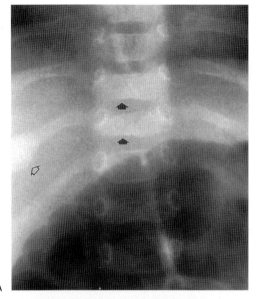

A

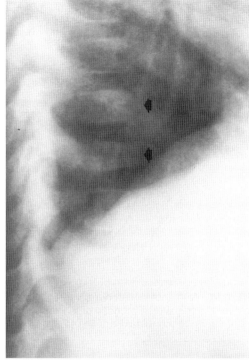

B

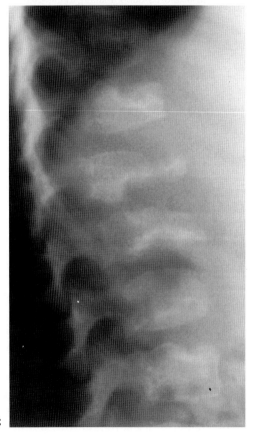

C

FIG. 7.12. Frontal **(A)** and lateral **(B)** views of the thoracolumbar spine show anterior compression of the tenth and eleventh thoracic vertebrae (*solid arrows*). Also evident is a healing fracture of the right seventh rib at the costovertebral junction (*open arrow*). **C:** Lateral view of a 5-year-old child with history of abuse in infancy shows anterior deformity of the vertebral bodies at multiple levels, reflecting old vertebral fracture.

verse and spinous processes, but it is relatively insensitive for vertebral body fractures.

Most inflicted spinal injuries occur in the lower thoracic and upper lumbar vertebrae, at the apex of an acute kyphotic angle resulting from hyperflexion (23,30,57,75,126). Occasionally, there may be a fracture/dislocation of the thoracolumbar spine with cord compression (26). Reports of fracture and/or ligamentous injury to the cervical vertebrae are rare, although spinal injuries in abused infants are presumably a result of violent shaking (65). Evidence exists, however, that cervical cord injuries may occur more frequently in shaken infants than previously recognized (36,65, 107). Prevertebral soft tissue swelling may be the only radiographic evidence of significant spinal injury. The craniocervical junction and upper cervical spine should be thoroughly evaluated with MRI in any shaken infant with an intracranial injury.

Variable anterior compression deformity of the vertebral body is usually present (Fig. 7.12A). The three histologic–radiographic patterns of vertebral body fracture are (a) pure compression of the anterior half of the vertebral body without disruption of the end plate; (b) compression fractures with extension into the end plate; and (c) combined lesions (54). The vertebral end plates are analogous to the metaphyseal–epiphyseal complex of the long bone, and end-plate injury often results in significant growth disturbance and persistent vertebral deformity (Fig. 7.12B) (136). More violent hyperflexion may be associated with disk rupture and herniation along the anterior margin or the anterior inferior margin of the vertebral end plates, resulting in a notched appearance. Uniform vertebral body compression is unusual in abused infants and should suggest weakened bone associated with intrinsic skeletal disease.

Injuries to the posterior vertebral elements most frequently involve the spinous process. These fractures are again related to severe hyperflexion and occur most frequently at or around the thoracolumbar junction (57). These fractures may be solitary or multiple,

and appear to result from avulsion of cartilage and/or bone at the attachments of the interspinous ligaments.

Skull

Cranial fractures are the second most common skeletal injury in abused children (88). The presence of a skull fracture indicates direct impact either from a blow to the head, or the rapidly moving head of a shaken baby brought up against a static object. Skull fractures are classified radiographically as simple nondisplaced linear fractures involving a single calvarial bone or complex multiple fracture lines (eggshell fractures), which may be displaced, comminuted, or widened (diastatic) (Fig. 7.13). Depressed skull fractures are uncommon in abused in-

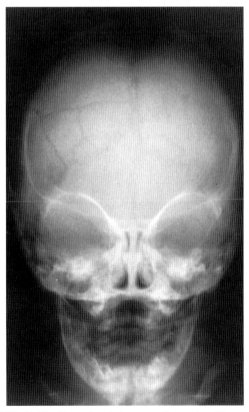

FIG. 7.13. Complex right posterior parietal "eggshell" fracture.

fants and young children, perhaps reflecting the inherent plasticity of the infant skull (88,89). The pattern of skull fractures as well as inconsistencies between the observed fracture and the alleged mechanisms of injury may be instrumental in confirming child abuse (110). Some investigators have suggested that complex fractures are more common in abused children (42), although this possibility has not been borne out in other reports (66). Skull fractures rarely result from accidental falls from up to 3 ft (39,76,129), and when they do occur are linear and uncomplicated.

Radionuclide scintigraphy (bone scan) is insensitive in identifying abuse-related skull fractures. Any patient undergoing CT scanning for head trauma should have images obtained at bone window settings to examine for unsuspected fractures. Fractures occurring in the same plane or at a shallow obliquity to the CT cut, however, may be undetectable.

Facial fractures constitute only 2% of all intentional injuries (131), despite the frequency of injury to the soft tissues of the face in abused children. Most such reported injuries involve the mandible or, less commonly, the maxilla, and are found in older children.

DATING FRACTURES

The capacity to determine the age of skeletal injuries is important in documenting child abuse. Discrepancy between the age of fractures and the clinical history of injury is often the first indication of inflicted injury in abused children, and the presence of multiple fractures of different ages is evidence of repetitive inflicted injury. Although precise dating of fractures is impossible, it is usually possible to define a relatively narrow time frame in which the injury is likely to have occurred; in general, the longer from the time of injury, the more imprecise is the dating process (18).

Dating fractures is based on the radiographic appearance of the soft tissues, periosteum, fracture line, and callus formation (95). Although there are well-established criteria for dating fractures, important differences exist between the pathophysiology of abuse-related fractures relative to usual accidental fractures in children. These differences are (a) abuse-related fractures occur predominantly in the infant younger than 2 years; (b) the fractures often reflect multiple episodes of trauma rather than a single incident; and (c) frequent delay in recognition and treatment of fractures results in additional repetitive injury to the original fracture site. The timetable and radiographic appearance for repair of fractures varies with the age of the child as well as the site and severity of injury. In general, the younger the infant, the more rapid the healing process. Understanding the stages of healing and histopathologic responses associated with skeletal injury is important in accurate dating of fractures.

The first phase of healing (induction stage) extends from the moment of injury to the appearance of new bone in the area of the fracture. The initial inflammatory response is usually associated with pain and swelling: with nondisplaced fractures, the inflammatory reaction may last only a few days. These infants may show no discomfort as early as 1 to 2 days after injury. Radiographically, initial findings are soft tissue swelling with displacement and obliteration of normal fat and fascial planes, which gradually recedes over the next 3 to 7 days (Fig. 7.6). The initially sharp acute fracture line gradually becomes less well defined as healing progresses.

The second phase of healing (soft callus stage) begins with subperiosteal new bone formation approximately 7 to 10 days after injury in infants, and slightly later (10 to 14 days) in older children. Recurrent injury at the same site within hours after initial trauma will produce more hemorrhage, but healing will then proceed normally. However, with repetitive injury more than 7 days later, additional bleeding and disruption of subperiosteal new bone leads to florid and exuberant callus formation (19). Similarly, fracture instability is associated with exuberant subperiosteal new bone and callus formation around the fracture site.

The third phase of healing (hard callus stage) occurs when subperiosteal and endosteal bone begins to convert to lamellar bone. In children, particularly infants, the hard callus stage begins at 14 to 21 days at the earliest and peaks at 21 to 42 days. Radiographically, progressive solid union is noted at the fracture site.

The final phase (remodeling stage) begins with gradual restoration of bony configuration and correction of deformity. Remodeling begins at 3 months, with a peak at ages 1 to 2 years.

The classic metaphyseal fractures of child abuse pose a special diagnostic problem in radiologic dating of fracture. Unlike diaphyseal fractures with subperiosteal hemorrhage and new bone formation, metaphyseal fractures most frequently do not disrupt the tightly adherent periosteum, and subperiosteal new bone formation will be absent or produce only a haziness of the adjacent cortex (19). More pronounced periosteal reaction is usually associated with periosteal shearing and/or more extensive injury to the metaphysis and displacement of the metaphyseal fragment (58). Radiologic–histopathologic studies have shown that healing of usual metaphyseal fractures is characterized histologically by significant thickening of the zone of hypertrophic cartilage in the physis, with extension of chondrocytes into the calcified primary spongiosa that may be detected radiographically as a radiolucent extension into the adjacent metaphysis (58). Because the relative rates of physeal growth of individual long bones are known, it may be possible to estimate more accurately the minimal age of a metaphyseal fracture based on radiologic appearance (98). Healing of metaphyseal fractures may also present radiographically with a sclerotic band as endosteal callus obscures the fracture line (19).

DIFFERENTIAL DIAGNOSIS

Before the diagnosis of nonaccidental injury as a result of child abuse can be estab-

lished, consideration must be given to possible preexisting medical conditions that may predispose structurally weak bones to injury with normal handling or minor trauma, and to disorders that may produce skeletal abnormalities that mimic the radiographic manifestations of inflicted trauma (Table 7.2) (12,37, 104,105). Although these conditions are the exception rather than the rule, they must be excluded before establishing the diagnosis of child abuse. Careful clinical and radiologic evaluation usually permits accurate differentiation of skeletal abnormalities associated with these conditions from the skeletal injuries of child abuse.

TABLE 7.2. *Child abuse: The differential diagnosis of skeletal injury*

Obstetric trauma
Prematurity
Nutritional/metabolic disorders
  Scurvy
  Rickets
  Renal osteodystrophy/secondary
   hyperparathyroidism
  Menkes' syndrome
Drug-induced toxicity
  Methotrexate
  Prostaglandin E
  Hypervitaminosis A
Infection
  Osteomyelitis
  Congenital syphilis
Neuromuscular defect
  Spinal dysraphism (myelodysplasia)
  Cerebral palsy
  Congenital insensitivity to pain
Neoplasm
  Leukemia
  Metastatic (neuroblastoma)
  Langerhans cell histiocytosis (histiocytosis X)
Accidental trauma
  Toddler fracture
Normal variant
  Physiologic periosteal new bone (infancy)
  Ossification center (acromial process)
Skeletal dysplasia
  Osteogenesis imperfecta
  Schmid/Schmid-like metaphyseal
   chondrodysplasia
  Metaphyseal dysostosis (Jansen type)
  Spondylometaphyseal chondrodysplasia
   (corner fracture type)
Miscellaneous
  Infantile cortical hyperostosis (Caffey disease)

Obstetric Trauma

Breech and other traumatic deliveries are a well-recognized cause of skeletal injuries in otherwise healthy neonates (22,27,82,84). Clavicular and humeral fractures occur most commonly with birth trauma. Both diaphyseal and metaphyseal fractures occur with the latter and are usually associated with breech positioning and difficult extraction. Congenital neuromuscular disorders, such as arthrogryposis, that are associated with contractures also may result in fractures in an otherwise uncomplicated delivery; fractures in such infants most frequently involve the lower extremities. Rib fractures are rarely the result of birth trauma, although they have been reported in at least one case with thoracic compression during midforceps delivery of a large neonate (less than 4,000 g) (106). Obstetric fractures heal rapidly with early callus formation.

Prematurity

The delicate osteopenic bones of premature infants are at increased risk for fractures during normal handling. In addition, acquired nutritional deficiencies and infections also contribute to bone fragility. Long-bone fractures and rib fractures are most frequently observed. Skeletal injuries in the premature infant are usually not clinically evident. The parent or caretaker during passive exercises may also inflict fractures (40).

Nutritional and Metabolic Disorders

Certain acquired nutritional deficiencies as well as inborn metabolic errors may have skeletal manifestations suggestive of abuse-related injuries.

Scurvy is a rare disorder in our modern world, although sporadic cases continue to be reported (43). Children with scurvy present with painful swollen limbs associated with radiographic evidence of extensive periosteal new bone formation as well as metaphyseal irregularity (Fig. 7.14). Fracture–separation of the distal femoral epiphysis may occur, reflecting the fibrous deficiency. The presence of a dense ring around an otherwise hyperlucent epiphysis (Wimberger's ring) is a typical finding in children with scurvy.

Rickets is associated with metaphyseal irregularity and splaying, widening of the physis, and occasional pseudofractures (Milkman fracture) (100). Periosteal reaction and new bone formation is common and occasionally is extensive (Fig. 7.15). The generalized distribution and symmetric pattern of skeletal involvement are distinguishing features of rickets.

Menkes' kinky hair syndrome is a rare congenital defect of copper metabolism associ-

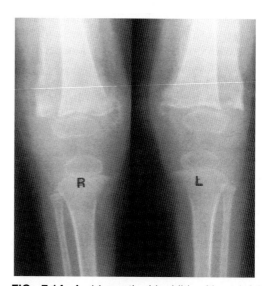

FIG. 7.14. A 14-month-old child with painful swelling of both legs has symmetric lateral dislocation of both femoral epiphyses with extensive periosteal new bone cloaking the distal femurs. The bones are generally demineralized with thin cortices. The growth plates are not widened, and the metaphyses are generally smooth. Dense zones of provisional calcification are evident. The femoral and tibial epiphyses are normally developed but have a relatively dense peripheral ossific rim (Wimberger's ring). (Courtesy of J.C. Hoeffel, Hôpital Jeanne D'Arc, Dommartin les Toul, France.)

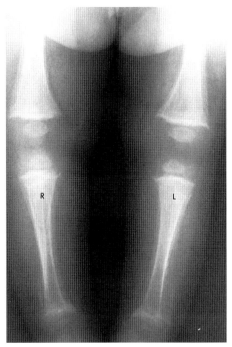
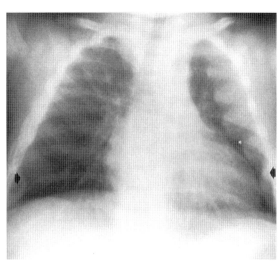

A   B

FIG. 7.15. A 6-month-old infant had failure to thrive because of intestinal malabsorption. The long bones **(A)** show generalized coarse demineralization with symmetric flaring and irregularity of the femoral and tibial metaphyses and periosteal new bone along the shafts of the long bones. The chest **(B)** also shows generalized skeletal demineralization with periosteal reaction and anterior enlargement of the ribs at the costochondral junction (rachitic rosary) (*arrows*).

ated with metaphyseal fractures and periosteal reaction, indistinguishable from abuse-related fractures. The presence of sparse "kinky" hair, calvarial wormian bones, anterior rib flaring, along with failure to thrive and developmental retardation, are distinguishing features of this condition.

Other congenital metabolic disorders such as mucolipidosis II (I-cell disease) may have radiographic features suggestive of abuse-related fractures. Again, the clinical and radiographic features suggest the correct diagnosis.

Drug-Induced Toxicity

A variety of therapeutic agents induce toxic osteopathies that resemble abuse-related lesions. The correct diagnosis is based on history of drug therapy.

Methotrexate therapy may be associated with an osteopathic condition characterized by periosteal reaction and impaction fractures of the metaphyses. Generalized and severe osteopenia is a prominent distinguishing feature of methotrexate toxicity.

Prostaglandin E therapy and hypervitaminosis A are associated with diaphyseal periostitis that may mimic skeletal trauma (Fig. 7.16). In addition, acute vitamin A toxicity results in increased intracranial pressure and sutural diastasis. A history of unusual vitamin intake or dietary habits and elevated serum vitamin A levels is diagnostic.

Infection

Osteomyelitis can result in metaphyseal irregularities and periosteal new bone growth that mimics metaphyseal and other fractures

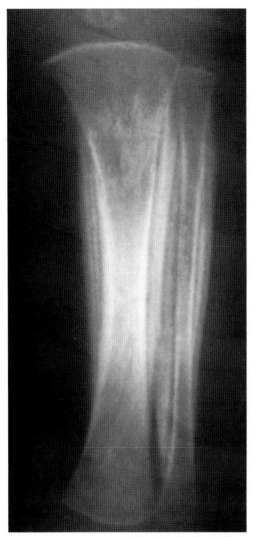

FIG. 7.16. A 3-month-old infant with congenital heart disease receiving prostaglandin E therapy has symmetric, uniform tibial and fibular diaphyseal periostitis. The metaphyses appear normal with smooth chondroosseous junctions.

in infancy. Involvement of the physis in meningococcal infection may result in shortening of affected limbs that is identical to long-term abuse-related traumatic sequelae.

Congenital syphilis usually manifests between ages 1 and 6 months with diffuse osteomyelitis that is characterized by symmetric metaphyseal irregularities and diaphyseal fractures associated with extensive diaphyseal periostitis resembling traumatic lesions (81). The diagnosis is suggested by the presence of focal erosion on the medial aspect of the proximal tibia (Wimberger sign) and is confirmed by serologic testing.

Neuromuscular Defects

Infants and children with a variety of congenital and acquired neuromuscular defects are at increased risk for accidental skeletal trauma. Spinal dysraphism and cerebral palsy are frequently associated with diffuse osteoporosis and contractures of the lower extremities. In such cases, fractures of the metaphysis and diaphysis may occur with routine handling or during physical therapy (13,40). Fracture risk is greatly exacerbated by cast immobilization, especially in patients undergoing surgery for hip subluxation. This surgery is often followed by body cast (spica cast) immobilization. This provides a stable environment for healing of the hip subluxation but leads to joint stiffness and increased osteoporosis. Experience suggests one in five of these patients will evidence a lower extremity fracture within 3 months of cast removal (124). Neurogenic sensory deficit with decreased or absent pain perception may result in nondisplaced fractures that go undetected for prolonged periods (35). As a result, these fractures lead to abundant callus formation. Given that these children are also at increased risk for child abuse because of their handicaps (32), it is essential to consider the possibility of maltreatment in any handicapped infant or child with unexplained fractures. Careful medical and social evaluation as well as strong family support is required in such situations.

Congenital insensitivity to pain is a neurologic syndrome associated with bizarre skeletal lesions (114). Radiographically, multiple fractures in different stages of repair in the absence of the history of trauma may at times be difficult to distinguish from child abuse (119). Careful clinical history and neurologic sensory examination will establish the correct diagnosis.

Skeletal Dysplasia

Osteogenesis imperfecta (OI) is an inherited disorder of connective tissue with deficiency of type I collagen leading to abnormal bone formation and increased bone fragility. As a result, trivial injuries may cause fractures in these patients (see also Chapter 9). Of all the various conditions invoked by parents and their legal representatives to explain inflicted fractures, OI is cited most frequently. It is therefore essential to be familiar with the classification of OI and the features that distinguish it from child abuse (2).

The simple classification of OI into congenita and tarda types fails to consider the complex and heterogeneous nature of this disorder. The current classification identifies OI as four major types, depending on age of onset of fractures, extraskeletal manifestations, and mode of inheritance (1). Infants with type I and II disease usually present no diagnostic problem and account for 80% of all cases of OI. Types I and II OI should not be confused with child abuse, because all children have blue sclerae and, with the exception of rare cases of type II OI with autosomal recessive or dominant new mutation inheritance, are autosomal dominant. Type II OI is lethal in the perinatal or neonatal period. Fractures associated with type I OI initially occur in the preschool period in most cases, although fractures may be seen in the neonate or at any time in childhood. Fractures heal at a normal rate, and their frequency declines after puberty. The bones are generally osteopenic within cortices. Rib fractures occur frequently. Bowing of the long bones of the lower extremities is characteristic, and wormian bones are present (Fig. 7.17). Stature is normal or near normal. Dentinogenesis imperfecta is variable, and children commonly have hearing loss or a family history of hearing impairment. By contrast, mild cases of type III and IV OI may be confused with child abuse. In both instances, sclerae may be normal, and with autosomal dominant new mutations, the family history of OI is negative. In type III OI, however, patients should have wormian bones and osteoporosis, which, along with other features of OI, should help identify the child with OI. Cases of OI IV pose greater diagnostic problems because skeletal involvement tends to be less severe than in type III disease. In these patients, however, a family history of wormian bones, osteoporosis, and characteristic clinical findings is often present. In rare cases of type IV OI, the potential for misdiagnosis exists. Given the rarity of this type of OI (1:1 to 3 million births), however, relative to the frequency of child abuse, the probability of error is minimal. It has been estimated that in a child younger than 1 year, with no family history and normal skull and teeth, the chance the fractures observed are related to type IV OI is less than 3 in a million (127). Although metaphyseal fractures may occur in OI, the onset is typically late in such children (8).

A variant form of OI, possibly related to a defect in copper metabolism, has been described as "temporary brittle bone disease," and has been proposed as a cause for multiple fractures including classic metaphyseal and rib fractures (20,25,101). However, the lack of clinical and laboratory data to support this work has called the validity of this proposal into question; and until scientific evidence firmly establishes the existence of this entity, it should remain strictly a hypothetical entity and not an acceptable medical diagnosis (3).

In most cases, accurate differentiation is possible based on correlation of data from the clinical history, physical examination, family history, and radiographic examination. In atypical cases, the availability of biochemical analysis of synthesis and structure may be instrumental in confirming the diagnosis of OI. This latter recourse is, however, rarely necessary, and routine dermal biopsy for children suspected to have been abused is unwarranted (51,120).

Unfortunately, children with OI also may be abused. In such cases, the diagnosis of child abuse may be made on the basis of fracture patterns typical of inflicted injury that are

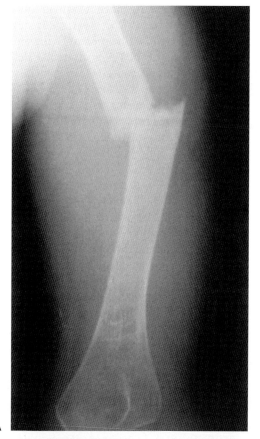

A

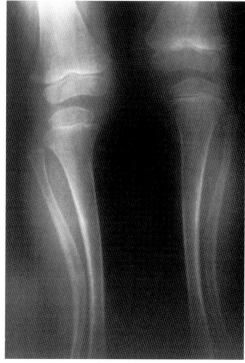

B

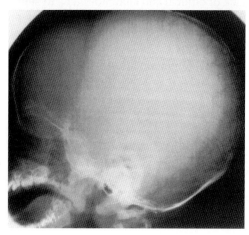

C

FIG. 7.17. An 18-month-old child with clinically short stature (osteogenesis imperfecta)
has a transverse fracture of the left humerus
(A) with symmetric tibial and fibular bowing
(B). The bones are generally demineralized
with thin cortices. The skull **(C)** shows multiple
sutural (wormian) bones.

inconsistent with the history and findings of the physical examination (74).

Schmid and Schmid-like metaphyseal chondrodysplasia is characterized by mild to moderate metaphyseal flaring, irregularity, and sclerosis, as well as by enlarged capital femoral epiphyses, coxa vara, and cupping of the anterior ribs (50).

Spondylometaphyseal dysplasia, corner fracture type, may also occur with metaphyseal fragmentation as part of the larger spectrum of dysplastic skeletal fractures (78). Similarly, Jansen-type metaphyseal dysostosis may manifest with metaphyseal irregularity and periosteal new bone resembling callus formation (37). Despite the striking similarity of the metaphyseal fragmentation in these patients to the abuse-related corner fracture pattern of metaphyseal injury, a misdiagnosis can be avoided if a careful family history is taken and a complete radiographic skeletal survey is obtained.

Neoplasm

Patients with leukemia and metastatic neuroblastoma can present with localized osteolytic lesions, periosteal new bone, and occasionally, pathologic fractures. In addition, the metaphyseal lucency that can be the initial skeletal manifestation of leukemia may be indistinguishable from incomplete or nondisplaced metaphyseal fractures. Nontraumatic leukemic lucencies are symmetric and generalized, however, and are noted without additional skeletal evidence of abuse (12). Careful clinical and hematologic evaluation will establish the diagnosis of neoplasm.

Langerhans cell histiocytosis (histiocytosis X) is a proliferative rather than a true neoplasm that occasionally is associated with long-bone or rib lesions complicated by an unsuspected pathologic fracture and periosteal new bone suggestive of child abuse. The diagnosis of histiocytosis is established by a complete radiographic skeletal survey with identification of appendicular and axial skeletal lesions that are typically lytic, without reactive sclerosis or periosteal reaction.

Accidental Trauma

Almost invariably, an incident or incidents of accidental trauma are described by the caretaker to explain the fractures and other injuries identified in cases of suspected or alleged child abuse. Frequent explanations include falls from bed or other pieces of furniture, dropping the infant, rough "play" by a parent or sibling, or being struck by a falling object (9,129). It would be useful in such cases to state that, based on scientific data, the fractures identified required a specific amount of biomechanical force to produce the observed injuries. With the exception of skull fractures, however, there is a paucity of experimental data relating to skeletal injuries in infants and children. With regard to skull fracture, the occurrence of fractures as a result of falls depends on the contact surface, drop height, and resultant gravitational force (g) (91). Some data indicate an increasing risk of skull fracture and concomitant intracranial injury with an impact force of greater than 50 g. A head-on fall to a concrete surface of 1 ft or more can generate an impact force of 160 g; at the same time, a 3-ft fall height is required to produce the same force with a packed dirt surface. Carpeted floors soften the impact even more.

Unfortunately, no such experimental data exist for appendicular and other axial skeletal injuries. Several reports, however, may prove helpful in determining the likelihood of extremity fracture occurring with accidental trauma (39,76,84,91). A study of 38 infants younger than 2 years with accidental falls from cribs (38 in.), beds (23 to 34 in.), and wagons (12 in.) showed that there were no appendicular or axial fractures other than a single simple skull fracture (91). Because most such falls are head first, variable soft tissue injury was limited to the head, and most children had no bruises or other cutaneous evidence of trauma. Another study of 81 children aged 5 years or younger with a fall height of 90 cm yielded similar results, with only one simple skull fracture and no appendicular fractures (39). It is evident from the results of these admittedly uncon-trolled studies that skeletal injuries in the pretoddler age (9 to 10 months) are rarely of accidental origin, and that any fracture in children in this age group must be given prompt and thorough evaluation for possible child abuse. It is equally evident that once the infant is ambulatory, the frequency of ac-cidental trauma resulting in skeletal injuries increases (133). Thus in the older infant and child with fractures that are not pathogno-monic of nonaccidental injury, differentia-tion between accidental and nonaccidental injury must be judged relative to the history of trauma and the patient's age, the presence or absence of other skeletal and nonskeletal injuries, and the child's general state of health. One suggested multidisciplinary ap-proach to distinguishing accidental from nonaccidental fractures is based on the use of established clinical and radiographic cri-teria for abuse-related injuries, an indepen-dent rating by the radiologist without clinical data, and a separate review by clinicians be-fore forming a consensus opinion (133). This retrospective analysis of clinical and radi-ographic data offers the potential for mini-mizing diagnostic errors resulting from busy outpatient clinics and emergency rooms as well as physician inexperience.

Normal Variant

Physiologic periosteal new bone is a reflec-tion of normal skeletal growth that appears along the shafts of the long bones in infants between ages 2 and 3 months and normally resolves by age 8 months: careful examina-tion of these areas is, however, necessary to exclude a coincidental fracture in abused in-fants (103,113). Metaphyseal spurring and cupping without fragmentation may also be seen in healthy infants and should not be con-fused with abuse-related fractures (63). In both cases, the radiographic changes are bilat-erally symmetric and are not associated with evidence of soft tissue injury.

Variation in the ossification of the scapular acromial process may also resemble an avul-sion fracture (56). These variants are localized to the inferior portion of the acromial process with well-defined margins, in contrast to acromial fractures, which frequently are asso-ciated with avulsive changes in the adjacent clavicle and abundant callus formation.

Miscellaneous

Infantile cortical hyperostosis (Caffey's disease) is an unusual condition of unknown etiology that is seen only rarely today. These infants, from ages 3 to 6 months, present with swollen, painful extremities, the appearance of chronic illness, and exuberant diaphyseal periostitis suggestive of child abuse. Absence of metaphyseal involvement and the presence of periosteal reaction involving the mandible establish the correct diagnosis.

SKELETAL INJURIES AS EVIDENCE OF CHILD ABUSE

If expert medical testimony is to be effec-tive in the documentation of abuse and subse-quent prosecution of the abusers, physicians and allied medical personnel must be able and willing to use radiographic and other findings of skeletal as well as nonskeletal trauma as evidence of inflicted injury. All too often, wit-nesses in legal proceedings in civil or criminal cases of child abuse are reticent when pre-senting radiographic evidence under oath. Al-though it is not possible to differentiate acci-dental from inflicted injuries in every case of suspected child abuse, there are patterns of in-jury and certain fracture types that are either pathognomonic or strongly suggestive of nonaccidental injury (Table 7.3). Although caution is important, the expert witness must unequivocally describe the presence and diag-nostic characteristics of skeletal injuries as evidence of child abuse (94).

Specific skeletal injuries that permit a de-finitive diagnosis of nonaccidental injury and abuse include metaphyseal–epiphyseal com-plex, thoracic, shoulder girdle, and vertebral fractures. The mechanical forces required to produce these fractures are not generated by

TABLE 7.3. *Specificity of skeletal injuries as evidence of child abuse[a]*

Specific fractures
  Metaphyseal–epiphyseal (<2 years of age)
  Thoracic cage
    Rib
    Sternum
  Shoulder
    Scapula
  Clavicle
    Medial (sternoclavicular)
    Lateral (acromioclavicular)
  Spine
    Vertebral body (anterior compression)
    Spinous process
Highly suggestive fractures/patterns
  Multiple: bilateral, symmetric
  Repetitive/different age
  Hands and feet
  Skull, complex fracture line
  Associated nonskeletal injury; intracranial, visceral
Nonspecific fractures
  Diaphyseal (shaft of long bone)
  Clavicular, midshaft
  Skull, linear

[a]In otherwise healthy infant/child without major trauma (i.e., vehicular)

simple accidental falls and normal handling in an otherwise healthy infant and child.

Other fracture patterns are highly suggestive of abuse and increase in specificity when there is a lack of adequate clinical history of trauma relative to the observed injuries. Included in these highly suggestive fractures are occult skeletal injuries; fractures inconsistent with accidental trauma given the age of the infant or history provided by caretakers; multifocal fractures of different ages, indicating repetitive episodes of trauma; or a pattern of concurrent skeletal and nonskeletal injuries.

Finally, some nonspecific fractures occur as the result of accidental trauma and are not by themselves specific evidence of abuse. Nonspecific fractures include single diaphyseal fractures of long bones, linear skull fractures, and midclavicular shaft fractures. To distinguish between accidental and inflicted injuries, these fractures must be considered within the context of patient age, history of trauma (or lack thereof), radiographic evidence of additional fractures, and other clinical findings suggestive of abuse (18).

REFERENCES

1. Ablin DS, Greenspan A, Reinhart M, et al. Differentiation of child abuse from osteogenesis imperfecta. *Am J Roentgenol* 1990;154:1035–1046.
2. Ablin DS. Osteogenesis imperfecta: a review. *Can Assoc Radiol J* 1998;49:110–123.
3. Ablin DS, Sane SM. Non-accidental injury: confusion with temporary brittle bone disease and mild osteogenesis imperfecta. *Pediatr Radiol* 1997;27:111–113.
4. Akbarnia BA, Akbarnia NO. The role of orthopedists in child abuse and neglect. *Orthop Clin North Am* 1976;7:733–742.
5. Akbarnia B, Torg JS, Kirkpatrick J, et al. Manifestations of the battered-child syndrome. *J Bone Joint Surg Am* 1974;56:1159–1166.
6. American College of Radiology. *ACR standards, standards for skeletal surveys in children.* Reston, VA: ACR, 1997:47–50.
7. Anderson WA. The significance of femoral fractures in children. *Ann Emerg Med* 1982;11:174–177.
8. Astley R. Metaphyseal fractures in osteogenesis imperfecta. *Br J Radiol* 1979;52:441–442.
9. Beals RK, Tufts E. Fractured femur in infancy: the role of child abuse. *J Pediatr Orthop* 1983;3:583–586.
10. Berdon WE. Battered children: how valuable are bone scans in diagnosis [Editorial]. *Appl Radiol* 1981;981.
11. Bergman AB, Larsen RM, Mueller BA. Changing spectrum of serious child abuse. *Pediatrics* 1986;3:113–116.
12. Brill PW, Winchester P, Kleinman PK. Differential diagnosis I: diseases simulating abuse. In: Kleinman PK, ed. *Diagnostic imaging of child abuse.* 2nd ed. St. Louis: Mosby, 1998:178–196.
13. Brunner R, Doderlein L. Pathological fractures in patients with cerebral palsy. *J Pediatric Orthop Br* 1996;5:232–238.
14. Caffey J. The parent-infant traumatic stress (Caffey-Kempe, syndrome battered babe) syndrome. *Am J Roentgenol* 1972;114:217–229.
15. Caffey J. Traumatic cupping of the metaphysis of growing bones. *Am J Roentgenol* 1970;108:451–460.
16. Caffey J. Multiple fractures in the long bones of infants suffering from chronic subdural hematoma. *Am J Roentgenol* 1946;56:163–173.
17. Cameron JM, Rae LJ. *Atlas of the battered child syndrome.* Edinburgh: Churchill Livingstone, 1975;20–77.
18. Carty HM. Fractures caused by child abuse. *J Bone Joint Surg Br* 1993;75:849–857.
19. Chapman S. The radiological dating of injuries. *Arch Dis Child* 1992;67:1063–1065.
20. Chapman S, Hall CM. Non-accidental injury or brittle bones. *Pediatr Radiol* 1997;27:106–110.
21. Conway JJ, Collins M, Tanz RR, et al. The role of bone scintigraphy in detecting child abuse. *Semin Nucl Med* 1993;23:321–333.
22. Cumming WA. Neonatal skeletal fractures: birth trauma or child abuse. *Can Assoc Radiol J* 1979;30:30–33.
23. Cullen JC. Spinal lesions in battered babies. *J Bone Joint Surg Br* 1975;17:364–366.
24. DeLee JG, et al. Fracture-separation of the distal humeral epiphysis. *J Bone Joint Surg Am* 1980;62:46–51.
25. Dent JA, Patterson CR. Fractures in early childhood:

osteogenesis imperfecta or child abuse? *J Pediatr Orthop* 1991;11:1984–1991.

26. Diamond P, Hansen CM, Christoferson MR. Child abuse presenting as a thoracolumbar spinal fracture dislocation: a case report. *Pediatr Emerg Care* 1994; 10:83–86.

27. Ekengren K, Bergdahl S, Ekstrom G. Birth injuries to the epiphyseal cartilage. *Acta Radiol* 1978;19:197–204.

28. Ellerstein NS, Norris KJ. The value of radiologic skeletal survey in assessment of abused children. *Pediatrics* 1984;74:1075–1078.

29. Feldman KW, Brewer DK. Child abuse, cardiopulmonary resuscitation and rib fractures. *Pediatrics* 1984;73:339–342.

30. Gabos PG, Tuten HR, Leet A, et al. Fracture-dislocation of the lumbar spine in an abused child. *Pediatrics* 1998;101:473–477.

31. Galleno H, Oppenheim WL. The battered child syndrome revisited. *Clin Orthop* 1982;162:11-19.

32. Gelles RJ. Child abuse and developmental disabilities. In: *Child abuse in developmental disabilities.* Washington, DC: DHEW Publication No. (OH-DS) 79030226, 1980:25–31.

33. Graif M, Sonntag VK, Rekate HL, et al. Sonographic detection of occult bone fractures. *Pediatr Radiol* 1988;18:383–385.

34. Gross RH, Stranger M. Causative factors responsible for femoral fractures in infants and young children. *J Pediatr Orthop* 1983;3:341–343.

35. Gypes MT, Newborn DH, Neuhauser EBD. Metaphyseal and physeal injuries in children with spina bifida and meningomyeloceles. *Am J Roentgenol* 1965;95: 168–177.

36. Hadley MN, Sonntag VK, Rekate HL, et al. The infant whiplash-shake syndrome: a clinical and pathological study. *Neurosurgery* 1989;24:536–540.

37. Haller JO, Kassner EG. The "battered child" syndrome and its imitators: a critical evaluation of specific radiological signs. *Appl Radiol* 1977;6:88–111.

38. Hedlund R, Lindgren U. The incidence of femoral shaft fractures in children and adolescents. *J Pediatr Orthop* 1986;6:47–50.

39. Helfer RE, Slovis TL, Black M. Injuries resulting when small children fall out of bed. *Pediatrics* 1977; 60:533–535.

40. Helfer RE, Scheurer SL, Alexander R, et al. Trauma to the bones of small infants from passive exercise: a factor in the etiology of child abuse. *J Pediatr* 1984;104:47–50.

41. Herndon WA. Child abuse in a military population. *J Pediatr Orthop* 1983;3:73–76.

42. Hobbs CJ. Skull fracture and the diagnosis of abuse. *Arch Dis Child* 1984;59:246–252.

43. Hoeffel JC, et al. Fracture separation of the epiphysis and scurvy. Congress of European Society of Pediatric Radiology, Budapest, Hungary, 1992.

44. Howard JL, Barron DJ, Smith GG. Bone scintigraphy in the evaluation of extra skeletal injuries from child abuse. *Radiographics* 1990,10.67 81.

45. Jaudes PK. Comparison of radiography and radionuclide bone scanning in the detection of child abuse. *Pediatrics* 1984;73:166–168.

46. Jaudes PK, Diamond LJ. The handicapped child and child abuse. *Child Abuse Negl* 1985;9:341–347.

47. Kahana T, Hiss J. Forensic radiology. *Br J Radiol* 1999;72:129–133.

48. Kempe CH, Silverman FN, Steele BF, et al. The battered child syndrome. *JAMA* 1962;181:17–24.

49. King J, et al. Analysis of 429 fractures in 189 battered children. *J Pediatr Orthop* 1988;8:585–589.

50. Kleinman PK. Schmid-like metaphyseal chondrodysplasia simulating child abuse. *Am J Roentgenol* 1991; 156:576.

51. Kleinman PK. Differentiation of child abuse and osteogenesis imperfecta: medical and legal implications. *Am J Roentgenol* 1990;154:1047–1048.

52. Kleinman PK. Diagnostic imaging in infant abuse. *Am J Roentgenol* 1990;155:703–713.

53. Kleinman PK. *Diagnostic imaging of child abuse.* St. Louis: Mosby, 1998;5–28.

54. Kleinman PK, Marks SC. Vertebral body fractures in child abuse: radiologic-histologic correlates. *Invest Radiol* 1992;27:715–722.

55. Kleinman PK, Merten DF. Section on radiology: diagnostic imaging of child abuse. *Pediatrics* 1991;87: 262–264.

56. Kleinman PK, Spevak MR. Variations in acromial ossification simulating infant abuse in victims of sudden infant death syndrome. *Radiology* 1991;180:85–86.

57. Kleinman PK, Zito JL. Avulsion of the spinal processes caused by infant abuse. *Radiology* 1984;151:389–391.

58. Kleinman PK, Marks SC Jr, Spevak MR, et al. Extension of growth-plate cartilage into the metaphysis: a sign of healing fracture in abused infants. *Am J Roentgenol* 1991;156:775.

59. Kleinman PK, Blackbourne BD, Marks SC, et al. Radiologic contributions to the investigation and prosecution of cases of fatal infant abuse. *N Engl J Med* 1989;320:507.

60. Kleinman PK, Marks SC, Adams VI, et al. Factors affecting visualization of posterior rib fractures in abused infants. *Am J Roentgenol* 1988;150:635–638.

61. Kleinman PK, Mars SC, Blackburne B. The metaphyseal lesion in abused infants: a radiologic histopathologic study. *Am J Roentgenol* 1986;146:895.

62. Kleinman PK, et al. Diagnostic performance of modern radiographic imaging systems in the detection of inflicted skeletal injury in infancy. *Am J Roentgenol* 1997;168(suppl):127.

63. Kleinman PK, Belanger PL, Karaellas A, et al. Normal metaphyseal variants not to be confused with findings of child abuse. *Am J Roentgenol* 1991;156:781–783.

64. Kleinman PK, Marks SC Jr. A regional approach to the class metaphyseal lesion in abused infants: the distal femur. *Am J Roentgenol* 1998;170:43–47.

65. Kleinman PK, Shelton YA. Hangman's fracture in an abused infant: imaging features. *Pediatr Radiol* 1997; 27:776–777.

66. Kleinman PK, Schlesinger AE. Mechanical factors associated with posterior rib fractures: laboratory and case studies. *Pediatr Radiol* 1997;27:87–91.

67. Kleinman PK, Marks SC Jr. A regional approach to the classic metaphyseal lesion in abused infants: the proximal humerus. *Am J Roentgenol* 1996;167:1399–1403.

68. Kleinman PK, Nimkin K, Spevak MR, et al. Follow-up skeletal surveys in suspected child abuse. *Am J Roentgenol* 1996;167:893–896.

69. Kleinman PK, Marks SC Jr, Nimkin K, et al. Rib fractures in 31 abused infants: postmortem radiologic-histopathologic study. *Radiology* 1996;200:807–810.

70. Kleinman PK, Marks SC Jr, Richmond JM, et al. In-

flicted skeletal injury: a postmortem radiologic-histopathologic study in 31 infants. *Am J Roentgenol* 1995;165:647–650.

71. Kleinman PK, Marks SC Jr. A regional approach to classic metaphyseal lesions in abused infants: the distal tibia. *Am J Roentgenol* 1996;166:1207–1212.

72. Kleinman PK, Marks SC Jr. A regional approach to the classic metaphyseal lesion in abused infants: the proximal tibia. *Am J Roentgenol* 1996;166:421–426.

73. Kleinman PK, Marks SC Jr. Relationship of the subperiosteal bone collar to metaphyseal lesions in abused infants. *J Bone Joint Surg Am* 1995;77:1471–1476.

74. Knight DJ, Bennett GC. Non-accidental injury and osteogenesis imperfecta: a case report. *J Pediatr Orthop* 1990;10:542–544.

75. Kogutt MS, Swischuk LE, Fagen CJ. Patterns of injury and significance of uncommon fractures in the battered-child syndrome. *Am J Roentgenol* 1974;121:143–149.

76. Kravitz H, Dreissen G, Gomberg R, et al. Accidental falls from elevated surfaces in infants from birth to one year. *Pediatrics* 1969;44(suppl):867–876 .

77. Krishnan J, Barbour PJ, Foster BK. Patterns of osseous injuries and psychosocial factors affecting victims of child abuse. *Aust N Z J Surg* 1990;60:447–450.

78. Langer LO Jr, Brill PW, Ozonoff MB, et al. Spondylometaphyseal dysplasia, corner fracture type: a heritable condition associated with coxa-vara. *Radiology* 1990;175:761–766.

79. Leonidas JC. Skeletal trauma in the child abuse syndrome. *Pediatr Ann* 1983;12:875–882.

80. Leventhal JM, Thomas SA, Rosenfield NS, et al. Fractures in young children: distinguishing child abuse from unintentional injuries. *Am J Dis Child* 1993;147:87–92.

81. Lim HK, Smith WL, Sato Y, et al. Congenital syphilis mimicking child abuse. *Pediatr Radiol* 1995;25:560–561.

82. McBride MT, Hennrikus WL, Mologne T. Newborn clavicle fractures. *Orthopedics* 1998;17:317–320.

83. Mellick LB, Reesor K. Spiral tibial fractures of children: a commonly accidental spiral long bone fracture. *Am J Emerg Med* 1990;8:234–237.

84. McClelland CQ, Heiple KG. Fractures in the first year of life: a diagnostic dilemma? *Am J Dis Child* 1982;136:26–29.

85. Merten DF. The battered child syndrome: the role of radiological imaging. *Pediatr Ann* 1983;12:867–868.

86. Merten DF, Carpenter BLM. Radiologic imaging of inflicted injury in the child abuse syndrome. *Pediatr Clin North Am* 1990;37:815–837.

87. Merten DF, Kirks DR, Ruderman RJ. Occult humeral epiphyseal fracture in battered infants. *Pediatr Radiol* 1981;10:151–153.

88. Merten DF, Radkowski MA, Leonidas JC. The abused child: a radiological reappraisal. *Radiology* 1983;146:377–381.

89. Merten DF, Osborne DR, Radkowski MA, et al. Craniocerebral trauma in the child abuse syndrome: radiological observations. *Pediatr Radiol* 1984;14:272–277.

90. Ng CS, Hall CM. Costochondral junction fracture and intraabdominal trauma in non-accidental injury (child abuse). *Pediatr Radiol* 1998;28:671–676.

91. Nimituyongskul T, Anderson LD. The likelihood of injuries when children fall out of bed. *J Pediatr Orthop* 1987;7:184–186.

92. Nimkin K, Kleinman PK, Teeger S, et al. Distal humeral physeal injuries in child abuse: MR imaging and ultrasonography findings. *Pediatr Radiol* 1995;25:562–565.

93. Nimkin K, Spevak MR, Kleinman PK. Fractures of the hands and feet in child abuse: imaging and pathologic features. *Radiology* 1997;203:233–236.

94. Norman MG, Smialek JE, Newman DE, et al. The post-mortem examination of the abused child: pathological, radiographic and legal aspects. *Perspect Pediatr Pathol* 1984;8:313–343.

95. O'Connor JF, Cohen J. Dating fractures. In: Kleinman PK, ed. *Diagnostic imaging of child abuse.* 2nd ed. St. Louis: Mosby, 1998:168–177.

96. Ogden JA. Injury to the growth mechanisms of the immature skeleton. *Skeletal Radiol* 1981;6:237–253.

97. O'Neill JA Jr, et al. Patterns of injury in the battered-child syndrome. *J Trauma* 1973;13:332–339.

98. Osier LK, Marks SC Jr, Kleinman PK. Metaphyseal extensions of hypertrophied chondrocytes in abused infants indicate healing fractures. *J Pediatr Orthop* 1998;13:249–254.

99. Oudjhane K. Occult fractures in preschool children. *J Trauma* 1988;28:858–860.

100. Patterson CR. Vitamin D deficiency rickets simulating child abuse. *J Pediatr Orthop* 1981;1:823–825.

101. Patterson CR, Burns J, McAllion SJ. Osteogenesis imperfecta: the distinction from child abuse and recognition of a variant form. *Am J Med Genet* 1993;45:187–192.

102. Pendergast NC, deRoux SJ, Adsay NV. Non-accidental pediatric pelvic fracture: a case report. *Pediatr Radiol* 1998;28:344–346.

103. Pergolizzi R Jr, Oestreich AE. Child abuse fracture through physiologic periosteal reaction. *Pediatr Radiol* 1995;25:566–567.

104. Radkowski MA. The battered child syndrome: pitfalls in radiological diagnosis. *Pediatr Ann* 1983;12:894–903.

105. Radkowski MA, Merten DF, Leonidas JC. The abused child: criteria for the radiologic diagnosis. *Radiographics* 1983;3:262–297.

106. Rizzolo PJ, Coleman PR. Neonatal rib fracture: birth trauma or child abuse. *J Fam Pract* 1989;29:561–563.

107. Rooks VJ, Sisler C, Burton B. Cervical spine injury in child abuse: report of two cases. *Pediatr Radiol* 1998;28:193–195.

108. Rossmuller B, Hahn K, Fischer S. Bone scintigraphy in non-neoplastic diseases in children. *Q J Nucl Med* 1998;42:133–147.

109. Roussey M, Le Francois MC, Le Marec B, et al. Cranial CT in child abuse. *Radiology* 1982;25:237–243.

110. Saulsbury FT, Alford BA. Intracranial bleeding from child abuse: the value of skull radiographs. *Pediatr Radiol* 1982;12:175–178.

111. Shand K. Epiphyseal separation of distal humeral epiphysis in an infant: a case report and review of literature. *J Trauma* 1974;14:521–526.

112. Shaw BA, Murphy KM, Shaw A, et al. Humerus shaft fractures in young children: accident or abuse? *J Pediatr Orthop* 1997;17:293–297.

113. Silverman FN. Unrecognized trauma in infants, the battered child syndrome, and the syndrome of Ambroise Tardieu. *Radiology* 1972;104:337–353.

114. Silverman FN, Gilder JJ. Congenital insensitivity to pain: a neurologic syndrome with bizarre skeletal lesions. *Radiology* 1959;72:176–190.

115. Silverman FN. The roentgen manifestations of unrecognized skeletal trauma in infants. *Am J Roentgenol* 1953;69:413–427.

116. Sinal SH, Stewart CD. Physical abuse in children: a review for orthopedic surgeons. *J South Orthop Assoc* 1998;7:264–276.

117. Singer J, Towbin R. Occult fractures in the production of gait disturbance in childhood. *Pediatrics* 1979;64:192–196.

118. Smith FW, Gilday DL, Ash JM, et al. Unsuspected costo-vertebral fractures demonstrated by bone scanning in the child abuse syndrome. *Pediatr Radiol* 1980;10:103–106.

119. Spencer JA, Grieve DK. Congenital indifference to pain mistaken for non-accidental injury. *Br J Radiol* 1990;63:308–310.

120. Steiner RD, Pepin M, Byers PH. Studies of collagen synthesis and structure in the differentiation of child abuse from osteogenesis imperfecta. *J Pediatr* 1996;128:542–547.

121. Stern L. The high risk infant and battering. In: *Child abuse in developmental disabilities:* essays. Washington: U.S. Department of Health, Education and Welfare (DHEW) Publication No. (OH-DS), 79–30226, 1980;20–24.

122. Strait RT, Siegal RM, Shapiro RA. Humeral fractures without obvious etiologies in children less than 3 years of age: when is it abuse? *Pediatrics* 1995;96:667–671.

123. Strouse PJ, Owings CL. Fractures of the first rib in child abuse. *Radiology* 1995;197:763–765.

124. Sturm PF, Almon BA, Christie BL. Femur fractures in institutionalized patients after hip spica immobilization. *J Pediatr Orthop* 1993;13:246–248.

125. Sty JR, Starshak RJ. The role of bone scintigraphy in the evaluation of the suspected abused child. *Radiology* 1983;146:369–375.

126. Swischuk LE. Spine and spinal cord trauma in the battered child syndrome. *Radiology* 1969;92:733–738.

127. Taitz LS. Child abuse and metabolic bone disease: are they often confused? *Br Med J* 1991;302:1244.

128. Tan TX, Gelfand MJ. Battered child syndrome: uncommon pelvic fractures detected by bone scintigraphy. *Clin Nucl Med* 1997;22:321–322.

129. Tarantino CA, Dowd MD, Murdock TC. Short vertical falls in infants. *Pediatr Emerg Care* 1999;15:5–8.

130. Tardieu A. Etude medio-legale sur les services et mauvais traitments exerces surdes enfants. *Ann Hyg Publ Med Leg* 1860;13:361–368.

131. Tate RJ. Facial injuries associated with the battered child syndrome. *Br J Oral Maxillofac Surg* 1971;9:41–45.

132. Tenebien M, Reed MH, Black GB. The toddler's fracture revisited. *Am J Emerg Med* 1990;8:208–211.

133. Thomas SA, Rosenfield NS, Leventhal JM, et al. Long bone fracture in young children: distinguishing accidental injuries from child abuse. *Pediatrics* 1991;88:471–476.

134. Thomsen TK, Elle B, Thomsen JL. Post-mortem radiological examination in infants: evidence of child abuse? *Forensic Sci Int* 1997;90:223–230.

135. Walker PL, Cook DC, Lambert PM. Skeletal evidence for child abuse: a physical anthropology perspective. *J Forensic Sci* 1997;42:196–207.

136. Wenger DR, Rokicki RR. Spinal deformity secondary to scar formation in a battered child: case report. *J Bone Joint Surg Am* 1978;60:847.

137. Worlock T, Stower M, Barbor P. Patterns of fractures in accidental and non-accidental injury in children: a comparative study. *Br Med J* 1986;293:100–102.

138. Youmans DC, Don S, Hildebolt C, et al. Skeletal surveys for child abuse: comparison of interpretation using digitized images and screen-film radiographs. *Am J Roentgenol* 1998;171:1415–1419.

8

Visceral Injury Manifestations of Child Abuse

Stephen Ludwig

Department of Pediatrics, University of Pennsylvania School of Medicine; and
The Children's Hospital of Philadelphia, Philadelphia, Pennsylvania

For many reasons, the visceral injuries that occur as the result of child abuse are the most lethal. Although head trauma accounts for the highest number of deaths, many head trauma victims survive their injuries. Abused children who sustain significant visceral trauma to the thoracic and abdominal organs frequently die before detection and treatment. These injuries are usually inflicted on young victims. There is often little chance or ability for the infant to prepare for or brace against the traumatic forces. Visceral injuries occur as the result of punching or kicking the child. In either situation, but particularly with kicking, tremendous forces are generated. Visceral injuries rarely produce immediately specific signs or symptoms that lead to prompt identification. Often there are no external signs because the traumatic forces are transmitted internally and leave no external markers. By the time the child develops hypotension and cardiovascular collapse and is brought to an emergency care facility, the assumption is made that there is a medical cause that requires standard cardiopulmonary resuscitation (CPR) rather than trauma resuscitation. Injury is often extensive, and recognition of it is often late; thus the lethality of visceral trauma is high.

This chapter explores the nature and extent of these injuries and focuses on the early identification with the hope that the outcome for this subgroup of abused children will be improved. Additionally, there is hope with the emergence of a number of pediatric trauma centers across the United States. The work of astute pediatric emergency physicians (32, 102) and pediatric surgeons (56) may make it possible for more of these children to survive so that the child abuse specialists will be able to advocate for their brighter futures.

INCIDENCE

Reported case series of children with all forms of trauma indicate that abdominal trauma is uncommon, but in a subgroup of those identified as having abdominal trauma, the data show an incidence of inflicted trauma of 4% to 15% (18,39,40,42,83,92,103,119, 120,124,125), depending on the site of data collection. Table 8.1 shows a listing of case series and the incidence of trauma ascribed to abuse. The estimates of inflicted trauma are conservative in any of these series, as there are cases of abuse that defy detection, as is known from the studies of all other forms of inflicted injury. Reviews of specific injury types [e.g., thoracic trauma (105), pancreatic trauma (4), liver trauma (118)] always reveal a definable but small segment of the cases due to an abuse etiology (Fig. 8.1). For example, O'Neill et al. (86) found an incidence of nine (8%) of 110 cases of abdominal trauma caused by abuse in a 1973 Nashville, Tennessee, series. Yammamoto (131) found that in a 1-year experience (1988) in Hawaii, with 4,623 trauma visits, only 77 involved the abdomen, and 31, the chest, and 201 of all injuries were thought to be abuse related.

TABLE 8.1. *Frequency of visceral injury due to child abuse in published literature*

Author	Year	Sample size	Injury type	Percentage abuse	Reference
O'Neill et al.	1973	9	Abdominal	—	86
Grisoni et al.	1984	12	Hepatic	10	41
Cooper et al.	1988	22	Abdominal	0.5	25
Ledbetter et al.	1988	156	Abdominal	11	65
Sivit et al.	1989	69	Abd/thoracic	20	11
Ng et al.	1997	12	Visceral	4	83
Yamamoto	1991	4,623	All trauma	4	13
Arkovitz et al.	1997	26	Pancreatic	19	4
Canty et al.	1999	79	Abdominal	19	19

Cooper et al. (25,26) surveyed 13,000 emergency department visits at two institutions in New York and Philadelphia and found 360 cases of abuse including 22 (6%) cases of major blunt abdominal trauma. Canty et al. (19) reported a large series of abdominal trauma cases collected over a 12-year period from a San Diego pediatric trauma center. The survey included 11,592 consecutive admissions from 1985 to 1997. There were 102 children with abdominal trauma. Twenty-three had penetrating trauma and 79 children blunt abdominal trauma. Of the 102 with abdominal trauma, 15 were victims of nonaccidental trauma. Based on a number of series over two to three decades, we can conclude that although abdominal and thoracic injuries occur infrequently (<1% of cases), there is a substantial frequency of abuse.

When analyzing the subgroup of fatal cases of trauma (12,50,70,114,129), the significance of abdominal and thoracic trauma becomes even more striking. Published series of child homicide cases invariably include a significant number of thoracoabdominal trauma episodes. The incidence of severe morbidity and mortality directly correlates with the interval between the time of trauma and the time when care is delivered. In abuse cases, this interval is usually prolonged, and thus the outcomes are poor.

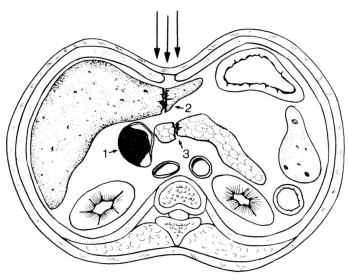

FIG. 8.1. Distribution of hollow viscous injuries. (From Kleinman PK. *Diagnostic imaging in child abuse.* Baltimore: Williams & Wilkins, 1987, with permission.)

In the study of Canty et al. (19), a period of 4 hours between traumatic event and identification was determined to be a significant predictor for increased mortality. Several studies documented the poorer outcome for abuse-related injuries as compared with similar severity injuries produced by noninflicted mechanisms.

CLINICAL PRESENTATION OF SPECIFIC INJURIES

The identification of inflicted visceral injury is difficult (31,45). There are several reasons for this, including the following:

1. Abuse victims are usually young and often unable to verbalize their complaints.
2. Children rarely expect and protect themselves from the traumatic force.
3. The traumatic force covers a larger percentage of body surface area and thus may involve more abdominal or thoracic structures.
4. The coverings of the visceral organs (i.e., abdominal muscles and thoracic cage) are more pliable and thus less likely to show external signs of the traumatic force such as bruising.
5. Parents are not forthcoming with history of injury.
6. Symptoms may not be manifested immediately.
7. Cardiovascular compensating mechanisms may initially work to blunt the effect of severe internal injury but eventually fail, and collapse occurs.
8. There is no single imaging study or laboratory test that is good for recognition of all injuries.
9. When other forms of more recognizable abuse predominate, for example, head trauma or multiple fractures, physicians have a falsely lower index of suspicion for abdominal or thoracic trauma.

Clinical presentations vary by site and type of injury, but the most common presentation is cardiovascular failure or collapse. Other less acute findings are found after a systematic evaluation in all cases of suspected abuse (33). Making a diagnosis requires the organized accumulation of data including a detailed history of injury, a careful and complete physical examination, selected laboratory and radiologic studies, and a sensitive observation of the interaction between the parents, child, and health care team. These four categories of data should be compiled and assimilated to determine if a reporting threshold of suspected abuse exists. More specific clinical findings are noted in the sections that follow.

THORACIC INJURY

Chest Wall Injury

Injuries to the chest wall included ecchymoses and contusions. These in themselves are not serious but serve as markers to more significant underlying pathology. In particular, bruises arrayed along the lateral aspect of the chest wall or back are significant as being signs for anterior and posterior rib fractures or for shaken impact central nervous system trauma (see Chapter 3). Anterior and/or posterior chest wall bruising are uncommon in accidental trauma and may be a marker for lateral rib fractures or cardiac contusions (see Chapter 7). In the series of Sugar et al. (117) of infants and toddlers with bruising, the incidence of chest wall or back bruising was extremely low, representing less than 2% of bruises, even in the group of children who were walking and most active.

Rib Fractures

Several case series of children with rib fractures indicated that child abuse is the most common cause of rib fractures if there is no clear history of motor vehicle crash or iatrogenic causes. Rib fractures are the most common sign of thoracic trauma (63). Rib fractures may also be a marker for intraabdominal trauma (82). Kleinman and Schlesinger (62) placed rib fractures in a category of fractures that makes them highly specific for abuse, particularly posterior rib fractures, an area that is generally protected by dense overlying muscles. In contrast, cases of lateral rib fractures may sometimes occur from falls, with very localized points of contact. Caution must be used in evaluating rib fractures in children with poor nutrition and prematurity, who seem to have rib fractures as a result of underlying metabolic bone disease. Certainly, osteogenesis imperfecta and other metabolic bone diseases must be considered when the young infant presents with rib fractures (63). Rickets also must be considered in the young child (younger than 2 years).

Children with rib fractures will be in pain and will have a period of crying and irritability. Rib fractures should be considered in the differential diagnosis of colic or unexplained crying. With extensive fractures, the child may show a change in respiratory pattern, breathing with short, shallow, rapid respirations.

There has been great controversy about the role of external cardiac compression as a causative factor for rib fractures. Studies indicate that although CPR might be a mechanism in older individuals with more brittle bones, it is not a factor in pediatric resuscitation performed by either trained or untrained personnel (32). Large case series have revealed only isolated case reports of lateral rib fractures after prolonged and vigorous CPR (17).

Healing rib fractures are easily visualized on standard radiographs of the chest (Fig. 8.2). In the acute phase, they are more difficult to see on radiographs. Coned-down views or tangential views may be helpful. If rib fractures are suspected but not visualized on the radiographs, a radionuclide bone scan may be more sensitive.

Hemo/Pneumothorax

The findings of blood and/or air in the pleural space may be a marker of trauma (75,105). Often there may be an associated rib fracture. Symptoms will depend on the degree of encroachment on the pleural space and the confinement of lung and shift of the mediastinum. Pneumomediastinum has also been reported as a manifestation of inflicted trauma (130). Standard chest radiographs in-

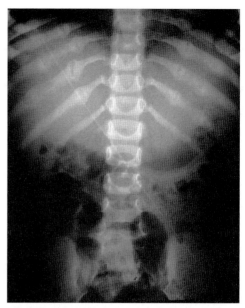

FIG. 8.2. Infant with multiple old rib injuries and gastric distention.

cluding posterior/anterior and decubitus films will show the hemothorax or pneumothorax.

Pulmonary Contusion

Pulmonary contusion is a rare inflicted injury (73). The findings are those of an oxygen deficit and associated changes in the respiratory pattern. The contusion may underlie an area of chest wall trauma. Radiographs reveal an area of increased density, usually in a peripheral lung field. McEniery et al. (73) reported an usual case of an infant with rib injuries and a pulmonary contusion resulting from a "bear hug."

Cardiac Trauma

Direct cardiac injury is rare in pediatric trauma and in particular in child abuse (68). In a series of cases reported by Dowd and Krug (29), there were only 184 children younger than 18 years reported. This study collected data from 16 centers over a 10-year period from 1983 to 1993. Three of the children were reported to have the injury as the result of assault, but there is no notation as to the relationship between the victim and the assailant. The clinical findings varied from chest pain to asystolic arrest. There were associated rib fractures in 23% and pulmonary contusion in 50.5%. A combination of diagnostic tests was used including electrocardiogram (ECG), echocardiography, and measurement of the MB band of creatine phosphokinase. Other blunt cardiac trauma case series have reported similar findings.

Suffocation

Suffocation may be the result of intentional injury or poor supervision (6). Suffocation has been identified as part of the Munchhausen syndrome by proxy (27) (see Chapter 14). The clinical findings may be very scant (53). The classic external manifestations such as contusions over the mouth and lips, scattered petechiae on the face and conjunctiva, and oropharyngeal bleeding are infrequently seen. Occasionally pulmonary radiographs reveal fluffy bilateral alveolar densities, findings consistent with a pattern of upper airway obstruction. The usual mechanism is occlusion of the mouth and nares. Suffocation also may occur from compression of the chest wall inhibiting respiration. Meadow (74) has reported on a series of suffocated children and underscores that many had been seen for medical attention with complaints of apnea, cyanosis, or seizures. There was a high mortality rate in this group and in the family history of sudden death or similar events in many of their siblings. Because the physical examination is often normal, these cases demand a high clinical suspicion, and some centers have instituted the practice of covert video surveillance in hospital rooms to investigate these suspicions. Undoubtedly, some cases of suffocation are ascribed to the inaccurate diagnosis of sudden infant death syndrome (SIDS) (104). There have been suggestions that the finding of intraalveolar pulmonary siderophages may be a marker for previous suffocation events (8).

Strangulation Injury

Although radiographically similar to suffocation, strangulation injuries (85) may have distinct external findings of contusions, ecchymoses, and muscle hematoma in the neck. Occasionally these markers may be seen externally, but in other instances can be seen only on autopsy when the skin is reflected, exposing the subcutaneous tissues. Strangulation also may occur when an infant's head is compressed or wedged between the bars of a crib or between the bed and the wall. Such cases demand a careful death-scene evaluation. Nixon et al. (85) from Wales have published an excellent case series of children with strangulation and suffocation injuries.

Acute Respiratory Distress Syndrome

Acute respiratory distress syndrome (ARDS) is still not well understood, even having been described in 1945 (2,38,91). However, after states of hypoxemia and/or hypotension, the syndrome may evolve. It has been associated with sepsis, pneumonia, near drowning, toxic ingestion, trauma, and other primary conditions (69). It may occur after trauma either to the head or abdominal cavity, suffocation, or strangulation. It often occurs in conjunction with circulatory shock. The radiographic findings are those of bilateral pulmonary infiltrates in the absence of cardiac failure. An increased oxygen requirement and a high mortality rate characterize the syndrome (89). In cases of ARDS without an apparent cause, consider child abuse as a possible etiology.

GASTROINTESTINAL–ABDOMINAL INJURY

Hypopharynx and Esophageal Injury

Hypopharynx and esophageal injury have been well recognized as part of the child abuse syndrome (72,79). Chapter 6 covers the maxillofacial and dental manifestations of abuse. A relatively common child abuse complaint is one of blood coming from the hypopharynx. In some cases, this is factitious and may be recognized by matching the blood produced on a bed sheet or bib with the infant's own blood type and finding them discordant. In other instances, one is able to find a specific lesion that has been produced by forcing objects into the child's hypopharynx or by insertion of the parent's finger into the oral cavity. Cases of esophageal injury have been reported (1) in which blunt-force trauma has caused perforation, or forced ingestion of caustics has caused erosive lesions. Oropharyngeal bleeding has been reported in up to one third of victims known to have been suffocated.

Hepatic Injury

Hepatic injury is perhaps the most serious and life threatening of the common intraabdominal injuries. The relative size and location of the liver make it a common end point for the force of a punch or a kick. Clinical manifestations and management will depend on the size of the laceration and its location (30,41). Some liver contusions will be contained by the liver capsule (6), whereas others will bleed more freely into the peritoneum (3). Symptoms may be evident immediately or may evolve over time as blood accumulates in the peritoneal cavity. Some injuries that initially appear stable may rebleed. This has called into question the ability of pediatric trauma scoring systems to be good predictors of this type of injury.

Measurement of liver enzymes is a good marker for significant injury. Hennes et al. (48) found that enzyme elevations [aspartate aminotransferase (AST), >450 IU/L; and alanine aminotransferase (ALT), >250 IU/L] were both sensitive and specific to find children with visible lesions on CT scan. If AST is elevated out of proportion to ALT, there may be an elevation of AST from muscle trauma. CT (121–123) is the best way to identify the location and extent of the liver trauma (Fig. 8.3). Beyond specific traumatic lesions, liver enzymes also may be elevated after a period of ischemia (36,87). This is a more diffuse injury that will not visualize on radiographic studies.

Coant and Kornberg (23) screened a group of children who had external markers for abuse. Liver enzymes, serum amylase, and urinalysis were obtained of all children. Four of the 49 children screened had elevation of the liver enzymes, and three of the four had liver lacerations on the CT scans despite the absence of any specific signs or symptoms referable to the liver. Although this work does not mandate the screening of all abused children for liver injury, it does raise a caution and a suggestion that a screen of a selected subset of children may be indicated.

Splenic Injury

Splenic injury also results from direct-force trauma being applied to the abdominal cavity, although this is a less common target than the liver because of its relatively protected location. Splenic injury should be suspected in any child who has left-sided chest wall injury. A splenic rupture in a child who is preambulatory should be considered abuse until proven otherwise. As with liver injury, the clinical manifestations may vary depending on the size and location of the laceration (103). The CT scan is the most accurate modality for visualizing the injury; however, ultrasound and nucleotide scans also have been successfully used (Fig. 8.4). Attempts at splenic salvage have been the mainstay of the therapeutic approach to this injury.

Pancreatic Injury

Pancreatic injury is another common child abuse injury (115). In a case series of 26 children with pancreatic injury from a Cincinnati pediatric trauma center (4), five were the result of child abuse. The other causes of injury included bicycle handlebar trauma, motor vehicle crashes, and falls. Most of the abused children had class I injuries, indicating contusion or laceration without pancreatic duct injury. The CT scan appears to be the most sensitive test to identify pancreatic injury. The

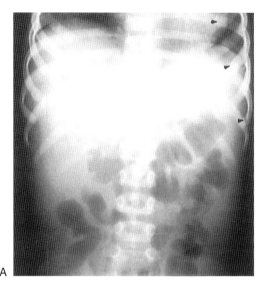

FIG. 8.3. A 21-month-old child was in shock, with a hemoglobin value of 8 g, after a "fall". Multiple abrasions and bruising of the face and abdomen were noted. **A:** Abdominal radiograph including the lower chest shows peritoneal fluid with bowel loops "floating" in the midabdomen, as well as multiple rib fractures *(arrows)*. **B:** CT scan shows a liver laceration *(arrow)* with a large hemoperitoneum. **C:** At a lower level, bright contrast enhancement of the bowel wall reflects hypovolemic shock *(arrows)*. Surgery revealed hemoperitoneum with a mesenteric laceration in addition to the liver laceration.

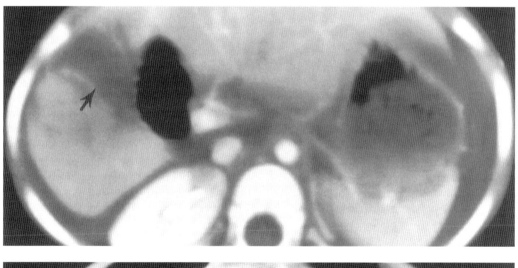

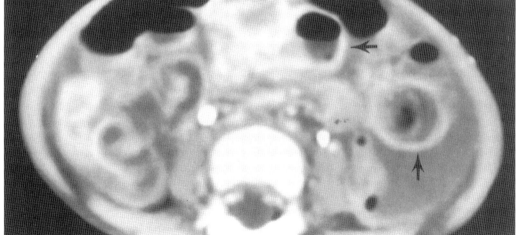

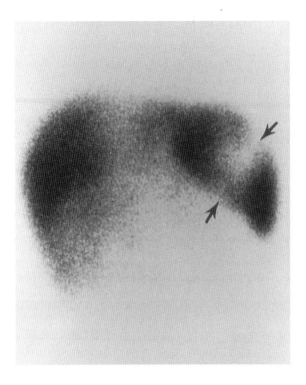

FIG. 8.4. A twelve-year-old boy was kicked in the abdomen by his father. Liver-spleen scintigram reveals a transverse laceration of the mid-spleen (*arrows*).

ultrasound appears to be less sensitive in diagnosing the acute injury but is very useful in finding and monitoring a pseudocyst of the pancreas (11,90,113) (Fig. 8.5). The measurement of serum enzymes also is an excellent marker of injury, but the level of the enzyme increase does not appear to correlate with the extent of injury. Unexplained pancreatitis in a young child is highly suggestive of unexplained trauma (28).

Stomach and Bowel Perforation

Stomach and bowel perforation have been reported to be the result of abuse in many instances (20,21,24,128,132). Many cases of stomach rupture (107,110) are complicated by the peritonitis that follows the soiling of the peritoneal cavity with gastric contents. Mortality is quite high in these cases. Bowel perforations may occur anywhere along the course of the intestine but most often tend to be located in the duodenum (84,126) because of its fixed position in the retroperitoneum and at the duodenal–jejunal junction. Symp-

toms may develop immediately or develop over time. There have been reports of cases that present in the subacute period because of the development of strictures (109). Of all the forms of abdominal trauma, bowel perforation is the most difficult to diagnose. A plain film series including flat and upright may show free air (132)(Fig. 8.6). Ultrasound may show free fluid in the peritoneal cavity. The CT scan also may show injury, but if there is high suspicion for the lesion, then laparotomy must be performed to localize the perforation.

With some small bowel injuries, there is hematoma without perforation (64,88). In such cases, an upper gastrointestinal contrast study (UGI) or more recently ultrasound (49) has been used to identify the thickened bowel wall lesion (34).

Anal–Rectal Injury

The rate of this anal–rectal injury remains low outside the group of children who are being sexually abused (see Chapter 10). Nonetheless, some children have been pun-

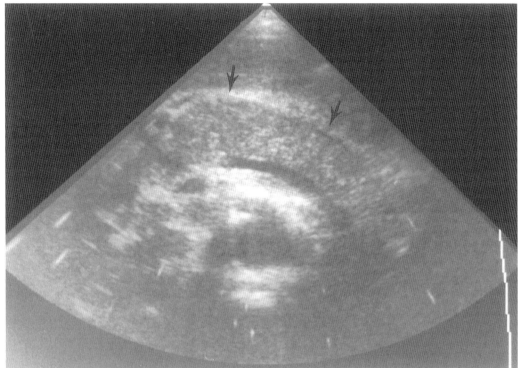

A

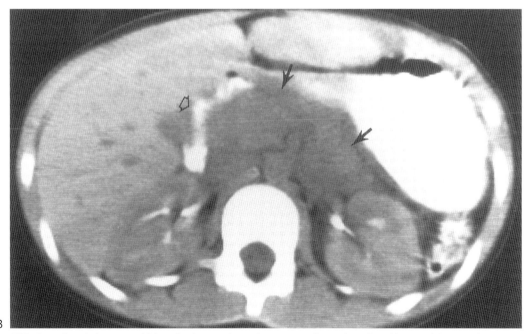

B

FIG. 8.5. An eight-year-old boy had emesis and severe epigastric pain without a history of trauma. He had multiple facial bruises. **A:** Transverse ultrasonogram of the epigastrium reveals a large, swollen pancreas (*arrows*) without laceration or pseudocyst. **B:** CT scan shows extensive pancreatic swelling (*solid arrows*) displacing and effacing the descending duodenum (*hollow arrows*).

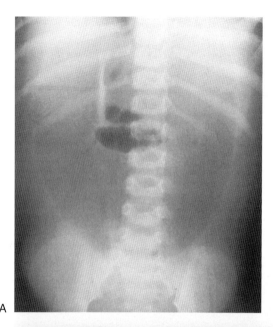

FIG. 8.6. A two-year-old child had acute onset of abdominal distention. Multiple bruises about the face and arms were noted. **A:** Abdominal radiograph reveals massive pneumoperitoneum. **B:** A lateral decubitus view shows an air-fluid level (*arrows*) with free peritoneal fluid.

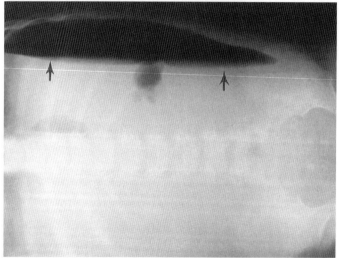

ished by insertion of foreign objects into the rectum or by forceful application of enemas. These children usually present with bleeding and/or pain. Rectosigmoidoscopy is the best way to survey the extent of injury and to document it. Stool cultures may be obtained to rule out infectious causes of rectal bleeding. Stool tests for the presence of blood also are a useful form of objective documentation.

Retroperitoneal Hematomas

Retroperitoneal hematomas also are rare and difficult to diagnose. They are mainly found when children seem to have the signs of ongoing blood-volume loss, and other more common sites have been ruled out.

Abdominal Vascular Injury

Abdominal vascular injuries also result in high rates of morbidity and mortality. Injuries vary from small venous mesenteric bleeds to disruption of the aorta or inferior vena cava (93). The extent of injury will determine the rate of onset of symptoms. Diagnosis may be difficult because of unrecognized traumatic etiology, a lack of specific tests, and the rapid progression of signs and symptoms. Localized ischemia may result in symptoms referable to one portion of bowel. A pattern similar to that of pneumatosis intestinalis (43) has been reported. Cases of chylous ascites and peritonitis also are documented in the literature (9,13).

URINARY TRACT INJURY

Renal and Urinary Tract Injury

Blunt force trauma may be injurious anywhere along the genitourinary tract from the kidneys to the tip of the penis (71,106,112). There may also be injuries to the blood supply to the kidney. Most renal, bladder, or urethral injuries will result in hematuria (46). If the child has more than 20 red blood cells per high-power field (rbc/hpf) on the urinalysis, a CT scan is indicated. Intravenous contrast studies, intravenous pyelography (IVP), and nuclear scan (59) are less useful but have indications if the patient is too unstable for CT or if a pedicle injury is suspected. Lack of hematuria may occur in rare circumstances such as a renovascular injury or a complete ureteral disruption. For lower tract and bladder injury, a voiding cystourethrogram (VCUG) may be the most informative study. Pelvic fracture may be a predictor of more serious abdominal and genitourinary injury (10).

Rhabdomyolysis

Rhabdomyolysis is an indirect form of renal injury (80,108). This results from massive muscle necrosis, and the breakdown products of muscle overload the kidney's ability to filter them. The result is heme-positive urine with the absence of any red blood cells on the microscopic urinalysis. The heme test is a false positive caused by myoglobin. Care must be taken to hydrate the patient, avoiding potassium-containing solutions lest the patient develop acute renal failure.

DIFFERENTIAL DIAGNOSIS

With all injuries and all cases of suspected abuse, a differential diagnosis must be considered (66,96). The symptoms of visceral trauma may be very protean and simulate many common entities such as gastroenteritis, viral hepatitis, or respiratory infection. Some of the other etiologies that closely mimic inflicted trauma and thus need to be contemplated include the following (97).

Lap-Belt Complex

In recent years, with the increased use of seat-restraint devices, some children have been improperly restrained by using a lap seat belt only. This has resulted in the identification of the lap-belt complex (5,37,81,98), a collection of injuries from the rapid deceleration of a child against a seat belt. The complex may include minimal abdominal wall bruising along with extensive intraperitoneal injury. The discordance between the external findings and the intraabdominal findings could cause the overdiagnosis of child abuse. Bowel perforations and vascular, renal, and lumbar vertebral lesions have all been reported. Magnetic resonance imaging is useful in delineating the vertebral and spinal cord injuries.

Falls

Falls have been reported as the cause of intraabdominal pathology. In taking the history, look for a body position or contact with an object that has a penetrating capacity. Falls down stairs have been well documented as causing minimal truncal injury (52). A child found at the bottom of a flight of stairs with bowel or vascular contusions or a laceration of the liver is likely to have been beaten before being thrown down the stairs.

Perforated Bowel Secondary to Appendicitis or Inflammatory Bowel Disease

Perforated bowel secondary to appendicitis or inflammatory bowel disease may mimic child abuse. There should be preceding history and signs and symptoms consistent with these diagnoses. However, particularly in the young child, signs and symptoms of nontraumatic bowel diseases may not be apparent.

Handlebar Injuries

Handlebar injuries may have a force that distends the abdominal musculature and concentrates the force on bowel, pancreas, or liver. Handlebar injuries may closely mimic the types of injury that result from abuse and are almost as common in terms of incidence in the preschool-aged child.

Glomerulonephritis or other causes of nontraumatic renal disease or minimal trauma hematuria are also potential traps for a child abuse misdiagnosis. When minimal trauma results in hematuria, make certain that a renal tumor or hydronephrosis is not making the kidney more vulnerable to bleed. Dark-colored or coke-colored urine may be the result of acid hematin, as is found in glomerulonephritis.

In considering the differences between inflicted trauma and noninflicted trauma, the following group characteristics tend to be true. When making the comparison, Ledbetter et al.(65) found that of the 156 cases of abdominal trauma, 89% had accidental trauma, and 11% were the victims of abuse. The abused group tended to be younger (median age, 2.6 months), had vague or changing histories of injury, had delayed treatment, had more hollow viscous injury and liver trauma, and had a mortality rate more than double that of the noninflicted group (Fig. 8.7). Other

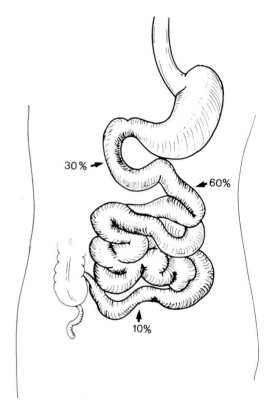

FIG. 8.7. Distribution of hollow viscus injuries. (From Kleinman PK. *Diagnostic imaging in child abuse*. Baltimore: Williams & Wilkins, 1987.)

factors to look for in the abuse group include healing injuries of different ages, old bruising in 50% to 90% of cases, and multiple forms of injury. Although these group differences are important factors to keep in mind, no single factor is sensitive or specific enough to be diagnostic of child abuse.

IMAGING STUDIES

With a plethora of imaging modalities, there is often confusion as to which test is the best one for a specific injury type (7,16,41, 47,54,57,58,60,61,76,77,78,101,121,122,123). Table 8.2 lists the modalities and their relative strong points. Any of the modalities are only as good as the technical quality of the study and the accuracy of the person interpreting the study. Some modalities such as ultrasonography are more dependent on the operator's skill

TABLE 8.2. *Child abuse injuries and imaging modalities*

Injury type	Radiograph	Ultrasound	CT scan	Nuclear scan	Other	References
Thoracic injury						
Rib fractures	X[a]			X		47, 77, 101
Hemo/Pneumothorax	X[a]		X			62, 63, 82
Pulmonary contusion	X		X[a]			130
Cardiac contusion			X	X	Echo-cardiogram	29, 99
Suffocation	X[a]					
Strangulation	X[a]					
ARDS	X[a]					14, 34, 44, 45, 58, 60, 76, 78, 101, 111, 121, 122, 123, 132
Abdominal injury						
Esophageal		X[a]	X[a]		Barium swallow[a]	1, 57, 67
Hepatic	X	X	X[a]	X		2, 67
Splenic		X[a]	X[a]			67
Pancreatic	X	X[a]	X[a]			113
Stomach/bowel	X	X	X[a]			16, 49, 64, 88, 116
Anal/rectal			X[a]			
Retroperitoneal		X	X[a]			
Urinary tract injury						
Renal		X	X[a]	X	Intravenous pyelogram	46, 59
Urethral					VCUG	
Vertebral/cord injury	X				MRI	

[a]Best modality.

IVP, intravenous pyelogram; VCUG, voiding cystourethrogram; MRI, magnetic resonance imaging.

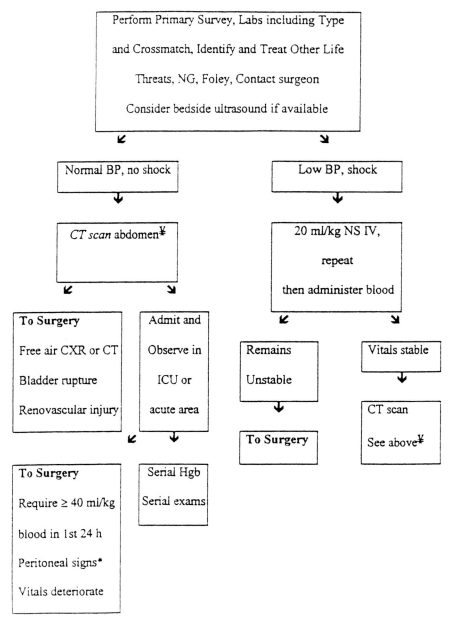

FIG. 8.8. Diagnostic evaluation of child with renal trauma. (From Rothrock SG, Green SM, Morgan R. Abdominal trauma in infants and children: prompt identification and early management of serious and life-threatening injuries. Part I: Injury patterns and initial assessment. *Pediatr Emerg Care* 2000;16:189–195).

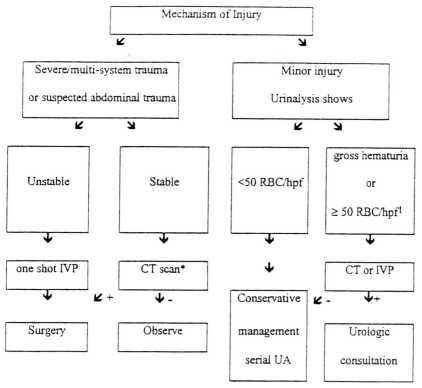

FIG. 8.9. Diagnostic evaluation of child with abdominal trauma. Part II: Specific Injuries and emergency department management. *Pediatr Emerg Care* 2000;16:189–195)

level and experience. The imaging modalities are constantly being refined, and the reader is urged to keep abreast of the most recent scientific literature. Figures 8.8 and 8.9 provide schemes for the immediate evaluations of patients who present with suspected renal trauma or abdominal trauma (94,95,100,102, 127). Note that the evaluation will depend on the clinical stability or instability of the patient. Bradin et al. (14) performed a retrospective study of abused children who underwent CT scan of the abdomen and compared the yield with those who had scans for motor vehicle injury. Their study showed that although CT scans were performed less frequently in abuse victims, they yielded a greater incidence and variety of significant abdominal injuries than did those in the motor vehicle crash controls.

LABORATORY STUDIES

Laboratory studies also are helpful in suggesting or confirming the diagnosis of visceral injury (48,51). A number of different tests may be used. The physician must be selective in the ordering and interpretation of studies. Positive laboratory studies are very helpful in the phase of case management that involves legal proceedings, as they have an element of scientific rigor and credibility that is helpful in describing and quantifying findings. Table 8.3 lists the available tests and their indications.

TABLE 8.3. *Laboratory tests and indications for detection of visceral trauma*

Test	Indication
CBC	Blood loss
Reticulocyte count	Chronic blood loss
Pulse oximeter	Decreased oxygenation
Serum amylase/lipase	Pancreatitis
AST/ALT	Liver trauma
Urinalysis RBCs	Renal trauma
Hematest stool	Bowel trauma
Hematest urine	Rhabdomyolysis
PT/PTT/Platelets	Bleeding disorder
Calcium/Phos/Alkaline phosphatase	Rickets/Metabolic bone disease
Creatine phosphokinase-MB	Cardiac trauma
ECG	Cardiac trauma
Blood type	Munchausen syndrome by proxy

CBC, complete blood count; AST, aspartate aminotransferase; ALT, alanine aminotransferase; PT, prothrombin time; PTT, partial thromboplastin time

FORENSIC CONSIDERATIONS

All of the standard protocols for forensic evaluation of abused neglected children include detailed examination of the thoracic and abdominal cavities and their contents. This is extremely important as the clinician may not see or be able to identify the nature and extent of the injury from external inspection or even from the information gathered by laboratory or radiographic studies. It also is important that histology specimens and microscopic studies be performed, as they may reveal old injury as well as acute new injury. Forensic examination by a competent and experienced pathologist is critical to the legal management of the child abuse case (15,35) (see Chapter 19).

In addition to forensic pathology evaluation, it is important to report cases promptly to police and child-protective services personnel. Site evaluations, recovery of evidence, detailed history taking, background searches, and review of other medical records may all be helpful in the complete evaluation of a specific case.

Another aid to the forensic process is photographs that are well taken, color balanced, and appropriately labeled. See Chapter 15 on photodocumentation. It also is important to document the findings that have been revealed by therapeutic interventions (55).

Finally, the most important adjunct to a sound forensic case is a complete, thorough, and accurate medical record. When a case involves visceral injury, there is often greater possibility for creating doubt to the benefit of a defendant. An accurate medical record that is complete and internally consistent is the best protection against a smokescreen obscuring justice (22).

CONCLUSION

Visceral injuries in the thoracic or abdominal cavity are rare in children, but when they occur, there is a significant risk that their etiology is nonaccidental trauma. The manifestations of visceral injury are many, and the signs and symptoms of each are varied. By keeping a high index of suspicion, the astute physician, by using a battery of laboratory tests and a wide array of radiographic modalities, should be able to make a prompt and possibly life-saving diagnosis. Delay in making the correct diagnosis and instituting prompt therapy has a high likelihood of resulting in severe morbidity or mortality. Education and collaboration between the pediatric trauma center and the regional child abuse specialists will result in lives saved as well as more improved medicolegal outcomes on behalf of the children served.

REFERENCES

1. Ablin DS, Reinhart MA. Esophageal perforation with mediastinal abscess in child abuse. *Pediatr Radiol* 1990;20:524.

2. Anzueto A, Melo J. Acute respiratory distress syndrome: liquid ventilation. *Respir Care Clin North Am* 1998;4:679.

3. Aoki Y, Nata M, Hashiyada M, et al. Laceration of the liver with delayed massive intra-abdominal hemorrhage: a case report of child abuse. *Nippon Hoigakv Zasshi Jpn J Leg Med* 1997;51:44.

4. Arkovitz MS, Johnson N, Garcia VF. Pancreatic trauma in children: mechanisms of injury. *J Trauma Injury Infect Crit Care* 1997;42:49.

5. Asbun HJ, Irani H, Roe EJ, et al. Intra-abdominal seatbelt injury. *J Trauma* 1990;30:189.

6. Baker SP, Fisher RS. Childhood asphyxiation by choking or suffocation. *JAMA* 1980;244:1343.

7. Beauchamp JM, Belanger MA, Neitzschman HR. The diagnosis of subcapsular hematoma of the liver by scintigraphy. *South Med J* 1976;69:1579.

8. Becroft DM, Lockett BK. Intra-alveolar pulmonary siderophages in sudden infant death: a marker for previous imposed suffocation. *Pathology* 1997;29:60.

9. Benhaim P, Strear C, Knudson MM, et al. Post-traumatic chylous ascites in a child: recognition and management of an unusual condition. *J Trauma Injury Infect Crit Care* 1995;39:1175.

10. Bond SJ, Gotschall CS, Eichelberger MR. Predictors of abdominal injury in children with pelvic fracture. *J Trauma* 1991;31:1169.

11. Bongiovi JJ, Logosso RD. Pancreatic pseudocyst occurring in the battered child syndrome. *J Pediatr Surg* 1969;4:220.

12. Bouska I. Causes of death in fatal cases of child abuse 1964–1988 [Czech] Priciny smrti letalnich pripadu tyraneho ditete zaleta 1964–1988. *Casopis Lekaru Ceskych* 1995;134:344.

13. Boyce BE. Chylous ascites. *Am J Dis Child* 1975;129:38.

14. Bradin SA, Mazur P, Gilbert J, et al. The yield of abdominal CT scan in the medical investigation of child abuse. *Pediatr Emerg Care* (in press).

15. Buchino JJ. Recognition and management of child abuse by the surgical pathologist. *Arch Pathol Lab Med* 1983;107:4.

16. Bulas DI, Taylor GA, Eichelberger MR. The value of CT in detecting bowel perforation in children after blunt abdominal trauma. *AJR Am J Roentgenol* 1989;153:561.

17. Bush CM, Jones JS, Cohle SD, et al. Pediatric injuries from cardiopulmonary resuscitation. *Ann Emerg Med* 1996;28:40.

18. Caniano DA, Beaver BL, Boles ET. Child abuse: an update on surgical management in 256 cases. *Ann Surg* 1986;203:219.

19. Canty TG Sr, Canty TG Jr, Brown C. Injuries of the gastrointestinal tract from blunt trauma in children: a 12-year experience at a designated pediatric center. *J Trauma* 1999;46:234.

20. Case ME, Naduri R. Laceration of the stomach by blunt trauma in a child: a case of child abuse. *J Forensic Sci* 1983;28:496.

21. Cassebaum WH, Carberry DM, Sefko P. Rupture of the stomach from mouth-to-mouth resuscitation. *J Trauma* 1974;14:811.

22. Chadwick D. Preparation for court testimony in child abuse cases. *Pediatr Clin North Am* 1990;37:955.

23. Coant PN, Kornberg AE, Brody AS, et al. Markers for occult liver injury in cases of physical abuse in children. *Pediatrics* 1992;89:274.

24. Cobb LM, Vinocour LM, Wagner CW, et al. Intestinal perforation due to blunt trauma in children in an era of increased nonoperative treatment. *J Trauma Injury Infect Crit Care* 1986;26:461.

25. Cooper A, Floyd T, Barlow B, et al. Major blunt abdominal trauma due to child abuse. *J Trauma* 1988;28:1483.

26. Cooper A. Thoracoabdominal trauma. In: Ludwig S, Kornberg A, eds. *Child abuse:* a medical reference. 2nd ed. New York: Churchill Livingstone, 1992:131–150.

27. Davis P, McClure RJ, Rolfe K, et al. Procedures, placement, and risks of further abuse after Munchausen syndrome by proxy, non-accidental poisoning, and non-accidental suffocation. *Arch Dis Child* 1998;78:217.

28. deRoux SJ, Prendergast NC. Lacerations of the hepatoduodenal ligament, pancreas and duodenum in a child due to blunt impact. *J Forensic Sci* 1998;43:222.

29. Dowd MD, Krug S. Pediatric blunt cardiac injury: epidemiology, clinical features, and diagnosis. *J Trauma Injury Infect Crit Care* 1996;40:61.

30. Dworkind M, McGowan G, Hyams J. Abdominal trauma: child [Letter]. *Pediatrics* 1990;85:892.

31. Evers K, DeGaeta LR. Abdominal trauma. *Emerg Med Clin North Am* 1985;3:525.

32. Feldman KW, Brewer DK. Child abuse, cardiopulmonary resuscitation, and rib fractures. *Pediatrics* 1984;73:339.

33. Fleisher G, Ludwig S. *Textbook of pediatric emergency medicine.* Baltimore: Williams & Wilkins, 1983: 2nd ed. 1988: 3rd ed. 1993: 4th ed. Baltimore: Lippincott Williams & Wilkins, 2000.

34. Foley LC, Teele RL. Ultrasound of epigastric injuries after blunt trauma. *AJR Am J Roentgenol* 1979;132:593.

35. Fossum RM, Descheneaux KA. Blunt trauma of the abdomen in children. *J Forensic Sci* 1991;36:47.

36. Garland JS, Werlin SL, Rice TB. Ischemic hepatitis in children: diagnosis and clinical course. *Crit Care Med* 1988;16:1209.

37. Glassman SD, Johnson JR, Holt RT. Seatbelt injuries in children. *J Trauma* 1992;33:882.

38. Goh AYT, Chan PWK, Lum LCS, et al. Incidence of acute respiratory distress syndrome: a comparison of two definitions. *Arch Dis Child* 1998;79:256.

39. Gonzalez R, Heiss WH, Rauh W. Blunt abdominal trauma caused by child abuse. *Monatsschr Kinderheilkd* 1987;135:692.

40. Gornall P, Ahmed S, Jolleys A, et al. Intra-abdominal injuries in the battered baby syndrome. *Arch Dis Child* 1972;42:211.

41. Grisoni ER, Gauderer MWL, Ferron J, et al. Nonoperative management of liver injuries following blunt abdominal trauma in children. *J Pediatr Surg* 1984;19:515.

42. Grosfeld JL, Ballantine TVN. Surgical aspects of child abuse (trauma-x). *Pediatr Ann* 1976;106.

43. Gurland B, Dolgin SE, Shlasko E, et al. Pneumatosis intestinalis and portal veingas after blunt abdominal trauma. *J Pediatr Surg* 1998;33:1309.

44. Haftel AJ, Rev R, Mahour GH, et al. Abdominal CT scanning in pediatric blunt trauma. *Ann Emerg Med* 1988;17:684.

45. Haller JA. Injuries of the gastrointestinal tract in children: notes on recognition and management. *Clin Pediatr* 1966;5:476.

46. Haller JO, Bass IS, Sclafani SJA. Imaging evaluation of traumatic hematuria in children. *Urol Radiol* 1984; 7:211.

47. Haller JO, Kleinman PK, Merten DF, et al. Diagnostic imaging of child abuse. *Pediatrics* 1991;87:262.

48. Hennes HM, Smith DS, Schneider K, et al. Elevated liver transaminase levels in children with blunt abdominal trauma: a predictor of liver injury. *Pediatrics* 1990;86:87.

49. Hernanz-Schulman M, Genieser NB, Ambrosino M. Sonographic diagnosis on intramural duodenal hematoma. *J Ultrasound Med* 1989;8:273.

50. Hodge D, Ludwig S. Child homicide. *Pediatr Emerg Care* 1985;1:3.

51. Isaacman DJ, Scarfone RJ, Kost SI, et al. Utility of routine laboratory testing for detecting intra-abdominal injury in the pediatric trauma patient. *Pediatrics* 1993;92:691.

52. Joffe M, Ludwig S. Stairway injuries in children. *Pediatrics* 1988;82:457.

53. Johnson P. Diagnosis of recurrent suffocation of children [Letter]. *Lancet* 1992;340:481.

54. Kane NM, Cronan JJ, Durfman GS, et al. Pediatric abdominal trauma: evaluation by computed tomography. *Pediatrics* 1988;82:11.

55. Kanter RK, Zimmerman JJ, Staus RH, et al. Pediatric emergency intravenous access. *Am J Dis Child* 1986; 140:132.

56. Kapklein MJ, Mahadeo R. Pediatric trauma. *Mt Sinai J Med* 1997;64:302.

57. Kaufman RA, Towbin R, Babcock DS, et al. Upper abdominal trauma in children: imaging evaluation. *AJR Am J Roentgenol* 1984;142:449.

58. Kaufman RA, Babcock DS. An approach to imaging the upper abdomen in the injured child. *Semin Roentgenol* 1984;14:308.

59. Kinmel RL, Sty JR. 99m Tc-methylene diphosphonate renal images in a battered child. *Clin Nucl Med* 1979; 4:166.

60. Kirks DR. Radiological evaluation of visceral injuries in the battered child syndrome. *Pediatr Ann* 1983;12:888.

61. Kleinman PK, Raptopoulos VD, Brill PW. Occult nonskeletal trauma in the battered child syndrome. *Pediatr Radiol* 1981;141:393.

62. Kleinman PK, Schlesinger AE. Mechanical factors associated with posterior rib fractures in abused infants. *Pediatr Radiol* 1997;27:87–91.

63. Kleinman PK. *Diagnostic imaging in child abuse.* Baltimore: Williams & Wilkins, 1987.

64. Kleinman PK, Brill PW, Winchester P. Resolving duodenal-jejunal hematoma in abused children. *Radiology* 1986;160:747.

65. Ledbetter DJ, Hatch EI, Feldman KW, et al. Diagnostic and surgical implications of child abuse. *Arch Surg* 1988;123:1101.

66. Ludwig S. Pediatric abdominal trauma. *Top Emerg Med* 1993:15:40.

67. Luks FI, Lemire A, St-Vil D, et al. Blunt abdominal trauma in children: the practical value of ultrasonography. *J Trauma* 1993;34:607.

68. Marino TA, Langston C. Cardiac trauma and the conduction system: a case study of an 18-month-old child. *Arch Pathol Lab Med* 1982;106:173.

69. Martino AR, Pfenninger J, Bachmann DC, et al. [Changes in the epidemiology of the acute respiratory distress syndrome (ARDS) in children] [Spanish] Cambios en la epidemiologia del sindrome de dificultad respiratoria aguda (SDRA) en niños. *Esp Pediatr* 1999;50:566.

70. Mayer T, Walker MJ, Johnson DG, et al. Causes of morbidity and mortality in severe pediatric trauma. *JAMA* 1981;245:719.

71. McAleer IM, Kaplan GW. Pediatric genitourinary trauma. *Urol Clin North Am* 1995;22:177.

72. McDowel HP, Fielding DW. Traumatic perforation of the hypopharynx: an unusual form of abuse. *Arch Dis Child* 1984;59:888.

73. McEniery J, Hanson R, Grigor W, et al. Lung injury resulting from a nonaccidental crush injury to the chest. *Pediatr Emerg Care* 1991;7:166.

74. Meadow R. Suffocation, recurrent apnea, and sudden infant death. *J Pediatr* 1990;117:351.

75. Meller J, Little A, Shermeta D. Thoracic trauma in children. *Pediatrics* 1984;74:813.

76. Merten DF, Carpenter BLM. Radiologic imaging of inflicted injury in the child abuse syndrome. *Pediatr Clin North Am* 1990;37:815.

77. Merten DF, Radkowski MA, Leonidas JC. The abused child: a radiological reappraisal. *Radiology* 1983;146: 377.

78. Mohamed G, Reyes HR, Fantus R, et al. Computed tomography in the assessment of pediatric abdominal trauma. *Arch Surg* 1986;121:703.

79. Morzaria S, Walton MJ, MacMillan A. Inflicted esophageal perforation. *J Pediatr Surg* 1998;33:871.

80. Mukherji SK, Siegel MJ. Rhabdomyolysis and renal failure in child abuse. *AJR Am J Roentgenol* 1987;148:1203.

81. Newman KD, Bowman LM, Eichelberger MR, et al. The lap belt complex: intestinal and lumbar spine injury in children. *J Trauma* 1990;30:1133.

82. Ng CS, Hall CM. Costochondral junction fractures and intra-abdominal trauma in non-accidental injury (child abuse). *Pediatr Radiol* 1998;28:671.

83. Ng CS, Hall CM, Shaw DG. The range of visceral manifestations of non-accidental injury. *Arch Dis Child* 1997;17:167.

84. Nijs S, Vanclooster P, deGheldere L, et al. Duodenal transection in a battered child: a case report. *Acta Chir Belg* 1997;97:192.

85. Nixon JW, Kemp AM, Levene S, et al. Suffocation, choking, and strangulation in childhood in England and Wales: epidemiology and prevention. *Arch Dis Child* 1995;72:6.

86. O'Neill A Jr, Meachum WF, Griffin PP, et al. Patterns of injury in the battered child syndrome. *J Trauma* 1973;13:332.

87. Oldham K, Guice KS, Kaufman RA, et al. Blunt hepatic injury and elevated hepatic enzymes: a clinical correlation in children. *J Pediatr Surg* 1984;19:457.

88. Orel SG, Nussbaum AR, Sheth S, et al. Duodenal hematoma in child abuse: sonographic detection. *AJR Am J Roentgenol* 1988;151:147.

89. Paulson TE, Spear RM, Peterson BM. New concepts in the treatment of children with acute respiratory distress syndrome. *J Pediatr* 1995;127:163.

90. Pena SDF, Medovy H. Child abuse and traumatic pseudocyst of the pancreas. *J Pediatr* 1973;83:1026.

91. Pfenninger J. Acute respiratory distress syndrome (ARDS) in neonates and children. *Pediatr Anaesth* 1996;6:173.

92. Philippart AI. Blunt abdominal trauma in childhood. *Surg Clin North Am* 1977;57:151.

93. Pisters PW, Heslin MJ, Riles TS. Abdominal aortic pseudo aneurysm after blunt trauma. *J Vasc Surg* 1993; 18:307.

94. Powell RW, Green JB, Ochsner G, et al. Peritoneal lavage in pediatric patients sustaining blunt abdominal trauma: a reappraisal. *J Trauma* 1987;27:6.

95. Ramenofsky ML. Pediatric abdominal trauma. *Pediatr Ann* 1987;16:318.

96. Reece RM, Grodin MA. Recognition of nonaccidental injury. *Pediatr Clin North Am* 1985;32:41.

97. Reece RM. Unusual manifestations of child abuse. *Pediatr Clin North Am* 1990;37:905.

98. Reid AB, Letts RM, Black GB. Pediatric chance fractures: association with intra-abdominal injuries and seatbelt use. *J Trauma* 1990;30:384.

99. Rodgers B. Trauma and the child. *Heart Lung* 1977; 6:1052.

100. Rothenberg S, Moore EE, Marx JA, et al. Selective management of blunt abdominal trauma in children: the triage of peritoneal lavage. *J Trauma* 1987;27:1101.

101. Röthlin MA, Naf R, Amgwerd M, et al. Ultrasound in blunt abdominal and thoracic trauma. *J Trauma* 1993; 34:488.

102. Rothrock SG, Green SM, Morgan R. Abdominal trauma in infants and children: prompt identification and early management of serious and life threatening injuries. Part I: injury patterns and initial assessment. *Pediatr Emerg Care* 2000;16:106–115. Part II: specific injuries and emergency department management. *Pediatr Emerg Care* 2000;16:189–195.

103. Saladino R, Lund D, Fleisher G. The spectrum of liver and spleen injuries in children: failure of the pediatric trauma score and clinical signs to predict isolated injuries. *Ann Emerg Med* 1991;20:636.

104. Samuels M, Southall D. Diagnosis of recurrent suffocation of children [Letter]. *Lancet* 1992;340:787.

105. Sarihan H, Abes S, Akyazici R, et al. Blunt thoracic trauma in children. *J Cardiovasc Surg* 1996;37:525.

106. Sawyer RW, Hartenberg MA, Benator RM. Intraperitoneal bladder rupture in a battered child. *Int J Pediatr Nephrol* 1987;8:227.

107. Schechner SA, Ehrlich FE. Case reports: gastric perforation and child abuse. *J Trauma* 1974;14:723.

108. Schwengel D, Ludwig S. Rhabdomyolysis and myoglobinuria as manifestations of child abuse. *Pediatr Emerg Care* 1985;1:4.

109. Shah P, Applegate KE, Buonomo C. Stricture of the duodenum and jejunum in an abused child. *Pediatr Radiol* 1997;27:281.

110. Siemens RA, Fulton RL. Gastric rupture as a result of blunt trauma. *Am Surg* 1977;43:229.

111. Sivit CJ, Taylor GA, Eichelberger MR. Visceral injury in battered children: a changing perspective. *Radiology* 1989;173:659.

112. Slosberg E, Ludwig S, Duckett J, et al. Penile trauma as a sign of child abuse. *Am J Dis Child* 1978;132:719.

113. Slovis TL, VonBerg VJ, Mikelic V. Sonography in the diagnosis and management of pancreatic pseudocysts and effusions in childhood. *Radiology* 1980;135:153.

114. Starc TJ, Langston C, Goldfarb J, et al. Unexpected nonHIV causes of death in children born to HIV-infected mothers. *Pediatrics* 1999;104:102.

115. Sternowsky HJ, Schaefer E. Traumatic pancreatitis with peripheral osteolysis suggesting child abuse [German]. *Monatsschr Kinderheilkd* 1985;133:178.

116. Strouse PJ, Close BJ, Marshall KW, et al. CT of bowel and mesenteric trauma in children. *Radiographics* 1999;19:1237.

117. Sugar NF, Taylor JA, Feldman KW. Bruises in infants and toddlers. *Arch Pediatr Adolesc Med* 1999;153:399.

118. Susom EM, Klotz D, Kottmeier PK. Liver trauma in children. *J Pediatr Surg* 1975;10:411.

119. Talbert JL, Felman AH. Identification and treatment of thoracoabdominal injuries in battered children. *South Med Bull* 1970;58:37.

120. Tank ES, Eraklis AJ, Gross RE. Blunt abdominal trauma in infancy and childhood. *J Trauma* 1968;8:439.

121. Taylor GA, Eichelberger MR. Abdominal CT in children in neurologic impairment following blunt trauma. *Ann Surg* 1989;210:229.

122. Taylor GA, Fallat ME, Potter BM, et al. The role of computed tomography in blunt abdominal trauma in children. *J Trauma* 1988;28:1660.

123. Taylor GA, Guion CJ, Potter BM, et al. CT of blunt abdominal trauma in children. *AJR Am J Roentgenol* 1989;153:555.

124. Touloukian RJ. Abdominal trauma in childhood. *Surg Gynecol Obstet* 1968;127:561.

125. Touloukian RJ. Battered children with abdominal trauma. *GP* 1969;40:106.

126. Tracy T Jr, O'Connor TP, Weber TR. Battered children with duodenal avulsion and transection. *Am Surg* 1993;59:342.

127. Velanovich V, Tapper D. Decision analysis in children with blunt splenic trauma: the effects of observation, splenorrhaphy, or splenectomy on quality-adjusted life expectancy. *J Pediatr Surg* 1993;28:179.

128. Vock R, Schellmann B, Schaidt G. Isolated injuries of intestinal tract due to body maltreatment [authors trans. from German]. *Z Rechtsmed J Legal Med* 1980; 84:155.

129. Wilske J, Eisenmenger W. Unnatural causes of death in children. *Offentl Gesundheitswes* 1991;53:490.

130. Woodruff WW III, Merten DF, Kirks DR. Pneumomediastinum: an unusual complication of acute gastrointestinal disease. *Pediatr Radiol* 1985;15:196.

131. Yamamoto LG, Wiebe RA, Matthews WJ. A one-year prospective ED cohort of pediatric trauma. *Pediatr Emerg Care* 1991;7:267.

132. Zahran M, Eklof O, Thomasson B. Blunt abdominal trauma and hollow viscus injury in children: the diagnostic value of plain radiography. *Pediatr Radiol* 1984; 14:304.

9

Conditions Mistaken for Child Physical Abuse

Jan Bays

Child Abuse Response and Evaluation Services, Emanuel Children's Hospital and Healthcare Center; and Department of Pediatrics, Oregon Health Sciences University, Portland, Oregon

A health care worker who discovers signs of child abuse is legally required to report the findings to child welfare agencies. Because the diagnosis of child abuse has serious consequences for the child, the family, and the suspected perpetrator, it is also the responsibility of the health care worker not to arrive at the diagnosis of abuse hastily, but to take a careful history, to perform a complete physical examination, and to order laboratory tests necessary to rule out conditions other than abuse. This chapter describes a variety of conditions that have been mistaken for child abuse.

CONDITIONS MISTAKEN FOR BRUISING RESULTING FROM CHILD ABUSE

"Normal" Bruises

Bruising is common in healthy, active children. In one study, 35% of normal children were reported to have bruises every other week (45). Two studies in America and England totaling more than 1,000 children younger than 3 years confirmed that bruises are rare in infants who are not yet mobile (20,138). From 40% to 50% of walking children had bruises over bony prominences on the front of the body, including the knee, anterior tibia, forehead, and chin. It was unusual for a child to have more than three bruises. "Normal" bruises were smaller than 10 mm. Bruises on the top of the head were uncommon and had a clear-cut origin, such as one girl who repeatedly pulled herself to stand, banging her head on the underside of a table. Significant bruises were not found after falls out of bed. Bruises of the soft tissues of the face, trunk, abdomen, or buttocks, and bruises of the hand were rare (20,138). Certain features of bruising suggest abuse: patterned bruises, injuries that do not fit the history or developmental stage of the child, multiple bruises of different ages, and bruises in unusual locations (102,116).

More than 60 reports are cited in the literature of children with conditions causing bruises that were confused with inflicted injuries (Table 9.1). These included dermatologic conditions, infections, coagulation disorders, and folk healing practices.

Dermatologic Disorders

"Mongolian" or Blue Spots

Mongolian spots or blue spots are the most prevalent skin condition confused with bruises (8,38,67,71,99,133,151,152). They are blue–grey areas of pigmentation overlying the sacral area, buttocks, back, legs, shoulders, upper arms, and, occasionally, the buccal mucosa (152). They are found in about 95% of black infants, 80% of Asian infants, 70% of Latino and American Indian babies, and 10% of white babies (61). Mongolian spots usually fade during childhood but occasionally persist into adulthood (70). Lay people or newly trained health care workers who are not familiar with this condition may report it as possible abuse,

TABLE 9.1. *Conditions mistaken for bruising resulting from abuse*

Reference	Age/Sex	Presentation	Referred as abuse?	Final diagnosis
Wickes (152)		Apparent bruising	Yes. Child protection called	Mongolian spots
Wickes (152)	5 mo	Apparent bruising both shoulders down to elbows, back, buttocks, ankles, and feet	Yes. Referred by physician as battered child	Mongolian spots (extensive)
Asnes (8)	6 mo M	Apparent bruises over back and buttocks	Yes. Nurse referred to doctor	Mongolian spots
Dungy (38)	2 cases, infants	Discoloration of back, hands, and feet	Yes. Day-care staff reported. Custody proceedings initiated	Mongolian spots
Oates (99)	2 yr	Extensive apparent bruising on back and buttocks	Yes. Reported to authorities	Mongolian spots (extensive)
Smialek (133)	Several cases	Evidence of apparent trauma to lower back	Yes	Mongolian spots, SIDS
Kaplan (67)	3 mo M	Apparent large bruises on back	Yes	Mongolian spots
Kirschner (71)	5 mo F	Discoloration of back, bruise under eye, blood from nose, death	Yes	Mongolian spot, SIDS, postmortem lividity
Kirschner (71)	5 mo F	Bruises of back, ankles, eyes, blood from nose	Yes	Mongolian spots, SIDS, postmortem purging
Wheeler and Hobbs (151)	5 cases	Apparent bruises	Yes	Mongolian spots
	3 cases	Apparent bruises	Yes	Capillary hemangiomas
	1 case	Apparent bruises	Yes	Prominent facial vein
	2 cases	Apparent bruises	Yes	Eczema
	1 case	Apparent bruises	Yes	Erythema nodosum
	1 case	Apparent bruises	Yes	Allergic periorbital swelling
	1 case	Apparent bruises	Yes	Bruises from dental treatment
	2 cases	Apparent bruises	Yes	Ink, paint, or dye on face
Tunnessen (145)	18 mo M	Apparent bruises	No. Abuse suspected until color wiped off	Dye from blue jeans
Lantner and Ros (75)	18 mo F	Blue discoloration on thighs and abdomen	No	Dye from blue jeans
Anh (7)	3 yr M	Ecchymoses on chest and back, death	Yes. Father jailed and committed suicide	Coining, influenza
Yeatman et al. (159)		Petechiae and purpura of chest and back	Yes. Referred by doctor for alleged trauma	Coining
Golden and Duster (47)	8 yr M	Petechiae, purpura over arms and ribs, coma, death	No	Coining, dengue fever
	8 yr M	Bruising on back, purpura of both lower extremities	Yes. Referred by school nurse	Coining, Henoch–Schönlein purpura
Du (36)	5 yr M	Large ecchymoses over neck and back, fever, seizures, ↓LOC	Yes	Coining
Du (36)	9 yr M	Ecchymoses on back	No	Coining
Silfen (130)	11 yr M	Erythematous patches on back	No. Questioned tactfully	Coining
Saulsbury and Hayden (124)	2 yr F	Purpuric lesions on back	Yes. Babysitter. Social services involved	Spoon rubbing
Leung (78)	3 yr M 7 yr F	Ecchymoses on back	No	*Quat sha* or spoon rubbing, Chinese folk treatment
Longmire (83)	11 mo F	Ecchymoses on trunk, fever, otitis media, hematuria	Yes. Confused with abuse until interpreter came	Coining, hematuria secondary to coining
Bryan (18)	11 mo F	Dramatic ecchymoses on trunk, hematuria	Yes. Confused with abuse until interpreter came	Coining, hematuria secondary to coining
Wheeler and Hobbs (151)	1 case	Apparent bruises	Yes	*Cao gio* or coining, Vietnamese folk treatment

TABLE 9.1. *Continued*

Reference	Age/Sex	Presentation	Referred as abuse?	Final diagnosis
Rosenblat and Hong (119)	8 yr M	Bruises on neck	Yes. Referred by teacher to child protection even though family explained practice	Coining
Asnes and Wisotsky (9)	8 yr M	Eight symmetric circular ecchymotic areas on back	Yes. Nurse referred	Cupping (learned in USSR)
Coffman et al. (26)	4 yr F	Apparent handprint bruises on back, loop-shaped marks on chest	Yes	Phytodermatitis from lime juice
Coffman et al. (26)	14 mo M	Apparent hand and finger print marks on chest and back	?	Phytodermatitis from lime juice
Schwer et al. (127)	10 mo M	Bruises of different ages on face, head, trunk, extremities and buttocks; old fracture of clavicle	Yes. Reported by emergency room physician	Hemophilia
O'Hare and Eden (102)	19 mo F	Florid periorbital ecchymoses and large forehead hematoma, widespread bruising of limbs and trunk without explanation	Yes. Referred by clinic for abuse	Low levels of factors II, VIII, IX
Wheeler and Hobbs (151)	3 yr M	Multiple bruises of different ages on arms, legs, and face	Yes	Hemophilia A
	3 cases	Widespread bruising	Yes	Idiopathic thrombocytopenic purpura
	1 case	Bruising	Yes	Hemorrhagic disease of the newborn
Carpentieri et al. (21)	4 mo M	Recurrent bruises, petechiae, failure to thrive, and anemia	Yes. Admitted to hospital for neglect	Vitamin K deficiency secondary to cystic fibrosis and malabsorption
Kaplan (67)	1 yr M	Generalized bruises	Yes	Vitamin K deficiency secondary to cystic fibrosis
McClain et al. (86)	2 yr F	Multiple contusions of different ages, death. Prior report of suspected abuse	Yes. Child protection involved	Acute lymphoblastic leukemia at autopsy
Brown and Melinkovich (17)	8 mo M	Red swollen ear, facial bruise, red swelling on forehead and arm	Yes. Reported by emergency room physician. Child protection involved	Henoch–Schönlein purpura
Waskerwitz et al. (148)	2 yr M	Ecchymoses and purpura over extremities, old burn on arm, father intoxicated	Yes. Mother accused father of abuse	Hypersensitivity vasculitis
Ragosta (110)	7 yr M	Linear bruises of different ages on face, back, chest, and arms	Yes. Suspicion of device used in punishment	Head lice with maculae ceruleae
Kirschner and Stein (71)	4 yr M	Multiple bruises, lethargy, fever, death	Yes	Meningitis, DIC
	2 yr F	Bruises on cheek and inner thighs, fever, death	Yes	Meningitis, DIC
	2 yr M	Bruises on buttocks and legs	Yes. "Severe beating"	Purpura fulminans
Adler and Kane-Nussen (4)	22 mo M	Bruises and target lesions on abdomen	Yes. Social services called to emergency room	Erythema multiforme
	23 mo M	Purpura on abdomen and trunk, bluish color on face and extremities, target lesions on face, abdomen, and legs	Yes. Child-protective services involved	Erythema multiforme

Continued

TABLE 9.1. *Continued*

Reference	Age/Sex	Presentation	Referred as abuse?	Final diagnosis
(*continued*)	3 yr F	Extensive purpura of body, rash of trunk and legs	Yes. Possible battering	Erythema multiforme
Owen and Durst (103)	6 yr F	Many bruises, multiple lacerations and scars over body	Yes. Two and one-half week hospitalization to rule out abuse	Ehlers–Danlos
Roberts et al. (117)	5 yr F	Extensive bruising on limbs and trunk, scars on legs	Yes. Doctor referred for battering	Ehlers–Danlos
Saulsbury and Hayden (124)	9 yr M	Multiple bruises, scars, nonhealing wounds	Yes. Referred by school to social services	Ehlers–Danlos. Father also affected
McNamara et al. (90)	10 yr M	Multiple, repeated, frequent ecchymoses of limbs and cheek. Scars on legs, forehead, cheek, and palm	Yes. School psychologist reported. Repeatedly questioned by school staff for 2 years	Ehlers–Danlos
Harley (55)	8 mo M	Multiple bruises and hematoma	Yes, placed in shelter care for several days	Hemophilia B
Harley (55)	2 yr F	Unexplained bruising	Yes, Sunday school reported, in custody for several days	Idiopathic thrombocytopenic purpura
Harley (55)	5 yr M	Multiple unexplained bruises	Yes, teacher reported; in shelter several days	Idiopathic thrombocytopenic purpura
Daly (31)	3 yr F	Bruises of legs and buttocks, limping	Yes, admitted to rule out abuse. Biopsy of lesions	Henoch–Schönlein purpura
Wetzel (150)	10 wk F	Bruises of legs and buttocks, intracranial and retinal bleeds, brain death	Yes	Vitamin K deficiency. Home birth, breast fed, no prophylaxis
Tanner (141)	9 cases	Strangers made accusations of abuse	No	Facial hemangioma

Wk, week; mo, month; yr, year; F, female; M, male; LOC, level of consciousness; DIC, disseminated intravascular coagulation; SIDS, sudden infant death syndrome.

particularly if they are unaware that a child is racially mixed. We hope that a consultant makes the correct diagnosis before legal steps are taken. This case, which occurred at the author's hospital, is typical.

A 3-month-old infant was seen in the emergency department late at night with fever and cough. A nurse observed the infant's mother slapping the 3-year-old sibling, and became concerned that the infant also had bruises on her buttocks. The nurse asked the father about the cause of the bruises, and he indicated they came from the mother. The infant was admitted largely because of concerns about abuse. The next morning, the child abuse consultant was notified and arrived to find a detective, a child-protection worker, and a uniformed officer ready to interview the family. The officer was equipped with handcuffs, a holstered gun, and a small dictionary to help translate in Spanish for the family, who spoke little English. The child abuse consultant asked to see the child alone first to avoid alarming the family unnecessarily in case the lesions were mongolian spots. The consultant identified classic mongolian spots. The father was asked about the spots and said, in Spanish, "She was born with those. Don't you know, all Latinos have those?" The law enforcement officers did not file a report, but the child-protection worker was asked to provide the family with education about appropriate discipline.

The possibility of abuse is likely to arise when the social situation is worrisome and an infant has mongolian spots that are numerous, overlapping, or in unusual locations. In questionable cases, the examiner should document the size, color, and location of the lesions and reexamine the infant in a week. Mongolian spots do not fade or change color in the manner of bruises.

Wickes and Zaidi (152) described a 5-month-old infant referred as a case of battering after the father murdered a sibling. The mother was hospitalized for psychiatric reasons. The infant had extensive "pigmentation over both shoulders extending up to the neck and nearly down to the elbow, two circular patches on the back and one in each loin, an irregular area over the sacrum and right buttock, and encircling lesions around the ankles involving the dorsum of each foot." Subsequent observation proved these, despite the alarming history, to be "blue spots."

Disorders of Blood Vessels and Collagen

Capillary hemangiomas have been mistaken for burns or bruises (151). In one study, 36% of parents of children with facial hemangiomas reported that strangers had made comments implying abuse (141).

Erythema multiforme (4), Henoch–Schönlein (HS) purpura (17,31), and hypersensitivity vasculitis (148) have been confused with battering. Children with erythema multiforme may suddenly develop unexplained red blotches that become ecchymotic. A careful search of the skin reveals typical target lesions, and the rash is seen to progress if the child is kept under observation. Laboratory workup is normal. Herpes simplex and *Mycoplasma* are the most common infectious causes of erythema multiforme. The lesions of HS purpura are usually confined to the lower extremities, but a biopsy may be necessary to make the diagnosis clear.

A worrisome social situation may heighten concerns about abuse in the presence of unexplained skin findings. Waskerwitz et al. (148) described a toddler with generalized swelling and scattered ecchymotic lesions over the extremities as well as an old burn scar on the arm. The father was intoxicated and began arguing with his estranged wife in the emergency department after she accused him of abuse. The child was admitted for protection and evaluation. He developed urticaria, which resolved with epinephrine therapy. A skin biopsy revealed leukocytoclastic angiitis.

Ehlers–Danlos syndrome is a hereditary disorder of collagen causing skin findings easily mistaken for abuse (90,103,117,124). The skin is velvety, hyperelastic, and fragile. Minor trauma can lead to ecchymoses, hematomas, pseudotumors, poor healing, and wide atrophic scars (Fig. 9.1). Bleeding studies are normal.

Owen and Durst (103) described a 6-year-old girl admitted to the hospital for a 2.5-week court-ordered child abuse evaluation after she sustained 20 lacerations, 15 requiring suturing. Eight visits to the emergency department for lacerations had occurred in the preceding 4 months. The parents reported that "following very minor trauma, she had frequent lacerations that were difficult to suture. Often the suture pulled through tissue, reopening the wound and sometimes necessitating reclosure." The child had typical features

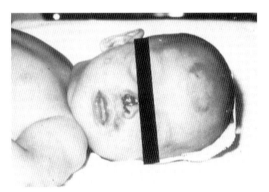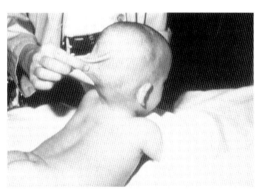

FIG. 9.1. Ehlers–Danlos syndrome mistaken for abuse. This child was admitted for plastic repair of an avulsion injury of the nose. Child abuse was suspected after a head injury occurred when only the mother was in the hospital room. An intern diagnosed Ehlers–Danlos. There was no family history. (Photo courtesy of Edward Zieserl, M.D.)

of Ehlers–Danlos syndrome with unusual facies, hyperextensibility of the skin and joints, and many wide, shiny thin "cigarette paper" scars. The mother stated that "India rubber skin ran in the father's family and he himself had it." The authors traced the disease back through five generations.

Dermatitis and Skin Staining

Phytodermatitis has been confused with skin pigmentation after bruises or burns resulting from abuse (26,32). This phototoxic reaction occurs when the skin is exposed to psoralens in the juice of certain plants and then to the sun. Authors of case reports described children who developed apparent "hand" or "loop" marks on their skin after being touched by adults who had squeezed limes for drinks at outdoor parties (Fig. 9.2). Plants that may cause phytodermatitis include lime, lemon, fig, parsnip, celery, and herbal preparations (91).

Eutectic mixture of local anesthetics (EMLA) cream is often used for topical anesthesia before procedures such as venipuncture, lumbar puncture, and dermatologic procedures. It can cause petechial or purpuric eruptions in infants and children, particularly those with preexisting eczema (19).

Millipedes produce a defensive secretion containing quinones that can produce blisters and a persistent mahogany-colored skin discoloration that might be confused with a burn (129).

Contact dermatitis also can be confused with abuse (Fig. 9.3). Pigmented lesions resembling healed burns or bruises have occurred after allergic reactions to rubber in tires, face masks, surf boards, squash balls, and the elastic bands of stockings and underwear (41).

Ragosta (110) described a child with multiple "bruises" of different ages on the face, back, shoulders, chest, and arms thought to be related to child abuse. The discovery of nits in the child's hair led to a diagnosis of maculae ceruleae. These purpuric lesions are produced by injection of an anticoagulant under the skin with hemosiderin deposition. When the lesions are caused by head lice, they are not by themselves suggestive of abuse or neglect. Maculae ceruleae are more often associated with the crab louse, however, and child sexual abuse should be suspected in a child with pubic lice anywhere on the body (128).

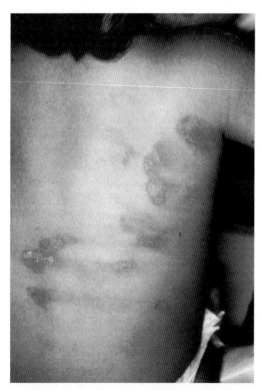

FIG. 9.2. Phytodermatitis mimicking hand prints or looped cord marks due to abuse. The lesions developed after exposure to lime juice. (Photo courtesy of R. Hansen, M.D.)

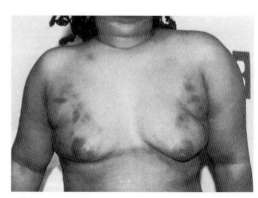

FIG. 9.3. Contact dermatitis in the distribution of a bra, confused with bruises due to abuse.

Ink, paint, or dyes on the face were mistaken for abuse in two children, one of whom was admitted to the hospital because of apparent bruising (151). Bluish discoloration of the skin related to dye "bleeding" from clothing has been confused with bruising from abuse or other serious medical conditions. The lesions are confined to areas exposed to the usually new, unwashed, black or blue clothing. Soap and water may not remove the discoloration, but alcohol is effective (56,75,77,145).

Coagulation Disorders

Hemophilia and von Willebrand's Disease

Coagulation abnormalities, both hereditary and acquired, can produce bruises confused with injuries resulting from abuse. Hereditary diseases include hemophilia and von Willebrand's disease. In 20% of new cases of hemophilia, the patient has no family history of the disease. The first evidence of hemophilia may be persistent bleeding or oozing after circumcision or other minor trauma. When the child begins to walk and fall, easy bruising and bruising on unusual locations may be seen. von Willebrand's disease and other platelet disorders are characterized by bleeding from mucous membranes, with epistaxis, melena or hematochezia, and petechiae (127).

A prolonged partial thromboplastin time (PTT) is seen in both hemophilia and von Willebrand's disease. The PTT is not very sensitive, however, and may be only minimally prolonged, even with factor VIII levels as low as 5% to 25% of normal. If hemophilia is suspected, actual assays of factors VIII and IX must be performed. If von Willebrand's disease is suspected, a bleeding time should be done. Surprisingly, there are only four case reports of children (ages 8, 10, 19, and 36 months) with multiple bruises who were found to have hemophilia after a mistaken diagnosis of abuse (55,102,127,151).

Abuse and Bleeding Disorders

It is important to remember that children with bleeding disorders are not immune from abuse. O'Hare and Eden (102) investigated the incidence of bleeding disorders in 50 children referred for suspected nonaccidental injury. A complete blood count (CBC), platelet count, prothrombin time (PT), PTT, thrombin time, fibrinogen, and bleeding time were performed for all children.

The diagnosis for one toddler was accidental trauma and a coagulation disorder, after low levels of factors II, VIII, and IX were noted. Two children were found to have sustained nonaccidental injury in association with a coagulation disorder. A 6-year-old girl with extensive bruising of the buttocks from being kicked by an adult also had an abnormal bleeding time and abnormal platelet aggregation. A 3-year-old girl with unexplained bruising of the chest and genitalia was diagnosed with von Willebrand's disorder.

Five children were found to have sustained nonaccidental injury and also had a laboratory abnormality of coagulation. A 2-month-old child with bleeding from a torn frenulum had been given salicylate by his parent. Four children, aged 4 months to 3 years, with abusive trauma, had a prolonged PTT at first assessment that resolved on repeated testing. The authors speculated that circulating thromboplastic substances from tissue injury may prolong the PTT. They concluded that ". . . non-accidental injury and bleeding disorders are in no way mutually exclusive. It is as potentially dangerous and unhelpful for the child and family to have an inappropriate diagnosis of non-accidental injury made when there is a bleeding disorder as it is for non-accidental injury to be dismissed. The child with a bleeding disorder is at particular risk from abuse . . . ."

Acquired Conditions: Idiopathic Thrombocytopenic Purpura and Leukemia

Several acquired conditions, such as idiopathic thrombocytopenic purpura (ITP) (55, 151) and leukemia (86), have been confused with abuse (Fig. 9.4). A CBC with differential, platelet count, PT, PTT, and bleeding time should be done in all cases of suggestive

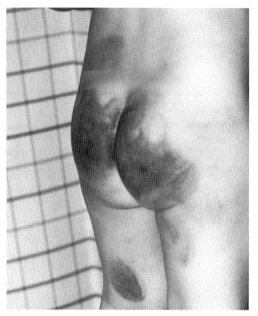

FIG. 9.4. Extensive ecchymoses after a mild spanking with a spoon in a 3-year-old boy with previously undiagnosed leukemia. The white blood count was 350,000.

or unexplained bruising. Many families who have abused their children use the excuse that the child or other family members bruise easily. In the face of such a history, a coagulation screen may clarify the diagnosis.

McClain et al. (86) described a 2-year-old girl who was found unresponsive in bed and died despite vigorous resuscitation efforts. Numerous bruises of different ages led to an investigation and autopsy. A report of suspected abuse had been made after the child was seen "covered with bruises" in a restaurant 1 month before her death. The maternal grandmother felt that the mother's boyfriend had injured the child.

Autopsy revealed massive splenomegaly with petechiae and contusions of various ages on the face, chest, abdomen, and lower legs, and focal hemorrhages of the anal mucosa. Extensive lymphoblastic infiltration was present in the liver, kidneys, heart, stomach, pancreas, bone marrow, and dura mater. Several days after the autopsy, laboratory results from samples drawn during resuscitation were reported, showing a hemoglobin of 1.8 g/dL, a hematocrit of 4%, a white blood cell count of 39,300/mm^3, a platelet count of 87,000/mm^3, and 100% lymphocytes on peripheral smear. Incredibly, 1 week before the child's death, she was seen by a physician for respiratory problems and was treated with antibiotics and bronchodilators. Apparently, the physician did not notice the child's bruises or evidence of anemia and leukemia.

Vitamin K Deficiency

Bruises related to acquired vitamin K deficiency have led to investigations of possible abuse (150,151). Hemorrhagic disease of the newborn can develop in 3- to 6-week-old breast-fed infants who did not receive vitamin K prophylactically at birth. Intracranial hemorrhage occurs in up to 50% of these children. Babies born at home are at risk, as they may not receive vitamin K or are given the less effective oral form (147). According to Krugman (personal communication, 1992), one such infant had subdural hemorrhages after being taken on a jolting ride on unpaved mountainous roads. Any disease associated with malabsorption of fat-soluble vitamins may manifest with easy bruising.

Carpentieri et al. (21) reported a 4-month-old infant with emaciation, delayed development, pitting edema, and a 2-week history of recurrent bruises. He was erroneously diagnosed as neglected until, by chance, a salty taste to his skin was noticed. Sweat chloride levels were elevated, and a test for fat malabsorption was positive. The final diagnosis was vitamin K deficiency resulting from malabsorption associated with cystic fibrosis. All of the child's symptoms and signs reversed with appropriate diet and administration of vitamin K.

Bruises can result from minor trauma after ingestion of anticoagulants such as warfarin. Accidental ingestion does occur, because some rodenticides containing warfarin have the appearance of candy (48).

Watts et al. (149) described a 7-year-old girl with bilateral occipital hemorrhagic infarcts after minor cerebral trauma. The child had residual bilateral third cranial nerve palsies and partial cortical blindness. Seven months later, she was readmitted with a large hematoma of the calf. PT and PTT were prolonged. Pellets of rat poison containing brodifacoum were found in a hole in the ceiling over the counter in the family kitchen. By 7 months after removal of the poison, the child's bleeding had stopped, and her coagulation times were normal. Seven months later, however, she began bleeding again, and once again had prolonged PT and PTT. Brodifacoum was found in rat droppings on the floor of the unkempt mobile home where the child lived. The family continued to deny the use of rodenticide. Ingestion of brodifacoum was judged to be accidental even though no other family members had abnormal clotting studies. The authors concluded that the child's visual handicap predisposed her to ingestion of food contaminated by brodifacoum or rat droppings.

Folk Medicine

A variety of Asian medical practices produce ecchymoses sometimes mistaken for bruises from abuse (54,84). The child's skin may be pinched or massaged by hand and rubbed or scratched with an implement like a spoon (*quat sha*) or coin (*cheut sah* or *cao gio*), resulting in a petechial or purpuric rash. Water, saline, hot oil, or tiger balm ointment may be applied to the skin during the procedure. Observation of the distinct dramatic and usually symmetric pattern of the bruises (Fig. 9.5) with a congruent history makes the diagnosis clear and avoids accusations of abuse (7,18,36,44,47,78,83,119,124,130,158,159). Microscopic hematuria has been reported after coining (83). Tragic results have occurred when coining was misdiagnosed as abuse. A Vietnamese father committed suicide after being jailed despite his explanations of how

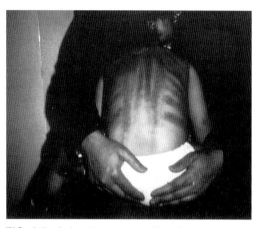

FIG. 9.5. Asian treatment with coining or spoon scratching produces patterned bruises sometimes mistaken for abuse. (Photo courtesy of K. Feldman, M.D.)

the coin-rubbing lesions on his son's back had occurred (7).

Keller and Apthorp (69) have objected to other authors' terming the bruises resulting from coining "pseudobattering," pointing out that "the definition of inflicted trauma should not be based on willful intent of those responsible . . . but specifically as trauma inflicted on a child by nonaccidental means." They recommended that physicians not report children traumatized through well-intentioned efforts to relieve pain and suffering, but that the physician be responsible for educating the family to prevent further trauma. Cultural sensitivity is important in assessing what inflicted injuries constitute abuse (113). It has been pointed out that Vietnamese immigrants were horrified to discover that Americans cut off a portion of the penis of most infant boys. The author experienced this dilemma recently.

A Southeast Asian infant was seen for a well-child visit. Three small circular burns were noted on the top of the ear pinna. The family explained that these marks were the result of a moxibustion treatment for ear pain. The pediatrician was about to begin a discussion of the unnecessary pain inflicted on the child by this well-intentioned folk treatment when she realized that she would soon inflict on the child three immunizations and a fingerstick. She postponed the discussion.

Cupping is an ancient therapeutic method practiced as recently as the 1940s in America and still used in Asia, Europe, Russia, and the Middle East. A heated cup is applied to the skin at specific points. As the cup cools, a vacuum creates suction on the skin, causing ecchymotic lesions that have been mistaken for bruising from abuse (9,43). Cupping and coining may have a counterirritant effect. An extreme form of this therapy is found in a report from Nigeria of a man with circular wheals and blistering who had hot jam jars containing hornets placed on his skin to relieve itching (143).

CONDITIONS MISTAKEN FOR BURNS RESULTING FROM ABUSE

Dermatologic Disorders

Several dermatologic conditions are associated with blisters that might be mistaken for abusive burns (Table 9.2). Phytodermatitis can cause erythema, blistering, and denudation of skin resembling abusive scald injuries (32). There are reports of nine children with impetigo mistaken for cigarette burns (68,99, 151). Dermatitis herpetiformis (154), diaper dermatitis (151), chilblain (151), drug eruption (151), mechanical abrasion (151), streptococcal toxic shock (97), and chemical burns also have been mistaken for abusive burns.

The skin lesions of dystrophic epidermolysis bullosa have been misdiagnosed as cigarette burns of the extremities. Siblings aged 3 and 4 years were evaluated by dermatologists and diverted from placement in foster care after two referring physicians had reported possible child abuse. The children had fresh erosions over bony prominences, including knees, elbows, knuckles, ankles, and forehead, with scarring and milium formation. Their mother, who had protested that she had trauma-induced blisters in childhood, had scars of the knees and elbows with "allopapuloid" lesions on her back (27). In mild forms of the disease, the only physical finding may be a dystrophic nail, or blisters only on the

acral bony prominences (Fig. 9.6). After one 8-year-old girl with epidermolysis bullosa was reported several times as a suspected victim of abuse, her mother was supplied with a medical report verifying her condition as inherited and not the result of battering (154).

Folk Treatment

Burns have been noted after folk treatment for illness or pain (54,84). In the practice of "cupping," alcohol is applied to the inner rim of the cupping glass and ignited with an alcohol-moistened pledget of cotton. The flame is extinguished before the cup is applied, creating a vacuum. If the alcohol is not fully burned away, skin burns can occur (122). An 11-year-old girl was seen with four circular areas of first-degree burn after such treatment (123).

Maquas are small deep burns intentionally inflicted for therapeutic purposes (Fig. 9.7). Hot metal spits or coals are applied to points near the site of disease or over a traditional "draining point." Twenty-six cases among adults were seen in a 5-year period at one Israeli hospital, most often in Bedouin patients, but also in Asian Jews, Arabs, Druses, and Russian Jews (118).

Moxibustion is a form of therapy related to acupuncture. Lighted sticks of incense, yarn, cigarettes, or cones of the herb *Artemisia* are burned near or on the skin at therapeutic points (Fig. 9.8) (39,76,113). When actual burns are produced rather than simple reddening of the skin, physicians should encourage parents to modify or abandon the practice.

Chemical or Accidental Burns

Chemical or accidental burns should be ruled out before abuse is diagnosed. A detailed history is essential. For example, lesions resembling cigarette burns have occurred in children exposed to the electrical current in an enuresis blanket (34). Butane and propane, which have replaced chlorinated hydrocarbons in aerosol sprays, can cause full-thickness burns from frostbite when children spray aerosols on their skin (74).

TABLE 9.2. *Conditions mistaken for burns resulting from abuse*

Reference	Age/Sex	Presentation	Referred as abuse?	Final diagnosis
Colver and Harris (27)	3 yr 4 yr	Apparent cigarette burns of knees, knuckles, ankles, and fore head with scarring	Yes. (Despite mother sayingshe had same problem)	Epidermolysis bullosa
Winship and Winship (154)	8 yr F	Blisters, scabs, and scars on face, hands, and feet, subungual bullae	Yes. By neighbors	Epidermolysis bullosa
	18 mo M	Sores and scars on trunk thought to be sunburn and cigarette burns	Yes. Father taken into custody	Epidermolysis bullosa
	8 yr M	Widespread bullous lesions	Yes. By social worker	Epidermolysis bullosa
	?	Apparent cigarette burns	?	Dermatitis herpetiformis
Oates (99)	4 yr M	Possible cigarette burns, circular lesions on arms	Yes. By county hospital	Impetigo
Kaplan (67)	4 yr M	Apparent cigarette burns, bullae with black centers on trunk	Yes	Bullous impetigo
Wheeler and Hobbs (151)	9 cases	Apparent cigarette burns	Yes. (Some children had been previous victims of abuse)	Impetigo
	3 cases	Apparent scalds	Yes. (One child was neglected)	Severe diaper rash
	2 cases	Apparent burns	Yes	Chilblain
	2 cases	Apparent burns	Yes	Mechanical abrasion
	1 case	Apparent burn	Yes	Fixed drug eruption
	13 mo M	Apparent scalds around both ankles (mother's history of vinegar exposure thought to be implausible)	Yes	Chemical burn, acetic acid (commercial strength)
Nunez and Taff (98)	3 yr F	Second- and third-degree burns of foot and ankle	Yes	Chemical burn, "Icy hot" balm
Dannaker et al. (32)	14 mo M	Apparent scalding, erythema, blisters, and denuded skin on cheeks, chin, and upper chest	Yes	Phytodermatitis, lime juice
Schmitt et al. (125)	8 mo F	Deep linear burn on arm, parents uncooperative	Yes. Foster care 6 mo	Car-seat burn (retrospective)
	8 mo M	Second-degree burns on side of foot	Yes. SCAN team consulted, not reported	Car-seat burn
	10 mo M	First- and second-degree burns of upper thigh	Yes. Public health nurse investigated	Burn from black safety strap on bicycle seat
	8 mo F	First- and second-degree burns of four digits and palm	Yes. Foster care 3 days	Car-seat burn (witnessed)
	5 mo F	Blister behind right ear, hygiene neglected	Abuse considered until additional information obtained	Burn on metal backpack tubing in hot car
Spencer and Grieve (134)	2 yr M	Since age 6 mo, burns to hands 3 times, deep cuts, bruises, and a skull fracture	Yes. Diagnosis made when sister found him touching iron without pain	Congenital indifference to pain
Sandler and Haynes (123)	11 yr F	Four circular first-degree burns on back	No	Cupping "ventosas," Latin American folk treatment
Zurbuchen (161)	8 yr M	Subcutaneous necrosis of thigh, skin graft required	Yes, mother addicted	Chemical burn from calcium chloride crystals in pocket

Wk, week; mo, month; yr, year; F, female; M, male; LOC, level of consciousness; DIC, disseminated intravascular coagulation; SIDS, sudden infant death syndrome; SCAN, suspected child abuse and neglect.

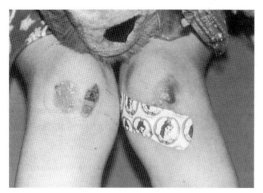

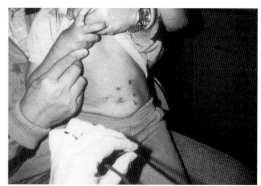

FIG. 9.6. Epidermolysis bullosa in a girl evaluated for possible abuse. There were additional lesions on the elbows, toes, and on the ankles under a shoe strap. (Photo courtesy of L. Keltner, M.D.)

FIG. 9.8. Moxibustion treatment resulting in abdominal burns in a Southeast Asian child.

Most burns to young children occur in the kitchen or bathroom. Accidental burns to the genitalia are commonly caused by children spilling hot liquids into their laps (93). Accidental burns to the back and buttocks are rare, and the history should provide a specific and adequate explanation. For example, a stove can tip over if a child climbs on an open oven door, and hot liquids spill onto the child's back (137). Walkers are a dangerous source of increased infant access to such hazards as hot fireplace screens, wood stoves, and cords dan-

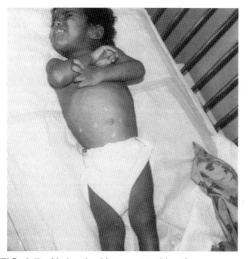

FIG. 9.7. Abdominal burns resulting from *maqua* treatment in a Saudi Arabian child with cerebral palsy. (Photo courtesy of R. Reece, M.D.)

gling from electric tea kettles (24). Even with an adequate accidental explanation for a burn, a report to child welfare authorities may be warranted, as in the case reports of children "unintentionally" injured when drain cleaner was hurled during domestic violence (15).

Circumferential burns of the extremities are usually abusive, but exceptions have been noted (Fig. 9.9). A 13-month-old boy was referred with apparent circumferential scalds around both ankles inadequately explained by the mother as resulting from exposure to vinegar. It was discovered that the vinegar was a commercial preparation of acetic acid with a pH of 1.5 used by the grandfather in a "pie and pea" stall. Elastic in the trouser legs held the caustic liquid at the ankle (151). In another example, a 3-year-old girl presented with circumferential second- and third-degree burns of the ankle and foot thought to be related to abuse. Further investigation revealed that the foster mother had applied Icy Hot analgesic balm to treat the child's sprained ankle in accordance with Latin American folk beliefs about treating a "cold" disease (sprain) with a "hot" remedy (98).

Calcium chloride, used as de-icing salt or dehumidifying agent, has caused burns mistaken for abuse. A boy who carried "white stones" in his pocket developed subcutaneous tissue necrosis on his thigh that required skin grafting (161). Accidental burns from hot car seats or bicycle or car seat belts have been confused with abuse. On a sunny day, dark upholstery or metal buckles rapidly heat to temperatures ca-

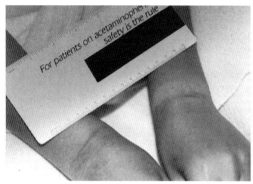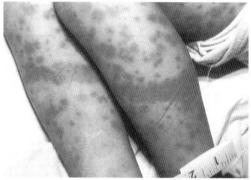

A B

FIG. 9.9. A: Rope burns due to abuse. The child was tied to a chair during anal sodomy. (Photo courtesy of P. Thomas, M.D.). **B:** Erythema multiforme in the distribution of sock elastic, resembling rope burns. (Photo courtesy of B. Lauer, M.D.)

pable of inflicting second-degree burns. Children aged 12 months or younger are particularly vulnerable, as they may not be able to move away quickly from the heat source (125).

CONDITIONS MISTAKEN FOR INTRACRANIAL BLEEDING RESULTING FROM ABUSE

Intracranial bleeding in children can be caused by accidental trauma, coagulation disorders, tumors, genetic defects, and vascular malformations. Inflicted trauma is the most likely cause of subdural hemorrhages in infants and young children. In one population-based incidence study, 21 of 100,000 infants younger than 1 year and 13 of 100,000 infants younger than 2 years had intracranial bleeding due to abuse (72).

The literature includes six descriptions of children with intracranial bleeding erroneously attributed to abuse, and later found to be related to other conditions (Table 9.3). None of these bleeds was subdural. Ryan and Gayle (121) reported a 6-week-old infant with vomiting and intraventricular and subarachnoid hemorrhage. A shaking–impact injury was considered. The infant bled at venipuncture sites and developed a large subgaleal hematoma at the site of an unsuccessful attempt at a scalp vein catheterization. A diagnosis of hemorrhagic disease of the newborn was made after it was found that the infant had not received vitamin

K prophylaxis at birth, had been exclusively breast-fed, and had prolonged PT and PTT. The baby died despite administration of vitamin K and fresh frozen plasma.

Other reports include a 6-week-old child with intracerebral hemorrhage related to an aneurysm (89) and a 10-year-old child with intracerebral hemorrhage from a brain tumor (68). Kaplan (68) described a 1-month-old boy with a bulging fontanelle and subdural fluid seen on computed tomographic (CT) scanning. Because the child had no external evidence of abuse, and the mother was nurturing and kept medical appointments, the assumption was made that the subdural collections had not resulted from abuse but were "benign subdural effusions," a diagnosis whose cause has yet to be adequately explained by those who posit it.

Prenatal and Perinatal Trauma

When a newborn presents with intracranial hemorrhage, the cause is usually birth trauma or perinatal disorders of coagulation (62). Breech birth and vacuum extraction can cause subdural and subarachnoid bleeding with significant sequelae. Bleeding due to birth trauma is typically in the posterior fossa, as opposed to bleeding due to abuse, which is most often frontal, parietal, and interhemispheric (100).

Abuse may be a cause of prenatal intracranial bleeding. Gunn and Becroft (50) reported

TABLE 9.3. *Conditions mistaken for intracranial bleeding resulting from abuse*

Reference	Age/Sex	Presentation	Referred as abuse?	Final diagnosis
Jocelyn and Casiro (62)	2 cases, neonates	Intraventricular hemorrhage, symptomatic after discharge home	Yes. Investigated but no proof	Unknown
McLellan et al. (89)	6 wk F	Seizures, pallor, screaming, bilateral RH, large intra-cerebral hemorrhage	Yes. Admitted with diagnosis of shaken baby	Aneurysm of right middle cerebral artery
Ryan and Gayle (121)	6 wk F	Vomiting, ↓ LOC, tense fontanelle, ↑ ICP, hemor-rhage into subgaleal space, ventricles, subarachnoid space and brain parenchyma	Yes. Possible shaken baby	Hemorrhagic disease of the newborn from vitamin K deficiency; death
Kaplan (67)	10 yr F	Brain dead, bilateral RH, intracerebral hemorrhage	Yes. "Misdiagnosed abuse"	Brain tumor at autopsy
	1 mo M	Bulging fontanelle, subdural fluid on CT scan	Yes. "Misdiagnosed abuse"	"Benign subdural effusion"
Guarnaschelli et al. (49)	2 mo M	Tense fontanelle, fixed pupils, arreflexia, seizures, bilateral subdural hemorrhages	Yes. "A variant of battered child"	Shaken to treat fallen fontanelle or *caida de mollera*
Wetzel (150)	10 wk F	"Brain dead," bruises on buttocks, small subdurals and retinal bleeding	Yes	Vitamin K deficiency. Home birth, breast fed, no prophylaxis

Wk, week; mo, month; yr, year; RH, retinal hemorrhage; LOC, level of consciousness; ICP, intracranial pressure; CT, computed tomography.

20 macerated stillborn infants with unexplained intracranial hemorrhages born to mothers from the Pacific Islands. Stephens et al. (136) described an American neonate with bilateral subdural hemorrhages of different ages and brain atrophy. In both reports, the authors proposed that the infants were victims of "abuse" *in utero,* injured when their pregnant mothers were beaten in episodes of domestic violence.

Folk Treatments

Can folk treatments cause intracranial hemorrhage in infants? Perhaps, but only if the forces used are sufficiently violent. Gunn et al. (51) described three live-born infants who had subdural hemorrhages *in utero* with no history of maternal trauma. Some evidence showed that bleeding had occurred before birth. Two infants had macrocephaly at birth, and one had subdural bleeding diagnosed sonographically 4 weeks before birth. The third had significant dilutional anemia at birth. Autopsy revealed a thick subdural membrane, indicating that the bleeding had occurred at least 10 days before birth. In the absence of evidence of *in utero* trauma, coagulation disorders, or vascular mal-

formations, these prenatal subdural bleeds remained unexplained.

The authors mentioned the possibility that a form of traditional Malaysian abdominal massage (*urut*) may have injured these infants *in utero.* The massage can be quite forceful, with the practitioner sometimes standing on the abdomen of the patient. *Urut* has been used to induce abortion and may have caused intestinal perforation in several adults (111).

There are two case reports of subdural bleeding attributed to *caida de mollera,* a folk treatment for "fallen fontanelle." A 2-month-old Mexican American boy was hospitalized, with pallor, a bulging fontanelle, and a right retinal hemorrhage. Lumbar puncture and subdural taps yielded large amounts of bright red blood. Two days before admission, his grandmother, a folk healer (*curandera*), treated him for *caida de mollera* or sunken fontanelle. Part of the treatment consisted of "holding the infant upside down by his ankles with his head partially immersed in boiling water, shaking him vigorously three times while slapping the soles of his feet. Following this procedure, the infant's fontanelle was no longer sunken." Skeletal survey was unremarkable. The infant developed severe cerebral atrophy and died 8 months later of pulmonary complications associated with severe spastic quadriparesis (49).

There is a belief among some Mexican Americans that an infant's fontanelle can drop if the child falls, is dropped, or has the nipple pulled out of its mouth too vigorously. If the fontanelle falls, the displaced part is felt as a rounded projection or *bolita* on the infant's palate, which prevents the child from feeding. The symptoms of fallen fontanelle are poor feeding, crying, and diarrhea and vomiting. To physicians, these symptoms and signs are diagnostic of dehydration from gastroenteritis.

The folk treatments for *caida de mollera* include pushing the palate upward, shaving, and applying a poultice or suction to the fontanelle. The infant may be held upside down, the crown of the head is dipped into water, and the soles of the feet are slapped.

Although physicians treating the infant just described in the early 1970s postulated that folk treatment caused the brain injury and termed this a "variant of the battered child syndrome" (49), another author recently has questioned this conclusion. She pointed out that there have been no further such reports in the intervening three decades and that the shaking in *caida de mollera* is gentle and not sufficient to cause intracranial bleeding (54).

Congenital Conditions

Although arteriovenous malformations (AVMs) are often mentioned in the differential diagnosis of intracranial bleeding, they are extremely rare in children younger than 2 years, when inflicted trauma is a more likely cause, and they are readily detected by imaging. AVMs occur most often in the brain substance and in the distribution of the middle meningeal artery (6,14).

Glutaric aciduria type 1 (GA 1) is a rare inborn error of catabolism of lysine and tryptophan. Subdural and retinal hemorrhages have occurred, sometimes repeatedly, in infants with GA 1 after minimal trauma. This condition is unlikely to be confused with abuse, as CT scans show widening of the sylvian fissure and frontotemporal atrophy, which presumably results in elongation and fragility of bridging veins. Subdural hemorrhage has not been seen in patients without cerebral atrophy. Patients with GA 1 also have macrocrania, developmental regression, delay in white matter myelination, and are not predisposed to fractures. Diagnosis can be made through metabolic assay of urine and blood (95,156).

Coagulation Disorders

Can intracranial bleeding be the result of coagulation abnormalities? Can brain injury result in coagulation abnormalities? The answer to both questions is yes.

A study of the records of 123 children with known hemophilia or von Willebrand's disease revealed 109 episodes of head trauma in 49 children, with five instances of intracranial bleeding. One was due to forceps delivery. The others were associated with skull fractures due to falls. There were three epidurals, one subarachnoid, and one subdural hematoma. All presented for evaluation within 24 hours, and none had associated injuries (33).

A review of more than 300 children with ITP found that episodes of major hemorrhage occurred when the platelet count decreased below 20,000/mm^3. Two children had intracranial hemorrhage, and both recovered without sequelae (92).

Head trauma in adults and children can be associated with abnormalities in coagulation. In one report of 147 children younger than 4 years with inflicted head trauma, 54% of patients with parenchymal damage and 20% of those without had abnormalities of clotting studies, most commonly prolongation of PT. The authors postulated that tissue factors are released from damaged brain cells and activate coagulation via the intrinsic pathway, sometimes resulting in disseminated intravascular coagulation. A full coagulation screen consisting of PT, PTT, TT, CBC, platelet count, fibrinogen, and fibrin degradation product (FDP) or d-dimer is recommended in all patients with suspected traumatic brain injury (60).

CONDITIONS MISTAKEN FOR HEMORRHAGE OF THE EYE RESULTING FROM ABUSE

Blunt injury, accidental or abusive, to the temporal region can result in unilateral periorbital ecchymosis. Although bilateral ecchymoses of the eyes are suggestive of abuse, they can be caused by an accidental injury to the forehead. Subconjunctival hemorrhages of limited size are present transiently after birth in 0.5% to 13% of newborns. Levin (80) stated that extensive subconjunctival hemorrhage after the first 1 to 2 weeks of life should be considered suggestive of abuse. Forceful coughing, vomiting, or Valsalva effect also can produce subconjunctival hemorrhage (94).

Nonabusive etiologies of retinal hemorrhages include severe accidental head trauma, severe compressive chest trauma, coagulopathies, blood dyscrasias, meningitis, severe hypertension, vasculitis, and throm-boembolic phenomena such as in bacterial endocarditis (37,79,80). Studies from the United Kingdom indicated that convulsions alone are not a cause of retinal hemorrhages in infants younger than 2 years (146).

Retinal hemorrhages occur in 20% to 30% of infants delivered vaginally and have even occurred during cesarean birth. These hemorrhages should resolve in the first week of life, rarely persisting as long as 6 weeks (79,80). Exposure to cocaine *in utero* may increase the incidence of birth-related retinal hemorrhages in newborns, and may delay their resolution (131).

In several reported cases, retinal hemorrhages were erroneously attributed to abuse (Table 9.4). A 2-month-old infant was found apparently dead in his pram. He was slapped repeatedly by the parents in an effort to revive him, and may have aspirated blood from an epistaxis. Fresh retinal hemorrhages observed in the hospital 10 minutes later were attributed to thoracic compression and hypoxia of the retinal vessels rather than to abuse (10). Another 6-week-old infant admitted for possible battering had had an intracerebral bleed

TABLE 9.4. *Conditions mistaken for hemorrhages of the eye resulting from abuse*

Reference	Age/Sex	Presentation	Referred as abuse?	Final diagnosis
Bacon et al. (10)	2 mo M	Apnea, slapped repeatedly to revive, fresh bilateral RH	Yes. Not reported after history obtained	RH produced by thoracic compression and hypoxia of retinal vessels
McLellan et al. (89)	6 wk F	Seizures, pallor, screaming, bilateral RH, large intra-cerebral hemorrhage	Yes. Admitted with diagnosis of shaken baby	Aneurysm of right middle cerebral artery
Riffenburgh and Sathyavagiswaran (114)	3 cases	RH seen at autopsy	N/A	MVA with severe head trauma
		RH seen at autopsy		Death 1 week after difficult forceps delivery
		RH seen at autopsy		Respiratory failure with CPR and damaging chest compressions
Wheeler and Hobbs (151)		Subconjunctival hemorrhages	Yes	Valsalva effect from coughing with pertussis
Mokrohisky and Kesselman (94)	11 yr M	Total subconjunctival hemorrhage, swelling and bruising of lids of both eyes	No. "Might have been confused with abuse"	Valsalva effect from straining to void with severe urinary retention
Wetzel (150)	10 wk F	Retinal hemorrhages, small subdurals, bruises of buttocks and legs, brain death	Yes	Vitamin K deficiency. Home birth, breast fed, no prophylaxis

Wk, week; mo, month; yr, year; F, female; M, male; MVA, motor vehicle accident; RH, retinal hemorrhage; CPR, cardiopulmonary resuscitation.

and retinal hemorrhages from a bleeding middle cerebral artery aneurysm (89).

Riffenburgh and Sathyavagiswaran (114) studied 77 pairs of eyes removed from children who had died of suspected child abuse. Forty-seven (61%) cases had retinal hemorrhages. Three of these had clear nonabusive etiologies. One had severe head trauma in a car accident, one died a week after a difficult forceps delivery, and the last had respiratory failure with damaging chest compression during attempts at resuscitation.

Accidental head trauma is an uncommon cause of retinal hemorrhage. No retinal hemorrhages were found in 50 children younger than 2 years with accidental head trauma who were studied by Alario et al. (5). Similarly, Duhaime et al. (37) found retinal hemorrhages in one (2%) of 44 children with accidental head injuries and in nine (38%) of 24 children with head injuries resulting from abuse. The one child with accidental injury and retinal hemorrhages died after a high-speed motor vehicle accident. Reece and Sege (112) found retinal hemorrhages in only 2% (five patients) of 233 accidentally head-injured patients and in 33% of the children with abusive head trauma. The patients with the retinal hemorrhages in the accident group all had been in major accidents accounting for the head injuries (motor vehicle crashes, fall from several stories, gunshot wound to the face).

Cardiopulmonary Resuscitation and Retinal Hemorrhages

Cardiopulmonary resuscitation (CPR) alone does not appear to be a cause of retinal hemorrhage (46). A prospective study (101) of 45 events of CPR in hospitalized children revealed only one infant with small punctate retinal hemorrhages. She had prolonged coagulation studies, a low platelet count, and had received 60 minutes of open cardiac massage. Kanter (66) also evaluated 54 children for retinal hemorrhage after CPR. Among five victims of trauma with retinal hemorrhage, four had other evidence of child abuse. The

fifth had been hit by a car, sustaining head and chest injuries. One 18-month-old child who had not sustained trauma also was found to have retinal hemorrhages. This child, found cyanotic and seizing at home, had arterial hypertension (190/120 mm Hg) after resuscitation. Both studies concluded that "retinal hemorrhage should not be attributed to the mechanical effects of cardiopulmonary resuscitation."

Confirmation for this view is found in a report of a 6-week-old infant with a nonaccidental crush injury to the chest causing injury to several ribs, pneumomediastinum, and lung contusion with diffuse alveolar damage. The father admitted he had crushed the baby to his chest in an attempt to stop him crying. This infant did not have retinal hemorrhage despite a compressive force sufficient to injure the lungs (88).

FALLS

Clinicians are often faced with a dilemma when a child presents with significant intracranial injury and a history of a fall. On the one hand, trauma is the leading cause of death in children, and falls are the third leading cause of trauma deaths in children 1 to 4 years old (53). On the other hand, in the absence of a history of significant trauma, such as a motor vehicle accident, child abuse is the most common cause of intracranial injury in children younger than 1 year (13,112). How does the clinician sort out accidental from nonaccidental causes?

Injuries Resulting from Short Falls

Several studies indicated that accidental falls from the height of a couch, bed, crib, or changing table only rarely cause a linear parietal skull fracture and almost never cause serious or life-threatening injury. This rule applies to simple gravitational falls onto a flat, somewhat resilient surface. Falls involving acceleration forces or entrapment in walkers, strollers, or crib rails can lead to more serious injury (52).

The initial studies on short falls were compiled as physicians first became aware that abuse might be a significant cause of head trauma in infants. In 1969 Kravitz et al. (73) found that, among 330 children injured in alleged accidental falls, only 10% had neurologic symptoms. There was one subdural hematoma. In 1977 Helfer et al. (57) reported on 246 children younger than 5 years who fell less than 5 feet. No child had serious injuries. Three sustained linear parietal skull fractures without central nervous system injury.

Billmire and Myers (13) reviewed CT scans of 84 infants younger than 1 year who were admitted to hospital with head injury. Accidental trauma (witnessed events with no discrepancies between physical findings and mechanism described) accounted for only one case of intracranial hemorrhage in an infant who was unrestrained in a motor vehicle accident. Retinal hemorrhages were not seen in any accidentally injured infants. In comparing the incidence of subdural hematomas in accidental head injuries with abusive ones, Reece and Sege (112) found that subdural hematomas were seen in only 10% of the accident group as compared with 46% in the inflicted-injury group. Subarachnoid hemorrhages were seen in only 8% of the accident group but in 31% of the abuse group.

Lyons and Oates (85) studied 200 children falling out of bed. They found no serious, multiple, visceral or life-threatening injuries. There was one simple skull fracture and one clavicle fracture. This and other studies indicated that child abuse should be suspected if significant visceral, thoracic, or non–skull fracture injuries are found in children who reportedly fall less than three stories (53).

Williams (153) reviewed 106 cases of falls in children younger than 3 years old. Only one death occurred from a fall of 70 feet. No life-threatening injuries occurred in falls from less than 5 feet. Three infants sustained small depressed skull fractures without loss of consciousness after falling between 4 and 5 feet onto an edged surface. The author concludes that "infants and small children are relatively resistant to injuries from free falls," and, that

when severe injuries or deaths are attributed to falls from a low height, child abuse is the likely etiology.

Chadwick et al. (25) reviewed 317 cases of falls in children. Only one death occurred in the group of 193 children who fell from heights of 5 to 45 feet. Seven deaths occurred in the 100 children falling less than 4 feet. All seven had other factors suggesting child abuse as the etiology, leading the authors to conclude that "when children incur fatal injuries in falls of less than 4 feet, the history is incorrect."

In a Missouri study (142) of 167 infants who fell vertically four feet or less (excluding acceleration injuries and walker-related falls), 18 were admitted with closed head injury. Sixteen of these had skull fractures. Seven had long-bone fractures and no other evidence of occult trauma on skeletal survey. Only two infants had intracranial bleeding. The initial history of a short fall was eventually replaced by a confession of abuse. One baby had been shaken, and the other hit by a stereo speaker thrown during domestic violence.

In summary, a history of an accidental fall of less than 5 feet is plausible if it results in either no injury, soft tissue injury with no neurologic sequelae (bruises or a "bump on the head"), or, rarely, if the infant impacts an edge, in a linear parietal skull fracture with no subdural bleeding and no central nervous system damage. Epidural bleeding may occur after an accidental skull fracture.

Our hospital staff requested a child abuse consultation when a 5-month-old infant was admitted with a skull fracture. The parents said that they had left the child in a church nursery during an evening service. After returning home, they noticed that the infant was fussy and had a small bump on the side of his head. They went immediately to the emergency department where an evaluation revealed an isolated linear parietal skull fracture, no intracranial blood, no other injuries, and no neurologic abnormalities. An investigation revealed that a teenage caretaker at church had been carrying the infant in an infant carrier with tubular metal edges. She dropped him onto a tile floor, impacting his head against the edge of the carrier. She reported this incident to the adult supervisor, but because the infant seemed uninjured at the time, no report was made to the parents.

Falls Down Stairs

Simple falls down stairs seldom result in significant head injury. In one series, only 2% of 363 children evaluated in an emergency department for falls down stairs sustained skull fractures. Nonaccidental injury should be suspected when a child presents with severe head injuries or multiple, truncal, or proximal extremity injuries and a history of an uncomplicated stairway fall (63).

When an infant falls while entrapped in a baby walker, however, skull fractures can occur, although serious sequelae are still rare. In one study, 95% of walker injuries involved falling down stairs, with 47% resulting in skull fractures (104). This increase in head injuries when walkers are involved may be related to the walker causing the infant's head to remain exposed and unprotected and also augmenting the energy of impact. A 23-month-old boy with large head size was found to have a large chronic subdural hematoma causing uncal herniation and midline shift. He had no evidence of bleeding disorders or child abuse. The child had fallen down a flight of stairs in a baby walker at age 6 months, with no apparent acute injury or sequelae. Because macrocephaly developed after the fall, the chronic subdural was considered a delayed sequela of the walker-related injury (35).

ABDOMINAL INJURIES CONFUSED WITH ABUSE

When children fall onto bicycle handlebars, serious intraabdominal injury can result, including rupture of internal organs or the aorta. Because the signs and symptoms of these impact injuries may not present for hours, and external bruising is frequently not present, there is some potential for confusion with injuries due to child abuse. The children who incur this kind of injury are usually old enough to give a history of a bicycle accident, however, unless they are unconscious (155).

CONDITIONS MISTAKEN FOR FRACTURES RESULTING FROM ABUSE

Table 9.5 is a list of reported cases of fractures erroneously attributed to abuse. An excellent review of the differential diagnosis of skeletal conditions resembling child abuse has been published (16).

Birth Injury

Fractures detected in infancy can present a difficult diagnostic problem. It is important to determine whether a fracture was the result of birth trauma or occurred after birth. Cumming (30) emphasized the importance of (a) knowing the fracture sites typical of birth injury, and (b) estimating the time of injury from radiographic signs of healing. He reviewed radiographs of 23 patients with fractures resulting from delivery. Patients with skull fractures and osteogenesis imperfecta (OI) were excluded. Fractures occurred at three sites: the clavicle, the humerus, and the femur.

Ten patients had fractures of the clavicle, all of the midshaft, with varying degrees of displacement, as a result of difficult vaginal deliveries. One infant had bilateral clavicle fractures. Six babies had fractures of the humeri, involving either the proximal or distal growth plates or the midshaft. Two resulted from breech deliveries, and four from cephalic deliveries. Seven infants had fractures of the femur. Five of the seven had meningomyelocele, and a sixth had severe neuromuscular deficit thought to be Werdnig–Hoffman disease. One child also had a tibial fracture. All the femoral fractures except one involved the midshaft. The patient with Werdnig–Hoffman disease had fractures through both distal femoral metaphyses.

Calcification of most birth fractures was apparent radiographically by 9 to 10 days. The au-

TABLE 9.5. *Conditions mistaken for fractures resulting from abuse*

Reference	Age/Sex	Presentation	Referred as abuse?	Final diagnosis
Bennani-Smires and Medina (12)	5 mo M	Subperiosteal new bone of diaphyses of humeri and legs, bucket-handle deformities of distal tibial metaphyses	No. (Had never left the) hospital	Copper deficiency from hyperalimentation
Helfer et al. (58)	10 mo M	Old fracture of humerus, swollen eye	Yes	Passive exercise incorrectly performed, accident to eye
Kirschner and Stein (71)	1 yr	Multiple skull fractures, respiratory arrest, death	Yes	Atypical suture lines, pneumonia
Horodniceanu et al. (59)	6 wk M	Swelling and pain of extremities, fracture of ulna with periosteal reaction	Yes. Admitted as battered child	Congenital syphilis
Fiser et al. (40)	5 wk F	Arms tender, no movement, bilateral humeral metaphyseal fractures with periosteal reaction, domestic violence	Yes. Admitted as battered child	Congenital syphilis
Kaplan (67)	3 mo M	Periosteal calcification, rash, poor hygiene	Yes. "Misdiagnosed abuse"	Congenital syphilis
	4 mo M	Fractured femur, epiphyseal and metaphyseal changes	Yes. "Misdiagnosed abuse"	Vitamin D–deficiency rickets
	4 yr F	Callus formation of tibias and femurs	Yes. "Misdiagnosed abuse"	Myelomeningocele, disuse atrophy, fall from wheelchair
	2 yr F	Spiral fracture of tibia	Yes. "Misdiagnosed abuse"	Accidental toddler's fracture
Wheeler and Hobbs (151)	1 mo	Fractured clavicle	Yes	Difficult birth
	5 mo	Bony injury to skull	Yes	Calcified cephalhematoma
	18 mo	Multiple fractures	Yes	Osteoporosis secondary to a neuromuscular disorder
		Painful swellings of lower extremities, suspected fractures	Yes	Caffey's disease
	9 mo F	Irritability and bulging fontanelle	Yes	Congenital hydrocephalus
		Prominent parietal eminence	Yes	Normal skull variant
		Prominent ribs, mother mentally ill	Yes	Scoliosis
		Suspected injury elbow	Yes	Osteomyelitis
Wright and Thornton (157)	19 mo M	Fractures of premastoid complex, ribs, femur, and tibia in 1.5 yr	Yes. In protective custody 2 times	Osteogenesis imperfecta
Paterson et al. (108)		Unexplained fractures	Yes. Child taken into protective custody 2 times	Osteogenesis imperfecta
Paterson and McAllion (107)		Unexplained fractures	Yes. Child in foster care 3.5 years before diagnosis made	Osteogenesis imperfecta
Gahagan and Rimza (42)	1 yr M	Fractures of femur, humerus, and ribs	Yes. New fractures occurred in foster care	Osteogenesis imperfecta
	9 yr F	Six fractures of fingers, tibia, and toe in 8 yr	Yes. Family observed by protective services until diagnosis made	Osteogenesis imperfecta
	16 mo M	Five fractures of tibias, radius, and fibula in 2 mo	Yes. Family history of osteogenesis imperfecta. Fractures occurred in care of sitter	Osteogenesis imperfecta and child abuse

Mo, months; yr, years; F, female; M, male.

thor concluded that "absence of calcification at a fracture site in an infant more than 11 days old suggests a postnatal accident, and since infants do not have accidents that no one knows about, the possibility of abuse must be considered." Brill and Winchester (16) agreed, stating, "Absence of callus at the site of a fracture after the age of 2 weeks is strong presumptive evidence that the fracture did not occur during delivery."

Clavicular fractures are a common birth injury, found in 1.7% to 3.5% of newborns. It is not unusual to miss a clavicle fracture during the newborn examination and then to detect a callus at the 2-week visit (65).

In contrast, rib fractures are an extremely rare birth injury. No rib fractures were detected in the series by Cumming (30). His findings are consistent with those of a prospective study by Rubin (120) of 15,435 births in which no rib fractures were seen. Injuries that were detected included 43 fractured clavicles, seven fractured humeri, and one skull fracture.

In a review of 25 infants with rib fractures, Thomas (144) found only one case in which the fracture was attributed to birth injury. The infant weighed 5,896 g at delivery by midforceps. At age 3 weeks, he was not using the right arm, and radiographs revealed healing fractures of the right fifth through seventh ribs posteriorly. One other infant with OI, who died at age 3 days, had fresh and healing fractures of all ribs bilaterally.

Rizzolo and Coleman (115) described rib fractures detected at 9 hours of life in a full-term infant weighing 3,300 g who was delivered after a vacuum-assisted delivery and moderate shoulder dystocia. Five fractures of the left posterolateral chest were noted, involving the third through seventh ribs. The fractures presumably occurred during delivery when the left rib cage passed under the pubic symphysis and the thorax was flexed upward during delivery of the rest of the body.

The infant had spent only 45 minutes with the mother, as the mother was a gestational diabetic and the baby was kept in the nursery for glucose monitoring. Even so, child abuse was explored, as the pregnancy was unplanned and unwanted, and the parents had

TABLE 9.6. *Risk, assessment profile for clavicle fracture as a birth injury*

Injury	Score
Infant weight >400 g	4
Shoulder dystocia present	3
Infant weight between 3,500 and 4,000 g	3
Midforceps used for delivery	3
Low forceps used for delivery	1
Fetal distress during delivery	1

A score of 5 or greater correctly predicted 50% of the injured group and a score of less than 5 predicted no injury in 94% of the comparison group (82).

separated 3 weeks before the baby's birth. No evidence of abuse was found, and the infant went home with her mother, remaining well through follow-up at age 1 year.

Levine et al. (82) developed a risk-assessment scale for fractured clavicle related to birth trauma after studying 13,870 term infants of whom 28 (two per 1,000) had this injury (Table 9.6). Rizzolo and Coleman (115) speculated that the same risk profile might apply to rib fractures.

Can rib fractures attributed to abuse be distinguished from those resulting from accidents? Schweich and Fleisher (126) reviewed the charts of 21 children hospitalized for rib fractures. Seventy-six percent were due to accidents, and 24% were attributed to abuse. The children with accidental injuries were significantly older than children subjected to abuse (mean age, 8 and 7/12 years; range, 2–15 years vs. mean age, 3 months; range, 0.5–7 months). Victims of accidental injury had histories of sudden forceful trauma, including motor vehicle accidents, falls from heights, and gunshots. Victims of abuse commonly presented with unexplained respiratory distress. The accidental group had fewer rib fractures (average, 3.3 fractures; range, one to eight) than the abused group (average, 11.8 fractures; range, three to 23).

Forceful Manipulation

Forceful, passive manipulation of an infant's extremities can cause fractures confused with abusive injuries. A 9-month-old infant was found dead in bed 5 hours after a feeding. Autopsy findings were consistent with sudden infant death syndrome. Radiographs revealed, however, three healing fractures, a left medial humeral epicondylar fracture, and bilateral midshaft fractures of the clavicles. Three forensic pathologists agreed that the injuries were intentionally inflicted. The case was reported and investigated as child abuse. The injuries were ultimately attributed to forceful "chiropractic" manipulation performed on the child by an aunt who had no formal training or certification in the field. In retrospect, the parents recalled that the child had cried during the manipulation and for days afterward had shown signs of pain and refused to pull up with his arms or get to his hands and knees. The histologic age of the fractures was consistent with the time of the manipulation (135).

Four infants with serious bony injury from passive exercise administered by adult caretakers were reported by Helfer et al. (58). Injuries in these four infants included a total of 27 fractures, 10 ribs, six humeri, four femurs, three ulnas, two ankles, one tibia, and one skull. Three of the babies had been born prematurely, and the exercises were prescribed by staff in the neonatal intensive care unit before discharge. When parents demonstrated their techniques to the staff, however, the amount of force used was significantly greater than what had been taught. A fourth infant was injured by a babysitter who viewed the child as handicapped and undertook the exercises on her own. Two infants had prior rickets of prematurity that had healed. None had other predisposing factors, such as prostaglandin therapy (see subsequent discussion).

The authors discussed the difficulty of distinguishing injuries related to abuse from those resulting from well-intentioned but overzealous passive exercise. They cautioned that because "we have not been able to find any documented evidence that short- or long-term outcome is improved (by these exercises) . . . those parents from a highly stressed environment with abusive potential or who have abnormal perceptions of their infants should not be provided with this potential method of abuse."

Metabolic, Genetic, and Infectious Conditions

Preterm or very low birth weight infants are more susceptible to fractures than are full-term infants for several reasons. They begin life with bones that are relatively undermineralized (35% bone mineral deficit in infants weighing <1,500 g) and are also more susceptible than are full-term infants to rickets. Preterm infants who have prolonged and complicated hospitalizations, particularly when lengthy periods of parenteral nutrition are required, are at greater risk of neonatal osteopenia. Studies showed, however, that premature infants given adequate amounts of calciferol, calcium, and phosphorus show accelerated mineralization of their bones, catching up to or exceeding term cohorts in bone-mineralization status by 16 weeks after delivery or by 60 weeks after conception (28).

Because children younger than 1 year are relatively nonmobile, identified fractures should prompt the clinician to look for evidence of either abuse or underlying host factors making a fracture more likely. Among 34 patients with 55 fractures in the first year of life, 56% were victims of abuse. In the nonabused group, 23% of the children had constitutional factors contributing to their fractures, including OI, cerebral palsy, osteopenia secondary to nutritional problems, Down syndrome, or chronic pulmonary disease, with rib fractures apparently resulting from postural drainage (87).

Drug or vitamin therapy can induce skeletal reactions causing confusion, with injuries attributable to abuse. Prostaglandin therapy for patent ductus can produce cortical proliferation along the diaphyses of long bones that could be confused with traumatic periostitis. Methotrexate therapy can induce osteoporosis with local periosteal reaction and fractures, particularly of the epiphyseal–metaphyseal area. Patients with hypervitaminosis A may have pain and swelling of the extremities and radiologic evidence of periosteal reaction of the diaphysis (109).

Several rare metabolic conditions are associated with bones that are easily fractured. Children with Menkes' kinky hair syndrome have been mistakenly diagnosed as victims of child abuse. They may exhibit failure to thrive, developmental delay, metaphyseal spurring and fractures, periosteal reaction, and subdural hemorrhages, all thought to be the result of copper deficiency. Bone biopsies in two patients have demonstrated abnormal bone collagen and lamellae, which might render bones more fragile. A 10-week-old child later diagnosed with kinky hair syndrome had multiple metaphyseal fractures and periosteal new bone formation of both humeri, femurs, tibiae, and fibulae. The hospital staff suspected child abuse, but, because at least one of the fractures occurred in the hospital, the parents threatened to take legal action against the hospital for negligence (3).

Fractures are rare in children with rickets and scurvy, but subperiosteal and metaphyseal calcification may mimic abuse-related injuries. Scurvy is rare compared with rickets, and can be distinguished from child abuse by characteristic bony changes (16). A good history, complete physical examination, and additional radiographic evaluation should point out potential causes of rickets, such as dietary imbalance, biliary atresia, osteopetrosis, and hypophosphatasia (109).

Phenobarbital and phenytoin can alter vitamin D metabolism, producing skeletal changes characteristic of rickets in up to 25% of patients taking these anticonvulsants. Seizure activity increases the risk of fractures, particularly when bone strength is diminished by rickets. Child abuse may be suspected, particularly when clinicians are aware that special-needs children are at increased risk of abuse or neglect, and a good history is lacking in a postictal, retarded, institutionalized patient. A comprehensive multidisciplinary evaluation may be necessary to differentiate rickets from abuse from rickets with superimposed abuse (160).

Skeletal lesions associated with congenital syphilis have been mistaken for abusive injuries (40,59). A 5-week-old infant was hospitalized with a tentative diagnosis of battered child syndrome after her mother, a victim of repeated episodes of domestic violence, brought the child to a clinic because she would not move her arms. Radiographs showed bilateral metaphyseal fractures of the humeri with periosteal reaction. Further radiographic evaluation revealed additional lesions compatible with congenital syphilis. The diagnosis was confirmed by serology, and treatment with penicillin led to complete healing (40).

Congenital indifference to pain is a rare autosomal recessive disorder that is easily confused with abuse. Patients can present with multiple bruises, burns, lacerations, fractures, and skeletal deformities from poor healing of unrecognized fractures. Surprisingly, the insensitivity to pain often passes unnoticed by clinicians. Injuries heal poorly, and a mistaken diagnosis of Ehlers–Danlos syndrome may be made. The tongue, lips, and fingers may be severely bitten, and teeth are lost early because of decay. Corneal damage can result from trauma to the eyes. Parents have described smelling burning flesh and finding their child casually leaning against a hot stove. Another child cut off the end of his tongue and brought it proudly to his mother! The neurologic examination is usually normal except for impaired corneal and gag reflexes, and absent or diminished sense of pain (16, 132,134).

Osteogenesis Imperfecta

OI is a group of rare heritable disorders of connective tissue resulting from abnormal collagen synthesis. Because OI is characterized by fragile bones, frequent fractures, and easy bruising, concerns of abuse may arise. Spiral or transverse fractures are most common, but metaphyseal fractures resembling abusive injuries also can occur (2,16). Several cases of OI mistaken for abuse have been reported (Table 9.5) (42,106–108,157). One case illustrates the need for multidisciplinary evaluation, including dental consultation, in cases of suspected OI.

A 3-year-old boy sustained a parietal hematoma and fracture of the premastoid complex requiring surgery after a fall off a porch at age 19 months. A routine chest radiograph revealed several healing rib fractures. No child abuse investigation was done until the child was readmitted 2 days after discharge with a femoral fracture. After 3 months in foster care with counseling and psychologic evaluations for his parents, he was returned home. Ten months later, he fractured his tibia in a fall to the floor while playing and was again taken into protective custody.

Although radiographs showed generalized osteopenia, OI was not considered until his pediatrician noted discolored teeth and requested dental consultation. His teeth were yellow–brown to gray with signs of excessive wear and enamel fracturing on the frontal incisors and radiographic evidence of bell-shaped crowns and wide pulp chambers. Further evaluation revealed distention of the lower rib cage, unusual skull shape, hyperelasticity of the joints, mild kyphoscoliosis, and hearing loss, confirming the diagnosis of OI (157).

OI is less common than child abuse. Type I is the most common form, occurring in one per 30,000 births. It is unlikely to be mistaken for abuse because it is characterized by blue sclera throughout life, short stature, dentinogenesis imperfecta, wormian bones of the skull, and late hearing loss. The peak ages for fractures are 2 to 3 years and 10 to 15 years (64). Types II and III are rare and are unlikely to be confused with abuse because extreme bone fragility leads to intrauterine or early infant deformities and death. Type IV OI also is rare, but it may be confused with abuse because bone fragility is variable, and sclera may be normal or become progressively less blue.

Paterson (105) surveyed 804 patients with OI in the U.K. and found that "in no less than 113 cases, parents had been accused at some stage of non-accidental injury," and in 18

cases, formal child abuse case conferences or care proceedings were initiated. In the worst case, a child was in out-of-home care for more than 3 years before OI was diagnosed (107). Paterson also wrote of evaluating 86 children with unexplained fractures suggestive of abuse. He postulated that these children had either OI or a new entity, "temporary brittle bone disease" caused by deficiency of copper or vitamin C. He did not document how these diagnoses were made. A list of characteristics of "temporary brittle bone disease" is worrisome in its overlap with characteristics of abuse and neglect: fractures, metaphyseal abnormalities, periosteal reaction, anterior rib changes, delayed bone age, vomiting and diarrhea, apnea, hepatomegaly, anemia, and prematurity (105).

Several authors have challenged Paterson's conclusion that OI is commonly mistaken for child abuse, pointing out that he arrived at the diagnosis of OI in many patients without characteristic radiographs, family history, or repeated fractures (23,140). Carty and Shaw (23) indicated that in Paterson's study of 78 patients with the diagnosis of OI subtype IVA, the incidence of skull fractures was high (28%), raising the possibility of misdiagnosis of OI for actual child abuse. Other authors pointed out that OI is rare, and only mild cases of new mutations of the rare OI types III and IV cause confusion (1,23,42). Taitz (139) calculated the probability of encountering a child younger than 1 year with OI and no other features or family findings of the disease as between one in 1 million and one in 3 million, or an annual incidence of one case every 100 to 300 years in a city of half a million people.

Gahagan and Rimza (42) reported a case that illustrates that OI and child abuse can coexist. A 16-month-old black boy incurred two fractures in 2 months while in the care of a babysitter: a fracture of the right distal tibia after falling down one step, and a chip fracture of the distal metaphysis of the left tibia after falling down five steps. A bone survey revealed four additional fractures of the long bones in different stages of healing. A radiologist thought the fractures were more typical of abuse than of OI. The mother stated that a sibling had OI. The patient had no bruises, and the sclera were not blue. Height and weight were at the fifth percentile. Skin biopsy confirmed OI type III or IV. A multidisciplinary child abuse team recommended that the child remain at home under supervision of child-protective services. No new fractures occurred after the change in babysitters.

OI should be considered in the differential diagnosis when medical staff are concerned that unusual or frequent fractures are related to abuse, if only in anticipation that this possibility may be raised in court. Consultation with a radiologist, geneticist, and dentist may be helpful. OI is unlikely in the absence of the features summarized in Table 9.7.

If OI is suspected, a punch biopsy of the skin should be sent to a regional research laboratory for analysis of collagen synthesis. Gahagan and Rimza (42) recommended,

> Biochemical studies to confirm or rule out the possibility of OI should be done in only children with repeat fractures when the history, physical examination, and clinical features are not typical of nonaccidental trauma . . . . If the child has other clinical manifestations of physical abuse, such as bruises not associated with the site of a fracture, intracranial injuries, or retinal hemorrhages, it is extremely unlikely that the fractures are due to OI. In these cases,

biochemical studies to rule out OI are probably not necessary. After a child has been placed in foster care, OI should be suspected if fractures continue to occur . . . the child who has multiple unexplained fractures in one environment and then has no further fractures when removed from that environment should be suspected of having nonaccidental trauma . . . child abuse could coexist with OI.

Because the results of collagen studies are not available for weeks to months, a multidisciplinary team may need to make decisions regarding safe temporary placement and supervision. Even after a diagnosis of OI is made, ongoing medical support and child-protective services involvement may be necessary to prevent further fractures (42).

OTHER CONDITIONS MISTAKEN FOR ABUSE

A few reports describe odd conditions confused with abuse (Table 9.8). One child referred with a diagnosis of traumatic alopecia related to abuse was found instead to have alopecia areata (151). Other nonabusive causes of patchy hair loss include tricotillomania, tinea capitis, and loose anagen hair syndrome. The last usually presents in 2- to 5-year-old girls with sparse blond hair that does not grow beyond the ear and can be pulled out without pain.

TABLE 9.7. *Features of osteogenesis imperfecta*

Repeated fractures
Osteoporosis
Thin cortices
Bowing and angulation of healed fractures
Blue sclera
Deafness or hearing impairment in second or third decade
Dentinogenesis imperfecta (discolored, translucent, worn teeth)
Wormian skull bones
Inverted triangle or tam-o'-shanter skull shape
Lax ligaments, hypermobility of joints
Excessive sweating, heat intolerance
Easy bruising, fragile skin
Short stature, growth retardation
Additional fractures in a protected environment
Family history of OI, bone deformity, repeated fractures, dentinogenesis imperfecta, or hearing impairment

Adapted from Ablin DS, et al.: Differentiation of child abuse from osteogenesis imperfecta. *Am J Roentgenol* 1990;154:1035. Brill PW, Winchester P. Differential diagnosis of child abuse. In: Kleinman PK. *Diagnostic imaging of child abuse*. Baltimore: Williams & Wilkins, 1987; and Jones KL. *Smith's recognizable patterns of human malformation*. 4th ed. Philadelphia: WB Saunders, 1988.

TABLE 9.8. *Other conditions mistaken for abuse or neglect*

Reference	Age/Sex	Presentation	Referred as abuse or neglect?	Final diagnosis
Oates (99)	6 wk	Two toes swollen and purple	Yes. Admitted for possible abuse	Hair tourniquet
Narkewicz (96)	1 mo M	Four edematous toes	Yes. Ongoing suspicion of abuse	Possible child abuse
	4 mo M	Swollen, red toe	No	Hair tourniquet
	3 mo M	Swollen, red toe	No	Hair tourniquet
Wheeler and Hobbs (151)		Apparent traumatic alopecia	Yes	Alopecia areata
Copeland (29)	15 mo M	Failure to thrive, sepsis from infected ulcer of face, death	Yes. Investigated as abuse	Panhypogamma-globulinemia
Kaplan (68)	12 yr F	Height and weight below 3rd percentile, flexion contractures of extremities, filthy, no speech, retarded	Yes	Severe retardation. Mother depressed and unable to care for child
	15 yr F	Height and weight below 3rd percentile, flexion contractures of extremities, lice, filthy, retarded, gained 15 lb in hospital	Yes. Mother had died at birth. Father chronic alcoholic encephalopathy	Microcephaly with severe retardation. Father unable to care for child
Carpentieri et al. (21)	4 mo M	Failure to thrive, bruises, apparent neglect	Yes. Admitted for neglect	Undiagnosed cystic fibrosis with malabsorption
Kaplan (67)	5 yr M	Failure to thrive, neglect	Yes	Severe cerebral palsy. Very difficult to feed. Gastrostomy tube used successfully
	1 yr M	Laceration with tourniquet applied for 18 h	Yes	Retarded mother's attempt at appropriate care

Wk, week; mo, month; yr, year; M, male; F, female.

On several occasions, a mistaken diagnosis of abuse has been made in children with edema and erythema of the toes, later found to result from a hair or thread wrapping around the digit (96,99). "Hair tourniquet" of the digits or penis is not rare and is usually accidental, but abusive injuries resulting from deliberate wrapping of an appendage have been described (11).

Copeland (29) described a 15-month-old child who was found dead with failure to thrive and sepsis from a large, foul-smelling ulcer of the face. The diagnosis was changed from abuse to panhypogammaglobulinemia after autopsy revealed an involuted thymus and depressed levels of immunoglobulins and complement.

Physiologic striae, caused by rapid growth, occur in about 5% of adolescents, typically on the buttocks, upper thighs, breasts, lower abdomen, and back. Striae on the lower back are oriented horizontally and have been mistaken for marks inflicted by cords or switches.

Before concluding that failure to thrive has resulted from parental dysfunction, other medical and social conditions must be eliminated. Carpentieri et al. (21) wrote of a 4-month-old child with growth retardation and bruises who was hospitalized for abuse and neglect but was found to have undiagnosed cystic fibrosis and malabsorption. Kaplan (67,68) described his experience with four cases of misdiagnosed neglect and failure to thrive that actually involved congenital conditions that made feeding extremely difficult, such as cerebral palsy and microcephaly, or parental limitations such as depression and retardation. He stated,

> Publicity from the press and television almost led to incarceration of the parents for crimes they did not commit . . . . The parents . . . had cared for their children to the best of their abilities for several years. . . . It is the duty of the physician to help distinguish among physical assault, neglect and congenital malformation. In some cases it may be necessary to defend not only the child but also the parents in family or criminal courts.

CONCLUSION

The number of reported cases of conditions confused with child abuse are surprisingly few relative to the overall incidence of detected abuse. Child abuse still remains under- rather than overdiagnosed. To avoid the morbidity and mortality associated with missed abuse, clinicians now recognize their obligation to report even suspected abuse. When abuse is diagnosed in error, however, significant emotional trauma can result to child, family, and suspected perpetrator. To avoid overdiagnosing child abuse, clinicians should exclude conditions commonly mistaken for abuse by careful history taking, thorough physical examinations, and when indicated, laboratory tests and consultation with specialists.

REFERENCES

1. Ablin DS, Greenspan A, Reinhart M, et al. Differentiation of child abuse from osteogenesis imperfecta. *Am J Roentgenol* 1990;154:1035–1046.
2. Ablin DS. Osteogenesis imperfecta: a review. *Can Assoc Radiol J* 1998;49:110–123.
3. Adams PC, Strand RD, Bresnan MJ, et al. Kinky hair syndrome: serial study of radiological findings with emphasis on the similarity to the battered child syndrome. *Radiology* 1974;112:401–407.
4. Adler R, Kane-Nussen B. Erythema multiforme: confusion with child battering syndrome. *Pediatrics* 1983; 72:718.
5. Alario A, et al. Do retinal hemorrhages occur with accidental head trauma in young children? *Am J Dis Child* 1990;144:445.
6. Allison JW, Davis PC, Sato Y, et al. Intracranial aneurysms in infants and children. *Pediatr Radiol* 1998; 28:223–229.
7. Anh NT. "Pseudo-battered child" syndrome. *JAMA* 1976;236:2288.
8. Asnes RS. Buttock bruises: mongolian spot. *Pediatrics* 1984;74:321.
9. Asnes RS, Wisotsky DH. Cupping lesions simulating child abuse. *J Pediatr* 1981;99:267.
10. Bacon CJ, Sayer GC, Howe JW. Extensive retinal haemorrhages in infancy: an innocent cause. *Br Med J* 1978;1:281.
11. Barton DJ, Sloan GM, Nichter LS, et al. Hair-thread tourniquet syndrome. *Pediatrics* 1988;82:925–928.
12. Bennani-Smires C, Medina J. Radiological case of the month: infantile nutritional copper deficiency. *Am J Dis Child* 1980;134:1155.
13. Billmire ME, Myers PA. Serious head injury in infants: accident or abuse? *Pediatrics* 1985;75:340.
14. Bills D, Rosenfeld J, Phelan E, et al. Intracranial arteriovenous malformations in childhood: presentation, management and outcome. *J Clin Neurosci* 1996;3: 220–228.
15. Bond S, Schnier G, Sindine M, et al. Cutaneous burns caused by sulfuric acid drain cleaner. *J Trauma* 1998; 44:523–526.
16. Brill PW, Winchester P, Kleinman PK. Differential diagnosis of child abuse. In: Kleinman PK, ed. *Diagnostic imaging of child abuse.* St. Louis: Mosby, 1998.
17. Brown J, Melinkovich, P. Schonlein-Henoch purpura misdiagnosed as suspected child abuse. *JAMA* 1986; 256:617.
18. Bryan CS. Vietnamese coin rubbing. *Ann Emerg Med* 1987;16:602.
19. Calobrisi SD, Drolet BA, Esterly NB. Petechial eruption after application of EMLA cream. *Pediatrics* 1998;101:471–473.
20. Carpenter RF. The prevalence and distribution of bruising in babies. *Arch Dis Child* 1999;90:363–366.
21. Carpentieri U, Gustavson LP, Haggard ME. Misdiagnosis of neglect in a child with bleeding disorder and cystic fibrosis. *South Med J* 1978;71:854.
22. Carty H. Brittle or battered? *Arch Dis Child* 1988;63: 350.
23. Carty H, Shaw DG. Child abuse and osteogenesis imperfecta [Letter]. *Br Med J* 1988;296:292.
24. Cassell OCS, Hubble M, Milling MAP, et al. Baby walkers: still a major cause of infant burns. *Burns* 1997;23:451–453.
25. Chadwick DL, Chin S, Salerno C, et al. Deaths from falls in children: how far is fatal? *J Trauma* 1991;31: 1353.
26. Coffman K, Boyce WT, Hansen RC. Phytodermatitis simulating child abuse. *Am J Dis Child* 1985;139:239.
27. Colver GB, Harris DWS, Tidman MJ. Skin diseases that may mimic child abuse. *Br J Dermatol* 1990;123:129.
28. Congdon PJ, Horsman A, Ryan SW, et al. Spontaneous resolution of bone mineral depletion in preterm infants. *Arch Dis Child* 1990;65:1038.
29. Copeland AR. A case of panhypogammaglobulinemia masquerading as child abuse. *J Forensic Sci* 1988;33: 1493.
30. Cumming WA. Neonatal skeletal fractures: birth

trauma or child abuse? *J Assoc Can Radiol* 1979;30: 30.

31. Daly KC, Siegel RM. Henoch-Schonlein purpura in a child at risk of abuse. *Arch Pediatr Adolesc Med* 1998; 152:96–98.

32. Dannaker CJ, Glover RA, Goltz RW. Phytodermatitis: a mystery case report. *Clin Pediatr* 1988;27:289.

33. Dietrich A, James C, King D, et al. Head trauma in children with congenital coagulation disorders. *J Pediatr Surg* 1994;29:28–32.

34. Diez F, Berger TG. Scarring due to an enuresis blanket. *Pediatr Dermatol* 1988;5:58.

35. DiMario FJ. Chronic subdural hematoma: another babywalker-stairs related injury. *Clin Pediatr* 1990;29: 405.

36. Du JNH. Pseudobattered child syndrome in Vietnamese immigrant children. *Can Med Assoc J* 1980; 122:394.

37. Duhaime AC, Alario AJ, Lewander WJ, et al. Head injury in very young children: mechanisms, injury types, and ophthalmologic findings in 100 hospitalized patients younger than 2 years of age. *Pediatrics* 1992; 90:179.

38. Dungy CI. Mongolian spots, day care centers, and child abuse. *Pediatrics* 1982;69:672.

39. Feldman KW. Pseudoabusive burns in Asian refugees. *Am J Dis Child* 1984;138:768.

40. Fiser RH, Kaplan J, Holder JC. Congenital syphilis mimicking the battered child syndrome: how does one tell them apart? *Clin Pediatr* 1972;11:305.

41. Fisher AA. Nonoccupational dermatitis to "black" rubber mix: part II. *Cutis* 1992;49:229.

42. Gahagan S, Rimza ME. Child abuse or osteogenesis imperfecta: how can we tell? *Pediatrics* 1991;88:987.

43. Garron DC. Cupping brings back memories [Letter]. *Lancet* 1988;1:310.

44. Gellis SS, Feingold M. Cao-gio: (pseudo-battering in Vietnamese children). *Am J Dis Child* 1976;130:857.

45. Gerrard JM, Duta E, Nosek-Cenkowska B, et al. A role for prostacyclin in bruising symptomatology. *Pediatrics* 1992;90:33.

46. Goetting MG, Sowa B. Retinal hemorrhage after cardiopulmonary resuscitation in children: an etiologic reevaluation. *Pediatrics* 1990;85:585.

47. Golden SM, Duster MC. Hazards of misdiagnosis due to Vietnamese folk medicine. *Clin Pediatr* 1977;16: 949.

48. Greeff MC, Mashile O, MacDougall LG. "Superwarfarin" (bromodialone) poisoning in two children resulting in prolonged anticoagulation. *Lancet* 1987;2: 1269.

49. Guarnaschelli J, Lee J, Pitts FW. "Fallen fontanelle" (caida de mollera): a variant of the battered child syndrome. *JAMA* 1972;222:1545.

50. Gunn TR, Becroft DMO. Unexplained intracranial haemorrhage in utero: the battered fetus? *Aust N Z J Obstet Gynaecol* 1984;24:17.

51. Gunn TR, Mok PM, Becroft DMO. Subdural hemorrhage in utero. *Pediatrics* 1985;76:605.

52. Haasbeek JF. Lower extremity compartment syndrome resulting from a toddler's bed. *Pediatrics* 1998;102: 1474–1475.

53. Hall JR, Reyes HM, Horvat M, et al. The mortality of childhood falls. *J Trauma* 1989;29:1273.

54. Hansen KK. Folk remedies and child abuse: a review with emphasis on caida de mollera and its relationship to shaken baby syndrome. *Child Abuse Negl* 1997; 22:117–127.

55. Harley JM. Disorders of coagulation misdiagnosed as nonaccidental bruising. *Pediatr Emerg Care* 1997;13: 347–349.

56. Harris CR, Evans D, Mariano C. Blue jeans hands syndrome [Letter]. *Ann Emerg Med* 1984;13:67.

57. Helfer RE, Slovis TL, Black M. Injuries resulting when small children fall out of bed. *Pediatrics* 1977; 60:533.

58. Helfer RE, Scheurer SL, Alexander R, et al. Trauma to the long bones of small infants from passive exercise: a factor in the etiology of child abuse. *J Pediatr* 1984;104:47.

59. Horodniceanu C, Grunebaum M, Volovitz B, et al. Unusual bone involvement in congenital syphilis mimicking the battered child syndrome. *Pediatr Radiol* 1978;7:232–234.

60. Hymel K, Abshire T, Luckey D, et al. Coagulopathy in pediatric abusive head trauma. *Pediatrics* 1997;99: 371–375.

61. Jacobs AH, Walton RG. The incidence of birthmarks in the neonate. *Pediatrics* 1976;58:218.

62. Jocelyn LJ, Casiro OG. Neurodevelopmental outcome of term infants with intraventricular hemorrhage. *Am J Dis Child* 1992;146:194.

63. Joffe M, Ludwig S. Stairway injuries in children. *Pediatrics* 1988;82:457.

64. Jones KL. *Smith's recognizable patterns of human malformation.* 4th ed. Philadelphia: WB Saunders, 1988.

65. Joseph PR, Rosenfeld W. Clavicular fractures in neonates. *Am J Dis Child* 1990;144:165.

66. Kanter RK. Retinal hemorrhage after cardiopulmonary resuscitation or child abuse. *J Pediatr* 1986;108:430.

67. Kaplan JM. Pseudoabuse: the misdiagnosis of child abuse. *J Forensic Sci* 1986;31:1420.

68. Kaplan JM. The misdiagnosis of child abuse. *Am Fam Pract J* 1984;30:197.

69. Keller EL, Apthorp J. Folk remedies vs child battering. *Am J Dis Child* 1977;131:1173.

70. Kikuchi I, Inoue S. Natural history of the mongolian spot. *J Dermatol* 1980;7:449.

71. Kirschner RH, Stein RJ. Mistaken diagnosis of child abuse. *Am J Dis Child* 1985;139:873.

72. Kotch JB, Browne DC, Dufort V, et al. Predicting child maltreatment in the first four years of life from characteristics assessed in the neonatal period. *Child Abuse Negl* 1999;23:305–319.

73. Kravitz H, Dreissen G, Gomberg R, et al. Accidental falls from elevated surfaces in infants from birth to one year of age. *Pediatrics* 1969;44:869–876.

74. Lacour M, Le Coultre C. Spray-induced frostbite in a child: a new hazard with novel aerosol propellants. *Pediatr Dermatol* 1991;8:207.

75. Lantner RR, Ros SP. Blue jeans thighs. *Pediatrics* 1991;88:417.

76. Lee STS. Anterior stenosis from joss stick burns. *J Laryngol Otol* 1990;104:497.

77. Leiferman KM, Gleich GJ. The case of the blue boy. *Pediatr Dermatol* 1991;8:354.

78. Leung AKC. Ecchymoses from spoon scratching simulating child abuse. *Clin Pediatr* 1986;25:98.

79. Levin AV. *Retinal hemorrhages in infants and young children.* Newsletter of the Section on Child Abuse

and Neglect, Elk Grove Village, IL: American Academy of Pediatrics, 1991.

80. Levin AV. Ocular manifestations of child abuse. *Ophthalmol Clin North Am* 1990;3:249.

81. Levin AV, Magnusson MR, Rafto SE, et al. Shaken baby syndrome diagnosed by magnetic resonance imaging. *Pediatr Emerg Care* 1989;5:181–186.

82. Levine MG, Holroyde J, Woods JR, et al. Birth trauma: incidence and predisposing factors. *Obstet Gynecol* 1984;63:792–795.

83. Longmire AW. Vietnamese coin rubbing. *Ann Emerg Med* 1987;16:602.

84. Look K, Look R. Skin scraping, cupping and moxibustion that may mimic physical abuse. *J Forensic Sci* 1997;42:103–105.

85. Lyons TJ, Oates RK. Falling out of bed: a relatively benign occurrence. *Pediatrics* 1993;92:125–127.

86. McClain JL, Clark MA, Sandusky GE. Undiagnosed, untreated acute lymphoblastic leukemia presenting as suspected child abuse. *J Forensic Sci* 1990;35:735.

87. McClelland CQ, Heiple KG. Fractures in the first year of life: a diagnostic dilemma? *Am J Dis Child* 1982;136:26.

88. McEniery J, Hanson R, Grigor W, et al. Lung injury resulting from a nonaccidental crush injury to the chest. *Pediatr Emerg Care* 1991;7:166–168.

89. McLellan NJ, Prasad R, Punt J. Spontaneous subhyaloid and retinal haemorrhages in an infant. *Arch Dis Child* 1986;61:1130.

90. McNamara JJ, Baler R, Lynch E. Ehlers-Danlos syndrome reported as child abuse. *Clin Pediatr* 1985;24:317.

91. Maurice PDL, Cream JJ. The dangers of herbalism. *Br Med J* 1989;299:1204.

92. Medeiros D, Buchanan GR. Major hemorrhage in children with idiopathic thrombocytopenic purpura. *J Pediatr* 1998;133:334–339.

93. Michielsen D, Van Hee R, Neetens C, et al. Burns to the genitals and perineum in children. *Br J Urol* 1996;78:940–941.

94. Mokrohisky ST, Kesselman NE. Valsalva effect may mimic child abuse. *Pediatrics* 1991;85:420.

95. Morris AAM, Hoffman GF, Naughten ER, et al. Glutaric aciduria and suspected child abuse. *Arch Dis Child* 1999;80:404–405.

96. Narkewicz RM. Distal digital occlusion. *Pediatrics* 1978;61:922.

97. Nields H, Kessler SC, Boisot S, et al. Streptococcal toxic shock syndrome presenting as suspected child abuse. *Am J Forensic Med Pathol* 1998;19:93–97.

98. Nunez AE, Taff ML. A chemical burn simulating child abuse. *Am J Forensic Med Pathol* 1985;6:181.

99. Oates RK. Overturning the diagnosis of child abuse. *Arch Dis Child* 1984;59:665.

100. Odita JC, Heibi S. CT, MRI characteristics of intracranial hemorrhage complicating breech and vacuum delivery. *Pediatr Radiol* 1996;26:782–785.

101. Odum A, Christ E, Kerr N, et al. Prevalence of retinal hemorrhages in pediatric patients after in-hospital cardiopulmonary resuscitation: a prospective study. *Pediatrics* 1997;99:e3.

102. O'Hare AE, Eden OB. Bleeding disorders and non-accidental injury. *Arch Dis Child* 1984;59:860.

103. Owen SM, Durst RD. Ehlers-Danlos syndrome simulating child abuse. *Arch Dermatol* 1984;120:97.

104. Partington MD, Swanson JA, Meyer FB. Head injury and the use of baby walkers: a continuing problem. *Ann Emerg Med* 1991;20:652.

105. Paterson CR. Osteogenesis imperfecta and other bone disorders in the differential diagnosis of unexplained fractures. *J R Soc Med* 1990;83:72.

106. Paterson CR. Osteogenesis imperfecta in the differential diagnosis of child abuse. *Child Abuse Negl* 1977;1:499.

107. Paterson CR, McAllion SJ. Child abuse and osteogenesis imperfecta. *Br Med J* 1987;295:1561.

108. Paterson CR, McAllion S, Miller R. Osteogenesis imperfecta with dominant inheritance and normal sclerae. *J Bone Joint Surg Br* 1983;65:35.

109. Radkowski MA. The battered child syndrome: pitfalls in radiologic diagnosis. *Pediatr Ann* 1983;12:894.

110. Ragosta K. Pediculosis masquerades as child abuse. *Pediatr Emerg Med* 1989;5:253.

111. Rahman MNG, McAll G, Chai KG. Massage-related perforation of the sigmoid colon. *Med J Malaysia* 1987;42:56.

112. Reece RM, Sege R. Childhood head injury: accidental or inflicted? *Arch Pediatr Adolesc Med* 2000;154:11–15.

113. Reinhart MA, Ruhs H. Moxibustion; another traumatic folk remedy. *Clin Pediatr* 1985;24:58.

114. Riffenburgh RS, Sathyavagiswaran L. The eyes of child abuse victims: autopsy findings. *J Forensic Sci* 1991;36:741.

115. Rizzolo PJ, Coleman PR. Neonatal rib fractures: birth trauma or child abuse? *J Fam Pract* 1989;29:561.

116. Roberton DM, Barbor P, Hull D. Unusual injury? Recent injury in normal children and children with suspected non-accidental injury. *Br Med J* 1982;285:1399.

117. Roberts DL, Pope FM, Nicholls AC, et al. Ehlers-Danlos syndrome type IV mimicking non-accidental injury in a child. *Br J Dermatol* 1984;111:341–345.

118. Rosenberg L, Sagi A, Stahl N, et al. Maqua (therapeutic burn) as an indicator of underlying disease. *Plast Reconstr Surg* 1988;82:277–280.

119. Rosenblat H, Hong P. Coin rolling misdiagnosed as child abuse. *Can Med Assoc J* 1989;140:417.

120. Rubin A. Birth injuries: incidence, mechanisms, and end results. *J Obstet Gynecol* 1964;23:218.

121. Ryan CA, Gayle M. Vitamin K deficiency, intracranial hemorrhage, and a subgaleal hematoma: a fatal combination. *Pediatr Emerg Care* 1992;8:143.

122. Sagi A, Ben-Meir P, Bibi C. Burn hazard from cupping: an ancient universal medication still in practice. *Burns* 1988;14:323.

123. Sandler AP, Haynes V. Nonaccidental trauma and medical folk belief: a case of cupping. *Pediatrics* 1978;61:921.

124. Saulsbury FT, Hayden GF. Skin conditions simulating child abuse. *Pediatr Emerg Care* 1985;1:147.

125. Schmitt BD, Gray JD, Britton HL. Car seat burns in infants; avoiding confusion with inflicted burns. *Pediatrics* 1978;62:607.

126. Schweich P, Fleisher G. Rib fractures in children. *Pediatr Emerg Care* 1985;1:187.

127. Schwer W, Brueschke EE, Dent T. Family practice grand rounds: hemophilia. *J Fam Pract* 1982;14:661.

128. Scott MJ, Esterly NB. Eyelash infestation by *Phthirus pubis* as a manifestation of child abuse. *Pediatr Dermatol* 1983;1:179.

129. Shpall S, Frieden I. Mahogany discoloration of the skin due to the defensive secretion of a millipede. *Pediatr Dermatol* 1991;8:25.

130. Silfen E, Wyre HW. Factitial dermatitis: cao gio. *Cutis* 1981;28:399.

131. Silva-Araujo AL, Tavares MA, Patacao MH, et al. Retinal hemorrhages associated with in utero exposure to cocaine. *Retina* 1996;16:411–418.

132. Silverman FN, Gliden JJ. Congenital insensitivity to pain: a neurologic syndrome with bizarre skeletal lesions. *Radiology* 1959;72:176.

133. Smialek JE. Significance of mongolian spots. *J Pediatr* 1980;97:504.

134. Spencer JA, Grieve DK. Congenital indifference to pain mistaken for non-accidental injury. *Br J Radiol* 1990;63:308.

135. Sperry K, Pfalzgraf R. Inadvertent clavicular fractures caused by "chiropractic" manipulations in an infant: an unusual form of pseudo-abuse. *J Forensic Sci* 1990; 35:1211.

136. Stephens RP, Richardson AC, Lewin JS. Bilateral subdural hematomas in a newborn infant. *Pediatrics* 1997; 99:610–612.

137. Still J, Craft-Coffman B, Law E, et al. Burns of children caused by electrical stoves. *J Burn Care Rehabil* 1998;19:364–365.

138. Sugar NF, Taylor JA, Feldman KW, et al. Bruises in infants and toddlers: those who don't cruise rarely bruise. *Arch Pediatr Adolesc Med* 1999;153:399–403.

139. Taitz LS. Child abuse and osteogenesis imperfecta. *Br Med J* 1987;295:1082.

140. Taitz LS. Child abuse and osteogenesis imperfecta. *Br Med J* 1988;296:292.

141. Tanner JL, Dechert MP, Frieden IJ. Growing up with a facial hemangioma: parent and child coping and adaptation. *Pediatrics* 1998;101:446–452.

142. Tarantino CA, Dowd MD, Murdoch TC. Short vertical falls in infants. *Pediatrics* 1999;105:5–8.

143. Thomas PS. Cupping brings back memories [Letter]. *Lancet* 1988;1:310.

144. Thomas PS. Rib fractures in infancy. *Ann Radiol* 1977; 20:115.

145. Tunnessen WW. The girl with the blue hands. *Contemp Pediatr* 1985;2:55.

146. Tyagi AK, Scotcher S, Kozeis N, et al. Can convulsions alone cause retinal hemorrhages in infants? *Br J Ophthalmol* 1998;82:659–660.

147. von Kries R, Gobel U. Vitamin K prophylaxis and vitamin K deficiency bleeding (VKDB) in early infancy. *Acta Paediatr* 1992;81:655.

148. Waskerwitz S, Christoffel KK, Hauger S. Hypersensitivity vasculitis presenting as suspected child abuse: case report and literature review. *Pediatrics* 1981;67:283.

149. Watts RG, Castleberry RP, Sadowski JA. Accidental poisoning with a superwarfarin compound (brodifacoum) in a child. *Pediatrics* 1990;86:883.

150. Wetzel RC, Slater AJ, Dover GJ. Fatal intramuscular bleeding misdiagnosed as suspected nonaccidental injury. *Pediatrics* 1995;95:771–773.

151. Wheeler DM, Hobbs CJ. Mistakes in diagnosing nonaccidental injury: 10 years' experience. *Br Med J* 1988; 296:1233.

152. Wickes IG, Zaidi ZH. Battered or pigmented? *Br Med J* 1972;2:404.

153. Williams RA. Injuries in infants and small children resulting from witnessed and corroborated free falls. *J Trauma* 1991;31:1350.

154. Winship IM, Winship WS. Epidermolysis bullosa misdiagnosed as child abuse. *South Afr Med J* 1988;73:369.

155. Winston FK, Shaw KN, Kreshak AA, et al. Hidden spears: handlebars as injury hazards to children. *Pediatrics* 1998;102:596–601.

156. Woelfle J, Kreft B, Emons D, et al. Subdural hemorrhage as an initial sign of glutaric aciduria type a: a diagnostic pitfall. *Pediatr Radiol* 1996;26:779–781.

157. Wright JT, Thornton JB. Osteogenesis imperfecta with dentinogenesis imperfecta: a mistaken case of child abuse. *Pediatr Dent* 1983;5:207.

158. Yeatman GW, Dang VV. Cao gio (coin rubbing): Vietnamese attitudes toward health care. *JAMA* 1980;244: 2748.

159. Yeatman GW, Shaw C, Barlow MJ, et al. Pseudobattering in Vietnamese children. *Pediatrics* 1976;58: 616–618.

160. Zeiss J, Wycliff ND, Cullen BJ, et al. Radiological case of the month. Simulated child abuse in drug-induced rickets. *Am J Dis Child* 1988;142:1367.

161. Zurbuchen P, LeCoultre C, Calza AM, et al. Cutaneous necrosis after contact with calcium chloride: a mistaken diagnosis of child abuse. *Pediatrics* 1998;102:596–601.

10

Medical Findings in Child Sexual Abuse

Martin A. Finkel and *Allan R. DeJong

*Center for Children's Support and Department of Pediatrics, University of Medicine
and Dentistry of New Jersey School of Osteopathic Medicine, Stratford, New Jersey;
*Pediatric Sexual Abuse Program, Thomas Jefferson University Hospital,
Philadelphia, Pennsylvania*

CHILD SEXUAL ABUSE

Sexual abuse of children was once regarded as an uncommon phenomenon. The "hidden pediatric problem" that Kempe referred to in 1977, however, refused to remain in hiding (166). As early as the latter half of the nineteenth century, three French physicians, Tardieu, Bernard, and Brouardel, had each tried to expose the problem. Near the turn of the twentieth century, Sigmund Freud initially tried to uncover it, but like children who attempt to disclose, he recanted and created a myth that children's accounts of sexual abuse were the result of childhood desires and fantasy. This myth was accepted more readily than was the truth. Child abuse reporting laws and the women's movement in the late 1960s and early 1970s helped to set the stage for increasing public and professional awareness of child sexual abuse. Official reports of child sexual abuse began to escalate in the United States throughout the 1970s, leading to Kempe's "call to arms."

Some early management approaches were patterned after adult rape crisis models; others used the social work or the mental health model. Rape crisis centers were poorly equipped to handle the social and psychiatric issues raised by child victims, and social work and mental health practitioners lacked appropriate medical back-up. Law enforcement was notably absent from either model. A multidisciplinary approach was developed, incorporating law enforcement and increasingly involving physicians who "specialize" in the evaluation of sexually abused children. Child Advocacy Centers evolved from this multidisciplinary approach and the desire to organize evaluation and services for sexually abused children in a child-friendly environment.

In the course of the last two and a half decades, we have witnessed awakening concern, increasing public awareness, and organized backlash about child sexual abuse. Statements like "children never lie" and "children always lie" have been shown to be myths. Management of sexual abuse began as an art, and the scientific basis for the art continues to be laid down. Physician comfort with the recognition of sexual abuse has increased, and our understanding of the variability of normal and abnormal physical findings has been extended. Knowledge regarding the epidemiology and management has grown rapidly and continues to evolve. In this chapter, we describe the areas of agreement and of controversy in the theory and practice in childhood sexual abuse.

Definition

We know of no universal definition of child sexual abuse. Most definitions cover a wide range of sexual activities, including situations with no physical contact. Kemp (166) defined child sexual abuse as the involvement of children and adolescents in sexual activities they do not understand, to which they cannot give informed consent, or that violate social taboos.

Some definitions focus on age differences (91,101) and others on the unwanted or inappropriate nature of the sexual contact (239). The most useful definitions emphasize the unwanted, manipulative, and exploitative factors while recognizing the importance of age or developmental level differences between participants (93,284,285). Chronologic age differences must be considered guidelines, because of individual variation in developmental maturation and the variation in age criteria for state statutory rape laws.

Normal and Abnormal Childhood Sexuality

Four general patterns of sexual behavior have been characterized: developmentally appropriate, inappropriate, developmentally precocious, and coercive. Developmentally appropriate behaviors are expected sexual behaviors of children at a particular developmental stage. Inappropriate sexual behaviors are sexualized behaviors that may be developmentally appropriate, like masturbation, but raise concerns when frequently done in public. Developmentally precocious behaviors are sexually intrusive behaviors such as attempts at intercourse in younger children without elements of force or planning. Coercive sexual behaviors are sexually abusive or offending behaviors that are planned and that use force or coercion (105,121,126).

Sexual behaviors appear during infancy and develop throughout childhood. An understanding of normal development of sexual behavior is helpful for distinguishing between normal and abnormal sexual activities (173). Normal sexual behaviors begin shortly after birth. Oral gratification appears to be the most important sensual experience for infants. Penile erections in young infants may be associated with bladder or bowel disten-

tion. Rubbing of the genitals during general body exploration may produce penile erections and vaginal lubrication within the first year of life. Genital self-stimulation is evident by the first birthday, particularly in boys, but becomes more apparent by 18 months in both sexes (123). Children learn to identify themselves as boys or girls by age 2 to 3 years and often enjoy displaying their nude bodies. Between ages 3 and 6 years, children understand the differences between boys and girls; masturbation is common, if not universal. They are exhibitionists; many enjoy being nude and undress in front of others (103). Young children like to touch not only their own bodies but also the genitals and breasts of their parents, siblings, and peers. Sex play with both same-sex and opposite-sex peers is common, which typically involves undressing and mutual touching. The child identifies with the parent of the same sex and flirts with the parent of the opposite sex. By age 6 or 7 years, children become more modest; overt sexual behaviors diminish with age, but they remain curious about sex, dirty words, and pornography (184,243). They may continue to "play doctor" and engage in sex play involving exposure, genital stimulation, and fantasy games (175). Much of their sex education at this age comes from the same-sex peer group; however, cross-gender sex play and genital touching and viewing within the nuclear family does occur (175,237). Parents often allow their children to come into their bed when sick or frightened, which might account for some of this contact (236), and bathing with a parent or sibling up to age 8 or 9 years is not unusual (238). With the onset of puberty and early adolescence, family-related exploration decreases. Homosexual peer group activity continues but is gradually replaced by heterosexual activity with peers by mid to late adolescence (243). However, some studies find that up to one fourth of adolescents initiate heterosexual sexual intercourse by age 12 years. National studies indicate that one third of ninth graders and two thirds of twelfth graders have initiated sexual intercourse (41). Certain sexual behaviors are unusual in children and should raise concerns about how the child learned the behavior. Behaviors seen in 1% or fewer of the children aged 2 to 6 years in day care were attempts to touch adults' genitals, attempting to make an adult touch their genitals, using objects to masturbate, and masturbation in a way to cause pain (187). Friedrich (104) studied parental reports of normal sexual behaviors in 1,114 children from 2 to 12 years old. Observed sexual behaviors peaked at age 5 years for both boys and girls and decreased with increasing age. However, asking others to do sex acts, trying to have intercourse, and putting their mouths on the genital areas of other children were rare in all age groups (106).

A specific sexual behavior can not be viewed in isolation when differentiating normal "sexual play" from problematic sexual behaviors. An evaluation must consider the child's affect, the detailed history, and the context of the activities. The answers to the following questions may help to differentiate sex abuse from sex play:

1. Is it consistent with the developmental level of participants?
2. Is it consensual or coercive?
3. What is the motivation of the participants?
4. Is some outside influence involved?
5. What is the age difference between the participants? and
6. What is the response of the child to the episode (62)?

Normal sexual activity during childhood typically involves consenting, developmentally appropriate activities that are mutually motivated by curiosity and pleasure involving peers in terms of cognitive level. Abusive sexual contact often involves coerced or pressured, developmentally inappropriate sexual contact among nonpeers, motivated by one participant's needs or an outside influence.

Theoretic Basis for Abuse

Children make perfect victims for sexual abuse. Children are taught to respect and obey authority figures, and usually adults can influence them with relative ease. They are naturally trusting and curious about everything, including sex. Children need affection and will actively seek out attention. Many abusers are attuned to this trust, curiosity, and need for affection, establish a rapport over time, and gradually undertake the process of victimization (11,26).

Sexual abuse is the product of complex factors involving the victim, the perpetrator, and the environment. Intrafamilial sexual abuse or incest is fostered by an environment that allows poor supervision or poor choice of surrogate caretakers, or fails to set appropriate sleeping arrangements and role boundaries (248). Likewise, extrafamilial sexual abuse is fostered by factors that increase the child's vulnerability. Children with unmet emotional needs are easier to victimize. Adolescent defiance and peer pressure place some children at increased risk of sexual abuse. The risk-taking child is even less likely to disclose the abuse out of fear of blame or punishment, or concern about angering or upsetting the peer group. Children with physical or developmental disabilities may be more vulnerable to abuse because of increased dependency on others, resulting from their handicaps (11).

Finkelhor (101) described four preconditions for sexual abuse. The first precondition is an abuser whose motivation to abuse children comes from "emotional congruence," often secondary to abuse as a child, sexual arousal by children, and the inability to have appropriate sexual relationships with peers. The second precondition is the ability of the abusers to overcome their own internal inhibitions or moral standards to abusing children. The third precondition requires overcoming external inhibitors to abuse, such as the protective parent or normal boundaries between family members or between children and adults in general. The final precondition is overcoming the resistance of the child through use of pressure, seduction, or coercion.

The process of sexual victimization usually occurs in the context of a relationship and is accompanied by behaviors designed to engage the child in the sexual activity and permit the abuse to go on over time. Initially, the child is targeted for victimization, and a nonsexual relationship is established. Typically, the sexualization of the relationship appears to take place gradually. The child's cooperation and silence are maintained through a variety of forms of coercion, often by exploiting a child's normal need to feel valued (26). Summit (257) used the term "child sexual abuse accommodation syndrome" to describe the process by which the perpetrator gains access to the child, initiates the abuse, and assures cooperation and secrecy, using threats or rewards. The child accommodates to the increased sexual demands with an increasing sense of betrayal and feelings of guilt, and may develop behavioral symptoms. The children who disclose often find an unsupportive response, which may lead to repeated attempts at partial disclosure. If the unsupportive reactions continue, the child's guilt is reinforced, and the child retracts the complaint of abuse. The child's false retraction is quickly accepted, leaving the child vulnerable to continued abuse (257).

Epidemiology

Incidence and Prevalence

Child sexual abuse is common, but there is little agreement on the actual incidence and prevalence. Three methods have been used to estimate the prevalence of child sexual abuse: studies of reported cases of sexual abuse, surveys of groups of adults about their childhood experiences with sexual contact, and surveys of children about sexual experiences. Reasons for the lack of agreement among the studies include the lack of a universal definition, variable research designs, sampling biases, and insufficient response rates to questionnaires (84,186). National data in the U.S. have been compiled annually since 1976 from reports to state child-protective service agencies. Substantiated cases increased dramatically from 1976 to 1986, but from 1986 to 1994, substantiated cases remained fairly stable (267). The number of reported cases have actually declined in recent years (54,272).

The National Incidence and Prevalence Study of Child Abuse and Neglect summarized data on child sexual abuse that was reported to child-protective services agencies and other service agencies during 1986 (NIS-2) and during 1993 (NIS-3). These surveys focus on cases involving abuse by caretakers and exclude many cases involving noncaretakers. The NIS-2 study concluded that 2.5 children per 1,000 are reported as sexually abused each year, a total of 155,900 cases annually. Whereas physical abuse reports increased 58% from 1980 to 1986, sexual abuse reports more than tripled (173,210). The NIS-3 study concluded that 300,200 children were classified as sexually abused. This rate was approximately double the rate from NIS-2, which parallels the increased rates for all forms of child abuse from 1986 to 1993 (246). However, based on prevalence data from other sources, there would be expected to be approximately 500,000 new cases each year in the U.S. (99). Relatively few data are available from self-reports from children. Two contemporaneous samples to the NIS-3 data are available for comparison from a telephone survey of a nationally representative sample of 10- to 16-year-olds and a nationally representative sample of households. Of 2,000 children surveyed, 10.5% reported ever experiencing attempted or completed sexual abuse, and 6.7% reported an experience in the past year (98). Of 1,000 parents polled, 1.9% reported they knew their child had been sexually abused in the past year, and 5.7% said their child had been previously sexually abused (108). Extrapolation from these data would suggest that 600,000 to 1.2 million children are sexually abused in the U.S. each year. Child victims surveyed as adults suggested that less than one third of sexual abuse is disclosed to anyone, and that only 2% to 6% of sexual abuse is reported to the police (91,101,239,285). Therefore, studies based on reported cases involve a nonrandomly selected sample of all cases. These reported data may be typical of abuse seen by medical, mental health, and social work professionals, but they may not accurately represent the nature of sexual abuse. Generalizations based on adult surveys also should be made with caution. Adult survey results vary significantly: from 2% to 62% of adult women and 3% to 16% of adult men were the victims of some form of sexual abuse during childhood (91,97,101,168,239,285). The wide variation in rates among surveys could result from methodologic differences or from different rates among selected population groups (285). Estimates (5) from reported cases that 1% of children will experience sexual abuse each year are more consistent with adult surveys reporting 6% to 24% occurrence of sexual abuse before age 18 years than are those reporting higher rates. Finkelhor (99) has concluded in his review of prevalence studies that a prevalence of 20% for women and 5% to 10% for men would be reasonable conservative estimates (99).

The number of reported cases escalated during the 1970s and 1980s (22,173,185,210). Greater public awareness and changes in legal and social attitudes to encourage reporting may be responsible for increasing numbers of reports rather than an actual increasing incidence of child sexual abuse (185). Unfortunately, methodologic differences make it difficult to compare early surveys of the incidence of child sexual abuse with more modern surveys. Studies from the 1950s by Kinsey (169) and Landis (178) found similar frequencies of child sexual abuse involving physical contact, 12% and 16% respectively. Almost all of Kinsey's adult subjects were born before 1929, and almost all of Landis's college coeds were born after 1929. In contrast, Russell (239) concluded that 28% of a random sample of women living in San Francisco mainly born after 1929 had experienced contact sexual abuse before the age of 14 years. In recent years, multiple surveys have been conducted in the U.S., Canada, Great Britain, Australia, and New Zealand, and show a lower rate of contact sexual abuse than was found by Russell, ranging from 8% to 15%. A national survey of women in the U.S. was conducted in 1991 by using criteria similar to those of Russell's study. This study had

a response rate of 92%, and resulted in prevalence rates between 15% and 26% for any type of child sexual experience and between 11% and 19% for contact sexual abuse (269). Another study was representative of the Canadian population as a whole and had a 94% response rate. Sexual abuse involving contact before age 14 years was reported by 10% of the female subjects in this sample (15). A *Los Angeles Times* survey conducted nationally in 1985 found that 24.6% of women responding were sexually abused before age 14 years, and that most of this abuse involved physical contact (97). Although findings from these studies differ as to the prevalence of abuse, both studies revealed no differences in the rate of abuse among older adults and younger adults who responded to the surveys. Therefore, these results provide a strong argument against a precipitate increase in the amount of sexual abuse in the recent past (85). These studies are further supported by data from two adult surveys conducted 10 years apart in Los Angeles County, showing no significant change in the prevalence rates between the two samples (286).

Presentation and Indicators

Victims of child sexual abuse can present in many ways. Recognition of sexual abuse requires a high index of suspicion and familiarity with the historical, physical, and behavioral indicators of abuse. Supportive documentation for sexual abuse usually requires careful search for indicators within all three categories (61). Many children are brought for medical evaluation after disclosure of abuse. Masked presentations of sexual abuse, however, are common. Some children present initially with physical or behavioral complaints and, on further investigation, the history of sexual abuse is obtained. Common masked complaints include genital symptoms, abdominal pain, constipation or rectal bleeding, straddle injury, pregnancy, and various other somatic and behavior problems (143, 247). Chronic or recurrent urinary tract infections may be another masked presentation

(22,61,247); however, symptoms mimicking a urinary tract infection are more common than actual urinary tract infections in sexually abused children (171,228). Although masked presentations do occur, most children who present for medical care because of anogenital complaints without verbal disclosure of abuse are not being sexually abused. Kellogg et al. (165) reported that 84% of 157 children referred for evaluations for suspected sexual abuse because of anogenital signs or symptoms alone did not have findings suggestive, probable, or indicative of sexual abuse.

Historical indicators are the most important in sexual abuse. A child's direct statement describing sexual abuse is the most definitive historical indicator of abuse. The child may also provide a history of abuse during evaluation of a particular physical problem or behavior problem. Both types of disclosures should be taken seriously and should be investigated. The verbal disclosure can be reinforced by a more detailed history providing details of the abuse, describing emotional reactions, feelings or sensations, and describing how the abuser used manipulation or coercion to gain cooperation and secrecy (248). The methods for obtaining the history of abuse are discussed further in a subsequent section.

Physical indicators of abuse may be used to corroborate the history of abuse. Some children, however, present for medical care because of physical injuries, sexually transmitted diseases (STDs), and pregnancy, yet may not be ready to disclose abuse. Some physical findings strongly suggest the need for further evaluation for probable sexual abuse even in the absence of a history. STDs in prepubertal children should be considered strong indicators of sexual abuse (40,132,212). The strength of the association between specific STDs and sexual abuse is discussed in detail subsequently. Pregnancy in the preadolescent or young adolescent and genital or anal injuries should always raise the suspicion of sexual abuse (22,61). However, both boys and girls may sustain anogenital injuries from nonintentional mechanisms that must be distinguished from inflicted injuries (30,69,161).

Some criteria for differentiating injuries related to sexual abuse from those resulting from accidental trauma are discussed in the section entitled Medical Evaluation.

Common behaviors are often categorized as behavioral indicators of child sexual abuse, although they may reflect the child's response to any emotional conflict. Many behaviors may be considered supportive evidence of sexual abuse, but should not be considered diagnostic of sexual abuse. Finkelhor and Browne (33,100) have provided reviews on both the initial and long-term effects of child sexual abuse. They suggest that the behavioral signs and symptoms of sexual abuse result from four traumatogenic features of the abuse: traumatic sexualization, betrayal, powerlessness, and stigmatization. Traumatic sexualization occurs because the child is rewarded for sexual behaviors, resulting in sexual acting-out behaviors in the child. Betrayal feelings occur because the abuser betrays the child's trust. Grief, depression, extreme dependency, anger, impaired ability to trust others, and regressive behaviors may result. A sense of powerlessness and hopelessness results from the control exerted by the perpetrator and is associated with anxiety, fear, phobias, nightmares, hypervigilance, and perception of self as victim, somatic complaints, running away, school problems, aggressive behavior, delinquency, vulnerability to subsequent abuse, or becoming an abuser. Stigmatization occurs because the child feels responsible for the abuse, which results in feelings of guilt, shame, isolation, lowered self-esteem, suicidal ideation, criminal behavior, and self-injuring behaviors, such as alcohol or drug abuse (94). However, there is no specific syndrome for sexually abused children and no single traumatizing process that can explain behavioral outcomes (167).

Empiric studies of child sexual abuse victims show that common initial reactions include fear, anxiety, depression, anger, hostility, poor self esteem, and inappropriate sexual behavior. Empiric studies with adult women who were victimized as children showed they were more likely to manifest depression, self-destructive behavior, anxiety, feelings of isolation and guilt, poor self-esteem, and a tendency to revictimization and substance abuse (33, 186,258). Psychosexual dysfunction, chronic pelvic pain, eating disorders, chronic gastrointestinal problems, and somatization have been described in adults (25). Posttraumatic stress disorder has been described in both child victims and adults who were victimized as children (65,100). Adolescent victims may have symptoms similar to those of younger children or exhibit reactions more typical of adult rape victims (14,38,86). Studies have suggested adolescent promiscuity, teen pregnancy, and prostitution to be associated with sexual abuse (73,105), but one long-term follow-up study showed only an increased risk of prostitution (278).

Studies of behavioral outcomes have shown no consistent relations between characteristics of the abuse and measures of outcome. Our understanding of factors that are predictors or positive and negative outcomes is limited; however, sexual abuse outcome is probably as much about parent–child relationships in combination with adverse life circumstances as it is about specific aspects of trauma (105). Both prior physical and prior sexual abuse have a significant effect on childhood sexual behaviors (104). Many children experience several types of maltreatment, and sexual abuse may not be the most important outcome variable when sexual abuse coexists with physical abuse and neglect (278). Paradise (217) concluded from a follow-up study of sexually abused girls that preexisting adverse psychological circumstances contribute significantly to persistent problematic behaviors after sexual abuse. The consequences of sexual abuse must be viewed in the hierarchy of experiences during childhood, considering both vulnerability factors and compensatory and resilience factors (46).

Behavioral indicators may lead to evaluation and disclosure in some cases, and may be used to support the verbal and physical evidence of abuse in other cases. The presenting symptoms of sexual abuse are often so general in nature, however, that caution must be exercised in interpreting the sensitivity and specificity of behavioral changes. Some children exhibit many behavioral symptoms; others show none. Likewise, similar behaviors can be seen among children experiencing physical or emotional abuse or other stressful life events (9,32,50).

Perpetrators

The adult perpetrator has no typical personality profile. The psychologic, economic, and demographic characteristics of the perpetrators show a wide variation. Many abusers are successfully employed, active in community affairs, and do not have prior criminal records. Many perpetrators were abused themselves during childhood. "Normal" heterosexual, bisexual, and homosexual adults can be abusers, although a sexual preference for young children is found among pedophilic offenders (22,34,173,263). Perpetrators are typically heterosexual and very rarely are homosexual or bisexual (157). Most perpetrators are male. Typically, the male acts alone, sometimes a male and female act together, and a female perpetrator probably acts alone in fewer than 10% of all cases (74,81,82,268).

Most perpetrators are previously known to the child, and typically hold some authority or trust position in relation to their victims. They gain the child's trust and maintain secrecy by rewards and threats, misuse of their authority positions, or misrepresenting the truth (34,37). Depending on the sample, and particularly on whether older adolescent victims are included, strangers make up only 10% to 25% of the perpetrators. Relatives are perpetrators in from 25% to 50% of cases, and 30% to 60% of the children are victimized by other individuals previously known to them (37,57,58,81,83,91,101,227,232,239, 253,264,269,284). Clinical samples often show relatively high percentages of relatives, but surveys of adults generally indicate relatively lower frequencies of abuse by relatives, and lowest frequencies by strangers (186). The older adolescent appears at highest risk of abuse by a stranger, yet most are abused by friends, acquaintances, or relatives. Different studies report fathers, siblings, uncles, or cousins are the most common perpetrators in incest or intrafamilial sexual abuse (62,91, 97,239,269,284).

Adolescents are perpetrators in at least 20% of cases, although some surveys reveal up to 50% of all offenders are younger than 18 years. Preadolescents may make up an additional 5% to 10% of all perpetrators (173, 210,263). The sexual acts range from genital viewing and fondling to intercourse. Some episodes are typical "date rape" or "acquaintance rape" situations in which the adolescent forces or pressures an adolescent peer into sexual activity (163). Other adolescent perpetrators engage younger children in sexual contact through misrepresentation of power or authority. Often these encounters are not isolated events, but represent a pattern of maladaptive sexual behavior (20,84,163,263). Many adolescent perpetrators are lonely, depressed, and socially isolated from their peers. Lack of disclosure or lack of intervention after disclosure allows them to continue to abuse other children. Siblings may be the most common group of victims, but other younger, extended family members also are common victims (62,84,92,263).

Victims

General Characteristics

Victims include boys and girls of all ages, races, and socioeconomic groups. Most reported cases involve girls. Boys typically represent about 20% to 25% and up to 40% of reported victims from some centers (173,141). In retrospective surveys of adults and college students, about one third of child victims are boys (91,97). One national survey of parents suggested identical rates of sexual abuse in boys and girls (108). Some abusers clearly show a preference for boys. Boys, however, may be more reluctant to report abuse than are girls because of implications of weakness or homosexuality (91,97).

Independent risk factors for child sexual abuse are not easy to identify. Reports from sexual abuse centers appear to reflect the population they serve, with variation in the racial and age distribution of the child victims and overrepresentation of lower socioeconomic classes (37,58,83,232,264). Many apparent risk factors relate vulnerability to unmet emotional needs in children (11,248). Poverty, drug abuse, alcoholism, unhappy family life, marital conflict, and poor parental attachment may increase the child's vulnerability to abuse. Although socioeconomic effects are not consistently demonstrated, children living in single-parent homes or with step-parents appear to be at significantly higher risk of sexual abuse (61,97,108,173,186,240). Male victims may be more likely to be abused outside the home and by nonrelated abusers. In clinical case series, boys tend to be younger than girls at the time of reporting, but the age of onset of abuse may be similar for both boys and girls. Boys may be more likely than girls to be covictimized by single or multiple abusers; girls appear more likely to be solo victims of a single abuser. Male perpetrators predominate, but boys are more likely than girls to be abused by a female perpetrator, with increasing risk of abuse by a woman with increasing age (141). Younger children are subject to more sexual abuse at the hands of family or caretakers, including female and male babysitters, and are probably less likely to experience sexual penetration than are older children (57,74,81,97,101,141,227,253, 268).

Infants and Young Victims with Physical Evidence but No Disclosure

Specific injuries or the presence of an STD in a young victim may strongly indicate that sexual abuse may have occurred. Some children disclose the abuse during the process of an appropriate history and physical examination (143,247); however, some children will not readily disclose that abuse occurred. These cases require further evaluation, because the child may not be ready to disclose the abuse when a physical problem causes a "premature" accidental discovery. The physician must report that the physical injury or infection is a strong indicator of abuse. Indicating that someone entrusted with the care of the child either abused the child or allowed the child to be abused permits investigation of the case under child abuse laws without naming a specific perpetrator.

Reporting suspected abuse is the first step. A thorough psychological evaluation may lead to disclosure. Involvement of child-protective services allows assessment of the home environment, caretakers, and the risk of further abuse. Even when a specific perpetrator is not identified, interventions may be directed toward making the child safe.

Preschool-Aged Children

Preschool children constitute the most underreported age group of sexually abused children (270). Detection of child sexual abuse typically relies on the disclosure of the abuse by the child. A child whose verbal communication skills are limited usually cannot verbalize what happened, where it happened, and who was involved. Even when a young child is able to verbalize that sexual abuse has taken place, his or her ability to provide a true and accurate account is often brought under question.

Most young children are victimized in their homes. The preschool-aged child also may be susceptible to victimization in day-care settings. A national study determined, however, that preschool aged children in day care had a lower risk of abuse than preschool children in their own homes (95). When abuse is disclosed by a child in a group setting, accounts of abuse by other children in the same setting, whether conflicting or identical, may be used to argue that the events have been fabricated. Coaching may be responsible for identical stories, and inconsistencies may be used to refute the initial complaint. Evaluation of possible group sexual abuse in preschool children requires extraordinary care and skill to collect accurate and complete verbal evidence while avoiding the "contamination" of each child with information obtained from other children. Early involvement of law enforcement is critical in these cases (95,192).

Preadolescents

School-aged and preadolescent victims are frequently abused by relatives, but their increasing circle of contacts allows increasing risk of abuse by known individuals who are not related (22,91). Children want to be accepted by their peer group. As their circle of friends expands, the older child or preadolescent may be victimized by new "friends" in new settings (86). Masked presentations may be more common in this age group (135,247).

Adolescents

Adolescent victims probably make up from one fourth to one half of all nonadult victims of sexual abuse (7,77,80,91,97,201,239,284). The potential for victimization increases when the child defies parental limitations or takes risks. Adolescents may be victimized by peers or by new "friends" of their peers (80,86). The victims find themselves "in over their heads" before they realize that the other individual is going to take advantage of them. The youngsters subsequently feel guilty for creating the at-risk situation, and may not disclose the abuse because of fear of being blamed or punished. The assumptions of contributory or shared guilt made by the victim are often reinforced by the words of the perpetrator and by the child's caretakers. In addition, the adolescent's interest in developing sexuality may make the child feel more guilty about the episodes (77,86).

Adolescents are particularly vulnerable to abuse by a peer-group acquaintance. "Date rapes" are common, and between 25% and 47% occur on the first date. The adolescent's guilt feelings about his or her inability to prevent the incident is mirrored in the typical response of the perpetrator, the child's parents, the police, and the judge or jury that the victim is somehow to blame (14,84). Furthermore, several studies have documented that both male and female subjects believe forced sex may be legitimate and acceptable in certain circumstances (7). This attitude compounds the guilt, and concerns about how their peer group would respond to the disclosure make adolescents reluctant to report abuse (77). Accusations of acquaintance or date rape often are met with counterclaims of consenting sexual activity. Consent to be with someone and to engage in other activities is not consent to have sexual intercourse or to be raped. Real consent requires knowing what is being proposed and understanding or being aware of the consequences and implications of the activity; it is an act of free will or choice and not done under misrepresentation, duress, or force.

Developmentally Disabled or Handicapped Children

Children and adults with developmental disabilities are potential victims of sexual abuse, but accurate data regarding their risk of abuse are not available. Some studies suggest their risk of sexual abuse is similar to that of nonhandicapped children; others note a slight increased risk; and still others report a significantly greater risk (75,206,261). Underreporting is a likely problem in these individuals because of certain aspects of their increased vulnerability and decreased communication skills (261). Vulnerability to abuse is increased by their degree of increased dependency on others. Victims are likely to be repetitively abused by family members and other known individuals who provide their basic needs. In the severely handicapped individuals, their extreme dependency in the institutional setting may increase their risk of abuse. The more mildly affected individual has a need to fit in and be accepted by the "normal" population. This need to fit in may lead them to do whatever they are told, increasing the risk of victimization. Children with disabilities that affect communication may be at particularly high risk for abuse. Communication with the

suspected victims must be maximized by using developmentally appropriate interviewing tech-niques that consider the specific communication disability of the child (75,206).

Allegations of Abuse within the Context of Custody Disputes

Physicians should view allegations or suspicions of child sexual abuse between separated parents as a serious problem that warrants thorough examination and evaluation by qualified professionals (52). Three types of reports are found in this context: sincere valid reports representing actual abuse, sincere valid reports resulting from misinterpretation of a child's statements or behaviors but abuse has not occurred, and deliberately fabricated false allegations. Estimates of the frequency of unsubstantiated sexual abuse claims in the setting of custody or visitation disputes range from 23% to 55% (52,122,214). Unsubstantiated or "unfounded" claims of sexual abuse are not synonymous with "false" claims. False allegations of sexual abuse when child custody is not an issue are considered uncommon, being reported in about 4% to 9% of all cases (160,214). The false recantation rate was 9% among a group of unselected child sexual abuse victims; however, whether the recantation of actual abuse is more or less common in custody disputes is not clear. Divorce and custody may be associated with higher risk of both true reports and fictitious claims of sexual abuse. Family dysfunction leading to divorce may take many forms, but family violence, substance abuse, and personality problems may be related to an increased risk of abuse (117). Sexual abuse does occur in this setting. Pending or actual parental separation results in strong emotions, unmet needs, and lack of supervision by the other parent, increasing the risk of abuse (262). False claims of sexual abuse also may occur, however, as an expression of the bitterness of feelings between parents, or because of the possible effect such claims may have on decisions about custody and visitation arrangements.

The issue of substantiating sexual abuse in custody disputes must be placed in perspective. From 23% to 55% of selected reports in the setting of custody disputes are unsubstantiated, whereas about 50% of all child sexual abuse reports investigated by child-protective services are not substantiated (52,84,160, 214). Substantiation rates for sexual abuse in custody cases may therefore be as high as or higher than rates for abuse not involving custody disputes. In addition, allegations of sexual abuse are unusual in child custody cases. In a review of 9,000 cases of disputed child custody from eight different court systems throughout the U.S., only 2% included allegations of sexual abuse. Only 14% of the accusations were determined to be deliberately false. The rate of substantiated abuse, however, was six times greater among the children in child custody disputes when compared with the substantiated abuse found in the 1988 Study of the National Incidence and Prevalence of Child Abuse and Neglect (262). False allegations of sexual abuse in the context of custody disputes do occur, but only in a minority of cases, and deliberate fabrication is unusual (52). Until empiric data are collected to show otherwise, the process of evaluating these cases should involve the same methods and criteria as are used for other cases of suspected sexual abuse (52).

Child Pornography and Prostitution

Child pornography and child prostitution are closely related. Pornography is often a sideline to prostitution, and both may be related to drug dealing (244). Child pornography may be used to help seduce victims into many forms of sexual exploitation, including prostitution. Sex rings may be established by abusers or by adolescents themselves for the purpose of supplying child pornography, child prostitution, or both to adult groups of varying numbers of participants (180,279).

Child pornography can be defined as any visual reproduction of the sexual abuse of children (244,266). Child pornography serves several purposes: to aid in recruitment of child victims, to document a pedophile's activities, and to make money. Child pornography may be used to lure children into sexual activity, to instruct them, and to ensure their continued participation and secrecy surrounding the sexual activity (244). Children shown these materials may have increased curiosity and decreased inhibitions, may become sexually aroused, or may be led to believe that this is acceptable behavior. Pedophiles commonly collect child pornography and other souvenirs of their victims. These collections provide a record of the child molesters' own relationships for continued self-gratification while supporting a need to validate and legitimize their behavior (181). Child pornography also allows child molesters to profit from their experiences. It allows individual molesters to communicate with each other, to trade with other molesters for new and different pornographic materials, to exchange victims for their sexual services, and to trade their original material to the producers of commercial child pornography (180). Although illegal in the U.S. and in many other countries, the production and distribution of child pornography has flourished as a multimillion dollar industry.

Child prostitution involves the sexual exploitation of children for profit and the use of minor children in sexual acts with adults where no force is present. The incidence of child prostitution in the U.S. is unknown, but with approximately 3 million youth running away from home, some experts suggest that 1 million or more are involved in prostitution each year (244,274). The association between juvenile prostitution and running away from home is strong: most child prostitutes are runaways, and most runaways who do not quickly return home learn to survive by exchanging sex for money, food, and shelter. Both male and female prostitutes often come from unstable or abusive homes (244,274).

Juvenile male and female prostitutes are different in several ways. Female prostitutes are recruited by pimps or by other female juvenile prostitutes. The pimps provide the recruits with food and shelter, protection, and emotional support in exchange for their full-time prostitution earnings (244). Male juvenile prostitutes are typically independent operators who are not governed by pimps. Males engage in prostitution for the money, the sexual excitement, and the adventure. In addition, they are less likely than female prostitutes to be arrested (274).

Organized sexual abuse often progresses from incest to "sharing" the child sexually with family and friends, selling the children outside the family, making and selling pornography, national and international traffic in children for child prostitution and pornography, predisposing the children to adult pornography and adult prostitution and revictimization (149). Computer-related sexual exploitation by "cyber pedophiles" has grown with the expansion of online services and the Internet. Sexual offenders use this "new" technology to meet their "old" needs to organize their collections of correspondence, pornography, and fantasy material; communicate with victims and other offenders; and acquire, create, and share child pornography. Children can be exposed to sexually inappropriate materials on the Internet, which include both legal and illegal activities. Producing or possessing child pornography, uploading and downloading child pornography, and soliciting sexual activity with children are generally illegal. However, sharing sexual fantasies, collecting and displaying adult pornography, disseminating "indecent" materials, and engaging in "cybersex" are usually not considered to be illegal (182).

Interventions should be focused primarily on the effects on the victims and secondarily on the crimes involved. Skilled law enforcement personnel should be notified as early as possible, however, to allow investigation of suspected sex rings or child pornography activities. Clinicians should address general issues of safety, the child's current level of cognitive and social functioning, and the impact of the abuse on the child and the family. Specific issues including sexualization of relationships, sexual identity, drug abuse, aggression, and posttraumatic stress may require

considerable attention, depending on the duration and the types of activities involved and the child's current level of functioning (180, 244,274).

MEDICAL EVALUATION

Medical Professional's Role and Diagnostic Considerations

The child-protection wheel has many cogs, and each serves an equally important function: each must be present for the wheel to turn smoothly. The medical diagnosis and treatment of residua to inappropriate sexual contact is only one of the many cogs of this wheel. The collective insights of many disciplines interacting with mutual respect and understanding of each other's capabilities and limitations are essential to ensure the best insights into what a child may have experienced when abuse is suspected. If medicine were the sole or dominant discipline, it would have the unenviable burden of responsibility for all decision making and the ultimate outcome.

The field of medical diagnosis and treatment of child sexual abuse has evolved over the last 20 years (14,39,58,74,75,112,139, 150,166,221,232,253,264,282). During this period, physicians have enhanced their knowledge and skills in evaluating children alleged to be abused (90). Physicians have had to define their role as part of the intervention system. Some clinicians see their role limited simply to referring suspected sexual abuse cases to a local or regional diagnostic center developed to serve the needs of these children. Others see an opportunity to participate actively in evaluating children and have learned much from the child-protection, law enforcement, and mental health communities regarding the needs of abused children. Each physician may define his or her role differently within his or her community.

The clinician has much to offer to the multidisciplinary team evaluating the alleged child sexual abuse victim. The medical examination is one of the first steps in addressing the diagnostic and therapeutic needs of the child suspected of being sexually abused. The physicians' diagnostic assessment must be the result of an objective and sound interpretation of the historical, behavioral, and medical examination findings. Clinicians experienced in evaluating children alleged to have been sexually abused are more objective and less influenced by independent variables (218,219).

The collective insights and shared decision making of the many disciplines involved in the initial assessment of the child is necessary to obtain as complete a picture as possible into what a child might have experienced and meet their needs for protection and treatment.

A successful medical examination requires technical skills and an understanding of the clinical presentation of child sexual abuse. The physician who understands the dynamics of how children are engaged in sexually inappropriate contact, the progression of the activities over time, the use of threats, the types of disclosure, and why children might recant will be best prepared to obtain as complete a medical history from the child as possible. This knowledge and the requisite skills necessary to obtain the history of the alleged inappropriate contact are essential. Clinicians must be as adept at obtaining the history and documenting the history as they are at obtaining cultures for STDs. It is much easier to obtain a culture than to listen to the emotionally charged histories that children provide. However, working with the sexually abused child has the potential for being enormously rewarding.

Children will present to the physician's office for an examination in a variety of ways. A parent may call after having observed behavioral changes in the child, or having been told of behavioral signs by a relative, friend, or schoolteacher. Physicians who have developed expertise in evaluating sexually abused children receive the bulk of their referrals primarily from child-protection or law enforcement agencies.

Clinicians who take an active role in examining sexually abused children must develop a relationship with their child-protection and law enforcement agencies. The clinicians' in-

volvement depends on not only their degree of interest, knowledge, and skill, but also the confidence that child-protection and law enforcement colleagues develop in the clinician.

The presentation of a sexually abused child is unlike that involving other acute pediatric diseases. Sexually abused children do not typically disclose their experiences or demonstrate behavioral signs and symptoms immediately after an episode of sexual contact (37, 38,91,122,248,257). Children who disclose shortly after a sexually inappropriate contact are more likely to have experienced their abuse by an extrafamilial perpetrator. Extrafamilial perpetrators are more likely to use force and restraint when engaging children in sexual activities, and thus these children are more likely to demonstrate acute signs of injury. Children presenting with acute injuries involving extragenital and anogenital sites are the least problematic to diagnose. Because most sexual contact with children does not follow the rape model, few children will present with acute injuries.

Most children are sexually abused by individuals who have ready access to them and are known, loved, and trusted by the child (41, 248,257). Thus for the most part, when children are engaged in sexual activities, the individual initiating the contact tends not to have a desire to harm the child physically. This is one aspect that differentiates the sexual abuse of children from classic rape. By contrast, when children experience physical abuse, there may have been some intent to harm the child physically (248). Most children who are physically maltreated have cutaneous or other manifestations of their abuse that suggest a nonaccidental etiology. In sexual abuse, the perpetrator's pathologic but effective strategy is to engage the child with as little discomfort as possible, which increases the likelihood of engaging the child again in the inappropriate contact. Although most children are not physically injured during sexual abuse, the individual engaging the child in the activities demonstrates a callous indifference to the emotional impact of the activities. Thus it is essential to understand the contextual framework in which children are engaged and maintained in sexual activities (101,166,248, 257). The clinician's diagnostic assessment is based on historical and behavioral details that at times are supported by confirmatory physical findings, forensic evidence, and/or STDs. When physical findings are present, they frequently are nonspecific and must be corroborated with historical details concerning the child's experience. When interpreting nonspecific findings, the relationship between these findings and the timing of the last contact must be considered objectively before concluding that a nonspecific finding is the residual to the alleged experience. The various dilemmas of interpretation are discussed in this chapter.

Historical Validation

The cornerstone of evaluating any medical problem is the medical history. The medical history determines how the physician will proceed with the examination and the scope of testing required. Few physicians would examine an adult patient without obtaining a history. It would be equally inappropriate to proceed with an examination of a child capable of talking without attempting to hear about the experience from the child directly. The child's history helps the physician to understand the child's experience, its context, and time frames of the events. Physicians are more likely to be able to diagnose a medical disorder if they understand not only the signs and symptoms of the disorder but also its evolution. To obtain a complete history, the physician should be familiar with the relevant mental health and social work literature on child sexual abuse. With this knowledge, physicians will understand how children are engaged and maintained in sexually inappropriate activities and begin to appreciate the clinical expression of their experience (93,96, 97,173,210,235,248,257,268).

A complete medical history should be obtained from the child's caretaker and include a birth, family, surgical, developmental, hospitalization, and medication history. It is important to recognize that the adult providing the history may have been unaware of the specific symptoms that the child may have had related to the sexual contact. Therefore, the gastrointestinal (GI) and genitourinary (GU) review of systems may not be complete until the child is spoken to independently.

Statements made by the child either spontaneously or elicited through nonleading questions must be preserved verbatim. The idiosyncratic statements of children provide the best insight into the child's experience and add context to the concern. The medical history obtained from the child may provide great insight into the spectrum of a child's experience and the potential for diagnosing either residual to injury or an STD. Child protection and/or law enforcement may have conducted an initial interview of the child before referring the child for diagnosis and treatment of any residual to the alleged sexual contact. The physician's medical history will focus on whether the child has been injured as a result of the alleged contact and will obtain historic details concerning signs and symptoms specific to the contact. Some of these details are obtained from the review of systems and medical history given by the accompanying parent.

Specific information about the alleged contact should be obtained by talking to the child independently. An appropriately obtained and documented medical history may meet the diagnosing and treating physician's exception to hearsay (204). The medical record should include verbatim documentation of both questions asked and the exact response of the child. Observations concerning the child's affect and behavior during the medical history are extremely important and may assist in formulating a clinical assessment. Mental health professionals are best equipped to interpret subtle changes in affect and behavior.

At times, it may be difficult to take a history from a child regarding sexually inappropriate experiences. The ability to listen to children talk about their experiences is not intuitive but rather a developed skill. The physician must appear empathetic but neutral when obtaining a history. As children talk, they also observe the physician's reaction to what they have to say. If the physician appears uncomfortable listening or is insensitive to the child's needs, the child may simply stop talking. Therefore it is critical that the physician be nonjudgmental and facilitating while keeping in mind that the questions posed must be presented in a nonleading manner.

Although physicians consider the sexual abuse of children abhorrent, a child experiencing inappropriate contact by someone that they love and trust may view the activity quite differently, particularly when the activity is presented in a "playful" or "loving" context. Children's responses to these experiences may be neutral, positive, or negative, depending on how the activities were represented to the child (190). Therefore the physician should not automatically presume that the child was psychologically damaged, embarrassed, or hurt by the experience (190,248). Young children are most likely to express confusion, excitement, or ambivalence and may be less likely to understand the inappropriateness and implications of the experiences.

When obtaining a history, it is important to understand that children who experience abuse have special emotional needs. Because of their abuse, they may have some difficulty developing rapport and trust with the examining physician. If the examiner is unhurried, nonjudgmental, and empathic, the child will be more likely to view the clinician as understanding and will therefore be more likely to share both the details of the events and the accompanying affective associations.

The purpose of the medical history is to gather information as well as to to impart information in the form of therapeutic messages. These messages also assist in relaying to the child that the physician understands what the child has experienced. For example, it is important for children to understand that they were incapable of consenting in an informed manner to the sexual contact that they have experienced. Many children who have been repeatedly engaged in an activity and receive rewards for participating have difficulty

in accepting that they are not responsible for having "allowed" the contact to happen. Unfortunately, such feelings may be reinforced when the child discloses abuse and the nonoffending parent responds by saying, "Why did you let him do it?"; "Why didn't you stop him?"; or "Why didn't you tell sooner?" Such responses make the child feel responsible for what has happened. When children are engaged in sexual activities, they are not given choices and are incapable of consenting to sexual activities. Children also are not empowered to stop the activities in which they are engaged.

Another extremely important message to impart is that the child did the right thing by telling and that he or she did not do anything wrong. This concept, coupled with a statement that this type of thing happens to a lot of children, helps decrease the sense of stigmatization, embarrassment, and isolation commonly seen after sexually inappropriate contact.

Abused children have experienced the abuse of power and authority (248,257). As a result, they may continue to behave, even after disclosure, in a manner reflective of their sense of powerlessness and remain at high risk for future abuse (94,96). Thus it is important to begin to empower children after their disclosure. This process can begin by simply asking the child what they want to happen now that they have disclosed. Children must be given the opportunity to begin to make choices that are in their best interest. Most children who purposefully disclose do so simply because they want the abuse to stop. Children frequently are fearful of the consequences of disclosure because of the overt or implicit threats used by the perpetrator to maintain secrecy. Secrecy facilitates repetition and removes accountability by the perpetrator (94,248,257). Children generally cannot conceive of the cascade of events that is precipitated by their disclosures. They cannot anticipate that the consequences of their disclosure may result in the prosecution of a family member, foster care placement for themselves, and possible abandonment by their nonoffending parent. All professionals involved in caring for abused children must be scrupulously honest and forthright when telling children what to expect after their disclosure. They should be encouraged to ask questions and assure them that they will be supported through the ensuing process.

The medical history should be documented with meticulous detail. As it is difficult for children to describe what they have experienced, the number of times a child must provide the details of the experience should be minimized. Memorializing the history with a hand-held tape recorder and/or videotape is an alternative to traditional contemporaneous handwritten notes. When a recording device is used, the child should always be informed and should consent. Young children enjoy speaking into a recorder and hearing their voices. Identifying information can be introduced on the tape. If the child prefers not to be taped, then that desire must be respected. Explain to children and adolescents that the purpose of taping is to help the doctor listen carefully to what they have to say and not spend time writing. Most children usually accept this explanation. Once engaged in the history, most children become unaware that they are being taped, and thus interference with their spontaneity is minimal. The added advantage of a video-recorded history is that it not only captures the child's verbatim statements as expressed in age-appropriate terminology, but also provides an opportunity to review and assess the accompanying affective and behavioral aspects of the statements. A recorded history is an excellent tool to use in self and peer critique, thus improving history-taking skills. Any recording of the history must be appropriately identified and kept in a manner that meets all standards of maintaining confidentiality.

Before proceeding with the history, the clinician should review with child-protection workers and law enforcement all previously conducted interviews. These interviews should be assessed for their thoroughness, which will assist in determining the scope of the medical history to be conducted. Children should be spoken to as soon after disclosure as possible, as early statements are generally more spontaneous.

In addition to reviewing the details of all prior interviews with the child, it is equally important to address the parental response since disclosure and to record any observations that the nonoffending caretaker may have made. The nonoffending parent can provide a wealth of information concerning the child's medical history and change in daily habits, as well as any behavioral changes and the child's statements that contributed to the suspicion that the child may have been abused. At the onset of the history, the child and parent may be seen together, but then each should be seen independently to address their individual concerns or worries. Many times, children and adolescents have unanticipated and unrealistic worries or concerns referable to their bodies as a result of what they have experienced. Addressing these issues is essential in identifying the possibility of an altered body image resulting from abuse. Children and adolescents frequently say that they feel that their body may have been injured, that people can tell simply by looking at them or by the way that they walk that they experienced a particular activity (94, 248). It is important to let children know that no worry or question is too silly or uninformed.

The young child must view the clinician as both nonthreatening and empathic if he or she is to separate from the parent. Every effort must be made by the clinician to create an environment in which the child will feel safe and understood. The clinician's history-taking style must be modified to meet the needs of the varying ages and developmental levels of children. Introductory statements might be as follows:

> Thank you for coming to see me today. I am a kid's doctor, and I talk to and look at a lot of kids your age, some older and younger, but a lot of kids just like you. I talk to kids when there is a worry or concern that they may have had something happen to them that might be confusing and difficult to understand. Some-

times it is by someone who they know and trust. I understand that that may of happened to you. Is that true?

Most children acknowledge these introductory comments by nodding affirmatively or saying "yes." At this point in the introductory comments that precede the history taking, it is an appropriate time to interject some important therapeutic messages. One of those messages is that they were brave for telling and that they did not do anything wrong. The next step is to explain that the purpose of the examination is to make sure that they are physically okay. Tell the child that it is equally important to see a "talking doctor." Explain that a "talking doctor" (psychologist/psychiatrist) is someone who understands how kids feel if they have had these things happen to them. This reference begins to set the stage for the mental health assessment by a child psychologist or psychiatrist.

Once the stage is set for the medical history to proceed, the physician should explain to the child in a developmentally appropriate way that they are being seen for the purpose of diagnosing and treating any effects of the alleged contact. One way to accomplish this is to explain to the children that when they have not felt well in the past and have gone to the doctor, the doctor asks them all kinds of questions. The doctor may ask them if their tummy hurts, if they have a fever, or their throat hurts. The reason the doctor asks these questions is because the doctor wants to know what's been going on so the doctor can decide what to look at, and whether tests or medication is needed to get them better. Then state, "I am going to ask you some questions about what happened, not to embarrass you or make it difficult, but to understand so I can take a look at you, do tests if necessary, and give you medication if needed."

The history should focus primarily on the specifics of what the child experienced and the context in which the alleged contact occurred. The child's history of the experience sets the stage to diagnose any residual to the alleged contact, whether it be acute or chronic injury, seminal products, or an STD. Children are told that the purpose of the examination is to make sure they are physically OK and to address any worries or concerns they may have about their body because of what happened.

Some children and adolescents find it difficult to verbalize their experiences. Using anatomic drawings, paper and crayons, or anatomically detailed dolls may facilitate the children's articulating or demonstrating their experience (29,118,276). Considerable research has been done in an effort to standardize the use of dolls and to establish the credibility of dolls as an interviewing instrument (276). When dolls were first introduced as a clinical tool, there was little instruction or standardization in interpretation of the results. Recent research has focused on normative play with these dolls in the non-abused pop-ulation, and has elucidated some of the inherent difficulties in interpreting the child's interaction with the dolls (29,151, 277). Anatomically detailed dolls can be of benefit in gaining information regarding the alleged sexual abuse.

Children use a variety of terms to describe their private parts. The terms a particular child uses for genital and anal anatomy need to be determined. If the child appears embarrassed, give the child permission to use his or her own words by telling the child that you have heard all kinds of names, some of which are silly, and some of which are embarrassing to say. Some children prefer writing the name down or whispering the name of their private parts.

The medical history should address the following issues: (a) how access to the child was achieved; (b) how the activity was represented to the child to engage the child in the activity, (c) progression of the activity(s) over time; (d) what rewards, threats, bribery, coercion, and/or intimidation was used to maintain the child in the activity(s) over time; (e) where the contact occurred; (f) the frequency of contact; (g) the child's description of how he or she felt when engaged in the contact; (h) specific details of what the child experienced and any discomfort associated with the events, including observations by the child in regard to bleeding, bruises, or ejaculate; (i) circumstances surrounding either accidental or purposeful disclosure; (j) to whom the disclosure was made and the response of that individual; and (k) what the child would like to happen now that the disclosure has occurred (192,248).

Depending on the child's developmental level and emotional preparedness to discuss what he or she has experienced, some or all of the details of their experience will be obtained. The physician should view the child's experience as a puzzle, gathering as many pieces as possible to glean the most accurate and complete picture. When questions are posed, they should be simple, unambiguous, and nonleading. Questions are of value only when they are not suggestive of the answer. Complex questions have the potential to confuse the child, and thus the child's response will be more difficult to interpret. Make sure the child understands the questions and feels free to ask for clarification if he or she does not understand. Using an open-ended style that progresses from the more general to specific eases the child into talking about his or her experience (123,151,189,192,248).

To achieve effective communication with child victims, the clinician must consider the following issues: (a) identifying and overcoming the child's fears and perceived consequences of the experience and subsequent disclosure; (b) understanding the coping strategies children use as a defense pattern; (c) appreciating that children provide the details of their experience in a fragmentary manner and may repress specific memories of their experience; (d) recognizing that, depending on developmental age, children will have varying abilities to communicate the frequency or time frame in which they experience the contact; and (e) becoming adept at providing options for children to answer questions in the most truthful and least threatening manner (158,192,204).

At each and every point of the history-taking process, the clinician must remember that the mental health and well-being of the child is paramount and more important than the specific details obtained. The physician should always consider that the impact of sexual experience is primarily psychological, and thus he or she must proceed with the sensitivity and empathy that these children need and deserve. The trusting relationship that should develop throughout the history will serve the physician well during the physical examination.

Physical Examination

All children alleged to be sexually abused should have a complete head-to-toe examination, even if the last alleged contact was months or years before, and the child feels fine. The history may have revealed that the child has an altered body image or feels that his or her body may have been injured in some nondescript way. Thus the examination has the potential to have considerable therapeutic value, even if acute or chronic signs of injury or STDs are not identified. The purpose of the physical examination is not only to diagnose and treat any "abnormality" as a result of the contact but, of equal importance, to reassure "normality," which may help the child achieve a sense of physical intactness.

Child-protective services and law enforcement often request physical examinations for their clients. They may need guidance from medical professionals in determining where to have the child examined as well as the appropriate timing for an examination. It is important to assure that a child does not have to undergo more than one physical examination. The initial examination must be conducted by a physician who both understands the needs of these children and can appropriately document the complete medical assessment. The courts consider the first examination of a child after a disclosure of sexual abuse to be for the purpose of diagnosis and treatment, and all subsequent examinations for the purpose of investigation. When an examination is deemed to be for the purpose of investigation, the diagnosing and treating physician's exception may not apply. The practical implication of this is that the screening examinations conducted by a primary care or emergency room physician unfamiliar with the needs of these children may limit the admissibility of a more competently obtained history and examination. When the circumstances dictate that a screening examination must be completed and the examining physician does not feel equipped to conduct a thorough assessment of diagnostic and treatment needs of the child, then a full examination must be deferred. Under these circumstances, the medical record should note that the child is being referred to a physician who can provide the specialized diagnostic and treatment needs. This set of circumstances is not dissimilar to the routine practice of requesting subspecialty consultation, with the ultimate diagnosis being rendered by the consultant.

Physicians should serve as the gatekeepers of medical services and determine where and when an examination is completed. The emergency department, a common point of entry for an examination, is generally the least appropriate environment for the first encounter, unless the hospital has appropriate personnel and equipment to serve the needs of these children.

Because most children do not disclose immediately after their last alleged sexual contact, the need for a rape kit, the diagnosis of acute genitourinary infections, STDs, and/or trauma is not usually the primary consideration. Thus most examinations are nonemergency and can be scheduled for an outpatient assessment after the initial child-protective service or law enforcement intervention.

Acute genital and anal injuries are infrequent, but when they do occur, an immediate examination is indicated. When a disclosure occurs, this timing provides the best opportunity to identify any acute as well as chronic residual to the contact, to treat medical problems, and to use a rape kit if there is reason to believe that seminal products or trace elements are present. When there is a need to use a rape kit, each component must be performed by personnel who are skilled in the collection and preservation of each compo-

nent. Under most circumstances, the child victim can identify the individual who has engaged the child in the contact. The information obtained from a rape kit can be helpful in confirming contact and an individual's identity.

Typically, when children present for examination after an alleged inappropriate sexual experience, either nonspecific findings or no residual to the contact is evident. When no acute signs of injury are present, the clinician must determine whether any chronic changes in genital or anal anatomy are present. Chronic residual to genital or anal trauma by definition will be evident long after the last sexual contact. Thus a delayed disclosure allows the scheduling of an examination in a nonemergency manner. The retrospective interpretation of changes in anal and genital anatomy and the inherent difficulties of such an assessment are discussed in another part of this chapter (88).

The disclosure of abuse precipitates a crisis for the family. Nonoffending parents frequently want an immediate answer as to whether the child's statements are true. Child-protective service, law enforcement, and parents may believe that the physical examination will confirm the contact and seek an immediate examination, usually either by their primary care physician or in the emergency department. To counter this misconception, the physician must determine the appropriate timing of the examination and explain to law enforcement and child-protection agencies and the nonoffending parent why deferring the examination may be in the best interest of the child.

As a rule, if the last episode of alleged contact occurred within 72 hours, an examination should be done immediately to identify and treat residual to the contact. Every effort should be made to see that the acute examination as well is conducted by someone with the appropriate skills and photodocumentation capabilities to avoid the child's being subjected to a repeated examination.

When more than 72 hours has passed since the last contact, the primary focus of child-protective service and law enforcement should be the initial coordinated interview. Once this is completed, the child can be referred for an assessment of the mental health impact of the contact, development of a therapeutic plan, and a medical examination. Concomitantly, the child-protection agency will be assessing the nonoffending parent and/or caretaker to determine if the safety of the child can be assured.

Preparation of the Child

Sexually abused children have been deceived, betrayed, and coerced into the sexual contact and may have considerable difficulty in developing trust. Completion of a thorough examination depends on the ability of the physician to anticipate and address the child's anxiety and fears. Because abused children have already experienced the abuse of power and authority, they should never experience the same by coercion, deceit, or the forced abduction of their legs by a "helping physician." A forced examination of an uncooperative child is universally unsuccessful and only results in a more frightened and less trusting child who is more difficult to examine in the future. If it appears that the child is unlikely to cooperate and there is no medically urgent indication for the examination, the examination should be rescheduled to a time when the child may be more receptive. When the presenting signs and symptoms suggest a need for an immediate examination and the child is uncooperative, sedation and/or examination under anesthesia is appropriate (220).

When children are fearful, there is usually an underlying basis that can be readily identified. Young children are most fearful of needles, being hurt, or the unknown. Each of these issues is addressed differently depending on the child's age (190). The purpose of the examination should be explained, telling the children how the examination will proceed and reassuring them that they can ask questions at any point if there is something that they do not understand. Wherever appropriate, the child and/or adolescent is given choices,

which assists the child in achieving a sense of control. Young children may prefer sitting in their mother's lap rather than being positioned on the examination table. Allow the adolescent patients to decide who will be with them during the examination. An adolescent, to protect the sense of privacy, may not want the mother in the room, particularly if the older child previously disclosed the experience to the mother, and she failed to intervene.

It also is important to address parental anxiety. The most common fear that parents express is that their young child will undergo an adult speculum and bimanual examination. Reassuring the parent that the prepubertal child will not have this type of examination relieves maternal anxiety and enables the parent to be supportive, comforting, and attentive to the child's needs during the examination.

Examination of the anogenital region should occur only in the context of a complete physical examination. When children are engaged in sexual activities, the contact is focused on their anogenital region. Implicitly, the message to the child who undergoes a head-to-toe examination is that all parts of his or her body are important. Although the physician, in examining the genitalia and anus, spends a significant amount of time, this component should be completed only as part of the natural progression of the head-to-toe examination. Extragenital signs of trauma, although less frequently present, are detected during a complete examination. Abused children may have had their general medical needs neglected, and the examination along with a complete review of systems and medical history serves to address their overall health needs and identify previously unsuspected medical problems.

The ability to perform a competent anogenital examination depends on the clinician's level of comfort, skill, and familiarity with the full spectrum of variations of normal anatomy. In one study, 77% of 129 physicians surveyed indicated they routinely examine the genitalia only 50% of the time, and 17.2% examine the genitalia less than 10% of the time. In that same study, only 59% of the examining clinicians correctly identified the hymenal membrane (174). Familiarity with children's genitalia occurs only when the genital examination is incorporated routinely into all health-maintenance assessments. Failure to do so limits the opportunities for a physician to develop a comfort level in conducting genital examinations and the recognition of subtle normal anatomic variations.

The examination of the child's private parts can be completed in the context of a routine health assessment as a part of providing anticipatory guidance regarding body safety. The anticipatory guidance concerning body safety can address car and bicycle safety as well as assessing the child's knowledge concerning private parts. The children might be asked if they know who is allowed to touch their private parts and under what circumstances. They may be instructed as to what to do if they are touched in a way that is not OK. Parents welcome this guidance as well as serving as a natural transition to the genital examination.

Positions

Only in the last 20 years has the medical literature become replete with descriptions of techniques to conduct a complete anogenital examination. Much of the literature has focused on examination positions in the prepubertal child (2,18,76,137,198,201). The optimal examination position(s) combined with a variety of techniques allow a full appreciation of the nuances of normal genital anatomy and the tissue changes that may reflect residual to trauma.

The position in which a child is most comfortable, most cooperative, and least embarrassed is the position that should be used initially. Frequently, a combination of the supine frog-leg and knee–chest positions maximizes observation of the hymenal membrane and structures of the vaginal vestibule (18). Small children are most likely to be comfortable when examined in the supine frog-leg position on the examination table or while being held in the caretaker's lap (Fig. 10.1). All chil-

dren and adolescents should be gowned and draped to protect their sense of privacy. Very young children are curious and may prefer not to be encumbered by a gown.

In the recumbent supine position, the child sits like a frog with her legs in full abduction and the feet in apposition. When using the separation technique, place the first and second fingers at the 10 and 2 o'clock positions, exerting gentle pressure until the labia separate and the hymenal membrane is visualized. With this technique, little or no tension is placed on the hymenal membrane (Fig. 10.2).

With the child in the frog-leg position, visualization of the structures of the vaginal vestibule is achieved with the use of labial separation with or without traction. The "traction technique" affords improved visualization of the hymenal orifice (198). Traction is most valuable in children who have redundant hymenal membrane tissue, as the mucosal surface's cohesive forces tend to obscure full visualization of the orifice. When using labial traction (Fig. 10.3) grasp the labia between the thumb and index finger of each hand and exert gentle traction in the posterior lateral direction. Steady tension may be necessary to overcome cohesive forces of a moist hymenal membrane, allowing the orifice to pop open. Before concluding that the edge of the orifice is rounded and/or narrowed, examine the child in the knee–chest position, which may allow a folded-over edge of tissue to flatten out, thus changing the initial impression of a narrow and rounded edge of the membrane.

In the prone knee–chest position, gravity allows the anterior vaginal wall to fall forward and any redundant tissue in the inferior quadrants of the hymen to thin out. The prone knee–chest position does have the advantage of facilitating visualization of the cervix if the hymenal orifice is of sufficient diameter and the patient is relaxed (76).

The prone knee–chest position (Fig. 10.4) is somewhat awkward and can be embarrassing for all but the youngest children. When using this position, prepare the child by asking if she has seen how babies sleep on their

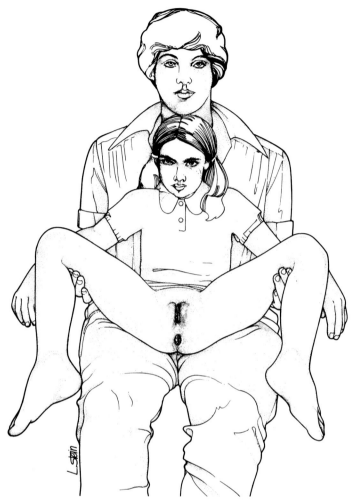

FIG. 10.1. Prepubertal child positioned in the lap of accompanying adult for genital and anal examination.

tummies with their behinds up in the air. Explain to the child that this is the position that you want her to be in, and have the accompanying adult assist in positioning the child. While the child is in this position, the clinician places the thumbs on the buttocks at the 10 and 2 o'clock positions and gently elevates the buttocks in a lateral and superior direction (Fig. 10.5) If the examiner is confident that complete visualization of all of the tissues has been achieved in the supine frog-leg position, it may not be necessary to examine the child in the prone knee–chest position.

The appearance of the hymenal membrane orifice may vary considerably depending on the examination position, state of relaxation, and degree of traction (18,198,216). McCann et al. (198) observed that the prone knee–chest position and the supine traction method proved superior to the supine separation technique for visualizing the hymenal membrane and its orifice. Maximal anteroposterior hymenal orifice diameters were obtained in the prone knee–chest position. Maximal transverse horizontal diameters were obtained in the supine position with traction. Variability

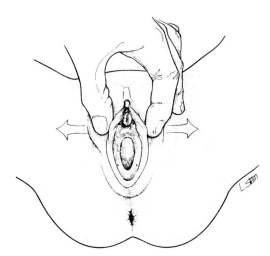

FIG. 10.2. Visualization of the structures of the vaginal vestibule assisted by placement of the fingers to separate labia, in the supine frog-leg position.

in measurements also is attributable to differences in the state of relaxation. This occurs because the hymenal membrane is attached laterally to the vaginal wall, and when the pubococcygeal muscles are tense, the vestibule is contracted, and the orifice may appear small; when relaxed, the orifice appears more dilated. The addition of labial traction provides another variable in measuring the maximal orifice diameter. The greater the traction, the larger the orifice might appear. The pas-

sage of an object such as a Foley catheter through the orifice and subsequent traction on the inflated balloon will result in even greater distention of the orifice.

The anus can be readily visualized in the knee–chest position. This knee–chest position may be uncomfortable for any child who has experienced anal penetration. Thus the left lateral decubitus (lateral knee–chest) or supine frog-leg with legs flexed onto the abdomen (supine knee–chest) are the best alternatives for examining either the male or female anus (Fig. 10.6).

The lithotomy position is most appropriate for examining the pubertal female child. Anticipate that the adolescent will feel vulnerable, anxious, and embarrassed in this position. For many adolescents, this may be the first genital examination since early childhood. To make this experience nonthreatening, take additional time, address anxieties and fears, explain throughout the examination what the adolescent should anticipate as one proceeds, and provide as much privacy as possible.

Once the patient is in the appropriate position for the examination, every effort must be made to minimize any discomfort. Children may be fearful of being touched by a cotton swab, because of a previous experience with throat cultures. A few simple steps can minimize the potential for causing discomfort. All

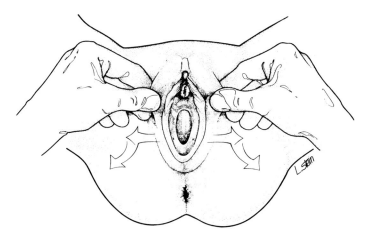

FIG. 10.3. Lateral and posterior traction of labia further facilitates visualization of structures of the vaginal vestibule, in the supine frog-leg position.

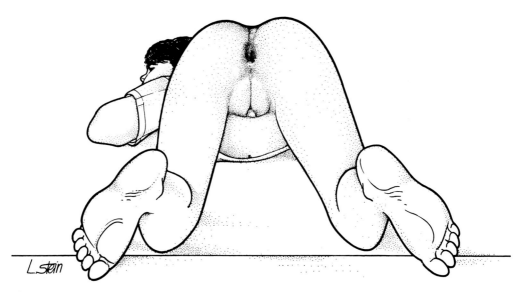

FIG. 10.4. Knee–chest position for genital examination of the prepubertal child to supplement the supine frog-leg position.

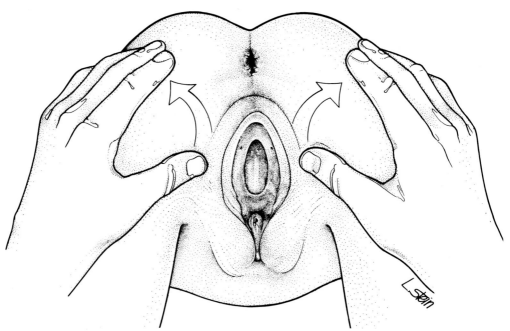

FIG. 10.5. Visualization of the structures of the vaginal vestibule while in the knee–chest position is facilitated by superior and lateral traction, as noted by hand placement.

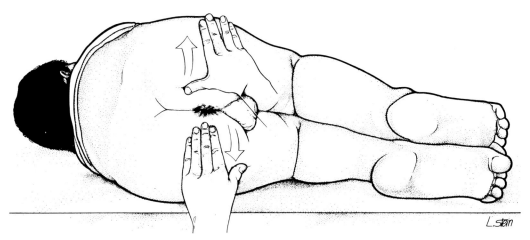

FIG. 10.6. Hand placement for separation of the buttocks to view external anal tissues with the child in the left lateral decubitus position.

visualization should be done before attempting any touching with cotton swabs. The unestrogenized hymenal membrane is very sensitive, and if touched directly, will cause discomfort. Therefore, when attempting to collect vaginal secretions for cultures, use urethral swabs (mini-culturette), which easily pass through a hymenal orifice of 2.5 mm or greater without touching the edge of the membrane or the external surface. A urethral swab moistened with sterile nonbacteriostatic saline before use will further reduce the chances of discomfort if the hymen is touched. Large cotton swabs are more likely to cause discomfort and should be avoided in prepubertal children. Before introducing the mini-culturette, separate the labia by applying pressure points with the second and third fingers of the left hand on each buttocks lateral to the fourchette. The downward and lateral pressure opens the vestibule for visualization. The pressure sensation of the index fingers on the buttocks will distract the child, and the swab can be introduced through the orifice to collect the specimen under most circumstances without touching the hymen. Alternatively, the clinician can pass a urethral catheter through the orifice and irrigate the posterior portion of the vagina with a few milliliters of saline. The vaginal wash is then plated on appropriate medium.

Generally, the examination of the prepubertal child is principally an external visualization facilitated by varying techniques of separation, traction, and positioning. Instrumentation of prepubertal children is rarely necessary. Use of a nasal speculum, as described in standard texts, is awkward and of limited value (55). Vaginal specula are reserved for pubertal children or prepubertal children who require an examination under anesthesia. Even removal of the most commonly found foreign body (toilet paper) can generally be achieved without a speculum or anesthesia with a simple irrigation technique.

An examination using a vaginal speculum is most appropriate for the pubertal child. Not all adolescents, however, undergoing an examination require a speculum and bimanual examination. If the clinical history suggests that penetration has occurred, a speculum examination is helpful in diagnosing intravaginal trauma, determining the maximal transverse orifice diameter, obtaining a Papanicoulaou (Pap) smear, and the collection of specimens for STDs.

To visualize the redundant edge of the estrogenized hymen completely before introducing a speculum, placing a moistened, large-diameter cotton swab run behind the inner aspect of the membrane circumferentially can help to identify any posttraumatic interruptions in the edge of the membrane. In the pubertal child, the use of labial separation and traction alone is generally inadequate to assess the maximal hymenal orifice diameter. Even a small-appearing hymenal orifice can dilate to a significantly larger diameter with the introduction of a speculum. This is due to the distensibility and elasticity of the estrogenized tissues. A speculum examination will assist in determining whether the transverse hymenal orifice diameter is sufficient to admit an object such as a penis. An adult vaginal speculum measures 35 mm in its diameter, exceeding the average transverse diameter of an adult erect penis.

Improving Visualization and Documentation

Once a child is comfortable and positioned for the examination, supplemental lighting, filters, and magnification can assist in optimizing visualization of all the details of the genital and anal tissues. Adequate lighting is a prerequisite to a thorough examination and any photographic or video documentation that should follow. Several inexpensive light sources, such as a goose-neck lamp, halogen procedure lights, and hand-held devices can be used, although they are usually inadequate to assure the consistent results that can be achieved by a light source attached to a colposcope or a fiberoptic scope with video capabilities. Moreover, the light created by inexpensive sources is insufficient for adequate photo documentation (231).

The genital tissues of prepubertal children are best examined with the use of magnification. Although this task can be achieved with a hand-held lens or the magnifying capabilities of an otoscope or ophthalmoscope, none of these methods is satisfactory. The least optimal choice is the otoscope or ophthalmoscope, in part because of a limited angle of view, a small lens, and a short working distance required between the child's genitalia and the examiner.

Astronomers view the heavens with a telescope, rarely relying on the naked eye. When visualizing all of the nuances of genital and anal anatomy, the physician's equivalent to the telescope is the colposcope. The first forensic application of this device was in 1981, when a Brazilian medical examiner, Wilmes Teixeira, reported his experience with this gynecologic instrument in examining 500 sexual assault victims (260). In this study, the colposcope was most useful in the pediatric age group. In 48.8% of the cases studied, the colposcope "clarified dubious diagnoses" made based on gross unaided visualization alone. In the total population of children and adults, clarification was facilitated in 11.8%. In 1986, Woodling and Heger (283) published their initial experience with the colposcope in the evaluation of children alleged to have been sexually abused. The colposcope has achieved widespread acceptance as the instrument of choice to improve visualization of the anal and genital anatomy and to document the examination (199,241). The colposcope provides an excellent light source with multiple or variable magnification capabilities. An alternative to the traditional colposcope is the fiberoptic scope that incorporates an excellent light source, variable magnification, a wide angle of view, along with videotape and print capabilities. Most fiberoptic scopes are a far less expensive alternative to the traditional colposcope but are limited by the lack of 35-mm photographic capabilities.

The traditional colposcope, outfitted with a 35-mm camera attachment, affords consistent and easy documentation of physical findings in either a slide or print format. Digital cameras provide some advantages over traditional film in that they allow immediate viewing of images and can be easily downloaded into a computer database or printed. Even the best digital cameras cannot capture the same spectrum of tonality that 35-mm film can. The best image can still be obtained with film. An alternative to a digital camera is to scan slide or color negative film. The scanned computer image that results will have a greater range of tonality and detail than could be obtained by a digital camera alone. Polaroid systems produce immediate images; however, they are generally of poor resolution and inadequate for reproduction. When a colposcope is not available, a macro focusing lens with 1:1 magnification capabilities and a ring flash can be used to document physical findings (231).

A colposcope with video capabilities has many advantages over still photography in the documentation of examination findings. Still photography provides only a moment-in-time, two-dimensional record of a given finding. The genital and anal tissues are dynamic, and video colposcopy assists in observing and recording the variable appearance of the tissues from moment to moment. Video colposcopy has the added advantage, particularly in prepubertal children, of allowing the child to observe exactly what the examiner is doing on the video monitor. For most children, this helps demystify the examination. Having a sense of control and participation throughout the examination at times comforts children who watch. Before a view of the child's genitalia, young children might find it fascinating to see their belly button or fingernail on the TV monitor. The child is then instructed to watch the monitor and observe the examiner's approaching finger before actually being touched. Children who are fearful of being touched by a cotton swab can be handed one and shown on the monitor where the examiner would like the swab placed. In this way, fearful children can collect their own specimens. Most pubertal children are not as curious and may not be interested in watching the examination on a monitor.

Video colposcopy is particularly advantageous for clinicians in a teaching institution. A teaching library is invaluable in demonstrating examination techniques and the full spectrum of genital and anal anatomy to residents and visiting clinicians. Residents participating in the examination of a child can review the tape in an unhurried manner out of the child's presence. Video colposcopy also allows instant replay for further study and interpretation.

A colposcope generally provides between four- and 30-fold magnification, depending on the individual manufacturer (87). The most useful range is between 4× and 15× magnification. Above 15× magnifications, both the angle of view and depth of the field are minimal. A colposcope equipped with an intraocular scale assists in obtaining an accurate measurement of the hymenal orifice diameter or the dimensions of specific abnormal findings. Colposcopes have built-in red-free filters that cast a green light, enhancing the appearance of the vascular pattern and the mucosa. A filter assists in the recognition of superficial abrasions of the mucosa of the vestibule and interruptions in the vascular pattern. Scar tissue also may be more apparent, as its avascular appearance contrasts with the surrounding vascularized tissues. The use of the red-free filter is preferential to the use of toluidine blue dye, which has been used to enhance the visualization of superficially abraded and lacerated tissues, but is unnecessarily messy, and the same observations can be made with a filter alone (183).

Photodocumentation of all abnormal findings should accompany every examination (89). Because of limitations of substantiating allegations of sexual abuse in the young child, establishing baseline documentation of anogenital anatomy may serve as a useful reference for those children who remain at risk. The adage, "A picture is worth a thousand words," applies to documenting findings that may be difficult to describe. The photograph memorializes findings of residual tissue damage from the alleged contact. As well, photographs can be used to obtain a second opinion, to demonstrate healing, to show the presence of STDs, as a teaching tool, and where appropriate, to demonstrate physical findings in court. From a practical perspective, 35-mm slides are inexpensive, readily developed, and easily printed if necessary. A camera fitted with a data back allows the imprinting of identifying information on the film plane and thus leaves no question as to the identity of the person represented in the image. Without a data back, an identifying slide preceding the sequence of photos should be obtained. It also is helpful to have the photographic laboratory imprint the slides sequentially. This simple technique maximizes the potential of maintaining the chain of custody. A Cyromedics

MM6000 video colposcope, with 35-mm slide camera, was used to obtain the genital and anal photographs illustrated in this chapter.

When extragenital signs of trauma are photographed, an accompanying ridged millimeter rule and gray scale (ABFO no. 2) should be included with the identifying name and date. This is critically important when bite marks are present. With a standard reference scale, an odontologist can determine whether the arch of a bite mark is that of a child or an adult (10).

Before photographing a child, explain that the only person who can take a picture of them with their clothing off is a doctor, with their mother or another trusted adult present. Reassure the child that the photograph will represent only a small part of his or her body, and that no one can identify them from the photograph. Ask the children if anyone has ever taken a picture of them with their clothing off. This question may uncover previously unsuspected pornography. Further questioning may include, "Have you ever seen any pictures of people with their clothing off?"; "Were any of the people in the photograph children"? Show the children the camera, whether hand-held or attached to a colposcope, and allow them to take a picture of their names and identifying information, such as date of birth and visit, if they so desire. Always respect the child's desire not to be photographed if expressed or sensed.

ANATOMY AND TERMINOLOGY

Familiarity with genital and anal anatomy and knowledge of descriptive terminology assists clinicians in enhancing their level of comfort in examining the sexually abused child and providing documentation in the medical record. The medical record must accurately reflect all of the nuances of the child's genital and anal anatomy in clear and descriptive terms. Before the American Professional Society on the Abuse of Children (APSAC) consensus statement on terminology in the medical evaluation of sexual abuse, there was some inconsistency in the manner in which findings were interpreted and described. It is important that clinicians involved in examining children speak the same language and describe normal and abnormal anatomic variations that exist from one child to the next by using the same terminology (Fig. 7) (Fig. 8). Documentation should be as specific as possible, and a term such as "normal genitalia" is of little descriptive value. The term "normal" does not take into account that the genitalia have many components, and the appearance of normal varies from child to child. Vulva, pudenda, and perineum also lack specificity and are of limited value. For example, vulva or pudendum feminum is a term that includes all of the components of the external visible genital structures, encompassing the mons pubis, labia majora and minora, clitoris, vestibule of the vagina, bulb of the vestibule, Skene's and Bartholin glands, and vaginal orifice. The perineum is the area between the thighs bounded by the vulva and anus in girls and scrotum and anus in boys (120,194,225,252,256).

Some anatomy texts cite the vagina as beginning at the vulva and extending to the cervix, whereas in others, the vagina extends from the cervix to the vestibule below (120,256). The vestibule is essentially a space that contains a variety of structures, each of which merits specific comment. The vestibule of the vagina encompasses the area bordered laterally by the labia minora, the clitoris superiorly, and the fourchette posteriorly. Within the vestibule, there are six perforations: urethra, periurethral ducts or Skene's glands, vaginal orifice, and greater vestibular ducts or Bartholin glands (225,252). The vaginal orifice is the perforation of the hymenal membrane.

The hymenal membrane is recessed in the vestibule, protecting it from direct trauma; hence the implausibility of injury to the membrane from athletic activity such as bicycling, horseback riding, or gymnastics. The common misconception that athletic activities result in injuries to the hymen has no scientific support. The rare impaling injury, when it occurs, is readily differentiated from

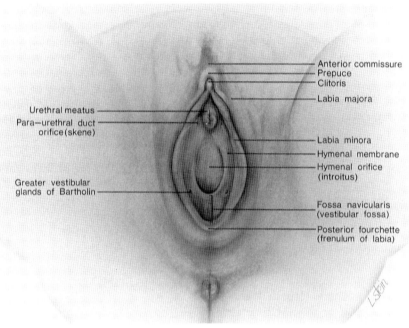

FIG. 10.7. Genital anatomy of the normal prepubertal female child.

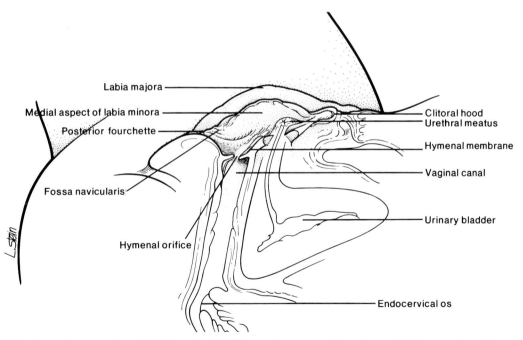

FIG. 10.8. Cross section of the female pelvis illustrating recessed position of the hymenal membrane at the entrance of the vaginal canal.

trauma resulting from the direct and premeditated introduction of a foreign body such as a digit or a penis into the vagina.

The internal surface of the hymenal membrane marks the beginning of the vagina. The hymenal membrane is attached laterally to the walls of the vagina and posteriorly to the floor of the vagina. The concave area between the posterior attachment of the hymen and the fourchette is the fossa navicularis. The posterior joining of the labia minora forms the fourchette. The labia majora, in most texts, are described as joining posteriorly to form the posterior commissure; however, other authors describe them as not joining but tapering off anterolaterally into the perineum (120, 194,225).

Another anatomically vague term is the introitus. Introitus is a generic term defined as the entrance to a canal or space (256). The term introital diameter has been used as a synonym for the opening in the hymen typically referred to as the vaginal orifice (277). To avoid confusion of terms, the opening in the hymenal membrane should be referred to as the hymenal membrane orifice or vaginal orifice rather than introitus.

Hymenal Membrane

"The most insignificant anatomic structure of the female without an analog in the male has assumed a social importance at variance with its almost neutral physiologic value or its potential influence upon health" (280). This vestigial remnant has merited mythologic, psychologic, sociologic, and now an amazing degree of medical notoriety as clinicians begin to take a twentieth century look at this tissue. "To say that this delicate piece of membrane is a far, from the nonphysical point of view, more important structure than any other part of the body is to convey but a feeble idea of the importance of the hymen in the eyes of the men of many past ages and even of our own times and among our own people" (280). Although this statement was made in 1912, there is little question that today the hymen has taken on new significance. Much of the

assessment of child sexual abuse has been focused on the appearance of the hymenal membrane orifice. Law enforcement, social workers, and parents may want to know if the hymen is "intact or broken," as if it were either impenetrable or a piece of china. Many professionals believe that the determination as to whether a child has been sexually abused will be answered by the mere examination of the hymen alone. In support of this desire to know, there is a volume of literature describing the appearance of the hymenal membrane in terms of both its normative state and changes due to injury (21,137,155,205,224).

The hymen was first described as an anatomic structure in reference to the genitalia by Andreas Vesalius, the father of modern anatomy, in the English literature in 1615 (251).

Before this time, the term hymen referred to an anatomically thin serous membrane, such as the pericardium or peritoneum (251). In Greek times, Hymen was the god of marriage, a beautiful youth carrying a marriage torch and nuptial veil (251). Embryologically, "the hymen develops as a result of the advancement of mesenchyme into the epithelial mass at the junction of the pelvic part of the urogenital sinus and the vaginal plate" (195). The external surface of the hymen is covered by urogenital sinus epithelium. Cells derived from the vagina cover the inner aspect of the hymen. The degree of vascularity and the amount of connective tissue between the epithelial layers vary considerably. The membrane is innervated and, in the prepubertal child, it can be exquisitely sensitive. Histologic studies of the fetal hymen note the presence of primary papillae with secondary branching (110). These papillae (excrescences) are most noticeable on the inner aspect of the hymen. It is possible that these microscopic papillae, when estrogenized, develop the fimbriated appearance so frequently seen in the pubertal child.

Many misconceptions concerning the hymen have developed over the years. The origin of these misconceptions is difficult to trace. Unfortunately, professionals have accepted many misconceptions as fact. One misconception is the existence of an entity known as congenital absence of the hymen. The authors frequently see a child on referral who "does not appear to have a hymen" and whose parents have been told that their child could have been "born without a hymen." Absence of the hymen cannot and does not exist on an embryologic basis as a sole congenital anomaly. It may be absent in the presence of other major urogenital anomalies, of which the least significant concern is the presence or absence of the hymen. If the GU tract is normally developed, the hymen is present. In a 1904 discussion concerning malformations of the hymen, Gelhorn noted (110), "Total absence of hymen, reports of which are found in older literature, have not been observed by modern authors, while not denying the possibility, consider this phenomenon exceedingly rare." Jenny et al. (155) examined 1,311 female newborns, all of whom had hymens.

Genital trauma can alter the appearance of the prepubertal and pubertal child's hymen in a variety of ways. In adult women, remnants of the hymenal membrane are referred to as carunculae hymenales. Microscopically, these carunculae are compact mounds of elastic and connective tissue that have lost their papillae (110). Carunculae hymenales do not exist in prepubertal children.

Over the last 20 years, there has been a limited but developing body of literature describing changes to the hymen in the prepubertal child resulting from trauma (77,88,183,201, 202). A full appreciation of the longitudinal changes in the hymen as a result of the influence of estrogen is yet to be elucidated. Clinically, the appearance of the estrogenized hymen is quite different from that of un-estrogenized tissues. The clinical challenge of estrogenized tissue is that it has a coloration similar to that of scar tissue and thus it can be difficult to identify healed trauma.

The appearance of the hymenal membrane is quite variable. Some aspects of the membrane such as the orifice configuration and the transverse and horizontal diameters are easily described and measured. Other charac-

teristics, such as thickness and the degree of elasticity or distensibility, which also are quite variable, present problems for objective quantification. Whenever the hymen and the hymenal tissues are described in the medical record, it is important to be as specific as possible concerning the character of the hymen and to avoid inaccurate and nondescriptive terms, such as marital, broken, virginal, or intact.

Many nonmedical professionals have the perception that the hymen is an impermeable membrane, and any opening is abnormal. An imperforate hymen is the only anatomic variant of hymenal configurations in which no opening is present. Distal vaginal atresia can be confused with imperforate hymen. Classically the imperforate hymen is diagnosed in puberty when the "amenorrheic" female presents with a midline abdominal mass and blue-domed appearance of the hymen (68). Before puberty, the imperforate hymen results in the formation of a mucocolpos. Other configurations of the hymenal membrane orifice are annular, crescentric, fimbriated, septate, or cribriform. Each of these types merits a brief discussion and is illustrated in the accompanying colpophotographic case slides. For an annular orifice to exist, hymenal membrane tissue must be present circumferentially. The orifice itself can be placed either centrally or ventrally. When the orifice appears crescentric, hymenal membrane tissue is not evident between approximately the 11 and 1 o'clock positions; the superior edge of the hymenal membrane interdigitates with the vaginal walls laterally, leaving a posterior rim of tissue that is variable in its width. When a band of hymenal membrane traverses an annular orifice, creating two openings, it is referred to as septate. This configuration is much different, however, from a septum of the vagina that extends posteriorly and divides the vaginal canal and may be associated with other congenital anomalies. When multiple openings are present in the membrane, the term cribriform is used, which means like a sieve (256). A hymenal membrane orifice with multiple finger-like projections on the edge of the membrane is referred to as fimbriated. These fingers most likely represent papillary excrescences (110,195). Suffice it to say that these projections frequently overlap, obscuring the orifice itself unless considerable labial separation and traction are applied. The degree of tautness of the membrane bridging the vaginal canal is variable and is dependent on the degree of relaxation of the patient when the membrane is examined. The terms redundant or folded also have been used to describe the membrane when it is not taut. The membrane's edge may have congenital clefts, external hymenal ridges, tags, bumps, or cysts. Supporting structures called pubourethral, pubovaginal, or pubococcygeal ligaments may be visible. Most apparent clinically are the pubourethral ligaments, sometimes referred to as periurethral supporting bands (21). Hymenal tags, which project from the margin of the hymen and prolapse over the edge of the membrane, were observed in 5.75% of 56 infants studied (205).

Longitudinal intravaginal columns (columnae rugarum) are present on the anterior and posterior vaginal walls (120). These columns are traversed by smaller columns, creating the rugae vaginalis (120). Berensen and Heger (21) described longitudinal external and intravaginal ridges in their study of the hymenal configuration of 468 neonates. They noted that the hymen in 80% of the newborns was annular, and in 19%, it was fimbriated; the remaining variations accounted for 1%. They also described the presence of anterior clefts in 34% of neonates with annular hymens. No posterior clefts were observed, further supporting concerns of most experts that interruptions in the integrity of the membrane's edge observed posteriorly are of posttraumatic etiology.

The appearance of the hymen in the newborn is influenced by maternal estrogen, and it changes when maternal estrogen effects diminish. Heger and Emans (136) suggested that removal of estrogen results in the apparent involution of tissue in the periurethral area, accounting for the discrepancy between the annular appearance of the hymenal membrane in 80% of newborns in their study and the impression that most young children have crescentric orifices. The reappearance of estrogen in puberty again changes the configuration of the orifice as periurethral hymenal tissue responds to estrogen. Longitudinal studies will elucidate hymenal changes secondary to estrogen. The hymenal membrane may have a localized cyst, which is differentiated from a bump by its fluid-filled appearance (203). In earlier reports, authors described bumps on the hymen as a posttraumatic finding, presumably as either a postinflammatory phenomenon or proliferative scar tissue. In these early case reports, histologic confirmation of observed findings was not used to support clinical observations.

The unestrogenized tissues of the hymenal membrane and the medial aspects of the labia minora and fossa are vascular and result in a diffusely reddened appearance. Many parents, when suspecting sexual abuse in their child, look at their child's genitalia, may incorrectly conclude that there is an abnormal degree of redness, and relate this finding to the clinician as prima facie evidence of abuse. Most parents who look at their child's genitalia do so after a bath in which the child has been sitting in a warm tub of water. As a sole indicator of abnormality, the degree of redness is not only difficult to quantify objectively but is also nonspecific. Moreover, without knowledge of the premorbid state of the genitalia, it is difficult to determine whether the vascularity is increased, decreased, or changed because of trauma unless accompanied by other signs of injury. Retrospective interpretation of changes in vascular patterns of the vestibular tissues without other stigmata and/or a history of genital trauma should be approached with caution. Traction can create midline blanching. Thus before interpreting a midline avascular area as scar tissue, the examiner must be sure that traction is not creating the observed finding. The frequency of congenital midline avascular interruptions of the external surface of the membrane or fossa is unknown. The vascular pattern of the external surface of the hymenal membrane and fossa is most commonly described as reticular, fine lacy, and symmetric. An interruption in the vascular pattern of the fossa that is interpreted as scar tissue should be accompanied by a history of significant trauma. Small 1- to 2-mm, ovoid translucent elevations that may be observed in the fossa generally represent lymphoid follicles and should be readily differentiated from vesicles or cysts (203). The study by McCann et al. (198) of genital findings in nonabused prepubertal children further elucidated a spectrum of normal variants.

Another characteristic of the hymenal membrane that has resulted in much interpretive debate is the hymenal orifice's transverse diameter measurement (2,39,116,136,215, 277). Early reference to the significance of a specific hymenal orifice diameter that, if exceeded, was strongly suggestive of sexual abuse, has been problematic. One author noted, "The findings presented indicate that in the absence of known perineal injury, the discovery of an enlarged vaginal opening (greater than 4 mm) correlates 3 out of 4 incidents to positive sexual abuse history given by the child" (39). This criterion alone cannot be considered evidence of sexual abuse. Subsequent commentary by Paradise (215) on the predictive accuracy of interpreting orifice diameters illustrates the limitations of a single measurement: "Most physicians would be relieved to have a single specific test for sexual abuse. Until we have this test, an over-emphasis on minute changes in the diameter of the hymenal opening will result in a number of children being identified as victims of sexual abuse, whereas a majority of sexual abuse victims with normal hymenal measurements will remain unidentified."

Clinicians are frequently asked to make a statement as to whether an object has been placed through a given hymenal orifice into the vagina. Measurements obtained during an examination have low predictive value and may not be helpful in determining whether penetration has occurred. Clinically the routine measurement of the anterior posterior and transhymenal hymenal orifice diameter may be of limited value.

Obtaining a maximal transverse and vertical diameter can be difficult because of the significant variability of the diameter depending on the examination position, degree of traction, and the state of relaxation of the child (Figs. 10.9–10.11). The most accurate way to obtain a measurement is through the calibrated intraocular scale of a colposcope. Calipers, millimeter rulers, and Glassifer rods are alternatives for obtaining these measurements. In determining the probability that an object was placed through a given orifice, it is helpful to know the diameter of objects that are commonly alleged to have been placed into the vagina. In our pediatric faculty, the average transverse diameter of the index finger at the distal interphalangeal joint was 15.6 mm. Although we could not find the supportive study concerning the average transverse diameter of an erect adult penis, Paul (221) has cited it to be 35 mm. Therefore, one would anticipate that if an object the size of a penis were introduced through the hymenal orifice of a prepubertal child, obvious residual should be apparent. All published studies note that the maximal transverse diameter in prepubertal children is less than or equal to 10 mm (18,77,116,136,215,216). Smaller-diameter objects, such as a digit, are less likely to result in residual damage.

Children frequently state that a given object was placed inside them, and yet there may be no confirmatory physical findings. The ability to differentiate "in" from "on" is a developmental task for which limited normative data exist. Children feeling pressure between the labia and over the fourchette and the periurethral/clitoral hood region may perceive a penis as being placed inside. This form of genital-to-genital contact is referred to as vulvar coitus. When vulvar coitus occurs, trauma to the fourchette, medial aspects of the labia, and the periurethral area may be obvious without signs of injury to the hymen, which is recessed and located at the entrance to the vagina. Genital-to-genital contact in the context of vulvar coitus does not necessarily result in trauma to the vestibular structures. If injury does occur, it is most likely to be su-

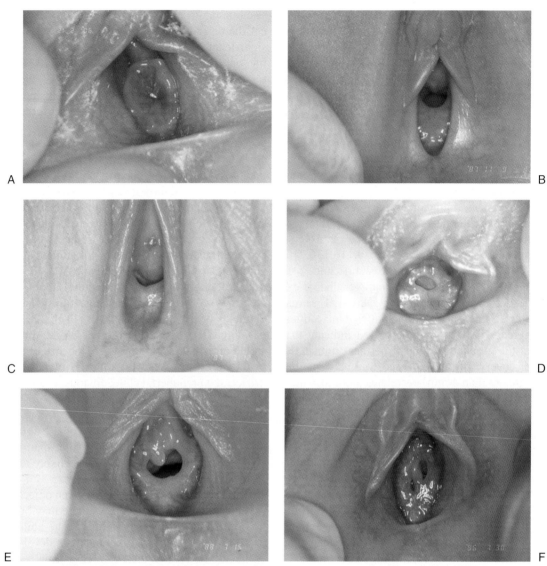

FIG. 10.9. Normal prepubertal anatomic variations. **A:** Fifteen-month-old girl has flared configuration to the annular orifice. Note thickened normal variation of the membrane. **B:** A 4 3/12-year-old girl has a crescentic orifice with thin sharply demarcated edge. External surface of the membrane has a lacy vascular pattern. Slight blanching in the fourchette results from traction. **C:** A 7.5-year-old girl with a crescentic orifice. The membrane has a less translucent and thicker appearance. Urethral meatus is apparent. **D:** A 2 4/12-year-old girl has a superior and eccentrically oriented annular orifice. External surface of the membrane is translucent. Labial traction is necessary to visualize the orifice. **E:** A 9 8/12-year-old girl has a prominent hymenal membrane projection of tissue at 11 o'clock with a small bump at 5 o'clock. Projection and bump may have been previously attached, forming a septum. **F:** A 5 7/12-year-old girl has a septum of the hymen, resulting in two orifices. Cohesive characteristics of moist tissue might obscure the presence of two orifices if traction is not used.

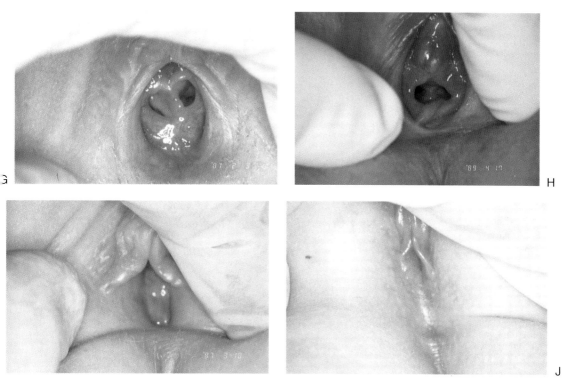

FIG. 10.9. *Continued.* **G:** A 5 7/12-year-old girl has a vaginal septum that bisects the annular orifice. Associated upper genital tract anomalies must be considered. **H:** A 6 10/12-year-old girl has a prominent hymenal tag prolapsing from the vagina through the orifice and onto the external surface of the membrane. **I:** A 2 11/12-year-old girl has no observable hymenal orifice with labial separation, traction, or positioning. **J:** A 4 6/10-year-old girl has acquired labial agglutination that obscures examination of structures of the vaginal vestibule. Small anterior separation of labia minora allows urine to escape.

perficial and heal without residual. A digit placed between the labia also may be perceived as being inside without findings of penetration through the orifice. In genital fondling, penetration of a finger is generally limited to the vestibule itself.

In prepubertal children, the hymen can appear to be thick and presumably elastic or thin and nonelastic. The extent to which the hymen is distensible in the prepubertal child is difficult to quantify clinically. The pubertal child's estrogenized hymen, however, is quite distensible, as evidenced by what may appear initially to be a small hymenal orifice that then readily admits an adult vaginal speculum without injury to the membrane itself. This observation also emphasizes that the absence of definitive findings of trauma to the hy-

menal membrane does not mean that an object could not have penetrated the orifice.

Muram (208) studied the relation between specific sexual acts and genital findings in cases in which all of the perpetrators admitted to the sexual contact. Specific findings of hymenal vaginal tears were found in 60% of the girls when the offender had admitted to vaginal penetration, contrasted to 23% when penetration was denied. Normal-appearing genital tissues or nonspecific findings were present in 39% of victims when penetration was admitted. A hymenal vaginal tear is defined as a laceration of the hymen extending to the posterior vaginal wall. An interruption in the integrity of the edge of the hymenal membrane extending to the floor of the vagina is specific to traumatic penetration. This find-

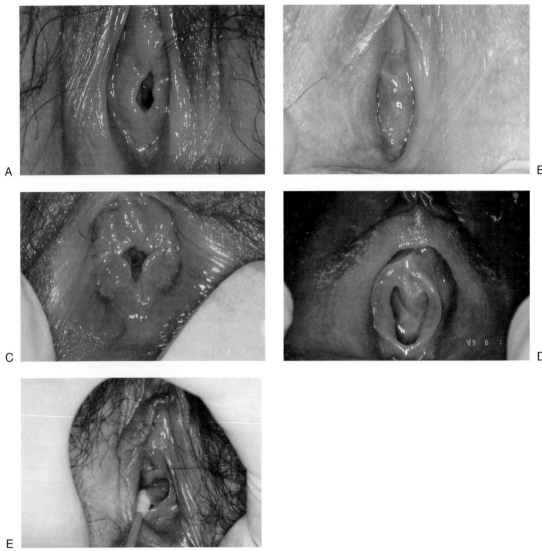

FIG. 10.10. Normal pubertal anatomic variations. **A:** A 12 4/12-year-old girl has an annular-config-ured orifice with minimal redundancy of tissue. Hormonal influence of puberty results in thickened, pinkish coloration, obscuring prepubertal vascular pattern. **B:** A 9 11/12-year-old girl has redundant tissue surrounding an anteriorly placed orifice. Although Tanner stage I, pubic hair estrogen effect of early puberty is evident. **C:** A 12-year-old girl with Tanner stage III anatomy. Multiple congenital clefts circumferentially lead to fimbriated or "frilly" appearance of hymen. Note that clefts do not extend to the vaginal wall. **D:** An 11 4/12-year-old with Tanner stage III anatomy. Note the flared appearance of the annular orifice, but no interruptions in the edge circumferentially. Elasticity of tissues is suffi-cient to admit a foreign body, such as a digit, without residual as alleged. **E:** A 14 2/12-year-old girl with Tanner stage IV anatomy. Prominent intravaginal longitudinal ridge (columnae rugarum) is at-tached to the internal surface of the membrane. When ridge attaches to membrane, it may result in the appearance of a bump on the external surface. Intravaginal ridges and small transverse ridges (rugae vaginalis) are normal anatomic structures. (Note: All pubertal children were examined in litho-tomy position unless otherwise noted).

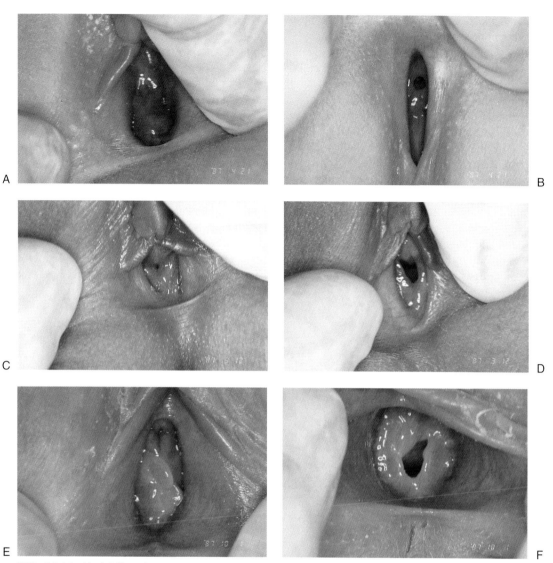

FIG. 10.11. Variability of appearance of genital tissues because of positional changes and relaxation. **A:** A 4 4/12-year-old girl in whom the hymenal orifice was not visualized with labial separation and traction in the supine frog-leg position because of redundant hymenal membrane tissue surrounding the orifice. This observation requires examination in the prone knee–chest position for improved visualization. **B:** Same patient as in **A**, examined in the knee–chest position. Note how gravity has resulted in redundant anterior tissue falling forward, allowing visualization of the annular orifice. **C:** A 4 2/12-year-old with a minute orifice visualized with labial separation. **D:** Same patient as in **C**, but note the different appearance of the orifice now that the child is relaxed. Relaxation is particularly important when attempting to assess the maximal transverse hymenal orifice diameter. **E:** A 9 11/12-year-old with Tanner stage II anatomy. With redundant estrogenized tissue, labial separation alone is insufficient to visualize hymenal orifice. **F:** Same patient as in **E** viewed with labial traction, which affords complete visualization of the hymenal orifice edge circumferentially. When labial traction is exerted, superficial tears of the fourchette may occur, particularly in prepubertal children.

ing is most commonly observed at the posterior rim of the hymen in the midline.

McCann et al. (198) studied the genital anatomy of 114 carefully selected, nonabused girls ranging in age from 10 months to 10 years. This study emphasized the frequency of normal or acquired genital findings that are not the result of abuse and the effect of examination technique and position on the varying appearance of a particular finding (Fig. 10.12).

Findings of erythema of the vestibule, periurethral bands, lymphoid follicles, urethral dilatation, labial adhesions, posterior fourchette midline avascular areas, friability of the fourchette, tags, notches, mounds and projections, and intravaginal columns and transverse ridges are common normal variants.

When an intravaginal column buttresses against the hymenal membrane edge, it may appear as a bump or mound on the edge of the hymen. Some examiners have interpreted bumps and mounds as a posttraumatic finding.

In 1989, White et al. (277) evaluated 242 children to ascertain whether the "vaginal introital diameter" (hymenal orifice) was useful in evaluating a child for sexual abuse. These clinicians concluded that a hymenal orifice diameter greater than 4 mm is highly associated with sexual contact in children younger than 13 years. In their nonabused subgroup of 23 children with a median age of 6 years, none was found to have a transverse diameter of greater than 4 mm. They also observed that

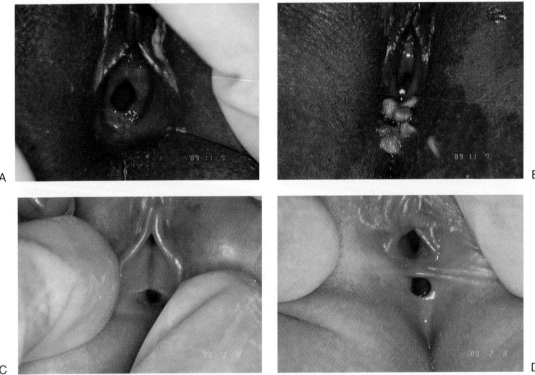

FIG. 10.12. Miscellaneous. **A:** A 5 2/12-year-old girl has erythema of the tissues of the vestibule. She had persistent vaginal discharge for 4 months and intermittent vaginal bleeding. **B:** Same patient as in **A** after irrigation of vagina with sterile water removed the tissue paper that was the nidus for persistent infection. **C:** A 4 7/12-year-old girl in whom the labial agglutination line is translucent. Agglutination obscures the appearance of the vaginal vestibule. **D:** A 4 4/12-year-old girl with labial agglutination that is thickened and was present longer than that in the patient in **C.** This child experienced genital fondling, and this agglutination may be the postinflammatory residual to this contact.

"introital dilation may not always occur with fondling or penile penetration: 27% of children who gave a history of sexual contact with penetration had a vaginal introital diameter of less than or equal to 4 mm." This finding raises a question as to whether these children had an accurate perception of penetration, as it is unlikely that an object could penetrate an orifice less than 4 mm without residual. For a digit or penis to penetrate through a hymenal orifice, a minimal transverse diameter is necessary. The diameter of a digit and a penis is many times the 4 mm proposed in this study. In the nonabused group, which ranged from ages 1 to 12 years, none had a transverse diameter greater than 4 mm. This fact also raises the question as to whether the measurements cited in this study were maximal diameters. A millimeter rule alone cannot be used to determine whether a child has been vaginally penetrated.

In a prospective study of symptomatic and asymptomatic sexually abused children, Emans et al. (77) found that sexually abused girls were more likely than asymptomatic control subjects to have increased friability of the posterior fourchette, attenuation of the hymen, scars, and synechiae of the hymen to the vagina. Sexually abused girls in this study, however, had a frequency of these findings similar to that found in the "genital complaint," presumably nonabused population. All children in the sexually abused group with hymenal tears gave a history of pain associated with vaginal penetration. The frequency of hymenal membrane clefts and bumps was similar in the sexually abused control and nonabused symptomatic groups. Rounding of the hymenal border in the absence of attenuation also was similar in all groups. It is interesting to note that scars and synechiae of the hymen were observed in the genital-complaint group without a history of genital trauma. This observation raises a cautionary note: before concluding that an avascular area is scar tissue, a history supportive of injury should be sought. It is possible that the "scars" noted in the nonabused group were avascular interruptions related to traction

blanching or a congenital fusion. It also is possible that those children with "scars" in the nonabused group had not disclosed prior abuse. Histologic confirmation of observed scar tissue was not obtained.

A cautionary note in regard to the term "attenuation." The definition of this term is "to make thin" (256). To apply this term correctly, the examiner must know that the posterior rim of the hymen was wider at some previous point in time and has since been narrowed. If the premorbid state is unknown, then the examiner should describe the observed finding as a narrow posterior rim and dispense with the term attenuated.

The 1999 guidelines of the American Academy of Pediatrics Committee on Child Abuse and Neglect note the following: "The diagnosis of child sexual abuse often can be made on a child's history. Physical examination alone is infrequently diagnostic in the absence of a history and/or specific laboratory findings. . . . Many types of abuse leave no physical evidence, and mucosal injuries often heal rapidly." Diagnostic findings in the AAP statement are categorized as (a) concerning but in isolation not diagnostic, (b) more concerning but in isolation not diagnostic, and (c) diagnostic with medical certainty. Included in the concerning findings are (a) abrasions or bruising of the inner thighs and genitalia, (b) scarring or tears of the labia minora, and (c) enlargement of the hymenal opening. More concerning findings include (a) scarring, tears, or distortion of the hymen; (b) a decreased amount or absent hymenal tissue; (c) scarring of the fossa navicularis; (d) injury to or scarring of the posterior fourchette; and (e) anal lacerations. Findings that confirm sexual abuse with medical certainty include (a) semen, (b) sperm, (c) acid phosphatase, and (d) positive culture for gonorrhea or positive serology for syphilis or human immunodeficiency virus (HIV) in absence of congenitally acquired infection (9).

Whether an acute or healed genital or anal injury is identified, it is incumbent on the clinician to obtain a complete history regarding the nature of the injury. When inflicted trauma is suspected, the essential components of the history include (a) the size and type of penetrating object; (b) the degree of discomfort associated with the event; (c) the number of episodes of contact; (d) associated symptoms (i.e., bleeding, dysuria); (e) whether treatment was sought and received; and (f) the interval of time between the last alleged contact and the time of examination. Key differences in the history of accidental trauma, such as a straddle injury, are that accidental injuries are more commonly observed by a third party, medical attention is sought immediately after the injury, a scene-of-injury visit confirms the plausibility of the injuries and the accompanying history, and the pattern of injury is consistent with the history (30,161). Of 161 accidental genital injuries reported in the literature, 3.7% involved the hymen. Impaling injuries do not always present with dramatic histories, and the resulting injuries can mimic those of sexual abuse (31). There is no support for the supposition that hymenal injuries are the direct result of either masturbation or the use of tampons (78). Again, the history

remains paramount in differentiating the cause of an injury.

Anal Anatomy

Consensus has been reached in regard to the appropriate descriptive terminology of the anus (Fig. 10.13). It is important to be as specific as possible when describing both normal and abnormal anal findings. The tissue overlying the subcutaneous external anal sphincter is the anal verge. The anal verge begins at the most distal portion of the anoderm and extends to the exterior margin of the anal skin. Within the loose connective tissue surrounding the external anal orifice is the external hemorrhoidal plexus of the perianal space. The anoderm extends from the anal verge to the pectinate or dentate line. There is a scalloped appearance to the anoderm at the point in which it interdigitates with the ampulla of the rectum because of the alternating rectal sinuses and columns. The external anal tissue generally has symmetric, circumferentially radiating folds

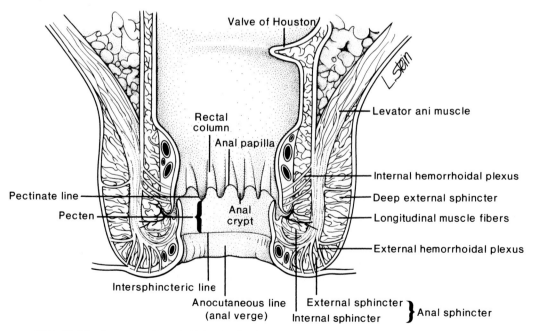

FIG. 10.13. Cross section of clinically significant structures of the rectosigmoid and anus.

known as rugae, formed by the corrugator cutis ani muscle (120).

Anal and Perianal Findings

Despite a consensus as to the appropriate descriptive terminology of anal anatomy, disagreement remains regarding the interpretation of anal findings and the frequency with which anal signs are observed. Contributing to the difficulty of interpreting the residual to anal trauma is the unquestionable ability of the external anal sphincter to dilate to accommodate a large bolus of fecal matter without injury to the tissues. Therefore, depending on the presence or absence of the following variables, a child may or may not have any residual to the introduction of a foreign body into the anus (Fig. 10.14). These variables are (a) size of object introduced, (b) presence or absence of force, (c) use of lubricants, (d) degree of "cooperativeness" of victim, (e) number of episodes of penetration, and (f) time interval since last alleged contact.

Hobbs and Wynn (139) reported that 40% to 50% of boys and girls with a history of anal penetration have abnormalities identified on examination. In the only article in the American literature specific to findings after anal abuse, 66% of 310 prepubertal children had normal-appearing perianal tissues (207). Acute anal injuries are easily recognizable and must be considered in light of the presenting history.

In attempting to understand the residual from chronic anal penetration, we searched the adult literature concerning reports descriptive of anal injuries in the consenting male homosexual population. No description of chronic sequelae could be found, except an anecdotal notation that "colleagues in genitourinary medicine tell me that even in adults admitting to regular anal intercourse, the anus may appear entirely normal" (47).

Of the physical findings considered to result from chronic anal penetration, the most controversial is the reflexive dilatation of the buttocks with separation. Hobbs and Wynn (140) have confidence in this particular sign

and state, "Dilatation over 0.5 cm without the passage of wind does not, in our experience, occur in normal children examined as described. The presence of stool visible in the rectum should not discount the significance of the finding." Hobbs and Wynne (140) reported this finding in 42% of sexually abused children with anal signs. Other authors have not found reflexive dilatation as prevalent in their series (47,201,255). In a nonabused population, McCann and Voris (201) observed that anal sphincter dilation occurred in 49% of children, and the mean anterior posterior diameter of the orifice was 1 cm, with a range of 0.1 to 2.5 cm. On its own, this sign should not be interpreted as abnormal. In the population of children specifically evaluated by Hobbs and Wynne (139) for anal abuse, 86% showed anal dilatations; 61%, fissures; 25%, venous congestions; 16%, scars; 16%, funneling; 7%, laxity; and 32%, other nonspecific signs. Hobbs and Wynn (140) noted, "Interestingly, few anal abused children (or their parents) communicated anal complaints to the doctor even when there was obvious physical abnormality."

McCann and Voris (201) observed that a variety of perianal findings seen in abused children also may be seen in nonabused children, thus highlighting problems with the sensitivity and specificity of soft tissue findings. Nonspecific findings noted by McCann et al. included perianal erythema (41%), increased perianal pigmentation (30%), venous congestion (73%), anal dilatation (49%), skin tags (11%), and "scars" (2%). Also described were congenital smooth areas in 26% of the children. These "smooth fan-shaped areas in the midline of the verge, either with or without depressions, appeared to be a congenital anomaly of the superficial division of external sphincter muscle fibers (201)." This particular finding has the potential to be misinterpreted as scar tissue. Once more, a history of injury must be obtained before concluding that scar tissue is present.

Posttraumatic skin tags of the anal verge must be differentiated from congenital skin

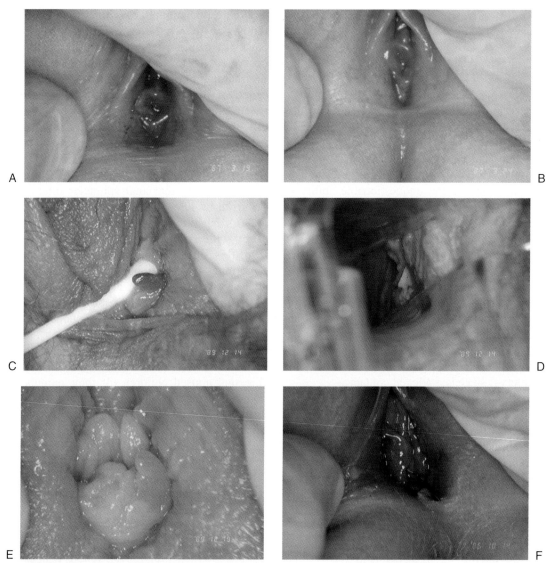

FIG. 10.14. Acute genital and anal trauma and healed residual. **A:** A 10-month-old girl has acute hemorrhage into the hymenal membrane and perihymenal tissues after attempted penetration. **B:** Same patient as in **A**, 5 days after acute injury. No residual is apparent because of healing of superficial injuries by regeneration of labile cells. **C:** A 13 10/12-year-old girl has acute hemorrhage into the fimbria of the hymenal membrane after penile penetration of the vagina. **D:** Same patient as in **C**, examined intravaginally with a speculum. Note the acute laceration of the vaginal canal (from 3 to 5 o'clock). **E:** Same patient as in **C** and **D**, 5 days later. Examination demonstrates complete healing of the injury to the membrane as well as the intravaginal mucosal laceration (not illustrated). **F:** A 19-month-old girl with prominent lacerations to the vaginal wall, membrane, and fourchette on postassault day 4 after penile vaginal penetration. Tissue edema and hemorrhage into tissues are evident.

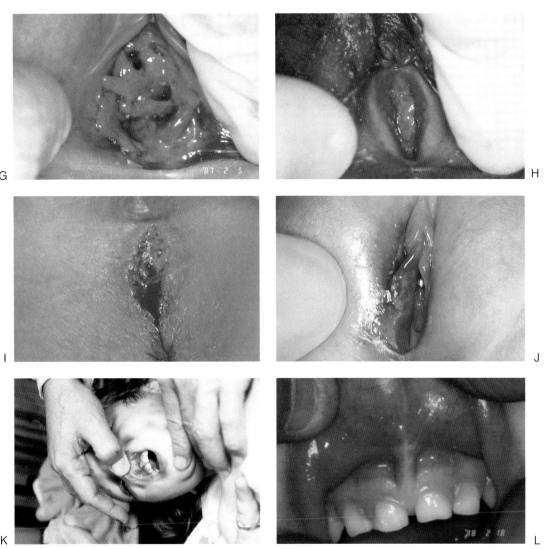

FIG. 10.14. *Continued.* **G:** Same patient as in **F.** Follow-up examination demonstrates healed residual to acute genital trauma, illustrating a marked difference from the appearance of acute injuries. Lacerated hymenal membrane remnants and scar tissue distort appearance in an unanticipated manner. Also evident are two condylomata at 7 o'clock position, emphasizing the need for continued follow-up of children at risk for contracting sexually transmitted diseases with long incubation periods. **H:** A 5 3/12-year-old girl with erythema and superficial abrasions to the medial aspect of the labia minora after vulvar coitus. Note the lack of signs of penetration through the hymenal orifice. **I:** A 2-year-old girl with acute laceration of the perineum and anal verge tissue at the 12 o'clock position after attempted penile anal penetration. **J:** A 6-year-old girl with an acute crush injury to the labia minora and majora after falling on a metal bar of a jungle gym. Note that the injury does not involve the hymenal membrane recessed in the vaginal canal. **K:** A 2 9/12-year-old girl has complete avulsion of the labial frenulum after physical and sexual assault. **L:** Same patient as in **K,** with the mother's fingers elevating the upper lip to reveal residual to the avulsion. The minimal amount of scar tissue demonstrates the difficulty in appreciating how extensive the initial injuries may have been by observing only healed residual.

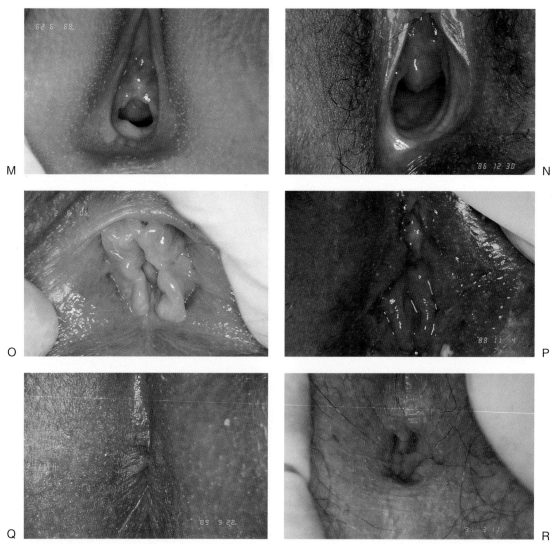

FIG. 10.14. *Continued.* **M:** A 4 4/12-year-old girl has healed interruption in the integrity of the hymenal membrane between 8 and 10 o'clock positions after painful digital penetration through the orifice. Lymphoid follicles are present in the fossa between 6 and 7 o'clock positions. **N:** A 12 5/12-year-old girl with Tanner stage II anatomy. Extremely narrowed posterior ring appears contiguous with the floor of the vagina. The child experienced repeated penile vaginal penetration. Premorbid appearance of the posterior rim is not observed. **O:** A 13 2/12-year-old girl with Tanner stage III anatomy. Healed residual to complete transection of the hymenal membrane at the 6 o'clock position. Scar tissue is evident at the base of the transection in the fossa. **P:** A 10-month-old girl after surgical repair of complete transection of the external anal sphincter after penile anal penetration. Rectal mucosa prolapsed because of tissue edema and decreased rectal tone. **Q:** Same patient as in **P** at final follow-up examination 10 months after acute injury. Note minimal distortion of the rugal pattern. With traction and flattening of verge tissues, a small avascular area remains. **R:** A 12.5-year-old girl has healed laceration of the anal sphincter at 10, 5, and 7 o'clock positions. Anus remains open without traction. Rectal tone is dramatically diminished, and no reflex constriction occurs.

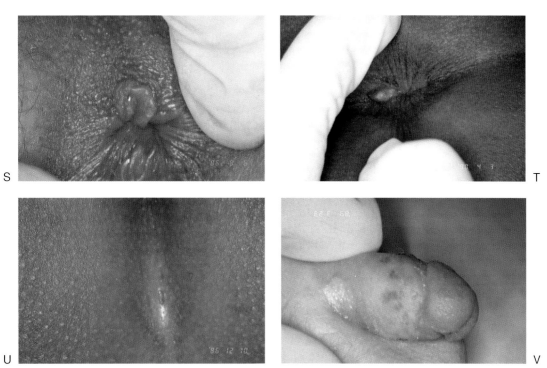

FIG. 10.14. *Continued.* **S:** A 14 3/12-year-old girl has a posttraumatic anal tag, the result of resorbed hematoma of anal verge tissue after penile anal penetration. **T:** A 4 5/12-year-old boy has a hypopigmented area in the anal verge with neovascularity apparent as granulation tissue continues to mature. **U:** A 3 9/12-year-old boy has superficial ulceration of the gluteal crease, which represents residual to the rubbing of the ventral side of a penis between the buttocks. **V:** A 3 5/12-year-old boy has circumferential bite marks to the shaft of the penis.

tags. Trauma to the anal verge may result in a localized collection of blood distorting the anal verge. After resorption of this hematoma, a small tag of loose skin may remain (222). Paul (223) proposed a triad of signs of frequent anal intercourse: (a) thickening of anal verge skin, with reduction or obliteration of anal verge skin folds; (b) increased elasticity of the anal sphincter muscle, allowing the introduction of three or more examining fingers with ease; and (c) reduction of the power of the anal sphincter muscle to contract with reduction of the anal grip. Paul cautioned that the absence of any one of the these features should raise doubt as to the diagnosis of frequent and long-standing anal penetration (223). The triad presented requires subjective judgments and a corroborating history reflective of chronic penetration to be given any

weight. Before accepting this triad as confirmatory of anal penetration, further study is needed. As stated previously, many variables exist that militate for or against the probability that residual will be present. Obviously, no experimental model can exist to document the residual of repeated introduction of a foreign body into the human anus with either mild, moderate, or excessive degrees of force. When clinicians testify to the presence of anal findings, however, they may be asked to give an opinion as to how much force and how many episodes of anal penetration were necessary to result in the observed residual.

Published studies are difficult to compare because of differing operational definitions that may include reliance on physical findings alone, history alone, or a combination of those factors to confirm penetration (141).

Children have difficulty in determining whether an object has been placed "in" their anal rectal canal. Pressure over the external anal verge tissues may cause a slight dilation of the anus and thus be perceived as "in" when, in fact, penetration into the canal *per se* did not occur. Therefore reliance on the child's perception of the experience as confirmatory of penetration should be approached with caution until further studies address the accuracy of a child's ability to differentiate "in" from "on" at varying developmental stages.

The most common object to penetrate the anus of a child is probably a digit. A digit could be readily introduced into the anus repeatedly without discomfort or residual. When reviewing a history of penetration, it is important to determine whether the child had any discomfort associated with the contact, the age-appropriate description of the experience, whether discomfort followed the event, and any associated observations concerning bleeding or the presence of ejaculate.

When examining the anus for residual to penetration, we believe that male patients are best examined in the left lateral decubitus position, a position in which they have not experienced the alleged abuse (Fig. 10.6). If a child has a history of chronic abuse, and no acute abnormalities are observed externally, anoscopy will provide little additional information and is not recommended. The digital rectal examination also provides little information to assist the examiner in determining if a child has been anally assaulted. If, however, on anoscopy or digital rectal examination the child provides a spontaneous utterance likening the experience to that of the penetrating event, this valuable disclosure information should be recorded as the child's verbatim statement. If the anus dilates, the presence or absence of stool should be noted. Reflex dilation of the anus with stool in the rectal ampulla is a normal response.

When acute signs of injury to the anal verge tissue are observed, anoscopy is then important to identify the presence of lacerations, petechiae, bruising of the anorectal canal, and seminal products. Surprisingly, external signs of trauma may be minimal in patients with significant acute internal injuries to the anorectal canal.

Male Genitalia

Anatomy of the male genitalia is rather straightforward. The medical records should document the following: (a) Tanner stage, (b) circumcision status, (c) retractability of foreskin if uncircumcised, (d) appearance of glans and frenulum, (e) urethral discharge, (f) any signs of injury to the glans or shaft of the penis, (g) the location of testes, (h) signs of scrotal trauma, (i) presence of hernias, and (j) inguinal adenopathy.

Injury to the male genitalia may include superficial abrasions to the shaft, petechiae, tears of the frenulum of the glans, bruising, and bite marks. When superficial injuries are present, an accompanying history of fondling, masturbation, and/or oral–genital contact is frequently present. Under most circumstances, there is no residual to these activities.

Residual to Sexual Contact

Patterns of Trauma

The difficulties associated with the retrospective interpretation of the residual to sexual contact have been discussed. Clearly, few physical findings represent definitive evidence of sexual assault (27). When a child presents with acute injuries, the pattern and extent of the trauma should be evident and documented. The spectrum of acute injury is variable, involving superficial mucosal abrasions and scratches to clear transecting lacerations of genital and anal structures (213). Superficial injuries and signs of irritation may be subtle and nonspecific. The extent of injury depends on many variables, most significant of which is the degree of force, the object used to inflict the injury, and the nature of the contact, with particular reference to whether "penetration" occurred.

The legal and medical definitions of penetration differ. The medical definition of penetration is "the passing into the deeper tissues or into a cavity" (256). From a strictly medical perspective, the term penetration in regard to the female genitalia implies the introduction of an object between the labia, through the hymenal orifice, and into the posterior portion of the vagina. As previously cited, children frequently state that an object was placed inside of them when corroborating evidence is not present. Most "penetration" of children is akin to the legal definition, which is "the insertion of the male part into the female parts to however slight an extent; and by which insertion the offense is complete without proof of an emission (28)." Certainly, any genital-to-genital or genital-to-anal contact is inappropriate, regardless of the depth of penetration.

In genital fondling of the female, the hand is usually placed over the mons pubis and the index and third finger separate the labia and enter the vaginal vestibule. Rubbing of the tissues bordering the vaginal vestibule may acutely demonstrate evidence of erythema, superficially denuded mucosa, abrasions/ scratches, and edema of the inner aspects of the labia minora and the periurethral area. Generally, fondling/penetration between the labia results in injuries between the 9 and 3 o'clock positions, with the child supine and less likely to involve the fourchette or fossa. Most fondling/digital penetration contact does not result in more serious trauma, but the forceful introduction of a finger into the vagina can result in significant trauma that will have residual.

Depending on the differential between the hymenal orifice size and the penetrating digit, the child may have either no residual from introduction through the orifice or a laceration of the membrane edge. Acute injuries to the hymen should be readily apparent, although injury to the hymenal membrane as a result of fondling is infrequent.

Children who are fondled and experience trauma to the periurethral area may complain of dysuria after the alleged event. This symptom is specific to irritation/inflammation of the distal urethra. If a history of dysuria is obtained in a nonleading and nonsuggestive

manner, it is valuable corroborating history of sexual contact and may be admissible in court. In a review of 105 cases meeting inclusion criteria, 23% of fondled children provided a history of postfondling dysuria. All of these children answered standard questions that were nonleading and nonsuggestive.

Dysuria also can be a posttraumatic event, occurring during vulvar coitus. This form of genital-to-genital contact also may be perceived by the child as penetrating. In vulvar coitus, the shaft of the penis is rubbed between the labia and can result in abrasions and bruising of the inner aspects of the labia minora. The penis can cause trauma to the periurethral/clitoral hood region and the fourchette as well. Because the hymenal membrane is recessed in the vaginal canal, vulvar coitus is not likely to result in injury to the hymenal orifice (Fig. 13). Berkowitz et al. (24) reported that trauma to the external surface of the hymenal membrane occurring within the context of vulvar coitus resulted in scar tissue, presumably creating a stenosis of a previously larger orifice, creating the appearance of an "acquired" imperforate hymen. Dysuria also may follow coitus. Dysuria associated with coitus is commonly referred to as honeymoon cystitis (193).

In sodomy, the dorsal side of the shaft of the penis may be rubbed over the external anal verge tissues, causing pressure perceived as penetration in the anorectal canal. When the shaft is rubbed between the gluteus over the natal cleft, it may result in superficial abrasions. This activity is commonly referred to by boys as "freaking." When either vulvar coitus or natal cleft rubbing occurs, the individual may ejaculate, and seminal products may be collected from the abdomen, inner thighs, buttocks, and back.

When an object forcefully penetrates into the vagina through the hymenal orifice in a young child, residual signs are generally obvious when examined acutely. This type of penetration will most likely result in a laceration to the edge of the membrane that extends to the vaginal floor. Most lacerations are seen between the 5 and 7 o'clock positions with the child supine but can be seen anywhere between the 3 and 9 o'clock positions. Forceful penetration also may result in lacerations to the fossa navicularis, the lateral walls of the vagina, and possible perforation of the posterior fornix into the peritoneum (222,223). Although most lacerations of the hymen stop at the floor of the vagina, some extend through the fossa and fourchette and into the perineal body. This type of injury is readily recognizable, and its full extent must be assessed with the child under anesthesia.

Accidental injuries to the genitalia do occur, and the pattern of trauma and the accompanying history are usually suggestive of its etiology (69,271). Most accidental injuries are the result of a child falling on a horizontal bar of a bicycle, jungle gym, or the classic "picket fence." The horizontal bar usually results in a crush injury of the clitoral hood/labia minora between the bar and the inner aspect of the thigh. This injury is usually unilateral. "Picket" injuries are more likely to be impaling. Occasionally, the forceful abduction of thighs results in a superficial laceration of the perineum. One report of injury to the genitalia occurred as a result of a seat belt (16). Masturbation is unlikely to result in any injuries to the genitalia other than localized erythema or superficial abrasions as the result of rubbing. Children do insert objects between the labia, but they rarely do so in a forceful way that would result in injury because of the exquisite sensitivity of the hymenal tissue.

Rubbing of the inner aspects of the labia occurring either in the context of vulvar coitus, genital fondling, or possibly masturbation can result in inflammation. Because of the close proximity of the inner aspects of the inflamed labia minora in prepubertal children, the mucosal surfaces may agglutinate. Labial agglutination is an acquired postinflammatory condition seen only in the prepubertal child and involves the thin unestrogenized vascular tissues of the inner aspect of the labia minora. The ability to examine the hymenal membrane may be compromised depending on the degree of fusion. The agglutination may extend from the fourchette to the clitoral hood, with only a minute opening for urine to escape, creating the appearance of an "absent" vagina. Although labial agglutination is a common finding in young children, its association as a residual to sexual abuse was described only recently (22,23,196). Caution should be exercised if agglutination is the only abnormal finding on examination. When agglutination is present, it can be medically dehisced by estrogen cream. "Gentle traction," as described in standard texts, should not be used because it results only in denuded edges that are painful and quickly readhere, making reexamination even more difficult.

Extragenital signs of trauma are infrequent in most cases of child sexual abuse. When they do occur, they usually occur within the context of "rape." If a child is forced to perform fellatio on an individual, tears to the labial frenulum and petechiae of the palate may be noted. Injuries reflective of force and restraint may be seen as ligature marks around the wrists and ankles. Bruising of the extremities may appear as grasp marks. Bite marks may be present on the neck, breast, buttocks, or inner thighs.

Retrospective Interpretation

Most children do not present for an examination immediately after their alleged sexual abuse; therefore few children will have acute signs of injury or evidence to collect. Thus the clinician is required to examine tissues that may demonstrate healed residual. Without knowledge of the premorbid appearance of the genital tissues, it is difficult to judge whether a particular finding is the direct result of sexual abuse. Several clinical scenarios can occur. First, the child may be seen long after the last episode of alleged contact, and thus only healed residual can be observed. Second, the child may have experienced genital or anal trauma resulting in residual and is being examined during the period of formation of granulation tissue and no obvious acute injury. Third, the child may present when nonspecific findings are present, and the physician must correlate the history of the alleged contact and the findings as residual to that contact. Finally, the child presents with acute signs of injury, the least problematic situation to evaluate. The pathology of healing is well understood (72,170). These principles of healing have only recently been applied to genital and anal injuries for a prospective look at how acute injuries heal (88,200). Observations by Finkel (88) on the healing chronology of genital and anal injuries have laid the foundation for our understanding of the retrospective interpretation of changes in genital and anal anatomy.

Most injuries to the genital and anal tissues are superficial and heal after a predictable pathologic process known as regeneration of labile cells. Regeneration involves four stages: (a) thrombosis and inflammation, (b) regeneration of epithelium over a denuded surface, (c) multiplication of new cells, and (d) differentiation into new epithelium. In the absence of new injury, this process proceeds at an approximate rate of 1 mm per 24 hours. Wound healing is usually complete in 48 to 72 hours, with differentiation of new epithelium within 5 to 7 days (72,170). This healing process is the basis for the clinical observation that obvious superficial injuries heal without any residual. Because most children disclose abuse more than 1 week after victimization, they will not have any confirmatory physical findings despite a history of being injured by the contact, unless the injuries are more serious and heal by the process of repair. Serious lacerating injuries, however, do heal with residual, which can be observed long after the alleged event. Deep wounds heal by the pathologic process known as repair, which leads to the formation of granulation tissue. This process also is predictable and involves the initial steps of regeneration but includes organization of the coagulated blood with the eventual formation of granulation tissue and its accompanying wound contraction. As macrophages begin to digest the fibrin clot, capillaries proliferate from the wound margins, and an amorphous gelatinous matrix forms, which is a substrate for the development of collagen fibrils. This young vascular connective tissue is "neovascularized." Only in this context is this term used appropriately.

Neovascularization should not be used to describe focal areas of increased vascularity. Neovascularity is a self-limited phenomenon in that it begins in the first several days of injury and continues until the wound has contracted. Mature granulation tissue takes several months to develop, accounting for the changing appearance of forming scar from red to pink to pale and then white.

When scars do form, they may distort the appearance of the genital tissues in unanticipated ways that make the retrospective appreciation of the extent of the acute injuries difficult, yet at times clearly recognizable (Fig. 10.13). Conversely, well-delineated acute lacerations that heal by secondary intention may be a fraction of their initial size when healed. Thus it may be difficult to conclude with certainty that they represent a scar without knowledge of the acute injuries, particularly in lacerations to the anus, because the external anal sphincter maintains the tissues in close approximation and usually results in a well-delineated narrow scar. Accompanying colposcopic case slides illustrate these observations (Fig. 10.13).

From a clinical perspective, it is impractical and unreasonable to perform a biopsy on genital and anal tissues that appear to be scar tissue for histologic confirmation. However, it is not unreasonable to obtain a thorough history concerning the nature of injuries and associated symptoms and to use caution before concluding that avascular areas of the genitalia/anus are scar tissue. When scar tissue is present, it is the residual to significant trauma, and a history reflective of significant injury should be obtainable. In very young children, a history may not be available, and the clinician may have to rely completely on clinical observations.

Whether the clinician finds healed residual or acute injuries, the wound characteristics should be described by using two points of reference from the midline. Both major and minor components of the injury should be described. For example, a superficially abraded contused laceration is a wound in which the most prominent feature is a laceration, followed by the next most prominent feature, bruising, and the least significant component of the wound, superficial abrasion.

Formulating a Conclusion

Formulating a diagnostic assessment warrants considerable thought. The clinician must consider: (a) historical details and behavioral indicators reflective of the contact, (b) symptoms that result from the contact, (c) acute genital/anal injuries and/or chronic residual, (d) forensic evidence, and (e) STDs. Throughout all aspects of the diagnosis and treating process, objectivity and an understanding of the limitations of clinical observations must be considered.

The following four common scenarios each require the formulation of a different diagnostic assessment:

1. The history/behavior is descriptive of inappropriate sexual contact; however, no diagnostic residual is evident;
2. The history/behavior is descriptive, and diagnostic findings are present that are reflective of the contact (i.e., trauma, STDs, and/or seminal products);
3. The history is diagnostic of inappropriate sexual contact without healed residua; and
4. The history/observations are limited, and although the behaviors observed by the parent have raised concern, there are insufficient historical or behavioral details to support a concern of inappropriate sexual contact.

Although the constellation of historical, behavioral, and examination findings will vary from case to case, the following serve as examples of how a diagnostic assessment could be formulated in each of the following common scenarios:

1. The history/behavior is descriptive of inappropriate sexual contact; however no diagnostic residual is evident.
   Example: The medical history presented by this 9-year-old girl reflects her experiencing progressive engagement in a variety of inappropriate sexual activities initially represented to her in a caring and loving context and progressing to use of threats to maintain secrecy. Although she did not complain of experiencing any physical discomfort after the genital fondling, oral–genital contact that she was coerced into performing, or the stroking of her uncle's genitalia, she has expressed a concern that merits attention. She told me that she was worried that people could tell that she had to do those disgusting things just by the way that people look at her. She provided a history of contact with what she described as "icky stuff" coming from her uncle's penis, placing her at risk for a sexually transmitted disease. I have evaluated this young lady for sexually transmitted diseases. Treatment and follow-up will be initiated should anything be positive. Her physical examination does not demonstrate any acute or chronic residua to the sexual contact nor would any be anticipated in light of her denial of discomfort associated with the contact. Her body image concern is common among children who experience sexual abuse. I do not believe there is any alternative explanation for this child's history of progressive engagement in sexual activities, threats to maintain secrecy, detailed description of a variety of sexually explicit interactions, and concerns about body image other than from experiencing such. The most significant impact of her inappropriate sexual experiences is psychological. She should be seen immediately by a clinical child psychologist to assess the impact of her inappropriate experiences and develop a therapeutic plan.

2. The history/behavior is descriptive of inappropriate sexual contact, and diagnostic findings are present that are reflective of the contact (i.e., trauma, STDs, and/or seminal products).
   Example: This 6-year-old girl provided a clear and detailed medical history reflecting her experiencing genital-to-genital contact and being coerced into placing her mouth on her father's genitalia. The geni-

tal-to-genital contact was perceived by her to involve penetration into her vagina. She provided a history of bleeding and pain after the genital-to-genital contact. Although the disclosure of her experiences occurred 1 month after the last contact, her physical examination demonstrates residual to such in the form of a healed transection of the posterior portion of her hymen, extending to the base of its attachment on the posterior vaginal wall. This finding is diagnostic of residual to the introduction of a foreign body through the structures of the vaginal vestibule, the hymenal orifice, and into the vagina. She did not complain of physical discomfort associated with the history of oral–genital contact, although she stated that her father peed in her mouth, placing her at additional risk for a sexually transmitted disease.

3. The history is diagnostic of inappropriate sexual contact without healed residua.

Example: This 5-year-old girl provided a detailed history reflecting genital-to-genital contact and discomfort associated with such. Although her perception of the genital-to-genital contact, as demonstrated on an anatomic model of the genitalia, involved penetration into her vagina, her examination indicates that any genital-to-genital contact that she experienced was limited to the structures of the vaginal vestibule. After the genital-to-genital contact, she provided a history of discomfort in the form of dysuria. Her review of systems was negative for any alternative explanation of dysuria. The symptom of dysuria temporally related to the genital-to-genital contact reflects trauma to the periurethral area as a result of rubbing. The trauma incurred to the distal urethra was superficial and has since healed without residual, as anticipated. The only way this young girl could know about the symptom of dysuria temporally related to the genital contact is by experiencing such.

4. The history/observations are limited, and although the behaviors observed by the parent have raised concern, there are in-

sufficient historical or behavioral details to support a concern of inappropriate sexual contact.

Example: At your request, I had the opportunity to examine this 2.5-year-old boy to diagnose and treat any residual to the concern that he may have been touched in a sexually inappropriate manner. This concern arose because of a genital rash, intermittent touching of his genitalia, and some resistance to having his diaper changed. Mom raised the question as to whether her son may have been touched in a sexually inappropriate manner to account for the genital irritation, increased genital touching, and resistance to have his diaper changed. Mom stated that she had been sexually abused by her father as a child and wanted to protect her son from the same. The maternal grandparents occasionally babysit for her son. His physical examination is positive for diaper dermatitis due to *Candida albicans.* The historical and behavioral details that have been provided are insufficient to confirm with medical certainty that this young man has experienced anything of a sexually inappropriate manner. The constellation of behavioral responses I believe are best attributed to his diaper dermatitis and not any sexually inappropriate contact. This child, as all children, should receive anticipatory guidance regarding body safety in an age-appropriate manner. Baseline documentation of the appearance of his anogenital anatomy has been obtained should there be any concern in the future. If so, this will serve as a useful reference. Mom will need to address some unresolved issues concerning her own experience and exercise caution in leaving her child in the care of any individual for whom she has concern.

Less common presenting scenarios include the following: (a) identification of a healed injury on examination with no prior suspicion of abuse for which no historical or behavioral indicators are presented; (b) a child presenting with a concern by a caretaker without historical or behavioral details to support the concern; and (c) the child with an unexplained STD. When the history and examination findings do not support each other, a statement that the examination is inconsistent with the history and an alternative explanation should be sought is most appropriate.

Concluding that a child's examination is "normal" or that "no evidence of sexual abuse" exists when the physical examination does demonstrate diagnostic findings fails to integrate historical, behavioral, and examination results adequately. The examples of conclusion scenarios presented in this chapter provide the greatest number of options for the physician to articulate clearly the findings and the significance of such. A

medical record that is detailed and clear in its conclusions reduces the likelihood that the clinician will need to appear in court. Conclusion options should also include a reference for the child to have a complete mental health assessment of the potential impact of the experience and the need to develop a treatment plan.

Sexually Transmitted Diseases

STDs, a common type of physical evidence and a common stimulus to the evaluation for child sexual abuse, may be the only physical evidence of sexual abuse in some cases (Fig. 10.15) (40,60,212,275). The infection or colonization may be symptomatic or asymptomatic. Sexually abused children are at risk for acquir-

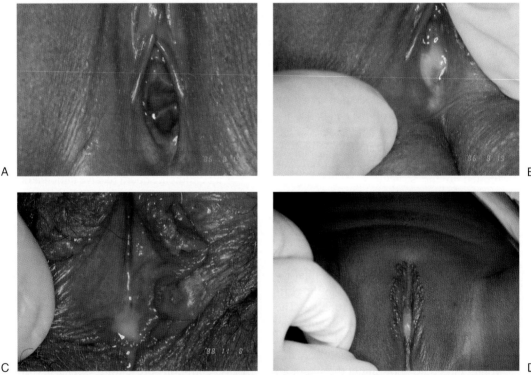

FIG. 10.15. A: A 4 4/12-year-old girl with copious vaginal discharge and erythema of the tissues of the vaginal vestibule. **B:** Same patient as in **A** after Valsalva maneuver, which results in making discharge more evident and easier to collect. This discharge was due to *Neisseria gonorrhoeae*. **C:** A 14 3/12-year-old girl has an ulcerative lesion of herpes simplex virus type II apparent at 4 o'clock position. Intravaginal lesions and discharge also are present. **D:** A 6.5-year-old girl in whom extensive condylomata acuminata line the outer aspects of the labia majora bilaterally.

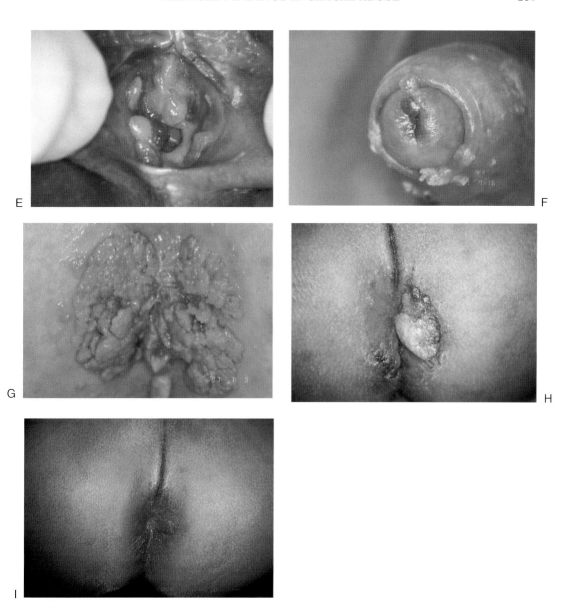

FIG. 10.15. *Continued.* **E:** Same patient as in **D,** with labial separation and traction. Condylomata completely distort and obscure the hymenal membrane. Note the significantly different appearance of the same wart type growing on the mucosal surface. **F:** 4 4/12-year-old boy with condylomata acuminata of the foreskin and urethral meatus. **G:** 1 5/12-year-old boy has extensive perianal condylomata obscuring the anal orifice as a result of the perpetrator rubbing a penis over external verge tissues. **H:** 2 5/12-year-old boy with a prominent discoid lesion of condyloma lata due to syphilis initially diagnosed as condylomata acuminata. **I:** Same patient as in **H** has reabsorption of condylomata following treatment for syphilis.

ing infections prevalent among sexually active adolescents and adults. STDs have been detected in approximately 1% to 30% of children examined for sexual abuse; however, the actual risk of acquiring sexually transmitted infections by child sexual abuse victims is unknown. The differences in the observed frequency of STDs in the children studied may be related to many variables: the type of sexual contact, the age of the child, the frequency of the abuse, the types of testing performed, the regional differences in the prevalence of STDs, and the percentage of children referred because of their symptoms of STDs. The incubation periods for the organisms and the timing of the examination after the abuse are critically important in detecting infections (19,131,133,148).

The Centers for Disease Control (CDC) suggests a general rule that, "The identification of a sexually transmissible agent from a child beyond the neonatal period suggests sexual abuse" (42). This general rule is appropriate; however, the amount of proof needed to overrule the suggestion of abuse is not the same for all diseases. The strength of the association between STDs and child sexual abuse varies from disease to disease (Table 10.1). Several factors must be considered when evaluating the strength of association between an STD and

child sexual abuse, particularly the age of the child and the specific disease identified. The disease must be diagnosed by using tests that have an acceptable degree of specificity in children. The physician should consider the possibility that the identified organism represents a perinatally acquired infection or an infection spread by fomites or nonsexual contact; however, the explanation that perinatal or nonsexual transmission for a specific disease is plausible does not mean it is correct. When no source of the organism is identified, it is not acceptable to conclude that the transmission must have been perinatal or nonsexual. Likewise, the inability to document a specific STD in a possible or suspected perpetrator does not rule out the possibility that this individual was the source of the child's infection.

Gonorrhea

Neisseria gonorrhoeae is the small gram-negative, oxidase-positive, diplococcal bacterium that causes gonorrhea or gonococcal infections. The incubation period is 2 to 7 days. Infections may be present with or without symptoms; infections of the throat (pharyngitis) and of the rectum (proctitis) are typically asymptomatic. If symptoms occur, they almost

TABLE 10.1. *Incubation, diagnosis, and implications of sexually transmitted diseases in prepubertal children*

STD	Incubation	Diagnosis	Relationship to sexual abuse
Gonococcal infections	2–7 days	Culture confirmed by two or more confirmatory tests	Certain[a]
Syphilis	10–90 days	RPR or VDRL confirmed by FTA-ABS or MHA-TP	Certain[a]
Chlamydial infections	Variable	Culture only; rapid techniques lack adequate specificity	Probable[a]
Human papilloma virus	1–9 mo (? 20 mo)	Inspection, application of acetic acid, or biopsy and viral typing	Probable[a]
Trichomoniasis	4–20 days	Wet mount of discharge, culture more sensitive	Probable[a]
Herpes virus-2	2–14 days	Culture with viral typing	Probable[a]
Herpes virus-1	2–14 days	Culture with viral typing	Possible
Bacterial vaginosis	7–14 days?	"Clue cells" on wet mount and positive "whiff" test	Uncertain
Genital mycoplasmas	2–3 weeks?	Culture	Uncertain
HIV infection	6 wk to 18 mo	ELISA confirmed by Western blot	Uncertain

[a]Except when perinatal transmission is documented.

always develop within a week of exposure. Vaginal discharge, if left untreated, may turn from purulent to serous and disappear in 2 months. Within 28 weeks of incubation, 90% of infected children are free of infection (145). Prepubertal genital infections are commonly associated with perineal pruritis, dysuria, or a purulent penile or vaginal discharge, but as many as 20% of patients are asymptomatic. Adolescents may present with cervical or urethral discharge, but up to one third of infections in adolescents are asymptomatic.

Reported rates of gonococcal infection range from 1% to 30% among sexually abused children (133,212). Accurate diagnosis of gonococcal infections can be made only by using Thayer–Martin or chocolate blood agar–based media, because the predictive value of Gram stains alone is not known in children. The laboratory must perform appropriate confirmatory tests, because similar bacteria, including *Moraxella catarrhalis, Kingella dentrificans, Neisseria meningitidis, N. lactamica,* and *N. cinerea,* can be misidentified as *N. gonorrhoeae.* In one study, 14 of 40 isolates for *N. gonorrhoeae* were shown to be falsely identified because confirmatory tests were not performed appropriately to exclude other bacteria (281). Positive cultures should be confirmed by two of the following methods: biochemical (carbohydrate utilization), direct fluorescence antibody, or enzyme substrate tests (4,42,281).

Culture results in suspected victims and suspected perpetrators require careful interpretation. Untreated asymptomatic gonococcal infection may persist for at least 6 months in untreated adults, and pharyngeal infections may persist despite treatment. Therefore repeatedly positive cultures do not necessarily mean repeated exposure and repeated abuse. Conversely, perpetrators who have taken commonly prescribed antibiotics for another infection may eradicate the gonococci and have negative cultures when they are subsequently screened as possible sources of the child's infection.

Spontaneous resolution of gonococcal infection without any antibiotic therapy commonly occurs within weeks to months of onset, and about 95% of all untreated infections resolve within 6 months. Blood tests for the presence of antibody to the organism are unreliable because of a high false-negative rate among recently infected individuals (3,102).

Routine cultures of the throat, rectum, and genital areas have been suggested for all sexually abused children regardless of history or symptoms (40,60). Routine cultures may detect clinically unsuspected infections. In one study, 532 sexually abused children younger than 14 years had routine cultures taken from all three body sites (60). Eleven of the 25 cases of gonorrhea detected were in children who had no symptoms of infection, including three of 12 prepubertal girls with vaginal infections, and eight infections were discovered at sites that had not been involved in the sexual contact, according to the child's initial history. Recent research has focused on using selective criteria for STD screening. These studies have found rates of gonococcal infection in abused children to be less than 3% (146,157,249). One study showed all six vaginal infections in prepubertal girls were symptomatic, and no isolated pharyngeal or rectal infections were identified (249). In another study, only 5% of prepubertal girls with vaginal infections (four of 84) did not have a vaginal discharge. The girls with asymptomatic infections would have been identified by using selective criteria for increased risk of STDs (147). Selective criteria are useful in girls; however, there are limited data on boys, who have typically asymptomatic pharyngeal and rectal infections (133).

Gonococci can survive up to 24 hours on fomites (toilet seats, towels) in moist purulent secretions. This fact raises the possibility of nonsexual transmission in some cases, although clear documentation of cases of nonsexual transmission is not available (212). Supportive evidence for nonsexual transmission was suggested by the authors of a study in 1927, who reported a hospital outbreak of 67 infants infected in the nursery over a 1-month period by an unknown source (145). Inadvertent prepubertal spread of *N. gonorrhoeae* by nonsexual contact or by sexual play has frequently been suggested, rarely described, and never rigorously documented.

Children with positive culture results may not be ready to disclose abuse; therefore, it is not appropriate to conclude that infection resulted from nonsexual contact. The physician should assume that prepubertal children with gonorrhea have acquired it by sexual contact and that most of these contacts were abusive. The ease of transmission of gonorrhea to children is unknown. In adults, the infection may be transmitted in as few as one of three sexual contacts with an infected individual. Contact with infected genital secretions is required for transmission; however, actual penile penetration may not be required (3,8,102).

Syphilis

Syphilis is detected in only none to 1.8% of reported victims of sexual abuse (60,133,212, 275). Like adults, abused children may present with asymptomatic disease, or symptomatic primary or secondary syphilis (114). Primary lesions or chancres are moist ulcerations with raised borders that may be mistaken for anal fissures or perianal cellulitis; secondary syphilis may be mistaken for a viral exanthem with a variable skin rash, classic lesions of the palms and soles, or flat-surfaced, raised perineal lesions known as condylomata lata (22).

Nontreponemal reagin tests such as the VDRL and the rapid plasma reagin (RPR) are commonly used for screening victims. Specific antibody tests for the organism *Treponema pallidum,* such as the fluorescent treponemal antibody, absorbed (FTA-ABS) or the microhemagglutination–*Treponema pallidum* (MHA-TP), must be done to confirm the screening test. The false-positive rate for both treponemal and nontreponemal tests in the general population is 1% to 2%. False-positive nontreponemal tests are obtained from patients with numerous conditions, including acute viral infections, atopic dermatitis, bacterial pneumonias, and after immunizations. Repeated testing is often required because of the long, variable incubation period, from 10 to 90 days (114). Although routine testing of all victims is usually recommended, the apparently low risk in abused children may support the idea of screening all adolescents but testing only children with a history of genital or perianal lesions, an exanthem, the presence of another STD, with known syphilis infection in the perpetrator, or who live in high-risk areas for syphilis (22, 133). Nontreponemal tests may yield negative results within months of treatment, and all are negative within 2 years. Treponemal tests remain positive for life. Only a negative treponemal test can be used to exclude a suspected perpetrator as the source of the child's infection (23).

Acquiring syphilis through blood transfusions is rare, and a few cases of facial lesions resulting from nonsexual transmission in children have been reported (145). Infections occurring in infancy may have resulted from prenatal exposure. Primary disease presenting after age 4 months or secondary disease presenting after the first year of life should not be considered congenitally acquired. Prepubertal children with primary or secondary stages of syphilis occurring beyond early infancy should be presumed to be victims of sexual abuse (142,176).

Chlamydial Infections

Chlamydia trachomatis or chlamydial infections are the most frequently recognized STDs in adolescents and adults (133). Rectogenital infection rates of 4% to 8% are typically reported among sexually abused children (127,144,229,245). Some infected prepubertal girls have a vaginal discharge; however, most chlamydial infections do not produce symptoms. The time period between sexual contact and onset of vaginal symptoms in children is unknown. Whether infections can relapse and the duration of persistent infection are not known; therefore it is difficult to determine when an infection was acquired (145).

Chlamydial infections are difficult to detect in children for several reasons. The estimated sensitivity of a single cervical swab culture ranges from 50% to 90%; isolation from vaginal pool swabs is expected to be lower. Recovery of the organism also depends on specimen handling before inoculation of the culture and which culture-confirmation techniques are used (132). Diagnosis in sexually abused children must be made by using a culture technique rather than the more commonly available rapid detection methods. Enzyme immunoassay (EIA) and direct fluorescence antibody (DFA) tests are extremely unreliable for vaginal or rectal specimens in children. These rapid detection methods can be used in the evaluation of cervical and urethral specimens in adults and conjunctival and nasopharyngeal specimens in infants with suspected chlamydial infection. Cross-reactivity with many common bacteria including *N. gonorrhoeae, Gardnerella vaginalis, Escherichia coli,* as well as other gram-negative enteric organisms and group A and B streptococci, make the results of anogenital samples extremely unreliable (130). DNA probe tests are not specific at anogenital sites in children, and they should not be used in any sexual abuse victims (42,133,134). A positive result of any rapid test for *C. trachomatis* in a low-prevalence group like sexually abused children may have an equal chance of being a true or a false positive. Nucleic acid amplification tests such as polymerase chin reaction (PCR), ligase chain reaction (LCR), and transcription-mediated amplification are approved for urethral, cervical, and urine specimens from adults, but potential false-negative and false-positive results and lack of data in children limit their application in sexual abuse. Because of the legal implications, only tissue cultures for chlamydia, confirmed by microscopic identification with fluorescent antibody staining, should be used in evaluating sexual abuse in children (132–134).

Perinatal maternal–infant transmission is common. As many as 50% to 60% of infants born to infected mothers acquire the infection or colonization, including 14% with subclinical rectal and vaginal colonization. Neonatal infections have been documented to persist for 12 months and may occasionally persist for as long as 3 years. Therefore positive cultures in children age 3 years or younger may occasionally represent persistent perinatal infections. Positive cultures in adolescents are also diffi-

cult to interpret. *C. trachomatis* was isolated from 18 of 127 female adolescent victims of sexual abuse; however, 16 of the 18 positive cultures were from previously sexually active adolescents. Therefore it may be correct to attribute many of the infections in this study to the prior consenting activity. Chlamydial vaginal infections beyond the first year of life are strongly associated with sexual contact. Some infections in preschool children, however, may represent persistence of perinatal infection, and many infections detected in adolescents may actually be the result of previous consensual sexual activity. The number of children with reported pharyngeal or rectal infections is too small to draw any conclusions about infections at these sites (35,130,133,145).

Human Papillomavirus

Human papillomavirus (HPV) infections are probably the most common STD in adults but are uncommon infections in children. The classic lesions characterizing this infection, condyloma acuminata or anogenital warts, are soft, irregular, multidigitated wart-like growths. Other common appearances of the lesions include small, flat, red, violaceous, or pigmented papules on the penile shaft, flat nondigitated cervical growths, and fine irregularities of the vulvar tissues called papillomatosis labialis. Most lesions occur in the perineal area, although they can be found on any moist skin areas or mucous membranes. Several levels of the GU tract may be involved simultaneously, and some lesions may be entirely internal, located inside the mouth, vagina, or rectum (6,59). Detection of subclinical disease is greatly enhanced by the application of 3% to 5% acetic acid to the perineum for several minutes; the subsequent presence of "acetowhite" patches is indicative of HPV infection (56).

Diagnosis is usually made by the typical clinical wart-like appearance of lesions and biopsy specimens, although more precise viral typing techniques can be used. There are over 70 different HPV types, but types 6 and 11 are most commonly associated with genital warts, with a smaller number of perineal lesions caused by HPV types 16, 18, and 31 (56). Viral typing allows comparison of the child's lesions and lesions from individuals with possible contact with the child (233).

Perinatal maternal–infant transmission is well documented, and the interval from exposure to development of the lesions is extremely variable (20 months in one case), with the average incubation period of 2 to 3 months in both nonsexually or sexually acquired infections (59). The role of perinatal transmission remains unclear. The presence of HPV DNA in infants born to infected mothers ranges from 1% to 77% and in uninfected mothers ranges from 1% to 50%, suggesting the possibility of nonsexual transmission from caretakers being important in the children of both HPV-positive and HPV-negative mothers (133). The most comprehensive prospective study of infants and toddlers presents a strong argument against perinatal transmission; women who were HPV DNA positive were just as likely as HPV DNA-negative women to have HPV DNA-positive infants and toddlers, and the HPV subtypes in infant–mother pairs were not concordant (273). Nonsexual transmission of common warts (usually HPV type 2) has been implicated in some of the typical perineal lesions in young children (48). DNA typing has demonstrated that 10% to 20% of children have anogenital lesions by skin HPV types (133). It cannot be assumed, however, that all perineal lesions caused by HPV type 2 or type 3 are acquired by nonabusive contact, because no correlation is found between the frequency of hand and genital warts. In addition, the common wart virus also could be spread from the infected hands of an individual through inappropriate genital fondling. The risk of acquiring HPV infection from cobathing and sexual play is unknown. Nonsexual transmission might have occurred in four cases in one series because of maternal history of genital warts and exposure to skin warts. Appropriate social and medical evaluation revealed sexual abuse in these four children, however. This report emphasizes the need for thorough investigation of sexual abuse in children with genital warts (135).

Early reports of genital warts in children documented fewer cases of sexual abuse, and in one third to one half, mode of transmission was unknown. More recent reports documented sexual transmission in more than 50% of the cases, with fewer cases in which mode of transmission was unknown. In one study, a confirmed history of sexual abuse was obtained from seven of nine children older than 3 years; no history could be obtained from any of the nine children aged 3 years and younger (125). In another study of patients referred to pediatric dermatologists, none of the infected children younger than 3 years was determined to be sexually abused. Whether some of these children were actually abused is not known. In the same study, however, 50% of children aged 4 years and older had proven sexual transmission (48). Asymptomatic HPV infection has been demonstrated by DNA probes and antibody techniques in up to 24% of oral mucosal samples in preschool children. The significance of this finding is unclear, because the source of the infection was not determined (153). The virus can remain latent in normal-appearing areas adjacent to the skin lesions. Therefore the appearance of new lesions up to several months after treatment may or may not be attributable to reexposure through continuing sexual contact. Viral transmission may occur from an individual without obvious lesions, so evaluation of possible sources of the virus must include a search for subclinical infections. The long and variable incubation period of the HPV and common subclinical infection make it difficult to identify the child's contact. Except for HPV infections appearing during the first 2 years of life, however, a high suspicion of sexual abuse is indicated (6,59). Children with anogenital warts should be screened for other STDs and interviewed in a developmentally appropriate manner for suspected abuse (13).

Trichomoniasis

Trichomoniasis and bacterial vaginosis are the most frequent infections acquired after sexual assault in adult and adolescent females

(19,133,156). *Trichomonas vaginalis* infection is uncommon in prepubertal girls and strongly suggests sexual abuse. Trichomoniasis is a common STD in adults, and infected male patients are typically asymptomatic. *T. vaginalis* infections are characterized by a purulent vaginal discharge, although asymptomatic infections can occur. It is not known how long children can be infected before developing symptoms (131). Infected mothers may transmit the infection to their infants during birth, and these infections can persist for up to 1 year (133). Trichomonas infections are rarely reported beyond infancy, however, except in postpubertal sexually active children and adults. The organism may be detected in a urine sample, but the diagnosis is usually made by microscopic examination of a wet mount of the vaginal discharge that reveals the causative protozoan in motion. Wet-mount preparations identify only 50% to 75% of cases detectable by using specific culture techniques (128). *T. hominis* is a commensal species inhabiting the bowel that must be distinguished from *T. vaginalis* (133). Nonsexual transmission is theoretically possible because the organism can survive up to several hours on objects or wet clothing, although no cases of proven fomite transmission have been reported (212). Therefore, trichomonas infections in prepubertal children beyond the first months of life are strongly suggestive of sexual abuse (159,275).

Herpesvirus Infection

Genital herpes infections are uncommon in children, and sexual abuse has been documented to be the cause in many cases (212, 245). Primary herpes genital infection is seen most frequently among sexually active adolescents and young adults. The risk of acquiring the infection through sexual abuse is unknown (131,133). Herpes simplex virus (HSV) infection is characterized by painful vesicular or ulcerated lesions involving skin and mucous membranes. The lesions, often accompanied by fever, appear after an incubation period of 2 to 20 days (mean, 6 days) after exposure. HSV type 1 infections usually occur in the mouth,

and most HSV type 2 infections occur in the genital area; however, HSV-1 or HSV-2 can be found at either location. Approximately 10% to 20% of herpes genital infections are due to HSV-1. Nonsexual transmission is not well studied, but HSV-1 infections are a fairly common childhood infection, usually involving only the mouth but occasionally the mouth and genital area simultaneously (109,162).

Although asymptomatic viral shedding is frequent in adults, routine HSV cultures are of little value in asymptomatic children. Cultures of active lesions may be positive in only two thirds of the cases, with vesicles having a higher yield than ulcerations. Suggestive lesions (vesicles or ulcerations) must be cultured and can be subtyped to distinguish HSV-1 from HSV-2 infections. In contrast, commercially available serologic tests for HSV antibody can document seronegativity but cannot consistently differentiate between HSV-2 and HSV-1 antibody. Epidemiologic studies in Nigeria and India have shown that 8.5% to 50% of children aged 1 to 10 years were seropositive for HSV-2, raising the possibility of, but not proving, contamination as the source of infection (145). No cases of fomite transmission have been documented, but HSV can survive for up to 4 hours on plastic, rubber, or metal surfaces (212). When a child has simultaneous oral and genital infection or when an infant or toddler has a caretaker with oral lesions, it may be reasonable to conclude that nonsexual transmission of genital lesions due to HSV-1 is the cause. The evidence suggests that except for transmission at birth, most HSV-2 genital infections are sexually transmitted (109,162).

Bacterial Vaginosis

Bacterial vaginosis (BV) appears to be a marker of sexual activity in adults, but children may acquire the infection through sexual and nonsexual means. BV (or nonspecific vaginitis) is a polymicrobial infection resulting from the replacement of *Lactobacillus* species with *Gardnerella vaginalis, Mycoplasma hominis,* and various anerobic organisms. Although *G. vaginalis* is one of the bacteria that may be involved in this infection, the presence or absence of this organism in a vaginal culture does not prove or disprove the diagnosis. Diagnosis requires both a microscopic examination of the discharge and simple chemical tests. The characteristic thin, grey–white to yellow vaginal discharge is examined microscopically for the presence of "clue cells," which are epithelial cells with clusters of bacteria adhering to the surface. A "whiff test" is performed by the addition of 10% KOH to the vaginal secretions, which results in a fishy or amine aroma in the presence of BV. Bacterial vaginosis has been defined as "definite" when both clue cells and a positive whiff test are found, and "possible" when one of the two tests is positive (145). A vaginal pH of more than 4.5 is present in postpubertal females with the infection, but vaginal pH is not a reliable criterion in younger girls. Gram-stained vaginal smears showing no lactobacilli and predominant gram-negative and gram-variable rods are sensitive and specific for BV in adults (133). One group of authors reported definite BV in four vaginal washings from 31 children obtained 2 or more weeks after sexual abuse in whom initial test results were negative (128). None of 23 specimens from nonabused girls was positive. The infection rate is increased after sexual contact, but this entity may be the most common cause of nonsexually transmitted vaginitis in children and adolescents (36,133). In a study of 26 girls younger than 14 years with symptomatic vulvovaginitis, the vaginal washings of nine (35%) had diagnostic tests positive for BV. Only three of these girls had a history of sexual abuse (131). The development of a new vaginal discharge after sexual abuse has been associated with BV, but the presence of this infection in a child may be attributed to either sexual or nonsexual transmission (36,128,133).

Colonization or asymptomatic infections with the genital mycoplasmas, *Mycoplasma hominis* (*genitalium*) and *Ureaplasma urealyticum,* strongly correlate with sexual activity in adults. Symptomatic infections are not common. Neither organism is clearly linked to vaginal infections, but *U. urealyticum* has been shown to be the cause of at least 10% of nonspecific urethritis in male patients (131). One controlled study of pharyngeal, anorectal, and vaginal colonization rates in abused and normal children with genital mycoplasmas has been reported (129). *M. hominis* was isolated from the anorectal and vaginal cultures of 23% and 34% of the 47 abused girls as compared with 8% and 17%, respectively, of the 36 controls. *U. urealyticum* was isolated from the anorectal and vaginal cultures of 19% and 30% of the abused girls as compared with 3% and 8% of 36 controls. No association was found between colonization with either organism and the presence of a discharge in these children. In summary, increased colonization has been demonstrated among sexually abused children for both *M. genitalium* and *U. urealyticum.* These organisms should not be considered significant markers for sexual abuse, however, because asymptomatic colonization also is common among nonabused children.

HIV Infection

The potential long-term risk of HIV infection among child sexual abuse victims is unknown, but it would be extremely unlikely for HIV infection to follow a single episode of sexual abuse. Sexual abuse has been implicated in cases of HIV infection (111,124, 188). Screening of victims for HIV infection seems most reasonable if the child gives a history of vaginal or rectal penetration by multiple perpetrators or an unknown perpetrator, or is symptomatic for HIV or any STD; or if the perpetrator is known to have HIV infection, is a known homosexual or bisexual, or is a known intravenous drug abuser (133). High prevalence of HIV infection regionally also may be considered a risk factor. Some experts recommend that all sexually abused children be screened for HIV, recognizing that many positive tests will result because of previously undocumented neonatal transmission (172). Screening of the perpetrator first, and then screening only a child whose perpetrator was positive for HIV is ideal, but this may not be a legal option in many states (22).

When testing is done within 2 weeks of exposure, a negative test provides information of prior HIV status only (152). If the initial test is negative, testing should be repeated at 6 weeks. Follow-up testing must be done at least 3 to 6 months after exposure because rarely, more than 6 weeks may elapse between exposure and seroconversion. The median interval from percutaneous or transfusion exposure is 3 weeks (19). The actual timing of follow-up specimens is not clear because no data are available on the incubation period after sexual assault in children. Screening for HIV infections is typically done by using EIA for HIV antibody. The predictive value of a positive test is low in a low-prevalence population. If the EIA test is positive, it is repeated, followed by a Western blot test or an immunofluorescence assay to distinguish between true and false positives (43). The issue of HIV infection should be addressed with every victim and his or her family, and regardless of the decision about testing, appropriate counseling support and follow-up should be provided (133,152).

Other Sexually Transmitted Diseases

Information is limited about other STDs and their association with sexual abuse of children. This lack of information is attributed to several factors: many have primarily nonsexual modes of transmission in children, some have a low prevalence among adults, and others are extremely rare in children. Ectoparasites including *Sarcoptes scabiei* (scabies), *Phthirus pubis* ("crab lice"), and *Pediculus* species (body lice) can be sexually transmitted, but close nonsexual contact is the predominant mode of transmission in children. *Molluscum contagiosum,* a poxvirus infection, has been linked to sexual activity in adults, but nonsexual transmission is common in both children and adults. Shigellosis, amebiasis, and giardiasis are known to be sexually transmitted, primarily among homosexuals. Hepatitis B virus infections are increased in homosexuals and heterosexuals with multiple partners. These findings, however, are not clear indicators of sexual abuse, because children develop these infections primarily through nonsexual contact with infected individuals. Lymphogranuloma venereum (LGV), granuloma inguinale, and chancroid are uncommon STDs in the U.S. and have not been reported in sexually abused children. LGV, caused by *C. trachomatis* subtypes L-1 to L-3, is a systemic infection that appears to be increasing in frequency among adults. Chancroid is caused by *Hemophilus ducreyi,* and dramatic increases in reported cases among adults in urban areas may lead to spread to children. Granuloma inguinale is suspected to be caused by *Calymmatobacterium granulomatis,* and is rare outside of the tropics (131).

Recommended Testing

Routine testing of all children who are suspected of being sexually abused is no longer recommended. Criteria for screening for STDs include historical and physical parameters associated with increased risk of infection (Table 10.2). The U.S. Public Health Services CDC recommends that the following tests for STDs be performed on selected, high-risk child sexual abuse victims: gonococcal (gonorrhea) cultures from pharyngeal, anal, and urethral or vaginal sites; chlamydial cultures from vaginal and anal sites in girls and anal and urethral sites in symptomatic boys; serology for syphilis, HIV, hepatitis B; examination for anogenital warts or ulcerative lesions; and in addition, for girls, culture or wet mount of vaginal secretions for microscopic examination for *Trichomonas,* and tests for BV. They recommend repeating all these tests in 2 weeks, and repeating the serologic tests in 12 weeks after the last abuse episode. The CDC recommends testing adolescents for gonorrhea and chlamydia from all sites of penetration or attempted penetration, testing for *Trichomonas* and BV, and

TABLE 10.2. *Collecting forensic specimens in sexual abuse*

1. Obtain 2–3 swabbed specimens from each area of body assaulted (for sperm, acid phosphatase, P 30, MHS-5 antigen, blood group antigen determinations). The number of swabs required depends on local laboratory. Most laboratories request air-dried specimens, which require drying for 60 min before they can be packaged
2. Mouth: Swab under tongue, and buccal pouch next to upper and lower molars. These areas are locations where seminal fluid is most likely to be persistent
3. Vagina: Use dry or moistened swab, or 2-ml saline wash. Remember that overdilution of secretions may produce false-negative results of tests for acid phosphatase. Secretions may also be collected with a pipette or eyedropper
4. Rectum: Insert swab at least ½ to 1 inch beyond anus
5. Specimens should be taken from any other suspicious site on the body. Saline- or sterile water–moistened swabs may be used to lift any stains suspected to be dried seminal fluid or blood. An alternate method is to scrape off the dried stains with the back of a scalpel blade into a clean envelope or tube
6. Make saline wet mount of specimens from all assaulted orifices and examine immediately for presence of motile and nonmotile sperm
7. Some forensic laboratories request a dry smear of each secretion sample using clean glass microscope slides; others prefer to prepare their own slides from swab specimens
8. Collect saliva specimen to determine the victim's antigen-secretion status. Saliva may be collected using 3–4 sterile swabs or a 2 × 2 gauze pad that the victim placed in the mouth
9. Obtain a venous blood sample from the victim for antigen-secretor status. This sample from the victim will be used in the analysis of the identity of the perpetrator
10. Save torn or bloody clothes or any clothing when semen staining is suspected, using Woods lamp. Semen may fluoresce with a blue or green color under the ultraviolet light of the Wood's lamp, although fluorescence under UV light is nonspecific. Various skin infections, congenital or acquired skin pigmentary changes and chemicals including systemic and topical medications, cosmetics, soaps, and industrial chemicals may fluoresce under UV light
11. If the victim was wearing a tampon, pad, or diaper during the assault or if a fresh tampon, pad, or diaper was used after the abuse, save this for analysis; seminal fluid products may be found on these items. Plastic bags should be used only on dry specimens and only if directed so by the laboratory. Sealed plastic may promote the growth of *Candida* and other organisms that might destroy some of the evidence
12. Save any foreign material found on removal of clothing. Fiber analysis or trace analysis may provide evidence that links the specimens to the perpetrator or the location of the abuse
13. Collect samples of combed pubic hair or scalp hair and fingernail scrapings. These procedures are often considered optional. Pubic hair, scalp hair, or skin fragments from scratching may be used to help identify the perpetrator. Control samples of the victim's body or scalp hair are collected for comparison. Usually it is recommended that the hairs be plucked rather than cut, although the additional trauma of plucking 10 to 20 hairs from a child may not be warranted unless foreign hair material is found on the child's body. Some protocols recommend considering cutting hairs or collecting plucked hairs at a later time if needed
14. Specimens should also be taken to screen for sexually transmitted diseases. The recommended procedures are detailed in the text. Swabs should **not** be air dried, because air drying kills the organisms and causes the cultures for these diseases to be falsely negative. Specimens for culture should be sent quickly to a microbiology laboratory for processing and not be included with the materials to be processed in the forensic laboratory

serologic testing for syphilis, HIV, and hepatitis B. Repeated testing should be considered at a 2-week follow-up, and repeated testing done for syphilis and HIV at 6, 12, and 24 weeks after the assault (43).

FORENSIC EVIDENCE COLLECTION AND INTERPRETATION

Forensic evidence is usually collected at the same time as the physical examination. The types of evidence sought include sperm, seminal fluid, and foreign materials on the victim's body surface or clothing. Such evidence is usually not found in child sexual abuse cases. Pregnancy and STDs have forensic significance but usually are not classified as forensic evidence.

Several general guidelines about evidence should be addressed before outlining a more specific approach to specimen collection (Table 10.3). First, specific details of collection, labeling, and packaging of specimens should be worked out with the laboratory processing the specimens. Second, a specimen-collection protocol should be used to

TABLE 10.3. *Persistence of forensic evidence in sexual contact*

Site	Type of evidence			
	Motile sperm[a]	Nonmotile sperm[b]	Acid phosphatase[c]	P 30[d]
Pharynx	½–6 h	6 h (?)	6 h (?)	No data available
Rectum	½–8 h	24 h	24 h (?)	No data available
Vagina	½–8 h	7–48 h	12–48 h	12–48 h
Clothing	<½ h	Up to 12 mo	Up to 3 yr	Up to 12 yr

[a]Rarely persist more than a few hours at any site. Lack of cervical mucus decreases sperm survival in prepubertal girls.
[b]Limited data on pharyngeal persistence. May persist indefinitely on clothing if kept dry and not washed.
[c]Limited data on pharyngeal and rectal persistence. May persist indefinitely on clothing if kept dry and not washed.
[d]May persist indefinitely on clothing if kept dry and not washed.

ensure that all appropriate specimens will be collected for both routine and nonroutine circumstances. Third, collection kits should be standardized, providing containers, collection devices, and checklists to assure proper collection of specimens. Fourth, the procedures for collecting specimens are best explained in advance to the child and the caretakers, because cooperation is key to the collection of proper specimens. Fifth, proper consent must be obtained from the parent and child before performing the examination and collecting evidence. Finally, the handling of collected specimens should be documented to maintain a "chain of evidence." Documentation includes limiting the number of personnel involved in handling specimens, and clearly recording the specimen handlers from the time of collection through the processing of the specimens in the laboratory (79,254).

Forensic evidence collection has been recommended when the examination occurs within 72 hours of acute sexual assault or sexual abuse (1,9). This recommendation is based at least in part on the fact that seminal fluid and other foreign substances are rarely recoverable in adults more than 72 hours after the last sexual contact. Specimens for STDs and pregnancy testing have forensic significance as well, but these specimens may be better collected more than 72 hours after sexual contact. Often, however, they are collected at the same time that "rape kits" or

evidence-collection kits are used. Those collecting and handling the specimens should wear gloves. These individuals should avoid contaminating body sites with secretions from distant sites, by collecting specimens carefully, and then removing remaining secretions or stains before sampling another site. The specific methods used to collect and transport specimens should be discussed with the laboratory personnel who will process the specimens. Individual laboratories may prefer synthetic rather than cotton swabs or other minor variations in techniques.

Numerous protocols recommend a Wood's lamp or ultraviolet light as an aid in identifing semen stains on skin or clothing. The fluorescing stains can be swabbed for forensic an-alysis. Semen will show white to yellow–green fluorescence under a Wood's lamp. Wood's lamp examinations have several shortcomings. The fluorescence of semen usually fades within 28 hours, yet semen may still be detectable by using sensitive forensic tests. Semen and urine fluoresce with the same color, and urine fluorescence persists for considerably longer (107). In addition, many products commonly found in the perineal area in children including Balmex, Desitin, Surgilube, and Barrier Cream will fluoresce under the Wood's lamp (242). Recognizing these limitations, the Wood's lamp may be of some help in identifying suggestive areas for more definitive testing (13).

Analysis of Specimens

Document Proof of Sexual Contact

Spermatozoa detected in specimens from body orifices provide strong evidence of sexual contact within the last 72 hours. Live, motile sperm are detected by using a saline wet mount and are the most tangible proof of recent ejaculation into the orifice. The specimen requires immediate analysis of because live sperm may be present for only 1/2 hour. The survival time of motile sperm is variable, depending on the body orifice in which it was deposited. Sperm motility rarely persists for more than a few hours. The mouth presents a particularly hostile environment because of the cleansing and digestive action of saliva, whereas motile sperm may be present occasionally up to 5 days in the cervix. Prepubertal girls do not produce cervical mucus, so the survival time of sperm in the vagina is shortened (216). Nonmotile or dead sperm are detectable for a longer time than are live sperm. Several studies suggest that sperm may be present for up to 12 to 20 hours and rarely up to 48 to 72 hours in the vagina after voluntary intercourse. About one half of specimens from the vaginal pool will have no detectable sperm within 24 hours of ejaculation. Sperm are rarely present more than 24 hours in rectal specimens. Persistence of sperm in vaginal and rectal sites, however, has been documented for up to 168 hours and 113 hours, respectively (5). Dry specimens from any site are quite stable, and sperm may be detected in stains on clothing for 12 months or longer (226,230,250,254).

Acid phosphatase is another important indicator of sexual contact. This enzyme is secreted by the prostate gland and is found in high concentration in semen, 130 to 1,800 IU/L, but is present in only very low levels, less than 50 IU/L, in vaginal secretions. Acid phosphatase is usually considered a more sensitive indicator of recent intercourse than is sperm, because in general, it is broken down less rapidly after sexual contact and may be detected for a somewhat longer period than sperm. Analysis for acid phosphatase, how-ever, should be considered complementary to identification of sperm. In individual cases, sperm may be detected in the absence of significant elevation of acid phosphatase. A marked elevation of the enzyme in vaginal secretions indicates intercourse within 24 to 48 hours; the level usually returns to normal in 72 hours. A negative test also can be consistent with a recent sexual contact with ejaculation, because levels may return to normal within 3 hours and as many as one half of the specimens will have undetectable levels within 24 hours. The level of acid phosphatase is typically elevated for an even shorter duration in the mouth (less than 6 hours) and in the rectum (less than 24 hours) but only estimates of the duration are available. Acid phosphatase has been detected in dried seminal fluid stains on clothing for at least 3 years after the deposition of the semen, and may persist indefinitely (5,222, 226,230,250).

Two other tests have been developed to detect the presence of seminal fluid residues, the P 30 and the mouse anti-human semen-5 (MSH-5) tests. P 30, or semen glycoprotein of prostatic origin, is a protein manufactured in the prostate gland that is secreted into the seminal fluid. High levels of P 30 are found in semen, ranging from 0.62 to 5.25 mg, with a mean of 1.55 mg/mL of seminal plasma. Levels of P 30 in seminal fluid in normal and vasectomized men are not significantly different. Only men produce P 30, and therefore, any amount found in the vaginal fluid, urine, or saliva of female patients is indicative of recent sexual contact. The amount of P 30 present declines to undetectable levels within 48 hours of ejaculation into the vagina. Therefore, a positive P 30 test from a vaginal fluid specimen means sexual contact has occurred within 48 hours. P 30 is a more sensitive test for the presence of seminal fluid than is acid phosphatase in the first 48 hours. Acid phosphatase, however, may be detectable in some vaginal specimens for longer than 48 hours. The protein is extremely stable when dried, and may be detectable for up to 12 years in dried seminal stains (119). The MHS-5 antigen detection test uses a monoclonal antibody probe technique for detection of seminal fluid. MHS-5 is a male specific protein produced only in the seminal vesicles and present only in semen. Standardized laboratory kits are available for this test; however, the test has not yet come into general use (138).

Laboratory tests for the presence of seminal fluid can be interpreted properly only if certain limitations are recognized. First, tests for sperm will be negative, but acid phosphatase, P 30, and MHS-5 tests are positive if the alleged perpetrator has aspermia or has had a vasectomy because the liquid portion of the seminal fluid is still produced and released. Second, the tests for sperm, acid phosphatase, P 30, and MHS-5 will be negative if ejaculation has not occurred or if a condom is used. Third, all tests may be negative despite immediate collection of specimens because of inadequate sampling, problems in handling and processing specimens, or if bathing, washing, or toileting activities have removed the ejaculate. Finally, all tests are likely to be negative if tests are obtained more than 48 to 72 hours after intercourse, because sperm, acid phosphatase, P 30, and MHS-5 are rarely detectable for more than 48 to 72 hours from body surfaces. Therefore we rarely attempt to recover seminal fluid from the body of the abuse victim more than 72 hours after the last sexual contact. Clothing worn during or immediately after the abuse may test positive more than 72 hours later, however, because seminal fluid products in dried stains can persist for a longer time.

Proving the Identity of the Perpetrator

Semen, blood, saliva, body hair, bite marks, and other materials occasionally found on the body of the victim may help to identify the perpetrator. The collection of this potential evidence is done as part of the routine evaluation of sexual assault victims presenting within 72 hours of the last sexual contact. Proper analysis of these materials requires the expertise of a forensic pathologist or a specialized crime laboratory.

Genetic markers can be used to identify the likely origin of body fluids. The basis of such identification is that approximately 80% of the general population are "secretors," and all body fluids of secretors including blood, semen, and saliva will contain genetically determined factors. The commonly assayed genetic markers are the ABO blood group antigens, the ten subtypes of the enzyme phosphoglucomutase (PGM), and the enzyme peptidase A. Some subtypes of individual genetic markers are common, whereas others are rarely seen in the general population. The frequency of particular combinations of subtypes of the genetic markers in the general population can be estimated. From this estimate, the chances of the body fluid being from a specific individual can be calculated. Although not so specific as fingerprinting, this process can be precise enough to provide strong evidence of the perpetrator's identity. Approximately 20% of the population are "nonsecretors," and genetic marker analysis provides little help in further characterizing the nonsecretor. Control samples of the victim's saliva and blood are required to determine which genetic markers represent the victim and which represent the perpetrator. Blood found on clothing or on the body of the victim may represent blood from victim or assailant, particularly if the victim had scratched or bitten the assailant and caused bleeding. Blood samples may be analyzed for genetic markers by using the same procedures as for other body fluids (171 226,234,254).

Body or scalp hair from the perpetrator occasionally may be may be found on the victim's body. Hair analysis requires the collection of suggestive "foreign" hair from the body of the victim, hairs collected from the alleged perpetrator directly, and the victim's own hair as a control. Because of the variability of hair types from different sites in one individual, multiple specimens from the alleged abuser and the victim must be collected from multiple sites. Microscopic analysis has limited specificity, and the laboratory can conclude in the majority of cases only that the sample is consistent with, inconsistent with, or inconclusive when compared with the perpetrator's hair. Similar microscopic comparison of foreign fibers found on the victim's body with known fibers from the perpetrator's house can help confirm the location of the abuse. Neutron activation analysis is a precise technique that can identify 18 variable components common to human hair and is almost as reliable as fingerprinting. Unfortunately, the instrument to perform this analysis is expensive and not widely available (254).

Bite-mark identification techniques can be used to determine the source of bite marks on the victim's body. Bite marks are rarely present, and accurate sampling and analysis are difficult. However, when good-quality pictures can be obtained of the bite marks, they may be as specific as fingerprints in identifying the perpetrator. Swabs from acute bite marks may contain saliva that can be analyzed for genetic markers. A forensic odontologist is the best resource for obtaining clear and convincing bite-mark evidence. A series of black-and-white and color photographs, showing overall orientation views and a series of close-ups, can be interpreted at a later date. A measuring scale should be included in the photographs, and the photographs taken at 90 degrees to each arch to avoid picture distortion due to the curvature of the skin (254,259).

DNA typing or profiling is the most specific development in the identification of the perpetrator of sexual abuse (113). This technique allows the identification of a specific individual through analysis of sperm, blood, hair root cells, or other tissue from the perpetrator found on the victim's body. Specific sequences of the DNA are identified in the tissue (i.e., sperm) collected from the victim's body, and compared with the unique sequence of DNA in tissue taken from the alleged perpetrator. Experts have debated the standards for forensic use of DNA typing, despite the extreme specificity of the results (12,177). The current technology for DNA typing has progressed to the point where the reliability and validity of properly collected, properly preserved, and properly analyzed DNA data should not be in doubt (209,211).

Most children evaluated for sexual abuse do not have forensic evidence. Studies focusing on highly selected groups of child victims reported 14% to 30% had positive tests for sperm or acid phosphatase (45,79,232,253). Authors of other studies suggest that only 2% to 5% of all sexually abused children evaluated have positive tests for sperm or acid phosphatase (58,63,264). Sperm and acid phosphatase are usually not detected in child sexual abuse victims, and frequency of detection is likely to be lower in unselected samples. Data on the use of testing for P 30 or MHS-5 in child sexual abuse victims are not yet available. Other forms of forensic evidence such as blood, hairs, fibers, or other foreign substances are reported in fewer cases than are sperm or seminal fluid (45).

Christian et al. (45) concluded that guidelines for evidence collection for adult sexual assault victims may not be appropriate for prepubertal victims. A total of 273 children younger than 10 years evaluated for suspected sexual abuse had rape kits performed by using selective criteria based on the history and physical examination. Some form of evidence was identified in 24.9%. More than 90% of the children with positive forensic evidence were seen within 24 hours, and all were examined within 44 hours of the assault. No swabs from any child's body were positive for blood after 13 hours or sperm/semen after 9 hours. After 24 hours, all evidence with the exception of one pubic hair was recovered from clothing or linens. Swabbing the child's body for evidence may be unnecessary after 24 hours. Because clothing and linens yield the majority of evidence, they should be vigorously pursued for analysis (45).

Forensic Evidence Summary

All children being evaluated for suspected sexual abuse should have a medical examination, although most examinations will not detect abnormal physical findings or provide positive forensic medical evidence that sexual contact has occurred. The forensic evidence is only as good as the collection process allows it to be. Using an appropriate protocol and documentation of proper handling of all evidence are essential. Delayed disclosure commonly associated with child sexual abuse limits the availability of forensic evidence. The identity of the offender can be suggested by forensic analysis of body fluid residues and other evidence, but body fluid residues or physical evidence must be present, and the expertise must be available to perform these tests. Most cases will not involve such information and analysis. The history of abuse is the most important evidence in matters of child dependency and criminal proceedings. Physical evidence that documents force or injury or documents sexual contact is helpful, but not necessary, for conviction of the perpetrator of sexual abuse. The presence of physical evidence does not assure conviction; however, the lack of physical evidence does not assure acquittal (63).

MANAGEMENT CONSIDERATIONS

Medical Intervention

The major medical interventions required involve therapy for STDs, emergency contraception, treatment of injuries, and certification of physical health. Interventions are often initiated at the first medical evaluation, but follow-up is recommended to maximize the effect of the interventions.

Prophylactic antibiotic therapy for sexually abused children is a controversial subject, but routine prophylaxis is not generally recommended (19,22,40,42,131,133,147,172,249). Routine prophylaxis is commonly offered to adolescents and adults for chlamydia, gonorrhea, trichomonas, and bacterial vaginosis as follows: ceftriaxone, 125 mg intramuscularly in a single dose, plus metronidazole, 2 g orally in a single dose, plus azithromycin, 1 g orally in a single dose or doxycycline, 100 mg orally twice a day for 7 days (42). Selective testing should be done for STDs in children as outlined previously. Specific therapy should be initiated if this testing reveals specific infections (Table 10.4). Ceftriaxone is the preferred treatment for proctitis, pharyngitis, and vaginal or urethral gonococcal infections by penicillinase-producing resistant organisms (PPNG) or organisms of unknown antibiotic sensitivity. Ceftriaxone is given in a single intramuscular dose of 125 mg. Ceftriaxone is effective in treating both gonorrhea and incubating syphilis. Spectinomycin (40 mg/kg) intramuscularly as a single dose (maximal dose: 2 g) can be given for penicillin-allergic individuals; however, incubating syphilis may not

TABLE 10.4. *Recommended therapy for sexually transmitted diseases*

Sexually transmitted disease	Therapy
Gonococcal infection	Ceftriaxone, 125 mg i.m. (≤45 kg), 250 mg i.m. (>45 kg)
	If allergic: spectinomycin, 40 mg/kg i.m. a single dose or trimethoprim/ sulfamethoxazole (SMX) (40 mg/kg/day SMX) × 5 days if treating pharyngeal infection in allergic individuals
Syphilis	Incubating: Ceftriaxone as above
	Early acquired (<1 yr): Benzathine penicillin, 50,000 units i.m. (maximum, 2.4 million units)
Chlamydial infections	<9 years old: Erythromycin, 50 mg/kg/day × 7–10 days
	≥9 years old: Tetracycline, 25–50 mg/kg/day × 7 days or doxycycline, 100 mg b.i.d. × 7 days
Human papillomavirus	Surgical excision, laser vaporization, cryosurgery, or applications of 75% trichloroacetic acid or podophyllin
Trichomoniasis	Metronidazole, 30–50 mg/kg/day × 7 days (maximum, 250 mg t.i.d.)
Genital herpes	Oral acyclovir, 200 mg 5 times a day × 7–10 days for initial episode
Bacterial vaginosis	Metronidazole, 15 mg/kg/day × 7 days (maximum 500 mg b.i.d.) or amoxicillin/clavulanic acid, 20–40 mg/kg/day amoxicillin × 7 days (maximum, 250 mg t.i.d.)

be controlled by this regimen. Cefixime, 400 mg orally as a single dose, has been recommended for uncomplicated gonorrhea infections in adults, where it is slightly less effective than ceftriaxone (97.1% vs. 99.1% cure rate). The safety and efficacy for gonorrhea in children is not known. Children and adolescents with primary or secondary syphilis should be treated with benzathine penicillin G, 50,000 units/kg, up to the adult dose of 2.4 million units as a single dose. Doxycycline, 100 mg twice a day, or tetracycline, 500 mg four times a day for 2 weeks, may be considered in nonpregnant penicillin-allergic individuals. Chlamydial infections should be treated in children younger than 8 years with 50 mg/kg/day (maximum of 2 g/day) of erythromycin in four divided doses for 10 to 14 days. Any child who weighs more than 45 kg can be treated with azithromycin, 1 g orally in a single dose. Alternative therapy for children 8 years or older is 100 mg/kg of doxycycline twice a day for 7 days. Trichomonas infections can be treated with metronidazole, 30 to 50 mg/kg/day, in divided doses to a maximum of 500 mg twice a day for 7 days. Adolescents may take metronidazole orally as a single 2-g dose. Bacterial vaginosis can be treated with 15 mg/kg/day of metronidazole, with a maximum recommended dose of 500 mg twice a day for 7 days.

Older children and adolescents may take metronidazole, 2 g orally as a single dose, or clindamycin, 300 mg orally twice a day for 7 days. Amoxicillin combined with clavulanic acid (Augmentum) has also been recommended in a dose of 20 to 40 mg/kg/day of the amoxicillin component in divided doses to a maximum dose of 400 mg twice a day. The therapy of anogenital warts is more complicated. Therapy is directed toward symptomatic warts, but often does not eradicate the infection, prevent recurrences, or decrease infectivity. Therapeutic methods include surgical excision for large lesions, cryotherapy with liquid nitrogen, laser vaporization, or local applications of either 75% trichloroacetic acid, 80% to 90% bichloroacetic acid, or 10% to 25% podophyllin. Two options are available

for patient-applied treatment of HPV lesions: pedofilox, 0.5% solution or gel, an antimitotic drug, and imiquimod, 5% cream, an immune enhancer that stimulates production of interferon and other cytokines. Inflammatory reactions are common, but often milder than with other agents. Pedofilox is applied to warts twice a day for 3 consecutive days each week for a total of 4 to 8 weeks. Imiquimod can be applied to warts at bedtime 3 times per week for as long as 16 weeks. Oral acyclovir may be given in a dose of 200 mg orally five times daily or 400 mg three times daily for 7 to 10 days for the first clinical episode of herpes genital infection in adolescents and older children. Oral acyclovir may shorten the duration of symptoms but has no effect on the risk, frequency, or severity of recurrences (42,131). HIV prophylaxis is a debated subject, with some sexual assault centers providing HIV prophylaxis in high-risk exposures if treatment can be initiated within 72 hours. The CDC states there is a lack of data on the efficacy of antiretroviral agents to reduce HIV transmission after a possible nonoccupational exposure. A recommendation cannot be made at this time on the basis of available information regarding the appropriateness of postexposure prophylaxis after sexual exposure to HIV (42). However, certain factors may influence a clinician to consider antiretroviral prophylaxis, including risk factors for HIV transmission, the regimen's toxicity, the ability to initiate medication within 72 hours of sexual contact, and the anticipated ability to adhere to the regimen (13).

Pregnancy risk and pregnancy prevention should be considered in all postmenarcheal girls. Although the risk of conception after unprotected coitus is negligible outside the 6 days before and 4 days after ovulation (<0.05%), the risk is as high as 14% to 17% from 3 days before to the day of ovulation. Unfortunately, many adolescents have irregular cycles, and few can pinpoint their ovulation days. Therefore all postmenarcheal girls should have a pregnancy test and be considered for pregnancy prophylaxis (216). Emergency contraception should be discussed with the adolescent if she is not pregnant and if less than 72 hours have elapsed since the assault. The most commonly used regimen is a combination of estrogen and progestin known as the Yupze method. The total dose of 200 µg of ethinyl estradiol plus 2.0 mg of norgestril can be given as two tablets of Ovral (0.05 mg ethinyl estradiol and 0.5 mg of *dl*-norgestril) given immediately, and an additional two tablets 12 hours later. Other combined pills can be used, and unit dose packaging is now available with the specific indication for emergency contraception. This treatment is 75% effective and reduces the pregnancy rate after unprotected intercourse to less than 2% if initiated within 72 hours of the sexual contact (22,115). Nausea (50%) and vomiting are common side effects, and antiemetics can be helpful. Menstruation occurs within 21 days in 95% of patients. If menstruation does not occur, both physiologic and psychological factors should be assessed (115,216).

Most acute genital and perianal injuries do not require surgical intervention. The primary therapy for acute injuries is maintaining proper hygiene. Sitz baths can be initiated after specimens for evidence and culture are collected to promote healing and to prevent secondary infections. Prophylactic broad-spectrum antibiotics are not generally indicated. Topical or oral antibiotics may be recommended for extensive injuries, but few data support their efficacy. Lubricating ointments or diaper creams may be helpful to reduce irritation. Nonstick dressings or absorbent pads may be considered in individual cases, but frequently changed cotton underwear may be sufficient. Small vulvar or perianal hematomas may be treated with pressure and ice packs. Large or enlarging hematomas or large lacerations may require a surgical or gynecologic consultation and treatment under anesthesia (61).

All children should have a follow-up appointment whether or not an acute injury or infection is present. In a child without initial injury or infection or with minor acute injury, this examination can be a time to reassure the child and the parents that no permanent phys-

ical damage has occurred. This "certification of physical wellness" may help some of the children avoid the "damaged goods" feelings commonly experienced by abused children. Children with more severe injury should be carefully followed up until healing is complete. They need assurance that residual scarring should not affect their health and functioning as adults.

Psychological Intervention

Numerous factors must be considered in assessing the child's responses to sexual abuse and need for treatment (19,118,164,189). Some data suggest that children may be more affected by abuse if they are abused for a longer duration, by a father or stepfather, with more force, by a male, or by an adult, or are victims who live in an unsupportive family or who are removed from their homes (51). Additional factors that may affect outcome relate to the child's age and stage of emotional and cognitive development, including aspects of the victim's perception, understanding, beliefs, and attitudes about the abuse (51). However, psychological outcome may have more to do with preexisting life circumstances, positive and negative, and individual vulnerability and compensatory and resiliency factors in the child than the characteristics of the abuse itself (46,104,217). At minimum, all sexually abused children should have a single follow-up visit after their initial evaluation with someone skilled in the assessment of emotional stress in the sexually abused child and his or her family. Assessment must consider the child's current psychosocial functioning, development, and family context. Many children may not require ongoing counseling. In such cases, the child and parents can be made aware of resources available for counseling if the need arises (248).

Treatment programs typically provide a variety of direct therapeutic and support services for the child and the family. The nature and sequence of treatment and services vary substantially depending on the specific needs of each case (164). However, services must be inclusive or coordinated, addressing victimization, perpetration, domestic violence, parent-al attachment, and family problems (121). Sexual behavior problems are particularly complex because both family factors and victims' sexual arousal and self-blame are important (126). Group therapy is often recommended for older children because it helps them realize that other children have had similar experiences (22,117). Maternal depression and parenting methods that are nonsupportive, rejecting, or controlling have a negative effect on child outcomes (67). Regardless of the family constellation and the perpetrator's identity, child sexual abuse is a crisis for the whole family. Children recover in the context of their families; the family can exacerbate the bad situation or facilitate recovery (51). Including protective caretakers in therapy is preferable. Individual, group, family, and parent therapy all have been used, but the modality used may be less important than the focus on the symptoms present (104).

Five primary areas must be addressed in each case. First, treatment should help the child feel safe. Second, counseling must also be considered for potentially abused or neglected siblings of the victim. Third, most families need help in dealing with the complexity and frustration of interventions. Fourth, therapy may be required to rehabilitate abusive parents and to improve overall parental and family functioning. Finally, therapy may be required to decrease the posttraumatic symptoms in the victim (118,189,191). Fear and anxiety tend to resolve more quickly than anger and inappropriate sexual behaviors. Therefore, the length of therapy is more a function of which symptoms are being treated (104). Cognitive behavioral therapy has been shown to reduce the symptoms of the posttraumatic distress disorder (67), depressive symptoms, and inappropriate sexual behaviors (49,66).

Legal Issues

Clinicians have an opportunity to collect certain forms of verbal and physical evidence that cannot be collected by other individuals (64). Physicians have four major legal responsibilities in child sexual abuse cases: appropriate reporting of suspected cases, examination of the child and collection of forensic evidence, documentation, and providing testimony as a fact or expert witness in court (17,179). The legal aspects of examination and evidence collection are discussed earlier in the chapter, and legal issues involved in criminal and civil court actions are discussed in another chapter. Therefore the focus of this section is on appropriate reporting and documentation.

Physicians are required to report suspected child abuse to the state child-protective service agency for further investigation in all 50 states. As mandated reporters, physicians are protected from suit by the alleged perpetrators if the suspicion proves to be unfounded. Physicians who fail to report suspected abuse may experience legal sanctions. Many states allow physicians to report suspected child sexual abuse by someone outside the family to either a law enforcement agency or to child-protective services. Most states require reporting to child-protective services if sexual abuse occurs within a family, by a nonfamily caretaker, or if it occurs because the parent has placed the child at unusual risk for abuse. If incest is suspected, most states require reporting to both child-protective services and law enforcement, because it is both a form of child abuse and a crime in most states (61,173). When behavior changes or a nonspecific history by a parent or child raises a concern in the absence of specific physical or laboratory findings, physicians may want to discuss such cases with their local or regional child abuse consultants as well as their local child-protective services agency before reporting. Some cases need to be reported because certain additional information is required to exclude the possibility of abuse. Physicians should remember that although they are not expected to perform a complete investigation before reporting, they should be able to articulate the reasons for their suspicion of abuse (9).

The legal implications of child sexual abuse demand careful documentation of the child's history, physical findings, and the collection of forensic materials. A medical record provides a description of medical care, serves as a means of communication among physicians, and is a legal document. As a legal document, the physician's records are accessible to both the prosecution and defense attorneys through a subpoena duces tecum, for presentation as evidence. Because the physician's record is created in the usual course of business, the physician's history of the abuse may be admissible when introduced under a business record exemption to the hearsay rule that would otherwise exclude hearsay evidence. Clear documentation of quotations in the child's own words and of factors that relate to the reliability of the child's statements can be one of the most important pieces of evidence of abuse. Good documentation, in some cases, encourages the perpetrator to confess, and in other situations, it provides the physician detailed information on which to base testimony in court (61,204). Particularly in civil or juvenile proceedings, a well-documented medical record may make it less likely that the physician will need to testify in court (9).

Prevention

Many efforts are directed toward identification of victims, and yet prevention is the ultimate goal in the management of child sexual abuse. Preventative efforts may be either primary, secondary, or tertiary. Primary prevention refers to approaches directed at the general population. Secondary prevention focuses on specific groups in the population who are considered at highest risk of abuse. Tertiary prevention involves intervention for the abused child, the perpetrator, and the family to lessen the emotional harm for the child and reduce the chances of repeated abuse (70,71). Primary preventive efforts are programs implemented in school systems and community organizations to teach children how to recognize abusive situations and how to respond assertively. Primary prevention programs have not provided an adequate solution

to the problem (265). Such programs are extremely variable in quality and quantity, and the positive and negative effects of these efforts have not been adequately studied. Some programs have found that the children do learn a few of the concepts presented, but whether this limited knowledge is translated into self-protective behaviors is not clear (54, 265). The learning is uneven, with older children 7 to 12 years of age and children with better self-esteem benefiting more. The most effective programs have shifted away from stressing the abstract concepts such as "good" touch and "bad" touch, and now emphasize building specific skills in such areas as assertive behavior, decision making, and communication (53). Further research is needed to explore what presentation styles, supplemental materials, and length of program are needed to allow children to incorporate the concepts taught into their behaviors (265). The most promising prevention programs are integrated into the school curricula, use developmentally appropriate curricula, and are presented in a simulating and varied manner. They emphasize the need for children to disclose any contact that makes them feel uneasy and allow adequate behavioral rehearsal of preventive strategies (54). Two potential benefits have been described. Anecdotal reports cite increases in disclosure during or after these programs, as children are provided with the message that it is all right to tell (70). Sexual abuse offenders themselves have stated that children who are taught about proper and improper touching, to say no to potential abusers, and to tell if they are abused are less likely to become victims (34). Most important, child abuse prevention can offer an opportunity for educators and parents to work together in creating safer environments for children. Training has resulted in more open discussions between parents and children and children and teachers (53). Parents should be encouraged to maintain open and trusting relationships so that the child feels comfortable telling the parent if "anything bad" should happen (71). These programs may have unforeseen costs, such as anxiety the children might feel or a hesitation of fathers about being physically affectionate toward their children. A few studies have revealed that some children are more leery of strangers and more uncertain about normal and abusive touches; some have even noted that a small percentage of participants experience more significant fear and anxiety. No study has documented that such effects last beyond the period immediately after the program (53,54).

Primary prevention could be incorporated by primary care physicians as sex and personal safety education during routine child care visits (154). Part of this anticipatory guidance should be to emphasize to parents that a child who is loved, is listened to, and has good self-esteem may be less likely to become a victim (34). Secondary prevention and educational and supportive services for high-risk groups have been used typically for the prevention of physical abuse. Specific efforts for sexual abuse prevention should also be directed toward children of substance abusers, children from single-parent or broken homes, children with neurobehavioral problems, and "latch key" children (70).

Tertiary prevention involves protective social service, counseling, and legal interventions after sexual abuse has been identified. Social service intervention involves social casework to monitor the family, providing family support services and initiating substitute foster care. Substitute foster care involves social service recommendations and the action of the civil or juvenile justice system to remove the child from home, monitor the child's placement, and reunify the family when it is feasible. This intervention also has its drawbacks, with overwhelming social service caseloads and lack of sufficient quality foster homes. Mental health interventions are often a major component of treatment programs, with counseling or psychotherapy for the child victim, for the nonoffending family members, and for the perpetrator (164,191). The potential impact of counseling is limited by a lack of self-motivation and adequate counseling services. Criminal prosecution and punishment of the perpetrator is perhaps the most controversial form of intervention. Prosecution demonstrates that the "crime" of child sexual abuse will not be tolerated, but whether it produces any general deterrent effect is unknown.

The efficacy of various primary, secondary, or tertiary efforts in preventing child sexual abuse has not been proven. Combinations of public and parent education, life skills development in children and young adults, support groups for vulnerable children and adults, and therapy for victims and their families may be expected to produce the best outcomes (54). Programs that teach children about sexual abuse and specific self-protective behaviors and anticipatory guidance during well-child visits may play a valuable role in providing improved parenting and self-protection skills. Physicians can help prevent child sexual abuse by being knowledgeable of community resources and by facilitating appropriate referrals. Some physicians may take a more active role in the evaluation and treatment of sexually abused children. Finally, all physicians should advocate public policies and social programs that help protect children and support families within their communities.

Multidisciplinary Team Approach

Effective assessment of the alleged child victim and intervention in the field of child maltreatment is the result of the collective insights of many professionals. The mechanism for achieving consensus and thus shared responsibility is the multidisciplinary team (MDT). Each discipline holds one piece of the puzzle, and until all of the interlocking pieces are joined, a full understanding of the child's experience and the needs of the victim and family will not be appreciated. The MDT is the mechanism to ensure improved coordination, better information gathering, and thus a more comprehensive assessment of an allegation. A comprehensive assessment assists in providing direction for the law enforcement, mental health, and the child-protection system to respond. When coordinated intervention occurs in a coordinated fashion, appropriate service needs can be identified early and delivered in a timely fashion.

The legal system can respond without compromising its focus and taking into account the needs of the victims and their families. Although valid statistics are lacking, the MDT is likely to lead to more successful prosecution when appropriate. The artificial turf issues in each discipline and the boundaries that exist to form the turf diminish with time, and all disciplines begin to interact to reflect a more global understanding of the system and the victim's needs.

Teams may be configured in many different ways with either a specific or a broad-based focus. Consultation teams that provide no direct client services may provide valuable input by reviewing case-management elements. Assessment and treatment teams have a specific client-based focus. Representatives of these teams can bring recommendations to the larger team for input into final disposition and service delivery (11,248). The issue of confidentiality must be addressed, with particular attention to how the team's discussions and recommendations are recorded. The confidentiality of the communication as well as discovery rules may vary from state to state.

The resources available within a given community in part define the members of the team. At a minimum, a representative from child protection, prosecutor's office, medicine, victim services, and mental health should be on the core team. The team can be expanded to include child-protection caseworker supervisors, resource-development specialists, deputy attorney general, and family court liaison. Representatives from the schools, local police, or a treating therapist can be invited to provide specific input that may be helpful to the team as needed (11). Other advantages, in addition to the basic case-management function of the team, include the ability to identify and address system problems, to provide a quality assurance assessment mechanism, and to educate fellow team members through formal or informal conferences to keep members current (11, 248). Teams provide an excellent opportunity

for clinicians to become involved in the child-protection system and to take a leadership role in their community. Medical clinicians functioning as a part of a team can educate team members concerning the scope of medicines' contributions in the field. In addition, medical clinicians can learn to appreciate the complexity of the system and then advocate for necessary changes that will positively affect children and their families, not achievable in the individual practitioners' offices. Working with abused children is gratifying and more than compensates for the emotionally difficult nature of this problem. Involvement of medical professionals in child protection is in its infancy. Clinicians who venture into this field can make significant contributions to the health and welfare of many children and their families.

REFERENCES

1. American College of Obstetrics and Gynecology. Sexual assault. *Int J Gynaecol Obstet* 1993;42:67–72.
2. Adams JA, Ahmad M, Philips P. Anogenital findings and hymenal diameter in children referred for sexual abuse examination. *Adolesc Pediatr Gynecol* 1988;1:123.
3. Alexander WJ, Griffith H, Housch JG, et al. Infections in sexual contacts and associates of children with gonorrhea. *Sex Transm Dis* 1984;11:156–158.
4. Alexander ER. Misidentification of sexually transmitted organisms in children: medicolegal implications. *Pediatr Infect Dis J* 1988;7:1–2.
5. Allard JE. The collection of data from findings in cases of sexual assault and the significance of spermatozoa on vaginal, anal and oral swabs. *Sci Justice* 1997;37:99–108.
6. American Academy of Dermatology. Genital warts and sexual abuse in children: American Academy Dermatology Task Force on Pediatric Dermatology. *J Am Acad Dermatol* 1984;11:529–530.
7. American Academy of Pediatrics Committee on Adolescence. Sexual assault and the adolescent. *Pediatrics* 1994;94:761–765.
8. American Academy of Pediatrics Committee on Child Abuse and Neglect. Gonorrhea in prepubertal children. *Pediatrics* 1998;101:134.
9. American Academy of Pediatrics Committee on Child Abuse and Neglect. Guidelines for the evaluation of sexual abuse of children: subject review [published erratum appears in *Pediatrics* 1999;103(5 Pt 1):1049]. *Pediatrics* 1999;103:186–191.
10. American Board of Forensic Odontology. Guidelines for bite mark analysis: American Board of Forensic Odontology. *J Am Dent Assoc* 1986;112:383–386.
11. American Prosecutors Research Institute National Center for Prosecution of Child Abuse. *Investigation*

and prosecution of child abuse. Alexandria, VA: American Prosecutors Institute, 1987.

12. Annas GJ. Setting standards for the use of DNA-typing results in the courtroom: the state of the art. *N Engl J Med* 1992;326:1641–1644.

13. Atabaki S, Paradise JE. The medical evaluation of the sexually abused child: lessons from a decade of research. *Pediatrics* 1999;104(1 Pt 2):178–186.

14. Bach CM, Anderson SC. Adolescent sexual abuse and assault. *J Curr Adolesc Med* 1980;1:12–15.

15. Badgley RF, et al. *Sexual offenses against children.* Ottawa, Canada: Minister of Supply and Services, 1984.

16. Baker RB. Seat belt injury masquerading as sexual abuse [Letter]. *Pediatrics* 1986;77:435.

17. Baum E, Grodin MA, Alpert JJ, et al. Child sexual abuse, criminal justice, and the pediatrician. *Pediatrics* 1987;79:437–439.

18. Bays J, et al. Changes in hymenal anatomy during examination of prepubertal girls for possible sexual abuse. *Adolesc Pediatr Gynecol* 1990;3:42.

19. Beck-Sague CM, Solomon F. Sexually transmitted diseases in abused children and adolescent and adult victims of rape: review of selected literature. *Clin Infect Dis* 1999;28(suppl 1):S74–S83.

20. Becker JV. What we know about the characteristics and treatment of adolescents who have committed sexual offenses. *Child Maltreat* 1998;3:317.

21. Berenson A, Heger A, Andrews S. Appearance of the hymen in newborns. *Pediatrics* 1991;87:458–465.

22. Berkowitz CD. Sexual abuse of children and adolescents. *Adv Pediatr* 1987;34:275–312.

23. Berkowitz CD, Elvik SL, Logan MK. Labial fusion in prepubescent girls: a marker for sexual abuse? *Am J Obstet Gynecol* 1987;156:16–20.

24. Berkowitz CD, Elvik SL, Logan M. A simulated "acquired" imperforate hymen following the genital trauma of sexual abuse. *Clin Pediatr Phila* 1987;26:307–309.

25. Berkowitz CD. Medical consequences of child sexual abuse. *Child Abuse Negl* 1998;22:541–550; discussion 551–554.

26. Berliner L, Conte JR. The process of victimization: the victims' perspective. *Child Abuse Negl* 1990;14:29–40.

27. Biggs M, Stermac LE, Divinsky M. Genital injuries following sexual assault of women with and without prior sexual intercourse experience. *CMAJ* 1998;159:33–37.

28. *Black's law dictionary.* 5th ed. St. Paul, MN: West Publishing, 1979.

29. Boat BW, Everson MD. Use of anatomical dolls among professionals in sexual abuse evaluations. *Child Abuse Negl* 1988;12:171–179.

30. Bond GR, Dowd MD, Landsman I, et al. Unintentional perineal injury in prepubescent girls: a multicenter, prospective report of 56 girls. *Pediatrics* 1995;95: 628–623.

31. Boos SC. Accidental hymenal injury mimicking sexual trauma. *Pediatrics* 1999;103(6 Pt 1):1287–1290.

32. Briere JN, Elliott DM. Immediate and long-term impacts of child sexual abuse. *Future Child* 1994;4:54–69.

33. Browne A, Finkelhor D. Impact of child sexual abuse: a review of the research. *Psychol Bull* 1986;99:66–77.

34. Budin LE, Johnson CF. Sex abuse prevention programs: offenders' attitudes about their efficacy. *Child Abuse Negl* 1989;13:77–87.

35. Bump RC. *Chlamydia trachomatis* as a cause of prepubertal vaginitis. *Obstet Gynecol* 1985;65:384–388.

36. Bump RC, Buesching WJD. Bacterial vaginosis in virginal and sexually active adolescent females: evidence against exclusive sexual transmission. *Am J Obstet Gynecol* 1988;158:935–939.

37. Burgess AW, Holmstrom LL. Sexual trauma of children and adolescents. *Nurs Clin North Am* 1975;10:551–563.

38. Burgess AW, Holmstrom LL. Coping behavior of the rape victim. *Am Psychiatry* 1976;133:413–418.

39. Cantwell H. Vaginal inspection as it relates to child sexual abuse in girls under thirteen. *Child Abuse Negl* 1981;7:171.

40. Centers for Disease Control and Prevention. Guidelines for treatment of sexually transmitted diseases. *MMWR* 1993;42(RR-1):1–111.

41. Centers for Disease Control and Prevention. Youth risk behavior surveillance–United States. *MMWR* 1996;45(SS-4):1.

42. Centers for Disease Control and Prevention. Management of possible sexual, injecting-drug-use, or other nonoccupational exposure to HIV, including considerations related to antiretroviral therapy: Public Health Service statement. *MMWR* 1998;47(RR-17):1.

43. Centers for Disease Control and Prevention. Guidelines for treatment of sexually transmitted diseases. *MMWR* 1998;47(RR-1):1–111.

44. Chadwick DL, et al. *Color atlas of child sexual abuse.* Chicago: Year Book, 1989.

45. Christian CW, Lavelle JM, De Jong AR, et al. Forensic evidence collection in prepubertal victims of sexual assault. *Pediatrics* 2000;106:100–104.

46. Cicchetti D, Toth SL. A developmental psychopathology perspective on child abuse and neglect. *J Am Acad Child Adolesc Psychiatry* 1995;34:541–565.

47. Clayden GS. Reflex anal dilatation associated with severe chronic constipation in children [see comments]. *Arch Dis Child* 1988;63:832–836.

48. Cohen BA, Honig P, Androphy E. Anogenital warts in children: clinical and virologic evaluation for sexual abuse [see comments]. *Arch Dermatol* 1990;126: 1575–1580.

49. Cohen JA, Mannarino AP. Intervention for sexually abused children: initial treatment outcome findings. *Child Maltreatment* 1998;3:17–26.

50. Conte JR, Berliner L. The Impact of sexual abuse on children: empirical findings. In: Walker LEA, ed. *Handbook on sexual abuse of children:* assessment and treatment issues. New York: Springer, 1988: 72–93.

51. Conte JR. Forensic and mental health issues in child sexual abuse. In: Krugman RD, Leventhal JM, eds. *Child sexual abuse: report of the twenty-second Ross roundtable on critical approaches to common pediatrics problems.* Columbus: Ross Laboratories, 1991:85–95.

52. Corwin DL, ed. Child sexual abuse and custody disputes. In: Krugman RD, Leventhal JM, eds. *Child sexual abuse: report of the twenty-second Ross roundtable on critical approaches to common pediatrics problems.* Columbus: Ross Laboratories, 1991:35–41.

53. Daro D. Child sexual abuse prevention: separating fact from fiction. *Child Abuse Negl* 1991;15:1–4.

54. Daro DA. Prevention of child sexual abuse. *Future Child* 1994;4:98–223.

55. Davies J. Anatomy of the female genital tract. In: Danforth D, ed. *Danforth's obstetrics and gynecology.* 6th ed. Philadelphia: Lippincott, 1990:1–39.

56. Davis AJ, Emans SJ. Human papilloma virus infection in the pediatric and adolescent patient [see comments]. *J Pediatr* 1989;115:1–9.

57. DeJong AR, Emment GA, Hervada AR. Epidemiologic factors in the sexual abuse of boys. *Am J Dis Child* 1982;136:990.

58. DeJong AR, Emment GA, Hervada AR. Sexual abuse of children: sex-race and age dependent variations. *Am J Dis Child* 1982;136:129.

59. DeJong AR, Weiss JW, Brent RL. Condyloma acuminata in children. *Am J Dis Child* 1982;136:704.

60. DeJong AR. Sexually transmitted diseases in sexually abused children. *Sex Transm Dis* 1986;13:123.

61. DeJong AR, Emans SJ, Goldfarb A. Sexual abuse: what you must know? *Patient Care* 1989;23:145.

62. DeJong AR. Sexual interaction among siblings and cousins: experimentation or exploitation? *Child Abuse Negl* 1989;13:271.

63. DeJong AR, Rose M. Legal proof of child sexual abuse in the absence of physical evidence. *Pediatrics* 1991;88:506.

64. DeJong AR. Impact of child sexual abuse medical examinations on the dependency and criminal systems. *Child Abuse Negl* 1998;22:645–652; discussion 653–660.

65. Deblinger E, McLeer SV, Atkins MS, et al. Post-traumatic stress in sexually abused, physically abused, and nonabused children. *Child Abuse Negl* 1989;13:403–408.

66. Deblinger E, Lippman J, Steer R. Sexually abused children suffering posttraumatic stress syndromes: initial treatment outcome findings. *Child Maltreat* 1996;1:310.

67. Deblinger E, Steer R. Maternal factors associated with sexually abused children's' psychosocial adjustment. *Child Maltreat* 1999;4:13–16.

68. Deuterman JL, Gabby SL. Imperforate hymen. *Illinois Med J* 1942;82:161.

69. Dowd MD, Fitzmaurice L, Knapp JF, et al. The interpretation of urogenital findings in children with straddle injuries. *J Pediatr Surg* 1994;29:7–10.

70. Dubowitz H. Prevention of child maltreatment: what is known? *Pediatrics* 1989;83:570–577.

71. Dubowitz H. Pediatrician's role in preventing child maltreatment. *Pediatr Clin North Am* 1990;37:989–1002.

72. Edwards LC, Dunphy JE. Wound healing in injury and normal repair. *N Engl J Med* 1956;259:224.

73. Elders MJ, Albert AE. Adolescent pregnancy and sexual abuse [see comments]. *JAMA* 1998;280:648–649.

74. Ellerstein NS, Canavan JW. Sexual abuse of boys. *Am J Dis Child* 1980;134:255–257.

75. Elvik SL, Berkowitz CD, Nicholas E, et al. Sexual abuse in the developmentally disabled: dilemmas of diagnosis. *Child Abuse Negl* 1990;14:497–502.

76. Emans SJ, Goldstein DP. The gynecologic examination of the prepubertal child with vulvovaginitis: use of the knee-chest position. *Pediatrics* 1980;65:758–760.

77. Emans SJ, Woods ER, Flagg NT, et al. Genital findings in sexually abused, symptomatic and asymptomatic, girls. *Pediatrics* 1987;79:778–785.

78. Emans SJ, Woods ER, Alfred EN, et al. Hymenal findings in adolescent women: impact of tampon use and consensual sexual activity. *J Pediatr* 1994;125:153–160.

79. Enos WF, Conrath TB, Byer JC. Forensic evaluation of the sexually abused child. *Pediatrics* 1986;78:385–398.

80. Everstine DS, Everstine L. *Sexual trauma in children and adolescents.* New York: Brunner/Mazel, 1988.

81. Faller KC. Characteristics of a clinical sample of sexually abused children: how boy and girl victims differ. *Child Abuse Negl* 1989;13:281–291.

82. Faller KC. A clinical sample of women who have sexually abused children. *J Child Sexual Abuse* 1995;4:3.

83. Farber SJ, et al. The sexual abuse in children: a comparison of male and female victims. *J Clin Child Psychol* 1984;13:294.

84. Feherenbach PA, et al. Adolescent sexual offenders: offender and offense characteristics. *Am J Orthopsychiatry* 1986;56:225.

85. Feldman W, Feldman E, Goodman JT, et al. Is childhood sexual abuse really increasing in prevalence? An analysis of the evidence. *Pediatrics* 1991;88:29–33.

86. Felice M, Grant J, Reynolds B, et al. Follow-up observations of adolescent rape victims: "rape may be one of the more serious afflictions of adolescence with respect to long-term psychosocial effects." *Clin Pediatr Phila* 1978;17:311–315.

87. Ferris DG, Willner WA, Ho JJ. Colpophotography systems: a review [published erratum appears in *J Fam Pract* 1992;34:25]. *J Fam Pract* 1991;33:633–639.

88. Finkel MA. Anogenital trauma in sexually abused children. *Pediatrics* 1989;84:317–322.

89. Finkel MA, Ricci LR. Documentation and preservation of visual evidence in child abuse. *Child Maltreat* 1997;2:322–330.

90. Finkel MA. Technical conduct of the child sexual abuse medical examination. *Child Abuse Negl* 1998;22:555–566.

91. Finkelhor DH. *Sexually victimized children.* New York: The Free Press, 1979.

92. Finkelhor D. Sex among siblings: a survey on prevalence, variety, and effects. *Arch Sex Behav* 1980;9:171–194.

93. Finkelhor D, Hotaling GT. Sexual abuse in the National Incidence Study of Child Abuse and Neglect: an appraisal. *Child Abuse Negl* 1984;8:23–32.

94. Finkelhor D, Browne A. The traumatic impact of child sexual abuse: a conceptualization. *Am J Orthopsychiatry* 1985;55:530–541.

95. Finkelhor D, Williams L, Burn N. *Nursery crimes: sexual abuse in daycare.* London: Sage Publications, 1988.

96. Finkelhor DH, Browne A. Assessing the long term impact on child sexual abuse: a review and conceptualization. In: Walker LEA, ed. *Handbook on sexual abuse of children: assessment and treatment issues.* New York: Springer, 1988:55–71.

97. Finkelhor D, Hotaling G, Lewis IA, et al. Sexual abuse in a national survey of adult men and women: prevalence, characteristics, and risk factors. *Child Abuse Negl* 1990;14:19–28.

98. Finkelhor D, Dziuba-Leatherman J. Children as victims of violence: a national survey. *Pediatrics* 1994;94(4 Pt 1):413–420.

99. Finkelhor D. Current information on the scope and nature of child sexual abuse. *Future Child* 1994;4:31–53.

100. Finkelhor D. The victimization of children: a developmental perspective. *Am J Orthopsychiatry* 1995;65:177–193.

101. Finkelhor DH, ed. *Child sexual abuse: new theory and research.* New York: The Free Press, 1984.

102. Folland DS, Burke RE, Hinman AR, et al. Gonorrhea

in preadolescent children: an inquiry into source of infection and mode of transmission. *Pediatrics* 1977;60: 153–156.

103. Friedrich WN, Grambsch P, Broughton D, et al. Normative sexual behavior in children. *Pediatrics* 1991; 88:456–464.

104. Friedrich WN. Clinical considerations of empirical treatment studies of abused children. *Child Maltreat* 1996;1:343.

105. Friedrich WN. Behavioral manifestations of child sexual abuse. *Child Abuse Negl* 1998;22:523–531; discussion 533–539.

106. Friedrich WN, Fisher J, Broughton D, et al. Normative sexual behavior in children: a contemporary sample. *Pediatrics* 1998;101:E9.

107. Gabby T, Winkleby MA, Boyce WT, et al. Sexual abuse of children: the detection of semen on skin. *Am J Dis Child* 1992;146:700–703.

108. Gallup Organization. *Disciplining children in America.* Princeton, NJ: 1995.

109. Gardner M, Jones JG. Genital herpes acquired by sexual abuse of children. *J Pediatr* 1984;104:243–244.

110. Gelhor G. Anatomy, pathology and development of the hymen. *Am J Obstet Dis Women Child* 1904;50:161.

111. Gellert GA, Durfee MJ, Berkowitz CD, et al. Situational and sociodemographic characteristics of children infected with human immunodeficiency virus from pediatric sexual abuse. *Pediatrics* 1993;91:39–44.

112. Giardino AP, Finkel MA. *A practical guide to the evaluation of sexual abuse in the prepubertal child.* Newbury Park: Sage Publications, 1992.

113. Gill P, Jeffreys AJ, Werrett DJ. Forensic application of DNA "fingerprints." *Nature* 1985;318:577–579.

114. Ginsberg CM. Acquired syphilis in prepubertal children. *Pediatr Infect Dis* 1983;2:232.

115. Glasier A. Emergency postcoital contraception [see comments]. *N Engl J Med* 1997;337:1058–1064.

116. Goff CW, Burke KR, Rickenbach C, et al. Vaginal opening measurement in prepubertal girls. *Am J Dis Child* 1989;143:1366–1368.

117. Goodwin J. Family violence: principles of intervention and prevention. *Hosp Commun Psychiatry* 1985;36: 1074–1079.

118. Goodwin J. Evaluation and treatment for incest victims and their families: a problem-oriented approach. In: Goodwon J, ed. *Sexual abuse.* Chicago: Yearbook, 1989:1–18.

119. Graves HC, Sensabaugh GF, Blake ET. Postcoital detection of a male-specific semen protein: application to the investigation of rape. *N Engl J Med* 1985;312:338–343.

120. Gray HT, ed. *Anatomy of the human body.* Philadelphia: Lea & Febiger, 1985.

121. Gray A, Pithers WD, Busconi A, et al. Developmental and etiological characteristics of children with sexual behavior problems: treatment implications [see comments]. *Child Abuse Negl* 1999;23:601–621.

122. Green AH. True and false allegations of sexual abuse in child custody disputes. *J Am Acad Child Psychiatry* 1986;25:449.

123. Green AH, ed. Overview of normal psychosexual development. In: Schetky DK, Green AH, eds. *Child sexual abuse:* a handbook for health care and legal professionals. New York: Brunner Mazel, 1988:12–21.

124. Gutman LT, St. Clair KK, Weedy C, et al. Human immunodeficiency virus transmission by child sexual abuse [see comments]. *Am J Dis Child* 1991;145: 137–141.

125. Gutman LT, St. Clair KK, Everett VD, et al. Cervical-vaginal and intraanal human papillomavirus infection of young girls with external genital warts. *J Infect Dis* 1994;170:339–344.

126. Hall DK, Mathews F, Pearce J. Factors associated with sexual behavior problems in young sexually abused children [see comments]. *Child Abuse Negl* 1998;22: 1045–1063.

127. Hammerschlag MR, Doraiswamy B, Alexander ER, et al. Are rectogenital chlamydial infections a marker of sexual abuse in children? *Pediatr Infect Dis* 1984;3: 100–104.

128. Hammerschlag MR, Cummings M, Doraiswamy B, et al. Nonspecific vaginitis following sexual abuse in children. *Pediatrics* 1985;75:1028–1031.

129. Hammerschlag MR, Doraiswamy B, Cox P, et al. Colonization of sexually abused children with genital mycoplasmas. *Sex Transm Dis* 1987;14:23–25.

130. Hammerschlag MR, Rettig PJ, Shields ME. False positive results with the use of chlamydial antigen detection tests in the evaluation of suspected sexual abuse in children. *Pediatr Infect Dis J* 1988;7:11–14.

131. Hammerschlag MR. Sexually transmitted diseases in sexually abused children. *Adv Pediatr Infect Dis* 1988; 3:1–18.

132. Hammerschlag MR. Chlamydial infections. *J Pediatr* 1989;114:727–734.

133. Hammerschlag MR. The transmissibility of sexually transmitted diseases in sexually abused children. *Child Abuse Negl* 1998;22:623–635; discussion 637–643.

134. Hammerschlag MR, Ajl S, Laraque D. Inappropriate use of nonculture tests for the detection of *Chlamydia trachomatis* in suspected victims of child sexual abuse: a continuing problem. *Pediatrics* 1999;104(5 Pt 1): 1137–1139.

135. Hanson RM, Glasson M, McCrossin I, et al. Anogenital warts in childhood [see comments]. *Child Abuse Negl* 1989;13:225–233.

136. Heger A, Emans SJ. Introital diameter as the criterion for sexual abuse [comment]. *Pediatrics* 1990;85:222–223.

137. Herman-Giddens ME, Frothingham TE. Prepubertal female genitalia: examination for evidence of sexual abuse. *Pediatrics* 1987;80:203–208.

138. Herr JC, Summers TA, McGee RS, et al. Characterization of monoclonal antibody to a conserved epitope on human seminal vesicle-specific peptides. *Biol Reprod* 1986;35:773.

139. Hobbs CJ, Wynne JM. Buggery in childhood: a common syndrome of child abuse. *Lancet* 1986;2:792–796.

140. Hobbs CJ, Wynne JM. Sexual abuse of English boys and girls: the importance of anal examination. *Child Abuse Negl* 1989;13:195–210.

141. Holmes WC, Slap GB. Sexual abuse of boys: definition, prevalence, correlates, sequelae, and management [see comments]. *JAMA* 1998;280:1855–1862.

142. Horowitz S, Chadwick DL. Syphilis as a sole indicator of sexual abuse: two cases with no intervention. *Child Abuse Negl* 1990;14:129–132.

143. Hunter RS, Kilstrom N, Loda F. Sexually abused children: identifying masked presentations in a medical setting. *Child Abuse Negl* 1985;9:17–25.

144. Ingram DL, White ST, Occhiuti AR, et al. Childhood vaginal infections: association of *Chlamydia tra-*

chomatis with sexual contact. *Pediatr Infect Dis* 1986;5:226–229.

145. Ingram DL, Controversies about the sexual and non-sexual transmission of adult STDs to children. In: Krugman RD, Leventhal JM, eds. *Child sexual abuse: report of the twenty second Ross roundtable on critical approaches to common pediatric problems.* Columbus: Ross Laboratories, 1991:14–28.

146. Ingram DL, Everett VD, Lyna PR, et al. Epidemiology of adult sexually transmitted disease agents in children being evaluated for sexual abuse. *Pediatr Infect Dis J* 1992;11:945–950.

147. Ingram DL, Everett VD, Flick LAR, et al. Vaginal gonococcal cultures in sexual abuse evaluations: evaluation of selective criteria for preteenaged girls. *Pediatrics* 1997;99:E8.

148. Ingram DL. The transmissibility of sexually transmitted diseases in sexually abused children: response to recommendations for a medical research agenda. *Child Abuse Negl* 1998;22:637.

149. Itzin C. Pornography and the organization of intra- and extrafamilial child sexual abuse: a conceptual model. In: Kantor JL, ed. *Out of the darkness: contemporary perspectives on family violence.* Thousand Oaks, CA: 1997:58.

150. Jaffee AC, Dynneson L, TenBensel RW. Sexual abuse of children: an epidemiologic study. *Am J Dis Child* 1975;129:689.

151. Jampole L, Weber MK. An assessment of the behavior of sexually abused and nonsexually abused children with anatomically correct dolls. *Child Abuse Negl* 1987;11:187–192.

152. Jason JM. Abuse, neglect, and the HIV-infected child. *Child Abuse Negl* 1991;15(suppl 1):79–88.

153. Jenison SA, Yu XP, Valentine JM, et al. Evidence of prevalent genital-type human papillomavirus infections in adults and children. *J Infect Dis* 1990;162: 60–69.

154. Jenny C, Sutherland SE, Sandahl BB. Developmental approach to preventing the sexual abuse of children. *Pediatrics* 1986;78:1034–1038.

155. Jenny C, Kuhns ML, Arakawa F. Hymens in newborn female infants. *Pediatrics* 1987;80:399–400.

156. Jenny C, Hooton PM, Bowers A, et al. Sexually transmitted diseases in victims of rape [see comments]. *N Engl J Med* 1990;322:713–716.

157. Jenny C, Roesler TA, Poyer KL. Are children at risk for sexual abuse by homosexuals? [see comments]. *Pediatrics* 1994;94:41–44.

158. Jones DPH, McQuiston M. Interviewing the sexually abused child. In: *The C. Henry Kempe National Center for the Prevention and Treatment of Child Abuse and Neglect.* Denver, Colorado; University of Colorado,1985.

159. Jones JG, Yamauchi T, Lambert B. *Trichomonas vaginalis* infestation in sexually abused girls. *Am J Dis Child* 1985;139:846–847.

160. Jones DPH, McGraw JM. Reliable and fictitious accounts of sexual abuse to children. *J Interpers Violence* 1987;2:27.

161. Kadish HA, Schunk JE, Britton H. Pediatric male rectal and genital trauma: accidental and nonaccidental injuries [see comments]. *Pediatr Emerg Care* 1998; 14:95–98.

162. Kaplan KM, Fleisher GR, Paradise JE, et al. Social rel-

163. Katz RC. Psychosocial adjustment in adolescent child molesters. *Child Abuse Negl* 1990;14:567–575.

164. Keller RA, Cicchinelli LF, Gardner DM. Characteristics of child sexual abuse treatment programs. *Child Abuse Negl* 1989;13:361–368.

165. Kellogg ND, Parra JM, Menard S. Children with anogenital symptoms and signs referred for sexual abuse evaluations. *Arch Pediatr Adolesc Med* 1998; 152:634–641.

166. Kempe CH. Sexual abuse, another hidden pediatric problem: the 1977 C. Anderson Aldrich lecture. *Pediatrics* 1978;62:382–389.

167. Kendall-Tackett KA, Williams LM, Finkelhor D. Impact of sexual abuse on children: a review and synthesis of recent empirical studies. *Psychol Bull* 1993;113: 164–180.

168. Kercher GA, McShane M. The prevalence of child sexual abuse victimization in an adult sample of Texas residents. *Child Abuse Negl* 1984;8:495–501.

169. Kinsey AC, et al. *Sexual behavior and the human female.* Philadelphia: WB Saunders, 1953.

170. Kissane, ed. Inflammation and healing. In: Kissane JM, ed. *Anderson's pathology.* 8th ed. St. Louis: CV Mosby, 1985:xx–xx.

171. Klevan JL, DeJong AR. Urinary tract symptoms and urinary tract infection following sexual abuse [see comments]. *Am J Dis Child* 1990;144:242–244.

172. Koop CE. *The Surgeon General's letter on child sexual abuse.* Rockville, MD: Department of Health and Human Services, 1988.

173. Krugman RD. Recognition of sexual abuse in children. *Pediatr Rev* 1986;8:25–30.

174. Ladson S, Johnson CF, Doty RE. Do physicians recognize sexual abuse? *Am J Dis Child* 1987;141:411–415.

175. Lamb S, Coakley M. "Normal" childhood sexual play and games: differentiating play from abuse. *Child Abuse Negl* 1993;17:515–526.

176. Lande MB, Richardson AC, White KC. The role of syphilis serology in the evaluation of suspected sexual abuse. *Pediatr Infect Dis J* 1992;11:125–127.

177. Lander ES. DNA fingerprinting on trial [see comments]. *Nature* 1989;339:501–505.

178. Landis J. Experiences of 500 children with adult sexual deviants. *Psychiatry* 1956;30(suppl):91.

179. Landwirth J. Children as witnesses in child sexual abuse trials. *Pediatrics* 1987;80:585–589.

180. Lanning K, Burgess AW. Child pornography and sex rings. *Federal Bureau of Investigation Law Enforcement Bulletin* 1984;53:10–16.

181. Lanning K. *Child molesters: a behavioral analysis for law enforcement.* Quantico, VA: Department of Justice, 1986.

182. Lanning KV. Cyber "pedophiles": a behavioral perspective. *APSAC Advisor* 1998;11:12.

183. Lauber AA, Souma ML. Use of toluidine blue for documentation of traumatic intercourse. *Obstet Gynecol* 1982;60:644–648.

184. Leaman KN, Knasel AL, ed. Developmental sexuality. In: MacFarlane K, Jones BM, Jenstrom LL, eds. *Sexual abuse of children:* selected readings. Washington, DC: U.S. Government Printing Office, DHHS, 1980: 14–19.

185. Leventhal JM. Have there been changes in the epi-

demiology of sexual abuse of children during the 20th century? *Pediatrics* 1988;82:766–773.

186. Leventhal JM. Epidemiology of sexual abuse of children: old problems, new directions. *Child Abuse Negl* 1998;22:481–491.

187. Lindblad F, Gustafsson PA, Larsson L, et al. Preschoolers' sexual behavior at daycare centers: an epidemiological study. *Child Abuse Negl* 1995;19: 569–577.

188. Lindegren ML, Hanson IC, Hammett TA, et al. Sexual abuse of children: intersection with the HIV epidemic. *Pediatrics* 1998;102:E46.

189. Long S. Guidelines for treating young children. In: MacFarlane K, ed. *Sexual abuse of young children.* New York: The Guilford Press, 1987:220–242.

190. Lynch L, Faust J. Reduction of distress in children undergoing sexual abuse medical examination. *J Pediatr* 1998;133:296–299.

191. MacFarelane K, Bulkley J. Treating child sexual abuse: an overview of program models. In: Conte DSJ, ed. *Social work and child sexual abuse*, New York: Howorth Press, 1982:145–157.

192. MacFarlane K, Kerbs S. Techniques for interviewing and evidence gathering. In: MacFarlane K, ed. *Sexual abuse of young children.* New York: The Guilford Press, 1987:68–98.

193. Macklin M. "Honeymoon cystitis" [Letter]. *N Engl J Med* 1978;298:1035.

194. MacNaulty AS. *British medical dictionary.* Philadelphia: Lippincott, 1961.

195. Mahran M, Salph AM. The microscopic anatomy of hymen. *Anat Rec* 1964;149:313–318.

196. McCann J, Voris J, Simon M. Labial adhesions and posterior fourchette injuries in childhood sexual abuse. *Am J Dis Child* 1988;142:659–663.

197. McCann J, Voris J, Simon M, et al. Perianal findings in prepubertal children selected for nonabuse: a descriptive study [see comments]. *Child Abuse Negl* 1989;13: 179–193.

198. McCann J, Wells R, Simon M, et al. Genital findings in prepubertal girls selected for nonabuse: a descriptive study. *Pediatrics* 1990;86:428–439.

199. McCann J. Use of the colposcope in childhood sexual abuse examinations. *Pediatr Clin North Am* 1990;37: 863–880.

200. McCann J, Voris J, Simon M. Genital injuries resulting from sexual abuse: a longitudinal study. *Pediatrics* 1992;89:307–317.

201. McCann J, Voris J. Perianal injuries resulting from sexual abuse: a longitudinal study. *Pediatrics* 1993;91: 390–397.

202. McCann J. The appearance of acute, healing, and healed anogenital trauma. *Child Abuse Negl* 1998;22: 605–615; discussion 617–622.

203. Merlob P, Bahari C, Liban E, et al. Cysts of the female external genitalia in the newborn infant. *Am J Obstet Gynecol* 1978;132:607–610.

204. Meyers JEB. Role of physician in preserving verbal evidence of child abuse. *J Pediatr* 1986;109:409.

205. Mor N, Merlob P, Reiner SH. Tags and bands of the female external genitalia in the newborn infant. *Clin Pediatr* 1983;22:122.

206. Morgan SR. *Abuse and neglect of handicapped children.* Boston: Little, Brown, 1987.

207. Muram D. Anal and perianal abnormalities in prepu-

bertal victims of sexual abuse. *Am J Obstet Gynecol* 1989;161:278–281.

208. Muram D. Child sexual abuse: relationship between sexual acts and genital findings. *Child Abuse Negl* 1989;13:211–216.

209. National Academy of Science. The evaluation of forensic DNA evidence: excerpt from the executive summary of the National Research Council Report [see comments]. *Proc Natl Acad Sci U S A* 1997;94:5498–5500.

210. National Center on Child Abuse and Neglect, Study Findings. *Study of national incidence and prevalence of child abuse and neglect.* Washington, DC: U.S. Department of Health and Human Services, 1988.

211. National Research Council Report. The evaluation of forensic DNA evidence: excerpt from the executive summary of the National Research Council Report [see comments]. *Proc Natl Acad Sci U S A* 1997;94:5498–5000.

212. Neinstein LS, Goldenring J, Carpenter S. Nonsexual transmission of sexually transmitted diseases: an infrequent occurrence. *Pediatrics* 1984;74:67–76.

213. Norrel MK, Benrub GI, Thompson RJ. Investigation of the microtrauma after sexual intercourse. *J Reprod Med* 1984;29:269.

214. Paradise JE, Rostain AL, Nathanson M. Substantiation of sexual abuse charges when parents dispute custody or visitation [see comments]. *Pediatrics* 1988;81:835–839.

215. Paradise JE. Predictive accuracy and the diagnosis of sexual abuse: a big issue about a little tissue. *Child Abuse Negl* 1989;13:169–176.

216. Paradise JE. The medical evaluation of the sexually abused child. *Pediatr Clin North Am* 1990;37: 839–862.

217. Paradise JE, Rose L, Sleeper LA, et al. Behavior, family function, school performance, and predictors of persistent disturbance in sexually abused children. *Pediatrics* 1994;93:452–459.

218. Paradise JE, Finkel MA, Beiser AS, et al. Assessments of girl's genital findings and the likelihood of sexual abuse: agreement among physicians self-rated as skilled. *Arch Pediatr Adolesc Med* 1997;151:883–891.

219. Paradise JE, Winter MR, Finkel MA, et al. Influence of the history on physicians' interpretations of girls' genital findings. *Pediatrics* 1999;103(5 Pt 1):980–986.

220. Parker RI, Mahan RA, Gingliano D, et al. Efficacy and safety of intravenous midazolam and ketamine as sedation for therapeutic and diagnostic procedures in children [see comments]. *Pediatrics* 1997;99:427–431.

221. Paul DM. The medical examination in sexual offenses. *Med Sci Law* 1975;15:154.

222. Paul DM. The medical examination in sexual offenses against children. *Med Sci Law* 1977;17.

223. Paul DM. What really happened to baby Jane? The medical aspects of the investigation of alleged sexual abuse of children. *Med Sci Law* 1986;26:85.

224. Pokorny SF. Configuration of the prepubertal hymen. *Am J Obstet Gynecol* 1987;157(4 Pt 1):950–956.

225. Pritchard JA, ed. Anatomy of the reproductive tract of woman. In: Cunningham FG, MacDonald PC, Grant NC, eds. *Williams Obstetrics.* 17th Ed. Norwalk, CT: Appleton-Century-Crofts, 1985:7–13.

226. Rapps WR. Scientific evidence in rape prosecution. *Univ Missouri Kansas City Law Rev* 1980;48:216.

227. Reinhart MA. Sexually abused boys. *Child Abuse Negl* 1987;11:229–235.

228. Reinhart MA. Urinary tract infection in sexually abused children. *Clin Pediatr Phila* 1987;26:470–472.

229. Rettig PJ, Nelson JD. Genital tract infection with *Chlamydia trachomatis* in prepubertal children. *J Pediatr* 1981;99:206–210.

230. Ricci LR, Hoffman SA. Prostatic acid phosphatase and sperm in the postcoital vagina. *Ann Emerg Med* 1982;11:530–534.

231. Ricci LR. Medical forensic photography of the sexually abused child. *Child Abuse Negl* 1988;12:305–310.

232. Rimza ME, Niggeman MS. Medical evaluation of sexually abused children: a review of 311 cases. *Pediatrics* 1982;69:8.

233. Rock B, Naghashfar Z, Barnett N, et al. Genital tract papillomavirus infection in children. *Arch Dermatol* 1986;122:1129–1132.

234. Roe RJ. Expert testimony in child sexual abuse cases. *Univ Miami Law Rev* 1985;40:97.

235. Rosenfeld AA, ed. Sexual abuse of children: personal and professional responses. In: Newberger EH, ed. *Child Abuse.* Boston: Little, Brown, 1982:57–89.

236. Rosenfeld AA, Wenegrat AO, Haavik DK, et al. Sleeping patterns in upper-middle-class families when the child awakens ill or frightened. *Arch Gen Psychiatry* 1982;39:943–947.

237. Rosenfeld A, Bailey R, Siegel B,et al. Determining incestuous contact between parent and child: frequency of children touching parents' genitals in a nonclinical population. *J Am Acad Child Psychiatry* 1986;25:481–484.

238. Rosenfeld AA, Siegel B, Bailey R. Familial bathing patterns: implications for cases of alleged molestation and for pediatric practice. *Pediatrics* 1987;79:224–229.

239. Russell DE. The incidence and prevalence of intrafamilial and extrafamilial sexual abuse of female children. *Child Abuse Negl* 1983;7:133–146.

240. Russell DE. The prevalence and seriousness of incestuous abuse: stepfathers vs. biological fathers. *Child Abuse Negl* 1984;8:15–22.

241. San Fillipo JS. Sexual abuse: to colposcope or not? *Adolesc Pediatr Gynecol* 1990;3:63.

242. Santucci KA, Kennedy KM, Duffy SJ. Wood's lamp utilization and the differentiation between semen and commonly applied medicaments. *Pediatrics* 1998;102:718.

243. Satterfield S. Common sexual problems of children and adolescents. *Pediatr Clin North Am* 1975;22:643–652.

244. Schetky DH, ed. Child pornography and prostitution. In: Schetky DH, Green AH, eds. *Child sexual abuse: a handbook for health care and legal professionals.* New York: Brunner Mazel, 1988:153–165

245. Schwarcz SK, Whittington WL. Sexual assault and sexually transmitted diseases: detection and management in adults and children. *Rev Infect Dis* 1990;12(suppl 6):S682–S690.

246. Sedlak AJ, Broadhurst DB. *Third national incidence study of child abuse and neglect.* Washington, DC: U.S. Government Printing Office, 1996.

247. Seidel JS, Elvik SL, Berkowitz CD, et al. Presentation and evaluation of sexual misuse in the emergency department. *Pediatr Emerg Care* 1986;2:157.

248. Sgroi SM. In: Books L, ed. *Handbook of clinical intervention in child sexual abuse.* Lexington, MA: DC Heath, 1982.

249. Siegel RM, Schubert CJ, Myers PA, et al. The prevalence of sexually transmitted diseases in children and adolescents evaluated for sexual abuse in Cincinnati: rationale for limited STD testing in prepubertal girls. *Pediatrics* 1995;96:1090–1094.

250. Silverman EM, Silverman AG. Persistence of spermatozoa in the lower genital tracts of women. *JAMA* 1978;240:1875–1877.

251. Skinner HA. *The origin of medical terms.* Baltimore: Williams & Wilkins, 1948.

252. Sloane E. *Biology of women.* New York: Wiley and Sons, 1985.

253. Spencer MJ, Dunklee P. Sexual abuse of boys. *Pediatrics* 1986;78:133–138.

254. Sproles ET. National Center for Prevention and Control of Rape. *The evaluation and management of rape and sexual abuse:* a physician's guide. Rockville, Md: U.S. Public Health Services, 1985.

255. Stanton A, Sunderland R. Prevalence of reflex anal dilatation in 200 children [see comments]. *BMJ* 1989;298:802–803.

256. *Stedman's medical dictionary.* 25th Ed. Baltimore: Williams & Wilkins, 1990.

257. Summit RC. The child sexual abuse accommodation syndrome. *Child Abuse Negl* 1983;7:177–193.

258. Swanston HY, Tebbutt JS, O'Toole BL, et al. Sexually abused children 5 years after presentation: a case-control study. *Pediatrics* 1997;100:600–608.

259. Sweet DJ, ed. Bitemark evidence: human bitemarks: examination, recovery, and analysis. In: Bowers CM, Bell GL, eds. *Manual of forensic odontology.* Colorado Springs: American Society of Forensic Odontology, 1995:118–137.

260. Teixeira WR. Hymenal colposcopic examination in sexual offenses. *Am J Forensic Med Pathol* 1981;2:209–215.

261. Tharinger D, Horton CB, Millea S. Sexual abuse and exploitation of children and adults with mental retardation and other handicaps. *Child Abuse Negl* 1990;14:301–312.

262. Theonnis N, Tjadin PG. The extent, nature, and validity of sexual abuse allegations in custody/visitation disputes. *Child Abuse Negl* 1990;14:301.

263. Thomas JN. Juvenile sex offender: physician and parent communication. *Pediatr Ann* 1982;11:807–812.

264. Tilleli JA, Turek D, Jaffee AC. Sexual abuse in children. *N Engl J Med* 1980;302:319.

265. Tutty LM. Child sexual abuse prevention programs: evaluating who do you tell. *Child Abuse Negl* 1997;21:869–881.

266. Tyler RPT, Stone LE. Child pornography: perpetuating the sexual victimization of children. *Child Abuse Negl* 1985;9:313.

267. U.S. Department of Health and Human Services, National Center on Child Abuse and Neglect. *Reports from the states to the National Center on Child Abuse and Neglect: Child maltreatment.* Washington, D.C., 1994.

268. Vander Mey BJ. The sexual victimization of male children: a review of previous research. *Child Abuse Negl* 1988;12:61.

269. Vogeltanz ND, Wilsnack SC, Harris TR, et al. Prevalence and risk factors for childhood sexual abuse in women: national survey findings. *Child Abuse Negl* 1999;23:579–592.

270. Walterman J, et al. Challenges for the future. In: Mac-

Farlane K, ed. *Sexual abuse of young children.* New York: The Guilford Press, 1987:316–329.

271. Waltzman ML, Shannon M, Bowen AP, et al. Monkey-bar injuries: complications of play. *Pediatrics* 1999; 103:e58.

272. Wang CT, Daro D, eds. *Current trends in child abuse reporting and fatalities: the results of the 1996 annual fifty states survey.* Chicago: National Committee to Prevent Child Abuse, 1997.

273. Watts DH, Koutsky LA, Holmes KK, et al. Low risk of perinatal transmission of human papillomavirus: results from a prospective cohort study [see comments]. *Am J Obstet Gynecol* 1998;178:365–373.

274. Weisberg K. *A study of adolescent prostitution.* Lexington, MA: Lexington Books, 1985.

275. White ST, Loda FA, Ingram DL et al. Sexually transmitted diseases in sexually abused children. *Pediatrics* 1983;72:16–21.

276. White S, Strom GA, Santilli G, et al. Interviewing young sexual abuse victims with anatomically correct dolls. *Child Abuse Negl* 1986;10:519–529.

277. White ST, Ingram DL, Lyna PR. Vaginal introital diameter in the evaluation of sexual abuse. *Child Abuse Negl* 1989;13:217–224.

278. Widom CS, Kuhns JB. Childhood victimization and subsequent risk for promiscuity, prostitution, and teenage pregnancy: a prospective study. *Am J Public Health* 1996;86:1607–1612.

279. Wild NJ. Prevalence of child sex rings. *Pediatrics* 1989;83:553–558.

280. Wile IS. The psychology of the hymen. *J Nerv Ment Dis* 1937;Feb.,1937:143–156.

281. Whittington WL, Rice RJ, Biddle JW, et al. Incorrect identification of *Neisseria gonorrhoeae* from infants and children. *Pediatr Infect Dis* 1988;7:3.

282. Woodling BA, Kossoris PD. Sexual misuse: rape, molestation, and incest. *Pediatr Clin North Am* 1981;28: 481–499.

283. Woodling BA, Heger A. The use of the colposcope in the diagnosis of sexual abuse in the pediatric age group. *Child Abuse Negl* 1986;10:111–114.

284. Wyatt GE. The sexual abuse of Afro-American and white-American women in childhood. *Child Abuse Negl* 1985;9:507–519.

285. Wyatt GE, Peters SD. Methodological considerations in research on the prevalence of child sexual abuse. *Child Abuse Negl* 1986;10:241–251.

286. Wyatt GE, Loeb TB, Solis B, et al. The prevalence and circumstances of child sexual abuse: changes across a decade. *Child Abuse Negl* 1999;23:45–60.

11

Conditions Mistaken for Child Sexual Abuse

Jan Bays

Child Abuse Response and Evaluation Services, Emanuel Children's Hospital and Healthcare Center; and Department of Pediatrics, Oregon Health Sciences University, Portland, Oregon

Child sexual abuse was not recognized as a common problem until the 1980s. The first article on child sexual abuse was listed in the Index Medicus in 1973; by 1987, 113 such citations were included (7). Studies indicated that 10% to 28% of children become victims of sexual abuse, making this a more common disease than pneumonia or urinary tract infection (39). As public awareness and reporting of suspected abuse has increased, so have requests to clinicians to evaluate their child patients for possible abuse. A mistaken diagnosis of sexual molestation can have traumatic and long-lasting consequences for the child, family, and suspected perpetrator. Clinicians, therefore, should be aware of medical conditions that can produce signs confused with child sexual abuse.

BEHAVIORAL CONDITIONS

A diversity of symptoms and behavioral changes have been linked with child sexual abuse (98), including difficulty sleeping, nightmares, unusual fears, sudden change in school performance, secondary enuresis (85) or encopresis (25), and sexualized behavior. This chapter does not cover the differential diagnosis of these symptoms. Clinicians should be aware that sexual abuse is only one possible explanation for such behaviors. For example, Yates (136) described four routes by which children may become eroticized, and suggested methods for differentiating these causes.

Caretakers and health care providers are sometimes uncertain about whether a child's sexual behavior is normal or suggestive of abuse. Information found in the Child Sexual Behavior Inventory can provide reassurance that certain behaviors are common in a child of a particular age. A child who exhibits sexual behaviors that are uncommon for the age and sex (e.g., putting their mouth on another's genitalia or asking others to engage in sexual acts) should be referred for further evaluation (44).

In addition, parental issues can cause confusion about possible child sexual abuse. These include mental illness, substance abuse, parental history of sexual abuse, unusual genital care practices, and hostile custody disputes (27,51,59,75). A clinician evaluating a child for possible abuse should take a careful history to detect these confounding factors.

DERMATOLOGIC CONDITIONS

Many parents become suspicious of sexual abuse on noting that their child has "a red bottom." Erythema of the anogenital area is a nonspecific sign with numerous causes: poor hygiene, diaper dermatitis, intertrigo, sensitivity to bubble bath and dyes used in toilet products, pinworms, and candidal infection. Anogenital erythema is often the presenting sign in a nonverbal infant who has returned from an overnight visit with a divorced father. The father may have avoided diaper changes for olfactory or aesthetic reasons or was wary of any genital contact lest allegations of abuse arise.

Bruises in the genital or anal area can also arouse suspicions of abuse. Any of the conditions described in Chapter 9 as causing bruises mistaken for physical abuse could also lead to mistaken diagnosis of child sexual abuse if the lesions occurred in the anogenital area. These include mongolian spots, Ehlers–Danlos syndrome, hypersensitivity vasculitis, meningococcemia, erythema multiforme, and bleeding disorders such as idiopathic thrombocytopenic purpura (8).

Phytodermatitis is a darkening of the skin that occurs when juices of plants such as limes, figs, or celery contact the skin with subsequent sun exposure. Apparent "loop marks" or "hand prints" have developed after adults who squeezed limes later touched children (28).

A 9-month-old child referred to our program for genital bruising was found to have purple stains from gentian violet applied to treat *Candida*. Dye "bleeding" from new black or blue clothing has also stained children's skin and caused consternation over abuse as well as other serious medical conditions. The dye may not wash off with water, but will wipe off with alcohol. In one case, numerous diagnoses were considered over a 2-day period by the parents (a dermatologist and an allergist) of a 10-year-old boy with blue discoloration of his hands and face. As his mother was observing his respiratory status as he slept, she realized that the color came from his new blue sheets (93).

Patients with Henoch–Schönlein purpura can present with pain, swelling, and hematoma of the penis or scrotum. In two reported cases, scrotal involvement preceded the characteristic rash by 36 hours (22).

The most common skin condition mistaken for sexual abuse is lichen sclerosus. The initial lesions are whitish or yellow papules that fuse to form white plaques. The skin becomes atrophic and thin, with fissuring and alarming subepidermal hemorrhages after such minor trauma to the anogenital area as wiping with toilet paper (Figs. 11.1–11.3). Lichen sclerosus usually occurs on the vulva and perianal

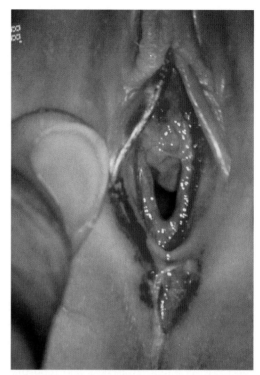

FIG. 11.1. Lichen sclerosus in an 8-year-old girl evaluated for sexual abuse after she had vaginal bleeding on returning from a 2-week visit with her divorced father. The subepidermal hemorrhages are characteristic.

region, producing a characteristic "hourglass," "figure of eight," or "keyhole" area of decreased pigmentation (Fig. 11.4). It also can occur at the urethral opening and cause phimosis in boys (21). Less often, it appears on the trunk, extremities, axilla, face, and neck. Despite its distressing appearance, lichen sclerosus is more often accompanied by itching or soreness than by actual pain, except when fissures cause pain with micturition or defecation or if lesions become infected. It may cause labial fusion, or in severe forms, atrophic genital scarring. Lichen sclerosus resolves spontaneously, usually during adolescence, in about one half of the cases. If the diagnosis is in doubt, a skin biopsy may be done (12,53,56,58,71,116,133).

Lichen sclerosus can occur in areas of trauma such as sunburn and at the site of pres-

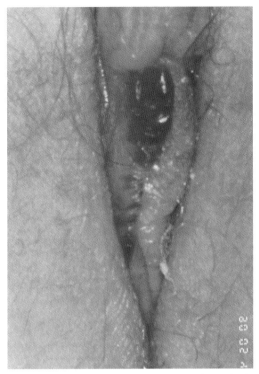

FIG. 11.2. Early lichen sclerosus with a single area of hemorrhage into the left labium minorum.

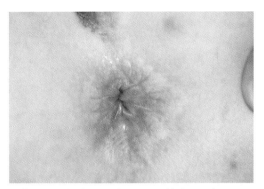

FIG. 11.3. Lichen sclerosus with hypopigmentation and fissuring of the perianal area.

simplex, lichen sclerosus, and impetigo (Fig. 11.5). Contact dermatitis can be triggered by soaps, fabric softener, bubble bath, toilet paper, dyes or sizing in clothing, or topical medication (60,133). Allergy to "black" rubber mix can manifest as dermatitis in areas in contact with underwear elastic (and also tires,

sure from waist or brassiere straps. Worsening of the condition has been related to tight clothing or riding a bicycle (58). Children with lichen sclerosus should be questioned about possible abuse, as the two conditions may coexist. It also is possible that the trauma of sexual abuse might bring out lichen sclerosus or worsen an existing case (56,58,71,115).

Authors of a retrospective review of 42 confirmed cases of lichen sclerosus in girls aged 3 to 15 years reported that the onset of the disease was associated with prior accidental injury in six cases and with sexual abuse in 12 (29%) cases. Two of the latter were "new" cases, uncovered by careful history and physical examination at the time of consultation. Five girls had evidence of autoimmune disease, arthritis, or serum autoantibodies (129).

A variety of dermatologic conditions cause rashes, pain, itching, bleeding, or fissures in the anogenital area. These include seborrheic dermatitis, atopic dermatitis, psoriasis, lichen

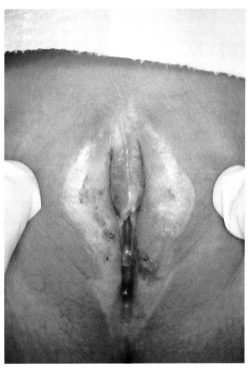

FIG. 11.4. Lichen sclerosus with striking hypopigmentation. (Photo courtesy of J. McCann, M.D.)

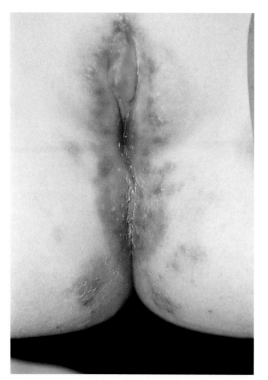

FIG. 11.5. Impetigo of the vulva autoinoculated from the ear.

scuba gear, wind-surfing boards, squash balls, rubber fingerstalls, elastic stocking tops, and rubber spectacle chains) (41).

Chigger bites can cause acute swelling, erythema, and pruritis of the penis. These insects are active during summer months in the southern and midwestern United States. Their bites may be confined to the penis (122). Scabies also can infect the penis, producing similar findings.

I evaluated a 5-year-old girl for suspected abuse. She was referred by her teacher and the school nurse because of open and almost continuous masturbation. The mother, who was not disturbed by this behavior, had restricted the child to masturbating in her room. The child stated that her vaginal area itched. In a private interview, she denied sexual abuse. She had patches of atopic dermatitis on the extremities. The genital examination was normal except for the hymen, which was pale and noticeably thickened. The child was referred to an allergist, who concurred with the diagnosis of

allergic reaction of the hymen. Treatment with antipruritic agents was successful in relieving the itching and stopping the "masturbation."

CONGENITAL CONDITIONS

Hemangioma of the hymen, vulva, vagina, or perineal body can be confused with erythema or abrasions resulting from sexual abuse (43,66). Hemangiomata may bleed or ulcerate, heightening concerns about possible molestation (Fig. 11.6) (8). A 5-week-old girl was treated for denuded erythematous areas of the labia and mons diagnosed as candida diaper dermatitis. Three days later, apparent healing of second- and third-degree burns of the labia were noted and confirmed by surgical consultation. The mother stated that the rash had appeared after the infant was left in the care of her father. A report of suspected abuse was filed, listing the father as the suspected perpetrator. One month later, the child

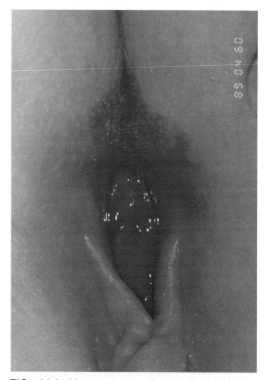

FIG. 11.6. Hemangioma of the posterior fourchette and perineal body mistaken for trauma due to abuse. The lesion blanched with pressure.

TABLE 11.1. *Common congenital genital structures in girls*

	McCann et al. (98)	Gardner (46)	Berenson et al. (9)
Ages and examination method	Prepubertal girls, supine and knee–chest, labial traction	Prepubertal girls, supine, labial traction, anesthetized	Neonates, supine, labial traction
Intravaginal ridges	90%	NR	56%
Midline avascular areas or lines	26%	27%	NR
"Tethers" of hymen to perihymenal tissue	16%	14%	86%[a]
Urethral dilation	15%	28%	NR
Hymen tags	24%	2%	13%
Septal remnants	19%	NR	NR
Hymen mounds or bumps	34%	11%	NR
Posterior fourchette friability	5%	6%	NR

NR, not reported.
[a]Includes periurethral support bands.

was found to have a capillary–cavernous hemangioma of the vulva corresponding to the original denuded area. Although the mother denied the previous existence of this lesion, old records indicted that a hemangioma of the labia majora with some denuded areas had been noted at the 3-week visit. The child abuse report was rescinded (94).

Congenital structures that should not be confused with scar tissue resulting from trauma include periurethral bands, hymenal tags, hymenal septa, septal remnants, intravaginal ridges, and tissue bridges or "tethers" between the hymen and perihymenal tissues (Table 11.1) (9,46,98).

Clefts in the hymen may be congenital or related to trauma. Position and configuration give clues as to origin. A shallow concavity with smooth borders occurring laterally and anteriorly may be congenital. A deeper, angular concavity found on the posterior or lateral hymen may be acquired (9,83).

Caution is advised in interpreting anogenital abnormalities in the midline; several midline congenital abnormalities have been recognized since clinicians began scrutinizing children's genitalia for signs of abuse. Anal skin tags have been seen after trauma from anal sodomy (112), but midline tags are a common congenital finding (Table 11.2). An-

TABLE 11.2. *Anal findings in normal, constipated, and abused children*

	McCann et al. (99)	Stanton and Sunderland (123)	Agnarsson et al. (3)	Clayden (26)	Hobbs and Wynne (56)
Subject number and type	N = 267, nonabused	N = 200, no abuse history	N = 136, referred for constipation	N = 129, referred for constipation	N = 337, evidence of abuse
Examination method	Knee chest	Unk	Supine or left lateral	Unk	Left lateral
Anal dilation	12%[a] 49%[b]	14%	19%[c]	15%	18%
Anal fissure	0%	2%	26%	NR	22%
Anal tag	11% (All but one in midline)	NR	5%	NR	3% (scars or tags)

NR, not reported; Unk, unknown, probably left lateral position.
[a]Observed for 1 min (knee–chest position).
[b]Observed up to 4 min (knee–chest position).
[c]Observed for 1 min (left lateral position).

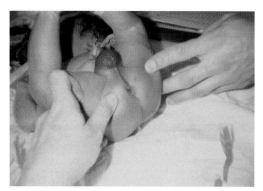

FIG. 11.7. Prominent median raphe. Perianal anatomic variations may occur in the anterior midline where this structure joins the anus.

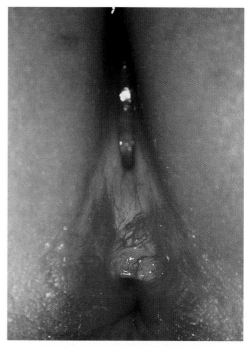

FIG. 11.8. Failure of midline fusion mistaken for trauma. Vascularity appears prominent due to pale mucosa at base of defect. Note anteriorly placed anus.

terior midline anal skin tags were found in 11% of nonabused children in one study (99). A median raphe, particularly in a girl, may be confused with scar tissue. In boys, the raphe is more obvious, as it runs without interruption along the underside of the penis, over the scrotum, and along the perineal body, tucking into the anus anteriorly (Fig. 11.7).

Failure of midline fusion is a term currently used for a congenital midline lesion that has been mistaken for scarring due to abuse (1). The genitalia are normal except for a midline defect extending from the fossa navicularis to the anus. The tissue at the base of the defect is pale with normal vascularity, and the skin edges bordering the defect are smooth (Fig 11.8). The several girls referred to our clinic with failure of midline fusion also have all had an anteriorly located anus. This is a congenital anomaly in which the anus is located anterior to the midpoint between the posterior commissure and the coccyx. When associated with refractory constipation and pain with defecation, it may require surgical correction (45). We have examined a few boys with similar, smaller lesions at the anal verge.

McCann et al. (99) noted a common congenital anomaly of the external anal sphincter that results in smooth, fan-shaped areas, with or without depressions, in the midline at the anal verge. In this study of 81 children, 26% had these smooth areas, which have been mistaken for anal scars, "funneling," or "thumbprints" characteristic of abuse (Fig. 11.9).

Another finding to interpret with caution is pale midline avascular streaks of the hymen, posterior vestibule, and posterior fourchette, particularly if all other genital findings are normal. In one study of 123 female newborns, 14% had white spots in the posterior vestibule, and 10% had white streaks extending from the posterior commissure into the posterior vestibule. The authors (82) termed these structures "linea vestibularis" (Fig. 11.10). Midline avascular areas were found in one fourth of prepubertal girls selected for nonabuse in two separate studies from Australia (46) and the U.S. (98). Other causes of avascular streaks in the posterior vestibule are scarring after trauma and partially resolved labial adhesions.

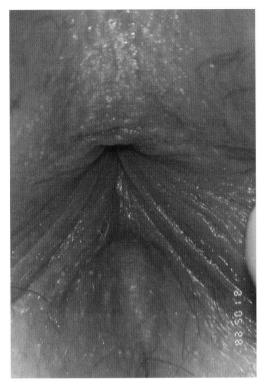

FIG. 11.9. Smooth, depressed, fan-shaped area in the posterior midline due to a congenital anomaly of the external anal sphincter.

Muram and Rau (104) described two infants with anomalies of the genitalia resulting from failure of the bulbocavernosus muscle to insert into the central perineal tendon and clitoris. One infant was erroneously diagnosed with sexual abuse. Findings included soft tissue masses in the labia majora that failed to converge anteriorly, absence of the posterior commissure, and poor definition of the fossa navicularis so the hymen appeared to arise out of vulvar skin. Other abnormalities possibly confused with injuries related to abuse include congenital pits (8), congenital cleft clitoris (8,120), labial hypertrophy (120), and congenital absence of the upper portion of the hymen (Fig. 11.11).

Because children with mental retardation or developmental delay are at higher risk of child abuse, their caretakers are understandably alert to signs of abuse. These children also may have congenital abnormalities or behaviors, however, that are easily confused with signs and symptoms of abuse. For example, multiple perianal nodules are seen in infants with systemic hyalinosis (49), the labia majora are absent in Escobar syndrome, and vaginal strictures are seen in dyskeratosis congenital syndrome (76). Clinicians evaluat-

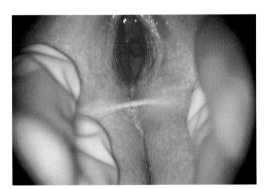

FIG. 11.10. Midline avascular streak or "linea vestibularis" of the posterior fourchette.

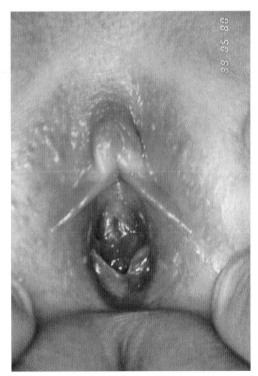

FIG. 11.11. Congenital absence of the upper half of the hymen. (Photo courtesy of R. Sewell, M.D.)

ing children with congenital anomalies for possible sexual abuse may need to consult references describing the many syndromes associated with anogenital anomalies (76).

URETHRAL CONDITIONS

Several urethral disorders can cause bleeding or confusing changes in anatomy potentially misdiagnosed as abusive in origin. These include urethral hemangioma (119), polyps (43), papilloma, caruncle (8), condyloma, and cysts, as well as ureterocele, sarcoma botryoides, ectopic ureter, prolapsed bladder, and urethral prolapse (Fig. 11.12) (73,96).

Patients with urethral prolapse can present with genital bleeding, dysuria, urinary frequency, or introital pain. Physical examination reveals eversion of the urethral mucosa in a rosette surrounding the meatus. The friable mass of tissue may ulcerate or become infected. It may obscure the anatomy of the hymen and be mistaken for abusive injury (72, 73,133).

A 5-year-old girl was brought to the emergency department after blood was found in the bathtub, in her underwear, and in her vaginal area. Physical examination showed erythema of the vulva, a blood clot in the introitus, and a laceration of the hymen. The child was placed in foster care. Three days later, she was seen at a sexual abuse clinic by the author and found to have a normal hymen with urethral prolapse and a tear in the urethral mucosa rather than the hymen. The child was treated and returned home.

Urethral prolapse occurs only in female patients and most commonly in prepubescent black girls. Antecedent episodes of increased intraabdominal pressure were documented in 67% of girls with urethral prolapse in one series, including straining with crying, coughing, or defecation. Sexual abuse was the cause in one patient. Other causes were burns, seizures, urinary tract infection, straddle injury, and strangury (96,133).

Girls with urethral prolapse should be questioned about sexual abuse, because genital trauma has been implicated in this condition. Forms of treatment range from a nonoperative approach, using antibiotics and topical steroids, to reduction of the prolapse and insertion of a catheter, to primary excision of the prolapse (72).

ANAL CONDITIONS

Perianal erythema and increased pigmentation are nonspecific findings not in themselves diagnostic of sexual abuse (99). Several reports exist of diseases producing perianal skin changes mistaken for sexual abuse trauma, including lichen sclerosus (Fig. 11.3), Crohn's disease (62), and hemolytic uremic syndrome (128).

Three children younger than 3 years were seen with reddening of the anus, venous dilation, and alternating contraction and relaxation of the anal sphincter after several days of bloody diarrhea. Sexual abuse was considered until signs of hemolytic uremic syndrome developed. In retrospect, the anal changes were thought to be due to *Escherichia coli* colitis (128).

Perianal fissures and scars may result from anal abuse (63,112). Abscesses and scarring in the anal area also may be caused by furuncles or by fistula in ano. Furuncles are common in infancy and respond to medical treatment. Fistula in ano results from devel-

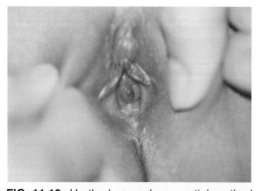

FIG. 11.12. Urethral caruncle or partial urethral prolapse in a 3-year-old African-American girl, causing bleeding and concerns about sexual abuse.

opmental abnormalities of the mucosal glands at the base of the anal crypt glands. They are more common in male patients (4:1), and usually manifest as a draining pustule in the first year of life. Rectal fissures sometimes accompany fistula. About 90% of fistulae in children do not respond to medical management, recur, and eventually require surgical excision (95). Anal fistulae or furuncles do not indicate sexual abuse.

Eversion of the anal canal has been described as a result of anal sodomy (63). This sign is not diagnostic of abuse, however, because it is associated with numerous conditions in children, including chronic constipation, acute diarrhea, cystic fibrosis, neurologic abnormalities, repaired imperforate anus, and rectal polyps (137).

Anal dilation as a sign of sexual abuse should be interpreted with caution (7,99). Hobbs and Wynn (63) observed anal dilation in 18% of victims of abuse and anal fissures in 22%. McCann's group (99), however, observed anal dilation in 49% of nonabused children after they had spent several minutes in the knee–chest position. A most remarkable example of anal dilation occurred in a healthy infant. The author was summoned by a nurse practitioner who was performing a well-child examination on the baby. He lifted the infant's legs, and we both gaped at the alarming degree of dilation of the external anal sphincter. As we were puzzling over how to interpret this finding, the internal sphincter opened, and the baby passed a large stool. The anal examination was subsequently normal.

Currently, anal dilation more than 15 to 20 mm in diameter without stool in the ampulla is considered a sign of anal sodomy, particularly if dilation recurs in different examining positions. Both external and internal sphincters should dilate. Causes of anal dilation mistaken for abuse include postmortem changes anal dilation (84), severe constipation (3,26, 63), and neurogenic patulous anus (118). A study of postmortem perianal findings in children revealed that anal dilation is common (77% of 50 cases). An exposed pectinate line, which can be confused with tears or fissures of the anal verge, was seen in almost half the cases (100).

During the course of a sex education class at school, a 14-year-old girl with myotonic dystrophy and developmental delay disclosed apparent sexual abuse by a male family member. A genital examination was normal, but she had a dilated and floppy anal sphincter with feces visible in the rectum. Reflex anal dilation was observed on parting the buttocks. The child had generally regular bowel habits with intermittent episodes of constipation treated with laxatives. The sexual abuse investigation was closed after information was obtained that five other children with myotonic dystrophy had similar abnormal anal signs, including anal laxity, perianal inflammation, fecal soiling, and reflex anal dilation (118).

Debate continues as to the types and frequency of anal findings attributable to chronic constipation. Table 11.2 summarizes studies on the frequency of anal dilation, fissures, and tags in nonabused children, abused children, and children referred to specialists for constipation (3,26,63,99,123).

TRAUMATIC CONDITIONS

Straddle Injuries

Injuries to the perineum can be classified as penetrating and nonpenetrating, intentional, and accidental. Straddle injuries, the most common injury to the genitalia, seldom involve penetration. Straddle injuries are associated with a history of an acute and dramatic fall onto an object such as a furniture arm or bar on a bike or play equipment. These injuries usually crush the soft tissue over a firm base, such as the pubic symphysis, the ischiopubic ramus, or the adductor longus tendon. Compared with injuries caused by abuse, straddle injuries are more often unilateral and anterior, causing damage to the external genitalia rather than the hymen or vagina (Fig. 11.13). Typically, bruising and swelling is noted of the anterior labia, clitoris, and periurethral tissue. Accidental injury to the internal genital structures or anus is rare, because they are protected by the bones of the

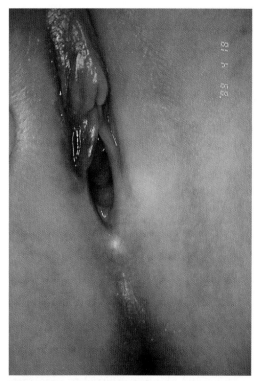

FIG. 11.13. Straddle injury to the right labium. The hymen was undamaged.

pelvis and the soft tissue of the buttocks and labia (8,77,103,130).

In a series of 100 children examined in an emergency department for straddle injuries, most had minor lacerations and abrasions of the genitalia. Among 72 girls, in 79%, the injury was to the labia majora or minora; in 16%, the injury was to the posterior fourchette; and 11% had hematoma of the vulva. Seven girls had injuries to the vagina and two had injuries to the hymen. Three girls had unintentional penetrating injuries caused by falls onto a plunger handle, a sharp fence post, and the exposed steering column of a bike. Five girls with injuries not accounted for by their histories eventually revealed sexual abuse. Among 28 boys, the most common injury was ecchymosis or minor laceration of the scrotum or penis. The authors listed factors that require investigation for sexual abuse. These are straddle injuries in nonambulatory children (younger than 9 months), extensive

trauma, coexisting nongenital trauma, and lack of correlation between history and physical findings [more specifically, perianal, vaginal, or hymenal injury without a history of penetrating trauma (34)].

Jones and Bass (77) reviewed perineal injuries in 463 children aged 13 years or younger seen over a 12-year period at a South African hospital. Accidents accounted for 57% of injuries. The leading cause was straddle injury on such objects as bicycle bars, beds, fences, concrete walls, and playground equipment. Other causes of accidental perineal injury were impalement, motor vehicle accidents, zipper injuries, and animal bites. Sexual or physical abuse accounted for 38% of perineal injuries. The most common genital injuries resulting from abuse were tears of the posterior fourchette and tears of the hymen. Four children were injured by forceful enemas, a highly regarded tribal treatment. Three had enemas administered by hosepipes, and one by a goat's horn. Two had third-degree perineal tears. Five percent of injuries could not be classified because the history was vague or unavailable.

Splitting injury to the midline anogenital structures can occur with sudden, violent abduction of the legs (64,86,112,130). A history of possible abuse should be taken, however; in one report of such injury, the cause was forced abduction of the legs during sexual abuse (40). Small fissures of the posterior fourchette can occur when the examining physician exerts traction on the labia (46). One physician describes watching as a mother caused an anal fissure by "violently opposing the child's buttocks" in an effort to demonstrate how other physicians had examined the child for possible abuse (4).

In a series of 56 prepubertal girls with unintentional perineal injury, only one had hymenal involvement. She had fallen at a park, abducting her legs. There was a pinpoint abraded area on her hymen (15). The author saw a 5-year-old girl with persistent genital bleeding after she fell "doing a split," on railroad ties on a school playground. She had been playing under adult supervision and denied sexual abuse. The child was examined under anesthesia and found to have a small laceration in the fossa navicularis.

Motor vehicle accidents can cause injuries to the genitalia (5,135). A 5-year-old girl was referred for possible sexual abuse when an emergency department physician noted bloody vaginal discharge after a motor vehicle accident. Her father, who was the driver of the car and had weekend custody, was referred to local authorities for investigation. Her injuries included a hematoma of the mons, abrasions of the labia, and a tear in the perineal body. The hymen was undamaged. The child denied sexual abuse. The injuries were attributed to an improperly worn seat belt, and the investigation was closed (5).

Water under high pressure, from activities such as water or jet skiing or from water slides, can cause serious penetrating injury to the vagina with little external evidence of trauma. These injuries are more common in parous women, but have been reported in prepubertal girls. Persistent vaginal bleeding after such activities requires an examination under anesthesia, which may reveal injuries requiring operative repair (89).

Labial fusion is a common condition in infants younger than 2 years. It is related to denudation and inflammation of the labial epithelium in contact with urine, stool, and diapers. A few millimeters of labial fusion is a common finding, observed in 39% of nonabused girls in one study (98). Extensive labial adhesion, with fusion leaving only a few-millimeter opening under the clitoris, occurs in fewer than 1% of girls (24).

Labial fusion may be secondary to atrophic or inflammatory conditions such as lichen sclerosus, vulvovaginitis, atopic or seborrheic dermatitis, varicella (11), or herpes (32). In older girls, the trauma of sexual abuse may cause labial fusion (11,97). Inquiries into possible abuse should be made if labial fusion is a new condition in a continent child several years out of diapers, with no predisposing skin condition, and if the adhesions are thick and resistant to treatment with topical estrogens.

Masturbation and use of tampons are often cited in the courtroom as causes of genital trauma. Tampons do not traumatize the hymen (33,134). Some authors stated that tampon use may increase the distensibility of the hymen from slight stretching (30), but Stewart (124) found no differences in the genital examinations of girls who did or did not use tampons.

Normal masturbation in girls is clitoral or labial and does not cause genital injury (64,67,134). Muram (103) mentions that minor abrasions may be caused by masturbation and that self-inflicted vulvar contusions may be seen in retarded girls. No genital or anal injuries were reported in a study of self-injurious behavior in 97 mentally retarded children aged 11 months to 21 years old (68). The authors warned that when anogenital injuries occur or foreign bodies are inserted into body orifices of children, particularly retarded children, child abuse should be considered.

Catheterization is another theoretic cause of genital trauma. No genital injuries were seen in 38 infants and children with neurogenic bladder who either catheterized themselves or had the procedure done by caretakers every 4 to 6 hours for a mean of 28 months (79). In some reports, boys developed hematuria (without external injury) after they inserted into their own urethras foreign objects such as a quartz crystal (117) and fishing line (37). Boys who inject bathwater into their own urethras may cause urinary tract infections (91).

Female circumcision can result in genital hemorrhage, infection, adhesions, or scars. This practice, encountered in patients of African or Middle Eastern origin, is classified as child abuse in some European countries. Adults participating in female circumcision have been prosecuted in France, but professionals in the United Kingdom are struggling with issues of cultural sensitivity and the fact that some 20,000 girls in that country could be added to "at risk" registers if female circumcision is classified as child abuse (69).

Anogenital Injuries in Boys

A review of rectal and genital trauma in boys compared physical findings in boys examined in the emergency department for accidental injury with the abnormal findings in a group of boys who were seen for suspected sexual abuse. The injuries were caused by falling or being caught on an object, by being kicked, shot, or being hurt by a toilet seat or bicycle. Accidental trauma resulted in lacerations or perforations of the scrotum or penis. No patient had anal injuries only. In contrast, the sexually abused group all had rectal lesions, none had scrotal injuries, and penile injuries were rare (80).

In two reported cases, genital injury occurred in boys who were injured in break dancing. One had a hematocele of the scrotum, and the other had a partial rupture of the bulbar urethra after a fall onto the corner of a coffee table (47).

Strangulation of the penis or clitoris by hair or fibers usually occurs accidentally (Fig. 11.14) (6,23,101,111,113). Careful inquiry should be made, however, as tourniquet injuries of the genitalia and digits have occurred as a result of physical or sexual abuse (35, 107). One 6-year-old boy with apparent paraphimosis began voiding through a fistula on the under surface of the penis at the coronal sulcus. Under general anesthesia, a fine nylon thread was found encircling the penis, tied in a knot that was buried by the healed skin on

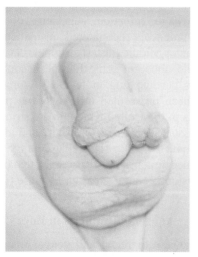

FIG. 11.14. Accidental tourniquet of an infant's foreskin by a hair.

the dorsal surface (57). A similar account is from 1832.

A 4-week-old infant was suckled by a nurse whom the family became dissatisfied with and dismissed. Two days afterward, Dr. G was sent for on account of painful swelling of the boy's penis, when he found a long hair five times wound and tied round the root of the penis. With great difficulty the hair was removed from the deep incision it had made . . . had it remained a short time longer, gangrene would inevitably have occurred. "Very probably," says Dr. G, "the nurse wished in this manner to revenge herself for her dismissal" (35).

Anorectal Injuries

Penetrating genital or anal injury can occur when children fall astride sharp objects (126). A Texas study of 16 cases of anorectal trauma in children younger than 16 years revealed that 80% of cases involved sexual abuse (13). Other documented causes of rectal injury or perforation include falls with impalement on broom or toilet-brush handles, pogo sticks, chair legs, bicycle seat poles, sprinklers, high-jump bars, and tree branches. Anal injuries in children also are reported from gunshot wounds, stabbings, motor vehicle accidents, coat hangers inserted by family members (for reasons not documented), and a swallowed fish bone that lacerated the rectal mucosa (13,74,114).

A report of small bowel evisceration apparently related to child abuse follows. A 4-year-old boy was transported by ambulance to an emergency department with the chief complaint of "bowel came out of bottom." An emergency laparotomy revealed a tear in the anterior rectosigmoid wall with prolapse of 15 cm of cecum and distal ileus. The child would say only that he had jumped on a toilet plunger while getting out of the bathtub. He also said that his 14-year-old sister had done something to him, but his mother had warned him not to talk about it. The sister had been the victim of two prior episodes of sexual abuse. Because the history was inadequate and the child had no evidence of external trauma, the injury was attributed to someone forcefully driving a long object into the rectum and sigmoid colon (114).

Suction drain injury occurs when children sit directly on uncovered swimming pool suction-drain vents capable of forming a strong vacuum. The child's perineum forms a firm seal, with relaxation of the anal sphincter and evisceration of the small intestine through tears in the anterior bowel wall. Associated injuries include perianal bruising and rectal prolapse (18,20). Less severe forms of anogenital suction injury might be mistaken for abusive trauma.

INFECTIOUS CONDITIONS

Certain sexually transmitted diseases (STDs) are considered diagnostic of sexual abuse if perinatal transmission has been excluded. These include syphilis, gonorrhea, and genital herpes. Mistaken diagnoses have been made, however, and certain cautions are advised. False-positive tests for STDs can occur.

A positive nontreponemal test for syphilis (RPR or VDRL) should be confirmed by a treponemal test (FTA). A positive culture for gonorrhea should be verified by at least two confirmatory tests. Whittington et al. (132) wrote that 14 of 40 specimens submitted to the Centers for Disease Control for confirmation as *Neisseria gonorrhoeae* had been misidentified by the referring laboratory. These mistakes resulted in initiation of sexual abuse investigations in eight cases and referral of 14 additional children for unnecessary examination or treatment. The organisms were correctly identified as *Branhamella catarrhalis, Kingella denitrificans,* and three species of nonpathogenic *Neisseria* commonly found in the eye, pharynx, and rectum.

There also are potential sources of error in identification of herpes simplex virus (HSV). Varicella manifesting on the vulva can cause confusion with herpes. Tzank smears do not distinguish herpes varicella from herpes zoster (17,60,70). Autoinoculation of HSV type 1 to genital sites is possible (81,106). Nonsexual transmission should be considered when children have concomitant oral lesions or herpetic whitlows. It also is possible, how-

ever, for HSV type 1 to be inoculated to the genitalia through oral sodomy (81).

Indirect tests for *Chlamydia* (DFA or EIA) are not appropriate for use in children because the predictive value is low (52); a positive indirect test must be confirmed by a chlamydial culture. Persistent carriage of perinatally acquired *Chlamydia* has been documented for more than 1 year in the infant vagina and rectum and for more than 2 years in the eye and pharynx (70).

Most vaginitis in children is not caused by STDs. Jenny (70) reviewed 22 nonvenereal causes of vulvovaginitis in children. *Shigella* vaginitis has been confused with gonorrhea and also with discharge resulting from a vaginal foreign body. Among 32 girls with *Shigella* vaginitis in one report, eight were suspected of having gonorrhea, and six had been treated erroneously for gonorrhea. Foreign body was considered in 22 girls, pelvic radiographs were obtained in 13, and three were examined under anesthesia. Vaginal discharge from *Shigella* is often bloody, but can also be watery, purulent, and any color from white to green. Diarrhea is not a common associated finding (105).

Streptococcal infection of the anus, vagina, and urethra may cause concern about abuse. Perianal streptococcal disease manifests as a painful or itchy rash sometimes associated with fissures, painful defecation, and blood-streaked stools (Fig. 11.15). The rash can be

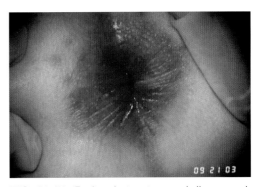

FIG. 11.15. Perianal streptococcal disease mistaken for abuse in day care. (Photo courtesy of C. Jenny, M.D.)

pink, red, or beefy red, with mucoid discharge or crusting. Fever is not present (87,88). In one study, 60% of children had positive throat cultures as well as positive anal cultures for group A β-hemolytic streptococci (GABHS) (87). The culture request must specify that GABHS is suspected, because rectal swabs are routinely plated on media hostile to streptococci. Intrafamilial spread may occur if bathwater is shared (87).

> A 2-year-old boy told his mother that his "bottom hurt" on returning from day care. His physician diagnosed anal trauma, and a day-care worker was interviewed by the police after the child said, "Mark hurt me." After the child was examined at a child abuse center, the diagnosis of perianal streptococcal cellulitis was made. On further questioning, the child said the day-care worker had hurt him when he was wiping after toileting. The pain apparently occurred because of preexisting anal irritation from the infection (8).

Patients with streptococcal balanitis can present with urethral discharge and/or erythema and swelling of the foreskin. The discharge may be thin and serous or thick and purulent. Sexual abuse was suspected in a 6-year-old boy who presented with symptoms due to streptococcal balanitis (90).

Streptococcal vaginitis causes erythema of the mucosal tissues and many types of discharge: thin, thick, serous, blood tinged, creamy, white, yellow, or green. The introitus and vaginal mucosa may be fiery red, edematous, and tender (48,108). A 1948 study of vaginal cultures from 286 children from infancy to age 14 years found that 13% grew hemolytic strains of streptococci (primarily group A), and 12% grew gonococci. Streptococcal vaginitis was sometimes associated with fever, pharyngitis, or scarlet fever (14).

Autoinoculation by contaminated nasopharyngeal secretions is the postulated mode of infection in most cases of GABHS anogenital infection (90). Identical streptococcal types have been isolated from pharyngeal and anogenital sites when both were infected (14,87). The possibility of transmission during oral sodomy by a perpetrator with GABHS pharyngitis, however, should be kept in mind (60,110).

Anogenital warts are considered sexually transmitted in adults, but in children, they may be acquired by other than sexual means. Evidence of autoinoculation of hand warts to the anal area has been provided by DNA typing (29,42). Vertical transmission within families also appears possible when bathwater, towels, bathing suits, or underwear are shared (10,29,109). As the incidence of human papilloma virus (HPV) infection in adults has increased, a parallel increase has occurred among children, attributable to perinatal transmission (29). Infection before birth, presumably bloodborne, also has occurred (125).

In one study of anogenital warts in children aged 10 months to 12 years, the etiology was reported to be unknown in 42%, vertical transmission in 42%, sexual abuse in 10%, and autoinoculation in 5%. How the authors placed patients in these categories is not clear, however, other than by examining the child and other family members for warts and by culturing for other STDs. No HPV typing was done (54).

Other authors have reported incidences of sexual abuse in children with anogenital warts of 10% (29), 27% (16), 50% (121), and 91% (61). Higher incidence is found when the evaluation includes a family investigation and interviews of the children. Nonsexual transmission is more likely when HPV is present in children younger than 3 years; sexual transmission is likely in older children.

Condyloma acuminata, caused by HPV, have been confused with condyloma lata, caused by syphilis (31,50,65). Perianal lesions of eosinophilic granuloma were mistaken for condyloma lata in a 2-year-old boy (19). A test for syphilis should be done in all children with apparent anogenital warts. Benign papillomatosis is a common finding in the fossa naviculari in adolescents and can be confused with HPV lesions (Fig. 11.16).

Microscopic evidence of sperm on a child's body, clothing, or in the urine, stool, or vaginal secretions is considered virtual proof of sexual abuse (if the child is not a pubertal male) (102,131). Even microscopic evidence of sperm can be mistaken, however, according

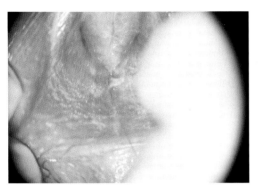

FIG. 11.16. Benign papillomatosis of the fossa navicularis in an adolescent. A Papanicolaou smear was negative.

to M.A. Finkel (personal communication, 1993). An investigation for possible abuse was launched when a child's stool specimen appeared to contain sperm. The investigation was closed when the Centers for Disease Control ultimately identified the specimen as *Myxosporidium,* a fish parasite with an appearance similar to that of sperm.

CONDITIONS CAUSING GENITAL ULCERS

Genital ulceration has a variety of causes, only some of which are related to sexual activity. Adler (2) categorizes genital ulcers by whether the ulcers are multiple or solitary, and painful or painless (Table 11.3). Multiple

TABLE 11.3. *Conditions causing genital ulcers*

Multiple	Solitary
Painful	
Herpes simplex (type 1 or 2)	Tuberculosis
Herpes zoster	Trauma
Beçhet's syndrome	Ulcerated hemangioma
Hemophilus ducreyi (chancroid)	
Yaws	
Stevens–Johnson	
Drug eruption	
Erythema multiforme	
Impetigo	
Folliculitis	
Furuncle ——————————————→	
Scabies (secondary infection)	
Candida	
Vincent's organism	
Jacquet erosive diaper dermatitis	
Granuloma gluteale infantum	
Balanitis/vulvitis	
Painless	
Secondary syphilis	Crohn's disease
	Carcinoma
	Lymphogranuloma venereum
←————→	Primary syphilis
	Tertiary syphilis (gamma)
	Reiter's syndrome
←————→	Granuloma inguinale
←————→	Leukoplakia
←————→	Lichen sclerosus
←————→	Carcinoma
	(Trauma)

Adapted from Adler MW. ABC of sexually transmitted diseases: genital ulceration. *Br Med J* 1983;287:1780, with permission.

painful ulcers are usually associated with herpes simplex. Cultures should be done to confirm the diagnosis of herpes and to differentiate type 1 from type 2. Herpes 2 infection appearing in the perinatal period may have been acquired at birth. Both types 1 and 2 can be transmitted through sexual abuse, but type 1 infection may be innocently inoculated by the child or by an adult with oral herpes. Herpes zoster rarely occurs in the genital area.

Scabies often occurs in the genital area in the absence of sexual abuse. It can involve multiple itching, painful ulcers if secondarily infected. Reiter's disease and Behçet's syndrome are multisystem diseases that rarely afflict prepubertal children. Both are characterized by painful oral and genital ulcers, arthritis, and ocular inflammation, conjunctivitis in Reiter's disease, and iritis in Behçet's. Because Reiter's disease can follow both STDs such as Chlamydia, and non–sexually transmitted infection such as Shigella, clinicians should be aware of the possibility of sexual abuse. (36,138). Other diseases producing multiple painful genital ulcers include Stevens–Johnson syndrome, erythema multiforme, and folliculitis, impetigo, drug eruptions, and Candida (2).

Ulcerations from Jacquet erosive diaper dermatitis are now rare because of the availability of good-quality cloth and disposable diapers. The disease is characterized by small, centrally ulcerated erythematous nodules on the concave surfaces in the diaper area. Hara et al. (55) reported a case in an 8-year-old girl with urinary incontinence because of ectopic ureters; she used toilet paper as an absorptive replacement for diapers. Granuloma gluteale infantum manifests with relatively large firm nodules on the convex portion of the diaper area. It may be related to use of topical steroids (55).

Three girls with genital ulcerations from Crohn's disease of the vulva have been reported (92). One case was evaluated for sexual abuse. An 8-year-old girl presented with a 16-month history of painless, nonpruritic vulvar erythema and edema. She had been examined by several physicians and treated unsuccessfully for contact dermatitis and candidiasis. An extensive evaluation for sexual abuse was unrevealing. Her perianal examination was reportedly normal. One month before admission, she developed bloody purulent perianal discharge. A 3.6-kg weight loss was associated with decreased oral intake because of fear of stimulating painful defecation. She had no growth retardation or other systemic symptoms.

Examination under anesthesia revealed a nontender red, firm, edematous vulva, a firm edematous clitoris, friable vaginal mucosa, and five fistulous openings in the perianal area. Cultures of the vagina and perirectum revealed no pathogens. Biopsies of the colon, rectum, and vulva showed many noncaseating granulomas and other features of Crohn's disease. Treatment with parenteral alimentation, prednisone, and metronidazole resulted in resolution of the vulvar and perianal abnormalities (92).

Oral ulcers and mucosal lesions can be caused by accidental trauma, infectious agents such as herpes and coxsackievirus, or oral sodomy. A South African study of 660 boys, ages 14 to 22 years, in reform schools found 19 boys with palatal lesions thought to be related to oral fellatio. The lesions were single or multiple, red atrophic patches on the central posterior palate. Seven boys were missing the front incisors, probably to facilitate oral sex. No lesions were seen in 600 control subjects from state schools (127).

Cellulitis or abscess of the labia majora is a rare infection in healthy girls and should lead to suspicion of an underlying immune deficit. Labial cellulitis or abscess, usually caused by *Pseudomonas,* was reported in six of 23 girls with chronic idiopathic neutropenia. It was the presenting manifestation in three patients. An evaluation for neutropenia also is warranted for patients with cellulitis of the perirectal area or groin (78).

Primary syphilis is the most common cause of painless genital ulceration. Because serologic tests for syphilis are not always positive when the ulcers of primary syphilis manifest, negative serologic tests should be repeated in 3 or 4 weeks if syphilis is suspected. Other causes of painless genital ulcers include lichen sclerosus, lymphogranuloma venereum, and granuloma inguinale.

Clinicians treating patients from tropical countries should be aware that yaws may be confused with syphilis. Endemic to tropical areas, yaws is caused by *Treponema pallidum pertenue,* a microorganism that cannot be distinguished serologically or microscopically from *Treponema pallidum pallidum,* the organism causing syphilis. Engelkens et al. (38) described a 3.5-year-old Indonesian boy with a 3-month history of ulcerated, crusted papillomatous lesions on the chin, neck, extremities, and prepuce of the penis. Dark-field examination of exudate from the skin lesions revealed many treponemes. His 8-year-old brother and his mother also had yaws. Yaws is transmitted by skin-to-skin contact, with early lesions occurring in extragenital sites, most often the lower limbs. The genital lesions of yaws have been confused with venereal syphilis.

CONCLUSION

As parents become better educated about the risks of sexual abuse, they are seeking consultation, education, and reassurance from their health care providers when anogenital conditions manifest. A mistaken diagnosis of sexual abuse can be traumatic to all concerned. To avoid this problem, clinicians should be familiar with the variety of conditions confused with child sexual abuse and confounding the diagnosis of STDs. Consultation with specialists in dermatology, surgery, urology, genetics, pathology, infectious disease, or child abuse may be prudent when the diagnosis is in doubt.

REFERENCES

1. Adams JA, Horton M. Is it sexual abuse? *Clin Pediatr* 1989;28:146–148.
2. Adler MW. ABC of sexually transmitted diseases: genital ulceration. *Br Med J* 1983;287:1780–1781.
3. Agnarsson U, Warde C, McCarty G, et al. Perianal appearances associated with constipation. *Arch Dis Child* 1990;65:1231–1234.
4. Baker RB. Anal fissure produced by examination for sexual abuse [Letter]. *Am J Dis Child* 1991;145:848–849.
5. Baker RB. Seat belt injury masquerading as sexual abuse. *Pediatrics* 1986;77:435.
6. Barton DJ, Sloan GM, Nichter LS, et al. Hair-thread tourniquet syndrome. *Pediatrics* 1988;82:925–928.
7. Bays J, Chadwick D. Medical diagnosis of the sexually abused child. *Child Abuse Negl* 1993;17:91.
8. Bays J, Jenny C. Genital and anal conditions confused with child sexual abuse trauma. *Am J Dis Child* 1990; 144:1319–1322.
9. Berenson A, Heger A, Andrews S. Appearance of the hymen in newborns. *Pediatrics* 1991;87:458–465.
10. Bergeron C, Ferenczy RR. Underwear: contamination by human papillomaviruses. *Am J Obstet Gynecol* 1990;162:25–29.
11. Berkowitz CD, Elvik SL, Logan MK. Labial fusion in prepubescent girls: a marker for sexual abuse? *Am J Obstet Gynecol* 1987;156:16–20.
12. Berth-Jones J, Graham-Brown RAC, Burns DA. Lichen sclerosus. *Arch Dis Child* 1989;64:1204–1206.
13. Black CT, Pokorny WJ, McGill CW, et al. Ano-rectal trauma in children. *J Pediatr Surg* 1982;17:501–504.
14. Boisvert PL, Walcher DN. Hemolytic streptococcal vaginitis in children. *Pediatrics* 1948;2:24–29.
15. Bond GR, Dowd MD, Landsman I, et al. Unintentional perineal injury in prepubescent girls: a multicenter prospective report of 56 girls. *Pediatrics* 1995;95: 628–631.
16. Boyd AS. Condyloma acuminata in the pediatric population. *Am J Dis Child* 1990;144:817–824.
17. Boyd M, Jordan SW. Unusual presentation of varicella suggestive of sexual abuse. *Am J Dis Child* 1987;141: 940.
18. Cain WS, Howell CG, Ziegler MM, et al. Rectosigmoid perforation and intestinal evisceration from transanal suction. *J Pediatr Surg* 1983;18:10–13.
19. Cavender PA, Bennett RG. Perianal eosinophilic granuloma resembling condyloma latum. *Pediatr Dermatol* 1988;5:50–55.
20. Centers for Disease Control. Suction-drain injury in a public wading pool—North Carolina, 1991. *MMWR* 1992;41:333–335.
21. Chalmers RJG, Burton PA, Bennett RF, et al. Lichen sclerosus et atrophicus: a common cause of phimosis in boys. *Arch Dermatol* 1984;120:1025–1027.
22. Chamberlain RS, Greenberg LW. Scrotal involvement in Henoch-Schonlein purpura: a case report and review of the literature. *Pediatr Emerg Care* 1992;8:213–215.
23. Chapman HL. Digital strangulation by hair wrapping. *Can Med Assoc J* 1968;98:125.
24. Christensen EH, Oster J. Adhesions of labia minora (synechia vulvae) in childhood. *Acta Paediatr Scand* 1971;60:709–715.
25. Clark AF, Tayler PJ, Bhate SR. Nocturnal faecal soiling and anal masturbation. *Arch Dis Child* 1990;65: 1367–1368.
26. Clayden GS. Reflex anal dilation associated with severe chronic constipation in children. *Arch Dis Child* 63:832–836.
27. Cobbs LW. A paranoid accusation of child molestation. *Hosp Pract* 1982;17:76A–76H.
28. Coffman K, Boyce WT, Hansen RC. Phytodermatitis simulating child abuse. *Am J Dis Child* 1985;139: 239–240.
29. Cohen BA, Honig P, Androphy E. Anogenital warts in children. *Arch Dermatol* 1990;126:1575–1580.

30. Colwell CA. The gynecologic examination of infants, children and young adolescents. *Pediatr Clin North Am* 1981;28:247–266.

31. Connors JM, Schubert C, Shapiro R. Syphilis or abuse: making the diagnosis and understanding the implications. *Pediatr Emerg Care* 1998;14:139–142.

32. DeMarco BJ, Crandall RS, Hreshchyshyn MM. Labial agglutination secondary to a herpes simplex II infection. *Am J Obstet Gynecol* 1987;157:296–297.

33. Dickenson RL. Tampons as menstrual guards. *JAMA* 1945;128:490–494.

34. Dowd MD, Fitzmaurice L, Knapp JF, et al. The interpretation of urogenital findings in children with straddle injuries. *J Pediatr Surg* 1994;29:7–10,

35. Dr G. Ligature of the penis. *Lancet* 1832;2:136.

36. Eldem B, Onur C, Ozen S. Clinical features of pediatric Bechet's disease. *J Pediatr Ophthalmol Strabismus* 1998;35:159–161.

37. Elder JS, Young LW. Radiologic case of the month: calcified vesical foreign body. *Am J Dis Child* 1986; 140:55–56.

38. Engelkens HJH, et al. Disseminated early yaws: report of a child with a remarkable genital lesion mimicking venereal syphilis. *Pediatr Dermatol* 1990;7:60–62.

39. Feldman W, Feldman E, Goodman JT, et al. Is childhood sexual abuse really increasing in prevalance? An analysis of the evidence. *Pediatrics* 1991;88:29–33.

40. Finkel MA. Anogenital trauma in sexually abused children. *Pediatrics* 1989;84:317–322.

41. Fisher AA. Nonoccupational dermatitis to "black"-rubber mix: part II. *Cutis* 1992;49:229–230.

42. Fleming KA, Venning V, Evans M. DNA typing of genital warts and diagnosis of sexual abuse in children. *Lancet* 1987;2:454.

43. French G, Johnson CF. Genital bleeding: two uncommon causes in patients referred to a sexual abuse clinic. *Clin Pediatr* 1994;33:38–41.

44. Friedrich WN, Grambsch P, Broughton D, et al. Normative sexual behavior in children. *Pediatrics* 1991; 88:456–464.

45. Fukunaga K, Kimura K, Lawrence JP, et al. Anteriorly located anus: Is constipation caused by abnormal location of the anus? *J Pediatr Surg* 1996;31:245–246.

46. Gardner JJ. Descriptive study of genital variation in healthy, nonabused premenarchal girls. *J Pediatr* 1992;120:251–257.

47. Gearhart JP, Lowe FC. Genitourinary injuries secondary to break dancing in children and adolescents. *Pediatrics* 1986;77:922–924.

48. Ginsberg CM. Group A streptococcal vaginitis in children. *Pediatr Infect Dis J* 1982;1:36–37.

49. Glover MT, Lake BD, Atherton DJ. Infantile systemic hyalinosis: newly recognized disorder of collagen? *Pediatrics* 1991;87:228–234.

50. Goldenring JM. Secondary syphilis in a prepubertal child: differentiating condyloma lata from condyloma acuminata. *N Y State J Med* 1989;89:180–181.

51. Goodwin J, Sahd D, Rada RT. Incest hoax: false accusations, false denials. In: Holder W, ed. *Sexual abuse of children:* implications for treatment. Englewood, Colorado: American Humane Association, 1983:37–45.

52. Hammerschlag MR, Rettig PJ, Sheilds ME. False positive results with the use of chlamydial antigen detection tests in the evaluation of suspected sexual abuse in children. *Pediatr Infect Dis J* 1988;7:11–14.

53. Handfield-Jones SE, Hinde FRJ, Kennedy CTC. Lichen sclerosus et atrophicus in children misdiagnosed as sexual abuse. *Br Med J* 1987;294:1404–1405.

54. Handley JM, Maw RD, Homer T, et al. Scissor excision plus electrocautery of anogenital warts in prepubertal children. *Pediatr Dermatol* 1991;8:243–245.

55. Hara M, Watanabe M, Tagami H. Jacquet erosive dermatitis in a young girl with urinary incontinence. *Pediatr Dermatol* 1991;8:160–161.

56. Harrington CI. Lichen sclerosus [Letter]. *Arch Dis Child* 1990;65:335.

57. Harrow BR. Strangulation of penis by a hidden thread. *JAMA* 1967;199:171.

58. Helm KF, Gibson LE, Muller SA. Lichen sclerosus et atrophicus in children and young adults. *Pediatr Dermatol* 1991;8:97–101.

59. Herman-Giddens ME, Berson NL. Harmful genital care practices in children: a type of child abuse. *JAMA* 1989;261:577–579.

60. Herman-Giddens ME, Berson NL. Dermatologic conditions misdiagnosed as evidence of child abuse [Letter]. *JAMA* 1989;261:3548.

61. Herman-Giddens ME, Gutman LT, Berson NL. Duke Child Protection Team: association of coexisting vaginal infections and multiple abusers in female children with genital warts. *Sex Transm Dis* 1988;15:63–67.

62. Hey F, Buchan PC, Littlewood JM, et al. Differential diagnosis in child sexual abuse. *Lancet* 1987;1:283.

63. Hobbs CJ, Wynne JM. Sexual abuse of English boys and girls: the importance of the anal examination. *Child Abuse Negl* 1989;13:195–201.

64. Hobbs CJ, Wynne JM. Child sexual abuse: an increasing rate of diagnosis. *Lancet* 1987;2:837–841.

65. Horowitz S, Chadwick DL. Syphilis as a sole indicator of sexual abuse: two cases with no intervention. *Child Abuse Negl* 1990;14:129–132.

66. Hostetler BR, Jones CE, Muram D. Capillary hemangiomas of the vulva mistaken for sexual abuse. *Adolesc Pediatr Gynecol* 1994;7:44–46.

67. Huffman JW, Dewhurst CJ, Capraro VJ. *The gynecology of childhood and adolescence.* 2nd ed. Philadelphia: WB Saunders, 1981:155.

68. Hyman SL, Fisher W, Mercugliano M, et al. Children with self-injurious behavior. *Pediatrics* 1990;85:437–441.

69. Jackson C. Female circumcision: should angels fear to tread? *Health Visitor* 1991;64:252–253.

70. Jenny C. Sexually transmitted diseases and child abuse. *Pediatr Ann* 1992;21:497–503.

71. Jenny C, Kirby P, Fuquay D. Genital lichen sclerosus mistaken for child sexual abuse. *Pediatrics* 1989;83: 597–599.

72. Jerkins GR, Verheeck K, Noe HN. Treatment of girls with urethral prolapse. *J Urol* 1984;132:732–733.

73. Johnson CF. Prolapse of the urethra: confusion of clinical and anatomic characteristics with sexual abuse. *Pediatrics* 1991;87:722–724.

74. Jona JZ. Accidental anorectal impalement in children. *Pediatr Emerg Care* 1997;13:40–43.

75. Jones DPH, McGraw JM. Reliable and fictitious accounts of sexual abuse to children. *J Interpers Violence* 1987;2:27–43.

76. Jones KL. *Smith's recognizable patterns of human malformation.* 4th ed. Philadelphia: WB Saunders, 1988.

77. Jones LW, Bass DH. Perineal injuries in children. *Br J Surg* 1991;78:1105–1107.

78. Jonsson OG, Buchanan GR. Chronic neutropenia during childhood. *Am J Dis Child* 1991;145:232–235.

79. Joseph DB, Bower SB, Colodny AH, et al. Clean intermittent catheterization of infants with neurogenic bladder. *Pediatrics* 1989;84:78–82.

80. Kadish HA, Schunk JE, Britton H. Pediatric male rectal and genital trauma: accidental and nonaccidental injuries. *Pediatr Emerg Care* 1998;14:95–98.

81. Kaplan KM, Fleisher GR, Paradise JE, et al. Social relevance of genital herpes simplex in children. *Am J Dis Child* 1984;138:872–874.

82. Kellogg ND, Parra JM. Linea vestibularis: a previously undescribed normal genital structure in female neonates. *Pediatrics* 1991;87:926–929.

83. Kerns DL, Ritter ML, Thomas RG. Concave hymenal variations in suspected child sexual abuse. *Pediatrics* 1992;90:265–272.

84. Kirschner RH, Stein RJ. The mistaken diagnosis of child abuse: a form of medical abuse? *Am J Dis Child* 1985;139:873–875.

85. Klevan JL, De Jong AR. Urinary tract symptoms and urinary tract infection following sexual abuse. *Am J Dis Child* 1990;144:242–244.

86. Kohr RM. Elevator surfing: a deadly new form of joyriding. *J Forensic Sci* 1992;37:640–645.

87. Kokx NP, Comstock JA, Facklam RR. Streptococcal perianal disease in children. *Pediatrics* 1987;80:659–663.

88. Krol AL. Perianal streptococcal dermatitis. *Pediatr Dermatol* 1990;7:97–100.

89. Kunkel NC. Vaginal injury from a water slide in a premenarcheal patient. *Pediatr Emerg Care* 1998;14:210–211.

90. Kyriazi NC, Costenbader CL. Group A beta hemolytic streptococcal balanitis: it may be more common than you think. *Pediatrics* 1991;88:154–155.

91. Labbe J. Self-induced urinary tract infection in school-age boys. *Pediatrics* 1990;86:703–706.

92. Lally MR, Orenstein SR, Cohen BA. Crohn's diseases of the vulva in an 8-year-old girl. *Pediatr Dermatol* 1988;5:103–106.

93. Leiferman KM, Gleich GJ. The case of the blue boy [Letter]. *Pediatr Dermatol* 1991;8:354.

94. Levin AV, Selbst SM. Vulvar hemangioma simulating child abuse. *Clin Pediatr* 1988;27:213–215.

95. Longo WE, Touloukian RJ, Seashore JN. Fistula in ano in infants and children: implications and management. *Pediatrics* 1991;87:737–739.

96. Lowe FC, Hill GS, Jeffs RD, et al. Urethral prolapse in children: insights into etiology and management. *J Urol* 1986;135:100–103.

97. McCann J, Voris J, Simon M. Labial adhesions and posterior fourchette injuries in childhood sexual abuse. *Am J Dis Child* 1988;142:659–663.

98. McCann J, Wells R, Simon M, et al. Genital findings in prepubertal girls selected for nonabuse: a descriptive study. *Pediatrics* 1990;86:428.

99. McCann J, Voris J, Simon M, et al. Perianal findings in prepubertal children selected for non-abuse: a descriptive study. *Child Abuse Negl* 1989;13:179–193.

100. McCann J, Reay D, Siebert J, et al. Postmortem perianal findings in children. *Am J Forensic Med Pathol* 1996;17:289–298.

101. Morgenstern J. Retention of urine, and edema of the penis from constriction of hairs. *Pediatrics* 1988;5:248–249.

102. Muram D. Child sexual abuse: genital tract findings in prepubertal girls. *Am J Obstet Gynecol* 1989;160:328.

103. Muram D. Genital tract injuries in the prepubertal child. *Pediatr Ann* 1986;15:616–620.

104. Muram D, Rau FJ. Anatomic variations of the bulbocavernosus muscle. *Adolesc Pediatr Gynecol* 1991;4:85–86.

105. Murphy TV, Nelson JD. Shigella vaginitis: report of 38 patients and review of the literature. *Pediatrics* 1979;63:511–516.

106. Nahmias AJ, Dowdle WR, Nab ZM, et al. Genital infection with herpesvirus hominis types 1 and 2 in children. *Pediatrics* 1968;42:659–666.

107. Narkewicz RM. Distal digital occlusion. *Pediatrics* 1978;61:922–923.

108. O'Connor PA, Oliver WJ. Group A beta-hemolytic streptococcal vulvovaginitis: a recurring problem. *Pediatr Emerg Care* 1985;1:94–95.

109. Pacheco BP, et al. Vulvar infection caused by human papilloma virus in children and adolescents without sexual contact. *Adolesc Pediatr Gynecol* 1991;4:136–142.

110. Palmer WM. Streptococcal vaginitis and sexual abuse [Letter]. *Pediatr Infect Dis* 1982;1:374–375.

111. Pantuck AJ, Kraus SL, Barone JG. Hair strangulation injury of the penis. *Pediatric Emerg Care* 1997;13:423–424.

112. Paul DM. The medical examination in sexual offenses against children. *Med Sci Law* 1977;17:251–258.

113. Press S, Schachner L, Paul P. Clitoris tourniquet syndrome. *Pediatrics* 1980;66:781–782.

114. Press S, Grant P, Thompson VT, et al. Small bowel evisceration: unusual manifestation of child abuse. *Pediatrics* 1991;88:807–809.

115. Priestly BL, Bleehen SS. Lichen sclerosus and sexual abuse [Letter]. *Arch Dis Child* 1990;65:335.

116. Priestly BL, Bleehen SS. Lichen sclerosus et atrophicus in children misdiagnosed as sexual abuse. *Br Med J* 1987;295:211.

117. Putnam N, Stein M. Self-inflicted injuries in childhood: a review and diagnostic approach. *Clin Pediatr* 1985;24:514–518.

118. Reardon W, Hughes HE, Green, SH, et al. Anal abnormalities in childhood myotonic dystrophy: a possible source of confusion in child sexual abuse. *Arch Dis Child* 1992;67:527–528.

119. Roberts JW, Devine CJ. Urethral hemangioma: treatment by total excision and grafting. *J Urol* 1983;129:1053–1054.

120. Rock JA, Azziz R. Genital anomalies in childhood. *Clin Obstet Gynecol* 1987;30:682–696.

121. Roussey M, Dabadie A, Chevrant-Breton O, et al. Condylomes acumines chez l'enfant. *Arch Fr Pediatr* 1988;45:29–34.

122. Smith GA, Sharma V, Knapp JF, et al. The summer penile syndrome: seasonal acute hypersensitivity reaction caused by chigger bites on the penis. *Pediatr Emerg Care* 1998;4:116–118.

123. Stanton A, Sunderland R. Prevalence of reflex anal dilation in 200 children. *Br Med J* 1989;298:802–803.

124. Stewart D. Tampon use and physical findings in sexually abused adolescents. Presented at the Fourth Annual Meeting of the North American Society for Pediatric and Adolescent Gynecology. Costa Mesa, CA: January 1990.

125. Tang CK, Shermeta DW, Wood C. Congenital condyloma acuminata. *Am J Obstet Gynecol* 1978;131:912–913.

126. Unuigbe JA, Giwa-Osagie AW. Pediatric and adolescent gynecological disorders in Benin City, Nigeria. *Adolesc Pediatr Gynecol* 1988;1:257–261.

127. van Wyk CW. The oral lesion caused by fellatio. *Am J Forensic Med Pathol* 1981;2:217–219.

128. Vickers D, Morris K, Coulthard MG, et al. Anal signs in haemolytic uraemic syndrome. *Lancet* 1988;1:998.

129. Warrington S, de San Lazaro C. Lichen sclerosis et atrophicus and sexual abuse. *Arch Dis Child* 1996;75: 512–516.

130. West R, Davies A, Fenton T. Accidental vulval injuries in childhood. *Br Med J* 1989;298:1002–1003.

131. Whitelaw JP. Clue to child sexual abuse [Letter]. *N Engl J Med* 1992;326:957.

132. Whittington WL, Rice RJ, Biddle JW, et al. The incor-rect identification of *Neisseria gonorrhoeae* from infants and children. *Pediatr Infect Dis J* 1988;7:3.

133. Williams TS, Callen JP, Owen LG. Vulvar disorders in the prepubertal female. *Pediatr Ann* 1986;15:588.

134. Woodling BA, Kossoris PD. Sexual misuse: rape, molestation and incest. *Pediatr Clin North Am* 1981; 28:481.

135. Wynne JM. Injuries to the genitalia in female children. *S Afr Med J* 1980;57:47.

136. Yates A. Differentiating hypererotic states in the evaluation of sexual abuse. *J Am Acad Child Adolesc Psychiatry* 1991;30:792.

137. Zempsky WT, Rosenstein BJ. The cause of rectal prolapse in children. *Am J Dis Child* 1988;142:338.

138. Zivony D, Nocton J, Wortmann D, et al. Juvenile Reiter's syndrome: a report of four cases. *J Am Acad Dermatol* 1998;38:32–37.

12

Failure to Thrive

*Deborah A. Frank, †Dennis Drotar, ‡John Cook, §Jennifer Bleiker, and
"Dorothy Kasper

*§Growth Clinic, Department of Pediatrics, Boston Medical Center; and *‡Department of Pediatrics,
Boston University School of Medicine, Boston, Massachusetts; †Behavioral and Pediatric Psychology
and "Ready Set Grow Program, Department of Pediatrics, Rainbow Babies' and Children's Hospital; and
†Department of Pediatrics, Case Western Reserve University School of Medicine, Cleveland, Ohio

Failure to thrive (FTT) is an imprecise term that refers to children whose growth deviates significantly from the norms for their age and gender (20). Traditionally, FTT was dichotomized into "organic failure to thrive," in which the child's growth failure was ascribed to a major medical illness, and "nonorganic failure to thrive," which was attributed primarily to psychological neglect or "maternal deprivation" (32,46,97,207).

This simplistic dichotomous conceptualization of FTT is obsolete (77). We now recognize that in all cases of "nonorganic" FTT, and in many cases of "organic" FTT, the proximate cause of growth failure is malnutrition, whether primary or secondary (34,35,77,78, 97,236). Malnutrition not only jeopardizes the child's growth, but also impairs immunocompetence and contributes to concurrent and long-term deficits in cognition and socioaffective competence (11,12,20,40,53,60,79, 88–91). The modern diagnosis and treatment of FTT focus on the assessment of and therapy for malnutrition and its complications (20,34,48,60,77,202,236). The needs of each child and family that are not thriving should be assessed along four parameters: medical, nutritional, developmental, and social. Before addressing the clinical care of any individual child and family, however, it is important to understand the ecologic context in which childhood malnutrition occurs in one of the world's richest nations.

ECOLOGIC CONTEXT

Food insecurity and hunger afflict millions of low-income American children, according to recent national surveys (107,147). Results of a national study of food security and hunger in the United States, released by the U.S. Department of Agriculture (USDA) in 1997, found that more than 15% of all households with children younger than 18 years were food insecure in 1995, and 4.9% were hungry. In this study, food-insecure households are defined as those unable to obtain reliably sufficient nutritious food for an active, healthy life (8,28). Hungry households are defined as those unable to obtain sufficient food to prevent all members from repeatedly experiencing hunger (198). The prevalence of food insecurity and hunger among minority households with children younger than 18 years, and single-parent households, is even higher. Among black and Hispanic households with children, 28.2% and 30.4%, respectively, were food-insecure, while 10.1% and 8.8% were hungry (8,31,38,39,74). These estimates are conservative, because homeless children and children living in homes without telephones were omitted from the survey.

The cumulative effects of days and weeks of inadequate diets are reflected in higher rates of short stature among low-income children participating in various national and state surveys, with rates approaching 10% of children with heights below the National Center for Health Statistics (NCHS) 5th percentile norms in most settings (55,106,127, 160,222). Thus children clinically identified as "failing to thrive," who are drawn disproportionately from low-income families, represent the extreme end of a spectrum of nutritional deprivation of children in or near poverty that often goes unrecognized by health providers in less extreme cases (22,34).

Poverty is the greatest single risk factor for FTT (31,127,152). By definition, the federal poverty level ($16,660 for an average family of four in 1998), set at three times the cost of a minimally nutritious diet, implies an income level inadequate for meeting children's needs for shelter, clothing, and food (19,31). Indeed, children living in families with incomes up to 185% of poverty are considered at nutritional risk (19,37,74,93,122). Recent studies have found that families in the U.S. need an income equal to at least 185% of the poverty level to achieve minimal economic self-sufficiency in the current environment of reduced social welfare assistance created by enactment of federal "welfare reform" legislation (49,50,165,182, 205,208). In addition to an insufficient budget for food purchases, economically disadvantaged families often lack access to supermarkets and live in homes lacking adequate food storage and preparation facilities (19,28,39,37, 74,223,234). As of this writing, social welfare policy changes, decreasing real wage levels, structural changes in U.S. labor markets, and changes in patterns of fertility, marital status, and living arrangements among the U.S. population have interacted to make children the most disadvantaged segment of American society (19,182,205,208). The proportion of U.S. children in poverty, and therefore at risk of FTT, has remained at or near 20% since 1981 (19,31,79). In 1998, more than 3 million more American children younger than 18 years were in poverty than were 20 years earlier in 1978, although during the 1990s, the U.S. economy experienced unprecedented growth, with unemployment consistently declining nationally (19,28,49,50,74).

Nevertheless, the economic circumstances of many poor families, especially poor single-mother families, worsened substantially over the period 1995 through 1997 (19,49,50). Primus et al. (182) found that while the disposable income of single-mother families in the lowest income quintile grew by nearly 14% from 1993 to 1995, it actually declined by 6.7% from 1995 to 1997. Sherman (205) found that the number of children living in families with incomes below one-half the poverty line increased by more than 17% between 1996 and 1997, with most of the increase occurring in mother-only families. Even though overall child poverty declined slightly over the period 1996 to 1998, the proportion of children younger than 6 years in poverty remained higher than 20% (19,28). For the poorest of the poor (families with incomes at or below 50% of poverty), economic conditions actually worsened during the 1990s (8,19,28).

While childhood poverty has increased throughout the 1980s and most of the 1990s, national programs designed to protect the health and nutritional status of low-income children have not been adequately funded to meet the growing need. Part of the increase in the depth of poverty amidst economic growth since 1996 has occurred among poor families with children and appears to reflect sharp decreases in the proportions of poor children and families receiving cash assistance and food stamp benefits. The percentage of poor children whose families receive cash assistance benefits decreased from 62% in 1994 to 43% in 1998. The percentage of poor children whose families receive food stamps dropped from 94% to 75% during the same period (28, 37–39,218). Nationally, more than a fourth (25.2%) of all poor children did not have health insurance in 1998, whereas 20% of all black and 30% of all Hispanic children were uninsured (33). Without health insurance, many of these children have limited access to the kind of preventive medical care that could detect and treat early growth failure.

The problem with child nutrition programs is twofold: first, the programs are not adequately funded to reach all those who are eligible; and second, the benefit levels for available programs are not adequate to meet the nutritional needs of recipients, particularly for rapidly growing infants and toddlers, and for children whose nutritional needs are increased by illness or prior nutritional deficit (as is the case for almost all children with the diagnosis of FTT) (8,28). In fiscal year 1998, food stamps provided maximal benefits of less than 80 cents per meal per person on average, so that many families relying on the program routinely run out of food near the end of the month (37–39,50). That same year, 52.8% of all Food Stamp Program recipients were children, and 81.8% of all food stamp benefits went to households with children (37,50).

The highly successful Special Supplemental Food Program for Women, Infants, and Children (WIC) is estimated by USDA to reach only 81% of all eligible women, infants, and children, whereas school breakfast is available to only about one in four children who receive school lunch (38,142,165,166,182). Although the WIC program food packages have been updated and improved over recent years, they are intended as only a supplement to the other food provided in the household, and thus provide less than 100% of the recommended daily allowances (RDAs) for a number of nutrients (142,182). For some WIC children in certain age groups, and many pregnant and postpartum mothers, the combination of WIC food and other food available in the household is insufficient to provide adequate nutrients (142, 182). Even with simultaneous participation in multiple programs (food stamps, WIC, school meals), many low-income families are unable to obtain enough food to avoid frequent episodes of food insecurity and hunger, and the chronic mild-to-moderate undernutrition that ensues (37,39,93,237).

To minimize the temptation to scapegoat families in clinical assessment and intervention, it is important to recognize that FTT often reflects economic conditions and changes in social policy that are far beyond the control of individual parents or health-care providers (122,134). Children also fail to thrive in spite of material adequacy in cases of severe parent–child interactive disorders, parental psychopathology, family dysfunction, or organic pathology. The impact of such problems on children's health increases dramatically in the context of poverty; lack of means to provide adequate care is often a major factor in the development of FTT (19,37,122). In our clinical experience, much FTT occurs in financial and social circumstances that would make it difficult for any parent to address successfully a child's physical and emotional needs. For this reason, true primary prevention of FTT, which is beyond the scope of this chapter, requires an end to the systematic deprivation of American families (31,37,38,122,172).

Family Risk Factors

Multiple family risk factors may interact with poverty to disrupt the child's caloric intake and trigger growth deficiency. Belsky's model of parental competence (15,59) provides a useful framework in which to consider family influences on growth deficiency. In this model, parental competence is influenced by three sets of factors: (a) parental resources, especially early developmental experiences and personality; (b) child characteristics, such as temperament, physical health, and illness; and (c) the family and social context of parent–child relations, including the parents' relationship, family social networks and resources, employment, and community resources (15, 57–59,93,100).

Parental Personal Resources

Early research efforts suggested that serious maternal psychopathology was not a powerful risk factor for FTT (139,140,177). Parental mood disturbances and/or adjustment problems, however, may affect the quality of parent–child interactions and hence the psychological outcomes of children who fail to thrive. Salt et al. (196) found that depressive symptoms, especially feelings of hopelessness, occurred more often among mothers of previously malnourished children than among mothers of comparison children. Depressive symptoms were more common in association with disadvantaged socioeconomic and home conditions. Polan et al. (175) also noted higher rates of affective and personality disorders among a small sample of mothers of FTT infants compared with controls, and suggested that maternal emotional status should be considered in planning intervention for this problem.

In a prospective study, Altemeier et al. (5) found that mothers of children who eventually developed FTT reported more problematic childhoods than did mothers whose children did not develop FTT. Maternal reports of being abused as a child correlated positively with subsequent FTT. Conversely, maternal perceptions of a happy childhood, that they were loved as a child, and that their parents were pleased with them, correlated negatively with the development of FTT (5). Benoit et al. (16) found that more mothers of FTT infants were classified as insecure in their attachment relationships compared with mothers of infants who grew at an average rate. Lack of resolution of mourning over the loss of a loved one was found in more mothers in the FTT group compared with controls. Mothers of children with FTT have reported high rates of physical abuse as children and as adults (5,235). Such psychological vulnerabilities in parental emotional resources could contribute to the development of dysfunctional parent–child relation patterns (61,66,175,177,187,181).

Child Characteristics

Children's physical and temperamental characteristics may contribute to the development of FTT by presenting parents with additional child-rearing burdens that tax their already strained emotional and economic resources (20,77,136). Pollitt and Leibel (178) suggested that lethargic, listless infant behavior might evoke less-responsive behavior from parents and contribute to FTT. As discussed in

detail later, prematurity and low birth weight impose additional caregiving burdens on parents. In addition, early childhood illnesses may also heighten risk for FTT (203).

Delayed or dysfunctional oral–motor development, as well as deficient signaling of needs during mealtimes, may contribute to FTT (155,189,192). Once a child begins to demonstrate deficient growth and nutrition, irrespective of the specific cause, the child's irritability and inconsistent social responsiveness may engender feelings of helplessness among parents as well as beliefs that the child is physically deficient or ill.

The Family and Social Context

Families of FTT infants have been identified as having lower economic levels, higher family stress, less available extended family for help with child-rearing, and greater social isolation than have comparison groups (22,129,139, 140,215). All of these factors could affect the family members' capacities to mobilize caretaking resources on behalf of the child. Relationship patterns also may be strained in some families of FTT infants (236). Drotar and Eckerle (64) found that mothers of FTT infants reported less supportive and cohesive family relationships than did families of comparison group infants. The quality of family relationships and organization may affect the timing, frequency, and consistency of reinforcement for feeding patterns and ultimately is reflected in the child's growth and health (59).

MEDICAL ISSUES IN EVALUATION AND TREATMENT

Family History

The assessment of FTT begins with a family history, focusing on issues such as consanguinity, developmental delay, atopy, human immunodeficiency virus (HIV) risk, and potentially growth-retarding familial illnesses such as cystic fibrosis, celiac disease, inflammatory bowel disease, or lactose intolerance. Height of both parents should be ascertained, as well as history of growth delay in childhood and timing of puberty. A familial pattern of short stature, or constitutional delay of growth, may obviate the need for extensive workup if the child is short but not underweight for height (125,131). Norms exist for correcting height percentiles for midparent height by using the National Center for Health Statistics (NCHS) grids (117). It is critical, however, to assess whether the parents themselves were malnourished as children, as is often the case among immigrant and low-income families. In such cases, the parents' stature does not provide an accurate indication of the child's genetic growth potential (84). Moreover, an experience of severe childhood deprivation may influence the parents' care-taking practices (75).

In addition to identifying biologic constraints on growth, a detailed family medical history may uncover significant psychosocial stressors. A chronically ill grandparent or sibling may divert the family's care-taking energies from the child who fails to thrive; FTT has been described in siblings of leukemic children (145). A family history of serious mental illness, intergenerational substance abuse, or developmental impairment also may be present (46). In our clinical experience, it is not unusual for a parent of a child who fails to thrive to have a history of an eating disorder in childhood, occasionally carrying the actual diagnosis of anorexia nervosa (2,195).

Perinatal Factors

After ascertaining family history, the medical assessment of a child who is not thriving should proceed to a detailed assessment of the child's prenatal and perinatal history by interview and, when possible, by review of neonatal records. This approach not only elucidates potential biologic risks to growth, but also may be helpful in identifying ongoing psychosocial risk factors that are concurrently influencing postnatal growth.

Low birth weight is a major predictor of later referral for FTT. In several clinical series, 10% to 40% of children hospitalized for FTT without a major medical diagnosis had a birth weight less than 2,500 g, compared with 7% of the general population (32,77,113,168, 202). In controlled studies of FTT that ex-

cluded infants with birth weights less than 2,500 g from their definition of FTT, infants later diagnosed as FTT still had lower birth weights than those who grew normally (178).

To evaluate accurately the impact of perinatal risk factors on later growth, a detailed history should be obtained covering the issues summarized in Table 12.1. It is critical to as-

TABLE 12.1. *Pregnancy and delivery*

Mother's reproductive history
Age
Cravidity/parity/abortions (spontaneous or induced)
History of pregnancy with identified parent
Conception planned or unplanned
Difficulties with fertility
Conceived while mother using contraception
Was abortion considered
Mother's nutritional status during pregnancy
Weight at conception
Pregnancy weight gain
WIC
Hypermesis
Mother's health habits during pregnancy
Cigarette packs per day
Alcohol
Prescribed drug use (particularly anticonvulsants)
Illicit drug use
X-rays
Occupational exposure
Complications of pregnancy
Infections/high fevers
Bleeding
Toxemia
Violence or Trauma
Labor and delivery
Vaginal or cesarean
Anesthesia
Maternal complications
Neonatal status
Gestational age
Apgars
Birth weight, length, head circumference (parameters and percentiles for gestation age)
Neonatal course
Mother and child separation
Need for special care
Duration of hospitalization for mother and chid
Complications: jaundice, respiratory, CNS, sepsis, necrotizing enterocolitis
Early feeding difficulties
Transfusions
Eye exam
Hearing exam

WIC, Special Supplemental Nutrition Program for Women, Infants, and Children; CNS, central nervous system.

certain not only the child's birth weight, but also gestational age, length, and head circumference at birth. Such data will identify prematurity as well as various patterns of intrauterine growth retardation that have prognostic implications for later growth.

Prematurity

Children born prematurely may be inappropriately labeled as FTT if the percentiles used for assessing growth parameters are not corrected for gestational age by subtracting the number of weeks the child was premature from the child's postnatal age at time of assessment. A statistically significant difference in growth percentiles will be found without such correction in head circumference until 18 months postnatal age, in weight until 24 months postnatal age, and in length until 40 months postnatal age (30). Even after such correction, infants with very low birth weights (less than 1,501 g) may remain smaller than infants born at term for at least the first 3 years of life (36). In these children, the distribution of mean height, weight, and head circumference is shifted downward relative to the NCHS norms so that the proportion of children with attained weight or height below the NCHS 5th percentile is increased (36). The rate of growth of such infants, however, should be the same as that of term infants of the same corrected age (36,134). Moreover, weight for length should be proportional despite somewhat lower fat stores (94). Thus formerly premature children who show depressed weight for height or whose growth progressively deviates from a channel parallel to the NCHS norms should be assessed carefully for a potentially correctable cause of growth failure. The neurologic, gastrointestinal, and cardiorespiratory sequelae of prematurity, as well as the behavioral disorganization characteristic of some premature infants, may all contribute to postnatal malnutrition. Growth difficulties should not be discounted in such children on the grounds that they were "born small." In addition to affecting the infant's behavior or physical growth potential directly, prematurity and low birth weight

also may act indirectly to increase the risk of growth failure by intensifying family stress and requiring early separation between parents and child for neonatal intensive care.

Intrauterine Growth Retardation

Size at birth reflects both the duration and the rate of growth during gestation. Infants whose rate of intrauterine growth is depressed are at risk for postnatal growth failure, regardless of gestational age. Intrauterine growth retardation (IUGR) is conventionally defined as birth weight less than the 10th percentile for gestational age. The degree of risk for postnatal growth failure after IUGR is not uniform, varying with both the cause of the IUGR and the pattern of relative deficit in length, weight, or head circumference at birth.

The best prognosis for postnatal growth pertains to infants with asymmetric IUGR, whose weight at birth is disproportionately more depressed than their length or head circumference. Such infants are at risk for FTT because they are often behaviorally difficult (4). With enhanced postnatal nutrition, however, they can manifest significant catch-up growth in the first 6 to 8 months of life so that later growth trajectories may be within the normal range (4,230). For such infants, early identification of growth failure and intensive nutritional and environmental intervention is critical because the potential for catch-up growth to repair the intrauterine deficit is maximal in the first 6 months of life (113,170).

Infants with symmetric IUGR, whose weight, length, and head circumference are proportionately depressed at birth, carry a relatively poor prognosis for later growth and development. A symmetric pattern of IUGR should alert the clinician to the possibility of chromosomal abnormalities, intrauterine infections, or prenatal teratogen exposure. For this reason, symmetrically growth-retarded children should be carefully scrutinized for dysmorphic features that may provide clues to syndrome diagnosis. Exposure to anticonvulsants, including hydantoin and valproate, may be associated with symmetric IUGR and dysmorphic features (108). Prenatal exposure to many legal and illegal psychoactive substances during pregnancy often contributes to symmetric IUGR, but the prognostic implications for later growth, particularly somatic growth, are variable (76). Because the issue of prenatal substance exposure and later growth potential is often raised in protective service cases, it warrants discussion in some detail.

Prenatal Exposure to Legal Psychoactive Substances and Later Growth

Although heavy use of caffeine prenatally is associated in some studies with depressed intrauterine growth, such use has no detectable effects on the later size of exposed infants (81). Some investigators have noted correlations between heavy cigarette exposure during pregnancy and statistically significant decrements in stature at school age, but the magnitude of the deficit (1 to 2 cm) is usually not large enough to trigger referral for FTT (146,194). Growth deficits persist from infancy to school age in children with dysmorphic features consistent with fetal alcohol syndrome, but not in children who were exposed yet are not dysmorphic (47,51,82). Length and head circumference are more depressed than weight in such cases (204).

Although fetal alcohol syndrome constrains postneonatal growth, clinicians also must remain alert to potentially treatable postneonatal medical and psychosocial factors that may be preventing children with fetal alcohol syndrome from attaining even their limited growth potential. As with very low birth weight infants, children with fetal alcohol syndrome in whom rate of growth deviates from their own previously established patterns should be evaluated meticulously (109). Neurologically based oral–motor difficulties are often associated with fetal alcohol syndrome and may limit caloric intake, unless gastrostomy tubes are placed (228). Even more commonly, the growth of children with fetal alcohol syndrome who remain in the care of mothers with active untreated alcoholism shows effects of inadequate care and

nutrition. Such children should not remain in conditions of profound deprivation on the grounds that they have fetal alcohol syndrome and "can't grow." Our clinical experience shows that with appropriate nutritional, neurodevelopmental, and psychosocial intervention, children with fetal alcohol syndrome can be brought into the normal range of weight for height, but remain short and microcephalic despite intervention.

Prenatal Exposure to Illicit Psychoactive Substances and Later Growth

The three most frequently used illicit drugs during pregnancy are marijuana, cocaine, and opiates. Unfortunately, few follow-up studies of exposed infants beyond the neonatal period have been performed. Infants who were exposed to marijuana during pregnancy tend to have a decreased weight and length, and sometimes head circumference, compared with unexposed newborns, probably because smoking marijuana, like smoking tobacco, increases maternal carbon monoxide levels, and decreases fetal oxygenation (80,247). However, in the only long-term follow-up study of prenatal marijuana exposure, conducted in a middle-class white sample, children with a history of prenatal marijuana exposure had weights and lengths significantly greater than their nonexposed peers, even after controlling for confounding variables (82,83). Therefore prenatal marijuana exposure is not a plausible biologic risk factor for later FTT.

In utero cocaine exposure is independently associated with decrements in gestational age, and with consistently lower birth weight, length, and head circumference (41,123,233, 247). At age 7 to 16 weeks, no difference was found in feeding behaviors between infants who were exposed prenatally to cocaine and those who were not exposed (163). If levels of exposure to cigarettes and alcohol are not controlled statistically, researchers have noted small but statistically significant decrements in head circumference, and in one cohort, in weight, among *in utero* cocaine-exposed children followed up until age 3 years

(41,121). However, in two studies that controlled statistically for the level of prenatal exposure to tobacco and alcohol, no negative effect of prenatal cocaine exposure was noted on weight, height, or head circumference (123,191). Accelerated rates of postneonatal weight gain have been noted after prenatal cocaine exposure (41,110,123). Therefore clinicians should not accept prenatal exposure to cocaine as a sufficient explanation for postnatal failure to gain weight.

Exposure to heroin or methadone *in utero* also has been linked to depressed birth weight, length, and head circumference, but follow-up studies of the growth patterns of these infants are not entirely consistent. Wilson et al. (238) reported that 3- to 6-year-old children exposed *in utero* to heroin were smaller in all growth parameters than were nonexposed social class controls. In most studies, however, smaller head circumference but few differences in somatic growth were noted when opiate-exposed infants were compared with children of the same social class without opiate exposure (52).

Growth failure in any child of a mother with a history of illicit substance use, particularly intravenous use, mandates assessment to rule out infection with HIV, because FTT is a common symptom in infected children (9,10). The quality of care the child is receiving at the time of referral also must be evaluated because continued parental substance abuse may be contributing to concurrent nutritional deprivation of the child. Even though *in utero* exposure to psychoactive substances may cause a decrease in birth weight, length, and head circumference, most such substances do not inhibit a child from showing postnatal somatic catch-up growth in response to adequate nutrition (76). Heavy prenatal exposure to alcohol or opiates may be associated with relative microcephaly, and fetal alcohol syndrome is characterized by persistent short stature. However, exposure *in utero* to the most commonly used psychoactive substances does not adequately explain a child who is underweight for height or one whose growth progressively deviates from a previously established trajectory.

Postnatal Medical Issues

Almost all severe and chronic childhood illnesses can cause growth failure. The mechanisms of such failure are multiple—enzymatic, metabolic, and endocrine in some cases, but also nutritional and psychosocial (132,174). Chronic physical problems that necessitate procedures such as gastrostomy or nasogastric feedings may impede the development of normal patterns of feeding.

Hospitalization should not be regarded as a diagnostic test for chronic illness (86). According to an old myth, environmentally deprived children ("nonorganic failure to thrive") grow in the hospital, whereas children with serious medical illnesses ("organic failure to thrive") will not. In fact, a positive growth response to hospitalization is a poor discriminant of major organic illness because both children with such illness and children with primary malnutrition will grow if given adequate caloric intake (23). Chronically ill children who do well in the hospital usually have complex technical, psychosocial, and nutritional needs that can be met by multiple shifts of highly trained medical personnel, but overwhelm parents who are not receiving adequate care-taking support at home. Conversely, unless the hospital provides specialized milieu therapy, usually not available on acute care wards, children with severe interactive feeding disorders or depression may deteriorate nutritionally in the hospital because separation from primary attachment figures and multiple caretakers may exacerbate their affective and behavioral feeding difficulties. Children who are simply underfed do well either in the hospital or in any setting when adequate calories are offered. Thus response to hospitalization in itself does not necessarily contribute to identifying the cause of FTT.

Whether in inpatient or outpatient settings, chronic illnesses severe enough to jeopardize growth usually can be ascertained from a meticulous history and physical examination (Tables 12.2 and 12.3). The list of occult med-

TABLE 12.2. *Child's postneonatal health history*

Immunizations
Allergies
Surgeries
Hospitalizations
Current medications
Midparent height
Consanguinity
Heritable conditions
Review of systems
   Weight loss
   Diarrhea/vomiting
   Dysphagia
   Snoring, difficulty with tonsils or adenoids
   Recurring pneumonia, otitis, or sinusitis
   Painful teeth
   Loss of previously acquired milestones
   Thrush/recurrent monilial rash
Pets
Travel
Passive tobacco exposure

ical conditions presenting as FTT is relatively circumscribed, and often these are identified during the review of systems (outlined in Table 12.2), focusing on infections and conditions that interfere with caloric intake or retention. In series of children hospitalized for

TABLE 12.3. *Physical examination*

Vital signs: blood pressure if over 2, temperature, pulse, respirations
General appearance: activity, affect, posture
Skin: hygiene, rashes, trauma (bruises, burns, scars)
Head: hair whorls, color and pluckability of hair, occipital alopecia, fontanel size and patency, frontal   bossing, sutures, shape, facial dysmorphisms
Eyes: ptosis, strabismus, fundoscopic where possible, palpebral fissures, conjunctival pallor
Ears: external form, rotation, tympanic membranes
Mouth, nose, throat: hydration, dental eruption and hygiene caries, glossitis, cheilosis, gum bleeding
Neck: hairline, masses, lymphadenopathy
Abdomen: protuberance, hepatosplenomegaly, masses
Genitalia: Malformations, hygiene, trauma
Rectum: fissures, trauma
Extremities: edema, dysmorphisms, rachitic changes, nails and nail beds
Neurologic: cranial nerves, reflexes, tone, retention of primitive reflexes, quality of voluntary movement

FTT of unknown origin, the most common previously undiagnosed illnesses are gastrointestinal, including chronic nonspecific diarrhea, gluten-sensitive enteropathy, food allergies, gastroesophageal reflux, cystic fibrosis, and lactose intolerance (18,73,116,118,207, 222). Immigrant children and children attending congregate day care or living in homeless shelters should be evaluated for giardiasis and other parasites and enteric pathogens if they have gastrointestinal symptoms such as diarrhea or abdominal pain, because these are common causes of malabsorption and growth failure (105,222). Outside the gastrointestinal system, clinicians should consider urinary tract infections and renal tubular acidosis as potentially clinically silent contributors to FTT. Subtle neurologic dysfunction manifested as fine and oral motor dysfunction also should be considered and ruled out (189).

Both overdiagnosis and underdiagnosis of "food allergy" can contribute to failure to thrive (193). In 1995 the European Academy of Allergy and Clinical Immunology created a standard terminology by which to assign a patient's reaction to a food (111,124). Only those reactions that are the consequence of an immune response [immunoglobulin E (IgE) mediated] to a food or food additive are clinically considered to be food allergies (124, 144), whereas a non–IgE-mediated immune reaction is classified as "adverse food reactions" or "food sensitivity" (124,130).

An exceedingly restrictive diet based on an imprecise or factitious diagnosis of food allergy may present as FTT (193). It is crucial that the cause of an apparent adverse reaction to a food be aggressively sought. Whereas negative skin tests are 95% accurate, positive tests are only 50% accurate and must be confirmed by history or a food challenge (124). It may take as long as 14 days to see a clinical response to an elimination diet. A double-blind, placebo-controlled food challenge is the "gold standard" for food allergy diagnosis, but may not always be practical in primary care settings (164). Alternative or additional methods such as radioallergosorbent (RAST) tests may be easier to obtain (115,164). The physician should be aware that *Helicobacter pylori,* other infections, and celiac disease may be manifested by the same symptoms as are food allergies (115,124,126,128,141). Conversely, 30% of atopic dermatitis in young children is triggered by food allergy, so that evaluation for food allergy should be considered in any child with FTT and eczema. Because children often "outgrow" their adverse reaction to a food by age 3 years, such evaluations should be repeated periodically so that the child's diet does not remain unnecessarily restricted (128,164,197).

In recent years, the differential diagnosis of FTT has expanded to include HIV infection. This diagnosis should be considered particularly in children whose mothers have a history of illicit psychoactive substance use, have had multiple sexual partners, or are sexual partners of substance-abusing or bisexual men. The diagnosis also must be ruled out in children of immigrants from areas where heterosexual transmission of HIV is endemic and when the child or mother or her sexual partner has had a blood transfusion (10).

In addition to primary illnesses that may be associated with secondary malnutrition and growth failure, the clinician must be alert to the medical complications of primary malnutrition, particularly recurring infections and lead poisoning. Malnutrition severe enough to produce growth failure also impairs immunocompetence, particularly cell-mediated immunity and the production of complement and secretory IgA (6,44,158). Recurring otitis media and gastrointestinal and respiratory illnesses are more common among children who fail to thrive than among well-nourished children of the same age (62,160,201,221,231).

Children who fail to thrive are often trapped in an infection–malnutrition cycle. With each illness, the child's appetite and nutrient intake decrease while nutrient requirements increase as a result of fever, diarrhea, and vomiting. In settings in which nutrient intake is already marginal, even when the child is well, cumulative nutritional deficits occur, leaving the child increasingly vulnerable to more severe and prolonged infections and

even less adequate growth. Commonly in developing countries and occasionally in developed countries, malnourished children succumb to fulminating infections.

Elevated lead levels correlate with impaired growth, even in the 5- to 35-mg/dL range (200). Here too, a negative cycle develops. Nutritional deficiencies of iron and calcium enhance the absorption of lead and other heavy metals (153). As lead levels rise, constipation, abdominal pain, and anorexia occur, leading to even less adequate dietary intake (224). In a recent study, 16% of children with FTT had lead levels high enough to warrant chelation (21).

Physical Examination and Laboratory Evaluation

The physical examination of the child who fails to thrive, summarized in Table 12.3, has three goals: (a) identification of chronic illness, (b) recognition of potentially growth-retarding syndromes, and (c) documentation of the effects of malnutrition. Some findings may be nonspecific and require elucidation by laboratory assessment; for example, hepatic enlargement may be seen with primary malnutrition, acquired immunodeficiency syndrome (AIDS), or underlying liver disease.

Laboratory evaluation should be restrained and guided by history and the findings of the physical examination. For example, a child who has no symptoms of cardiorespiratory distress and no heart murmur does not need an electrocardiogram. Basic laboratory studies should be used to identify derangements caused by malnutrition and to rule out the few potentially occult diseases just described (112). All children should have a complete blood count, assessment of lead and free erythrocyte protoporphyrin levels, urinalysis, and a tuberculin test. Iron deficiency is a common finding. If the child does not respond promptly to nutritional intervention, blood urea nitrogen or creatinine and serum electrolytes should be measured. These tests also are mandatory in children with vomiting or diarrhea, clinically obvious dehydration, or third-degree malnu-trition, which is often associated with hy-pokalemia. In children with severe anthropo-metric deficits, it is useful to obtain an albumin level to assess protein status and to determine alkaline phosphatase, calcium, and phosphorus levels. A depressed alkaline phosphatase value suggests zinc deficiency; an elevated level, especially if associated with a depressed phosphorous value, is sug-gestive of rickets (17). HIV testing, sweat tests, and stool assessments for *Giardia* should be performed in epidemiologically at-risk populations (6,9,10). RAST or skin testing for food allergies should be consid-ered in children with FTT and atopic der-matitis, as well as for those with a history of rash, urticaria, or vomiting and diarrhea re-curring after ingestion of selected foods. In a child with FTT and vomiting not explained by food allergies and not responsive to em-piric management, radiographic, pH probe, and endoscopic studies to rule out anatomic intestinal abnormalities, gastroesophageal reflux, and esophagitis may be indicated, particularly among children with neurologic impairments and unexplained respiratory symptoms (116). For short children with weight proportionate to height, bone-age ra-diographic studies of the wrists and knees are helpful in discriminating those who are constitutionally short (bone age equals chronologic age and is greater than height age) from those with growth hormone or thy-roid deficiencies or chronic malnutrition (bone age equals height age and is less than chronologic age) (169,174).

Careful physical examination will usually identify untreated dental cavities and ab-scesses that make eating and chewing painful and lead to inadequate caloric intake (1,29). Large tonsils and a history of chronic snoring and recurring otitis/sinusitis warrant radio-logic study of the upper airway and possibly a sleep study because severe tonsillar–ade-noidal hypertrophy may cause growth failure through mechanical feeding difficulties and intermittent hypoxia (199). Furthermore, it is important to observe a feeding because subtle oral–motor difficulties may interfere with di-etary intake in children with otherwise sub-clinical neurologic abnormalities (155,189).

Medical Management

The pediatric health care provider should play an ongoing role in the management of children who fail to thrive. Children must be seen more frequently than is dictated by rou-tine health management schedules to monitor their growth and development in response to interventions. Weekly visits are often neces-sary at the beginning of diagnosis and treat-ment. Meticulous management of concurrent chronic illness is essential, enlisting and coor-dinating assessments in as many disciplines as necessary. Lead poisoning, if identified, should be treated according to standard proto-cols (226).

The health provider must take an aggres-sive stance to interrupt the infection–malnu-trition cycle. In addition to all immunizations routinely recommended by the American Academy of Pediatrics, the influenza vaccine and newly licensed pneumococcal vaccine should be considered for children with sec-ond- and third-degree malnutrition and for those with recurring respiratory infections (6). Families should be instructed to seek care at the first signs of infection so that immedi-ate workup and treatment are provided. Re-curring otitis or sinusitis are indications to consider antibiotic prophylaxis with sulfisox-azole or amoxicillin, but the clinician must be alert to break through infections with resistant organisms. Referral for otolaryngologic as-sessment is warranted if prophylaxis is inef-fective (201). In addition, for each episode of acute illness, the clinician should provide spe-cific instruction about appropriate diet during and after the illness to try to maintain and re-pair nutritional status. A child should never receive a clear liquid diet for more than 24 hours (222).

Hospitalization is indicated for severely malnourished children, for children with seri-ous intercurrent infections, for those whose safety is in question, or if a special combination of disciplines or diagnostic procedures is necessary and can be assembled most efficiently inside the hospital. In many centers, the availability of interdisciplinary outpatient clinics for the diagnosis and management of FTT has greatly reduced the need for hospitalization (173). Referral for specialized inpatient or outpatient assessment should be considered, however, for any child who has not responded to 2 or 3 months of intensive management in a primary care setting.

NUTRITIONAL EVALUATION AND TREATMENT

The major components of a nutritional history for a child who is failing to thrive are summarized in Table 12.4. The assessment should focus not only on current feeding practices, but also on the development of feeding since birth. Often a child's growth failure is triggered by a shift in feeding practices. For example, the shift from soy formula to whole milk at age 12 months, as mandated by the WIC program, may trigger FTT in a severely lactose-intolerant or milk protein–allergic child (244). In many children, feeding struggles and growth failure begin with the introduction of solid foods at age 5 to 7 months. In rare instances, the introduction of gluten-containing cereals triggers celiac disease and growth failure. Thus comparison of the lifelong feeding history with the growth curve can provide diagnostic clues to the nutritional risk factors in FTT.

In assessing current feeding practices of the child who fails to thrive, the clinician should ascertain when, where, how, and by whom the child is fed, as well as what the child is fed and why. Comprehensive assessment of feeding problems requires a combination of methods such as structured interviews with primary caregivers and direct observation of the child's response to feeding in multiple situations. Parents should be asked to fill out a checklist of possible behavioral feeding problems (e.g., spitting out food, tantrums during meals, food refusal), to supply a few days of food-intake records, and to indicate how the parents have tried to manage the child's problems (148,149,

TABLE 12.4. *Nutritional evaluation protocol*

Interview
Feeding history adjusted for age
  Breast or formula
  Age solids introduced
  Age switched to whole milk
  Food allergy or intolerance
  Vitamin or mineral supplements
Current feeding behaviors
  Difficulties with sucking, chewing, or swallowing
  Frequency of feeding
  Who feeds
  Where fed (alone or held, with or separate from family, lap or high chair)
  Finickiness, negatism
  Perceived appetite
  Pica
Caretaker's nutrition knowledge
  Difficulties with English or literacy
  Adequacy of developmentally appropriate nutrition information
  Unusual dietary belief (religious or food fad constraints on permitted foods): are some foods perceived as dangerous?
Adequacy of financial resources for food purchase
  Food stamps: how much/month for how many people
  WIC
  Adequacy of earned income
  Benefits: Transitional Aid to Needy Families (TANF), Supplemental Social Security Income (SSI)
  Recent change in food budget (cuts or increases in benefits, new mouths to feed, job gain or loss)
  Familiy's knowledge of how to budget food purchasing
Material resources for food preparation and storage
  Refrigeration
  Cooking facilities
  Running water
  24-Hour dietary recall: was yesterday typical?
Food frequency

WIC, Special Supplemental Nutrition Program for Women, Infants and Children.

156). In some hospital settings, detailed monitoring and record keeping of specific child behaviors that interfere with feeding can be used (171,187). To minimize the influence of uncontrolled variables on the child's behavior, such observations should be conducted in a highly standardized fashion (i.e., in the same place, at the same time, with the same staff). Parental interactions with and response to their children during mealtimes also should be assessed to determine the interrelationship among specific child problem behaviors, parental responses, and antecedent cues.

Ideally, history should be supplemented by a home-based feeding observation that will elucidate not only interactive or mechanical feeding difficulties but also the material conditions of the home and family routines (176).

Heptinstall et al. (114) found that inconsistent timing of the presentation of meals and dysfunctional mealtime procedures, such as solitary meals without supervision, occurred more frequently in growth-deficient children than in normal controls. Common sources of difficulty in the timing of feedings include infrequent feedings (restricting a toddler to three meals a day), constant feedings (grazing), and lack of a consistent feeding schedule. Children are often fed in inappropriate settings, which may or may not be under the parents' control. For example, children in welfare motels or homeless shelters may have to be fed sitting on the floor or the bed because there is nowhere else to sit. Conversely, many parents can be encouraged to put the child in a high chair, when one is available, and not to position the child in front of the television or other distractions during feeding. A hammer-lock hold in a parent's lap is usually ineffective and uncomfortable for both parent and child. A home observation also will elucidate the affective tone of the feeding process and identify dysfunctional interactions, such as interrupting the feeding too often to clean the child, struggles over the child's efforts to feed independently, or inappropriate coaxing or threatening of the child. Efforts should be made to identify all the different caretakers (relatives, neighbors, daycare providers, etc.) involved in feeding the child to enlist these individuals in improving the child's nutritional intake.

Serious deficits in age-appropriate feeding behavior such as chewing, self-feeding, use of utensils, swallowing, or sucking may benefit from intensive behavioral training programs using procedures such as shaping, fading, and modeling to teach novel behaviors (e.g., chewing for a child who has had prolonged pureed feedings) or to enhance adaptive feeding responses (148,149). Disruptive behaviors such as tantrums, expelling food, selective food refusal, attempting to leave the table or

high chair, throwing food, whining, or crying may improve after application of learning-treatment methods such as extinction, time-out, and the contingent application of reinforcers, such as parental attention (187). Inappropriate parental responses such as coaxing, threatening, or "giving in" to the child's demands by terminating the meal or allowing the child to eat only preferred items reinforce these maladaptive behaviors and should be modified (65).

Many parents benefit from substantial preparation and instruction before feeding training and continuous support and guidance throughout. In some cases, serious feeding problems may be best treated in an inpatient setting until the child's behavior improves to the point that parents can learn the procedures that maintain the behavior change (42,148, 149,171,192).

In addition to how the child is fed, the clinician must ascertain what the child is fed and why. The family's level of nutritional knowledge and dietary beliefs should be assessed. American parents and children are continually bombarded with nutritional misinformation from television and other commercial sources, urging them to spend their scarce food resources on expensive heavily sweetened or salted foods of low nutritional quality (71,206). Certain groups of parents, particularly adolescents, and those who are intellectually limited, illiterate, or unable to speak English, are particularly likely to lack adequate information regarding nutritionally sound feeding practices. Immigrants are at risk unless they are able to obtain culturally appropriate foods. Most ethnic diets are adequate, but when traditional foods are unavailable, immigrants may not know what to select from the foods available in American markets. Parents also may offer children an inadequate, strictly vegetarian diet because of adherence to unusual dietary practices prescribed by a nontraditional religion or food fads, such as macrobiotics (246). Parents seeking to prevent obesity or cardiovascular disease also may inadvertently cause their toddlers to fail to thrive by overzealous enforcement of a low-fat "prudent diet" appropriate for adults but not for growing children (183). Restricted diets imposed because of actual or presumed food allergies often are not adequately supplemented with alternate sources of calories and micronutrients, with consequent nutritional deficiencies (124,193).

As discussed in the introduction to this chapter, the family's economic resources for food purchase, food storage, and food preparation must be tactfully ascertained. Finally, a 24-hour dietary recall and 7-day food frequency are essential in determining the quality and quantity of the child's diet. Common findings among children with FTT include excessive intake of juice, water, tea, or carbonated and sweetened beverages, which depress appetite but provide few nutrients. In addition, fruit juices high in fructose or sorbitol have been associated with malabsorption and osmotic diarrhea in some cases of FTT (45,216). Low-income families may have particular difficulties in meeting the needs of children with restricted and, therefore, more expensive diets as in the cases of multiple food allergies, lactose intolerance, or gluten-sensitive enteropathy (128,154).

Anthropometric Assessment

Serial anthropometric assessments are critical to the management of FTT. Initial measurements form the basis for triage and calculation of caloric needs (see subsequent discussion), as well as providing some prognostic information for later developmental potential. Frequent follow-up assessments also provide the clearest indication of the effectiveness of intervention.

Children referred for FTT must be measured in a standard fashion by trained personnel using the same scale at each measurement, according to published protocols for obtaining accurate and reproducible anthropometric measurements (20,101,219,241). Infants should be weighed naked, and young children should wear underwear only.

The relationship of the child's weight and height to each other and to standard norms is used to identify both the chronicity and the severity of nutritional deficit. By international consensus, the NCHS growth charts are used to evaluate the growth of infants and preschool children, regardless of ethnicity (103,106,241). Revised growth charts, anticipated in the near future, will eliminate the discontinuity between recumbent length and standing height, and provide percentile lines above and below the 5th and 95th percentiles (103). These will be available on the Internet at http://www.cdc.gov/nchswww.

Weight for age, the most powerful predictor of mortality, provides a composite measure of past and present nutrition and growth, reflecting both current and previous insults (137). When constitutional, endocrine, and genetic factors can be ruled out, depressed height for age is considered a manifestation of the cumulative effects of chronic malnutrition (234). In contrast, depressed weight for height indicates acute and recent nutritional deprivation (234). The revised NCHS norms will provide weight-for-height graphs for children up to age 6 years, as well as body mass index (BMI) norms for children older than 2 years (103,106,241). Children at highest risk are those for whom both weight for height and height for age are depressed, indicating acute malnutrition superimposed on a chronic problem.

By definition, most children labeled as FTT have weights or heights at or below the lower percentiles on the NCHS charts, so that additional calculations are necessary to quantify the severity of nutritional risk. A useful clinical technique, initially devised by Waterlow et al. (99,131,232) is to categorize the child's malnutrition as first (mild), second (moderate), or third degree (severe) by dividing the child's current weight for corrected age, and for current height by the median value ("the standard") for that parameter on the NCHS grids. To assess the severity of chronic malnutrition, height for age is assessed in the same way (Table 12.5). Children with third-degree malnutrition (weight for age less than 60% of standard, or weight for height less than 70% of standard) are in acute danger of severe morbidity and possible mor-

TABLE 12.5. *Percent medial as indicator of severity of nutritional deficit*

Grade of malnutrition	Weight for age	Height for age	Weight for age
Normal	90-110	>95	>90
First degree (mild)	75-89	90-94	90-89
Second degree (moderate)	60-74	85-89	70-79
Third degree (severe)	<60	<80	<70

tality from their malnutrition and should be hospitalized (see Table 12.5). At present, the standard NCHS growth charts are cross-sectional for monitoring weight gain over time, and therefore do not fully illustrate the magnitude of changes in a child's weight relative to height (242). Calculating a patient's Z-score will reflect how far from the mean a child veers, thus giving a more accurate calculation of how malnourished the child is in comparison to a healthy child of that gestational age. However, such a detailed calculation is often not pragmatic in a clinical setting because not every physician has access to a computer at the time of the child's visit.

The goal of nutritional intervention in FTT is to achieve catch-up growth, that is, growth at a faster than normal range for age so that the child's relative deficit of body size is restored. If the child with an established growth deficit simply resumes growth at the normal rate for age, relative deficits persist compared with children of the same age who have always grown normally. To assess whether catch-up growth is occurring, the clinician must be aware of age-specific changes in normal growth rates, as summarized by Guo et al. (104); these are not altered by the new edition of the NCHS norms (103). In the first 3 months of life, median weight gain averages 26 to 31 g a day; from 3 to 6 months, 17 to 18 g a day; from 6 to 9 months, 12 to 13 g a day; from 9 to 12 months, 9 g a day; and from 12 months onward, 7 to 9 g a day. A minimal goal for catch-up growth is two to three times the average rate of weight gain for corrected age. Thus a 1-year-old child who is gaining 30 g a day is showing excellent catch-up growth, whereas a 1-month-old child who also is gaining 30 g a day is growing at only the normal rate for age and will not repair existing deficits. The goal for catch-up growth must be continually revised as the child matures.

Principles of Nutritional Treatment

To achieve catch-up growth, the underweight child must receive nutrients in excess of the normal age-specific requirements of the recommended daily allowances (RDA) (162). Daily caloric needs for catch-up growth in calories per kilogram can be estimated as follows: kcal/kg = 120 kcal/kg × median weight for current height current weight (kg) (151).

In most cases, according to this calculation, children require 1.5 to 2 times the expected intake for their age to achieve optimal catch-up growth (35,151,187). Protein intake should be enhanced in similar proportions to permit maximal growth (151).

Nutritional rehabilitation must address the child's needs for micronutrients as well as calories and protein. Iron deficiency, with or without associated anemia, is seen in as many as one half of all children presenting with FTT (21). Vitamin D–deficiency rickets also has been described (17). Even among children whose micronutrient stores are adequate at initial presentation with FTT, the demand of rapid tissue synthesis during catch-up growth may produce nutritional deficiencies. Whether or not zinc status can be measured, zinc supplementation should be provided to meet the RDA because such supplementation has been shown to decrease the energy cost of weight gain (27,34,230). A multivitamin supplement containing the RDA for all vitamins and for iron and zinc should, therefore, be prescribed routinely for children with FTT during nutritional rehabilitation, with additional supplementation of iron or vitamin D to therapeutic levels in children with iron deficiency or rickets (54). Use of a once-a-day vitamin supplement also is useful to reduce pressure on caretakers to assure that their child is receiving a completely balanced diet. Caretakers no longer have to worry whether their child is eating green beans or other low-calorie vegetables as a source of vitamins and can focus solely on ensuring adequate intake of calories and protein.

In general, it is not possible for a child to eat twice the normal volume of food to obtain the nutrient levels necessary for catch-up growth. Instead, the child's usual diet must be fortified to increase nutrient density, for example, by providing formula of 24 to 30 calories per ounce rather than the standard 20 calories per ounce. A prepackaged 30-calorie per ounce preparation for children aged 1 to 6 years is now commercially available. Like investigators in the Third World, we have found this preparation to be well accepted, well tolerated for rapid weight gain, and effective when its cost can be subsidized by health insurance or other mechanisms (161). Because the formula does not require parental preparation and is often perceived by families as "medicine" exclusively for the use of the FTT child, it can be used effectively in high-risk families who otherwise have difficulties in preparing appropriately enriched diets for their child. Detailed protocols for other methods of dietary supplementation have been published elsewhere (187). The participation of an experienced pediatric nutritionist is critical in developing a dietary regimen appropriate for each child.

The process of refeeding to promote catch-up growth must be undertaken with some circumspection in children with third- and severe second-degree malnutrition. If high food intakes are provided at the beginning of nutritional resuscitation, these children may develop vomiting, diarrhea, and circulatory decompensation (151,231). To minimize these complications, such children should, for the first 7 to 10 days of treatment, be restricted to the normal dietary intake for age, offered as frequent small feedings. The intake may then be gradually advanced over the next week to a diet that meets the calculated requirements for catch-up growth. Moderately and mildly malnourished children may be offered food ad libitum, while calorie counts are maintained. Once a baseline of spontaneous intake is established, preferred foods may be enriched to bring dietary intake to catch-up levels.

Depending on the severity of initial deficit, 2 days to 2 weeks may be required to initiate catch-up growth (35). Less severely malnourished children who are not hospitalized should be monitored at least weekly as outpatients during this phase. Accelerated growth must then be maintained for 4 to 9 months to restore a child's weight for height (35,161). Biweekly to monthly outpatient visits for weight checks, adjustment of diet, and treatment of intercurrent medical problems are essential during this period. Intake and rates of growth spontaneously decelerate toward normal levels for age as deficits are repleted. Because weight is restored more rapidly than height, caretakers may become alarmed that the child is becoming obese. They should be reassured that the catch-up growth in height lags behind that in weight by several months, but balance will occur if dietary treatment is not prematurely terminated (23,26, 173). In our program, the anthropometric criterion for discharge from a specialized outpatient program is when the child is able to maintain weight for height above the 10th percentile and a normal rate of weight gain for age (see previous section) on at least two assessments, 1 month apart, on a normal diet for age (i.e., the weight-for-height deficit is repaired, and the child no longer requires an especially enriched diet to sustain normal growth).

PSYCHOSOCIAL ISSUES IN EVALUATION AND TREATMENT

Psychologic Assessment

As shown in Table 12.6, a wide range of psychological functions, including both intellectual and socioemotional development, may be affected by growth deficiency, malnutrition, and associated risk factors, and should be documented in a comprehensive assessment approach (58,96). Psychological assessment is best construed as a continuing process

TABLE 12.6. *Comprehensive psychosocial assessment of failure to thrive*

Area of assessment	Method of assessment	Information obtained
Psychologic status, cognitive development	Bayley Scale of Mental Development (13,14), Fagan (70)	Intellectual strengths and deficits relative to age norms
Social and affective-responsiveness	Behavioral observations; Bayley Infant Behavior Record, rating scale (149,150)	Child's degree of social withdrawal: response to objects
Behavior during feeding	Behavioral observations and rating scales	Presence of behavioral feeding problems and skill deficits
Parent-child relationship	Observations of mother-child interaction (237)	Strengths and deficits in parent-child relationship
Family environment		
Stimulation provided by family members	Observation of interaction with child; Home Scale (34)	Level of stimulation provided
Family structure	Interview about family tree	Quality of family functioning and stability
Family resources	Interview about finances	Level of family resources and depletion
Family stress: relationships and support	Interview	Level of family stress: strengths and problems in family functioning
Parental beliefs about FTT	Interview	Parental beliefs about causes and consequences of FTT (54)

FTT, failure to thrive.

that begins with an initial or baseline assessment at the time the child's growth deficiency is first noticed and includes sequential assessments to assess the child's short- and longer-term responses to intervention (58). One important purpose of assessment is to document the functional impact of the child's FTT, malnutrition, and associated risk factors on cognitive development and behavior. The second is to monitor the effects of treatment.

Intellectual Development

Children who experience prolonged malnutrition and/or chronic FTT appear to be at risk for intellectual deficits severe enough to affect their learning potential (64,66,90,209, 210). The severity of developmental impairments varies substantially, however, among preschool and school-aged children with histories of early FTT (7,40,55,56,90,92,159, 186,213,214). Studies have underscored the central importance of a history of serious malnutrition as well as the quality of the home environment and educational experience in predicting the cognitive development of affected children in later life (25,64,69,88–92, 119,157,159,245).

Standardized infant assessment tests provide objective information concerning the child's mental age and strengths and weaknesses in intellectual functioning (13,14,57, 58). When available, measures of infant information processing, such as the Fagan test, are especially helpful for infants whose lack of responsiveness or significant motor limitations compromise their performance on the Bayley record (70). Cognitive assessment data can be used to develop a program of stimulation that can be initiated in the hospital and/or planned for the child's ongoing follow-up. In addition, sequential assessments of cognitive development are especially helpful to document progress in test performance after initial nutritional or psychological intervention and to plan additional interventions (65).

Intellectual assessment can be a productive means of involving the parents of FTT children in their child's treatment planning (65). Observing their child's assessment helps parents to appreciate the nature of their children's intellectual strengths and weaknesses. When parents have observed developmental testing, it is also easier and more productive to discuss the pattern of their child's intellectual strengths and deficits with them. We find also if parents are invited to discuss their child's development and participate in the evaluation, they are less defensive about the overall evaluative process.

In evaluating the child's development, the clinician should pay careful attention to the potential effects of the child's nutritional state on his or her response to test items. Infants who have experienced nutritional and/or stimulus deprivation are often withdrawn, which may severely limit their capacity to respond at least initially (53). For this reason, intellectual tests given early during the hospitalization, when the child is unresponsive, may underestimate intellectual potential. Conducting the assessment soon after the hospital admission and repeating it before discharge (taking into account practice effects) should provide a more predictive estimate of intellectual potential than one assessment (68). In addition, just as the child's progress in physical growth can be evaluated through the use of the growth grid, the child's intellectual progress can be monitored through the use of repeated assessments; however, assessment of the child's current intellectual level does not shed light on the causes of deficits or on developmental prognosis, with the exception that extremely low scores are more predictive than are those within the normal range (229).

Socioemotional Development

Children with FTT are at risk for deficits in their socioemotional development. Although no one pattern of behavioral disturbance is associated with FTT, deficits in social responsiveness, affect, activity level, and avoidance of social contact have been noted by many observers (43,63,66,67,87,178,180,181,185). Polan (175) found that children with FTT consistently demonstrated less positive affect in a range of situations than did normally growing children, and that acute and chronic malnutrition were associated with heightened negative affect.

Children with early histories of FTT have a higher incidence of insecure attachments characterized by anxious, avoidant, or disorganized behavior than do children with normal patterns of growth (48,100,213). Valenzuela (225) suggested that the combination of

the negative effects of malnutrition on children's reactivity to stress, coupled with the impact of such behaviors on the responsiveness of caregivers, might result in a vicious cycle that could eventually culminate in the development of a behavioral disorder. Controlled studies of children with early histories of FTT are consistent with this hypothesis, in that they suggest a continuing risk to socioemotional development beyond the point of initial diagnosis of FTT (62). Areas of particular vulnerability among children with early histories of FTT and malnutrition include the ability to contain impulses and to organize their behavior (11,12,67,78,88–92,186).

Because multiple areas of psychological development may be affected, a comprehensive assessment of several behavioral domains, including social responsiveness, affect, and response to feeding, is generally necessary for children with FTT. Structured instruments can be used to guide such observations. Rating scales such as the Bayley Infant Behavior Record (IBR) assess the child's affective responsiveness and response to tasks during testing, and rating scales have been developed to assess clinically relevant aspects of FTT children's behavioral style (e.g., persistence, social responsiveness) during testing and play situations (13,14,239,240). A comprehensive assessment of the child's behavior and emotional development can be used to generate a profile of behavioral strengths and deficits to guide treatment planning and evaluation of the child's progress. Ordinarily one would expect improvement in the FTT child's social responsiveness and affect after nutritional treatment. Some children, however, continue to demonstrate significant deficits in responsiveness and/or problems in feeding that pose a salient burden to their caregivers and hence should be addressed in specialized intervention.

Assessment of the Family Environment

In addition to assessing the impact of FTT and associated risk factors on the child's psychologic development, it also is necessary to assess aspects of the family environment (relationships, resources, and parent–child interaction) that would be expected to influence the child's response to medical and psychologic intervention, as shown in Table 12.6. Given the impact of parent–child relationships on child development, observations of the parents' interactions with the child in a range of situations (feeding, teaching the child a skill, or free play) provides a useful method of assessment (3, 190). The patterns of parent–child relationships associated with FTT are complex and heterogeneous (3,34,148,149,184,185). Deficient stimulation is one typical pattern; conflict and parental reinforcement of deviant behavior is another (148,149,185). Several methods of assessment are available (34,148,149). The Home Observation for Measurement of the Environment (Home) Inventory is a reliable and valid measure of the level of stimulation provided to the child in the family environment (34). Short questionnaire forms of the Home Scale are used in pediatric practice to assess the quality of the home environment.

One of the difficulties in assessing parent–child interaction in a hospital or clinic situation is that the child is removed from his or her home environment, and it is difficult to create a naturalistic setting for assessment. It may be possible, however, to use play or feeding situations to approximate important interactions. To make effective judgments about strengths and problem areas in parent–child relationships, clinicians must have extensive experience with a wide range of FTT infants and their parents (85). In many respects, the identification of strengths in the family–child relationship that one can build on in an intervention is every bit as important as is documenting deficits. When available, obtaining observations of the parent–child relationship in the home setting provides valuable information that can be used to gauge the family's ability to respond to intervention.

The quality of relationships within the family, including the relationships and interactions of other family members with the child, can have an important influence on the child who fails to thrive. For this reason, specialized methods of clinical assessment are needed to assess family feeding and cultural practices; routines and organization; finances; the quality of maternal relationships with other family members; and family members' perceptions of the causes, influences, and consequences of the child's FTT (64,65). Clinical interviews are especially useful in helping family members share their ideas about what may be influencing the child's feeding, physical growth, and development, and to provide a context in which to observe fathers' and other family members' interactions with their children (64,65). Because parents' appraisal of their child as physically ill, quiet, or demanding may influence their interactions with the child, it also is instructive to assess parents' perceptions of their children's needs for interaction and nurturance.

Interviewing families concerning potentially sensitive areas of parental beliefs, family relationships, and patterns of caretaking is a difficult task because family members often become defensive about such inquiry. We find that participation in the process of constructing a genogram, a detailed and expanded family tree, is a useful way to help family members share their impressions of family history and current relationships.

INTERVENTION

The clinical management of FTT should be approached as a chronic condition requiring long-term multidisciplinary follow-up, with exacerbations and remissions expected. In our experience, successful intervention requires active team involvement from the time of referral of a pediatric health care provider, a pediatric nutritionist, a social worker, and professionals with expertise in behavior, development, and family function. The initial focus of interdisciplinary management is assessment of the child and family for purposes of planning treatment. Subsequently, the focus concerns intervention and ongoing monitoring of the child's progress. In an optimal team approach, professionals interact frequently and directly with the family and with each other, ideally in the context of scheduled weekly clinic visits and periodic case conferences. In addition, we find regular home visits by one or several of these professionals are effective to gather diagnostic information and to provide ongoing support and guidance for the family (24,77).

The first priority must be to stabilize the child's acute medical problems and nutritional deficits, and to enhance as much as possible the material conditions of the home and family resources by helping parents to use federal feeding programs, referring to local emergency relief programs, and providing advocacy around housing, heat, and other survival issues. Certainly, medical care and nutritional resuscitation alone are not sufficient to deal with the developmental and emotional deficits that constitute the major long-term morbidity in children who have had malnutrition in early life. For this reason, we find it useful to distinguish between (a) a core intervention plan, which includes identification and treatment of the child's medical problems, nutritional treatment, advice to parents about nutrition, pediatric follow-up, and attempts to stabilize issues such as heating and housing; and (b) specialized interventions, such as parent training, family counseling, or behavioral treatment of feeding problems, which are necessary to address specific problems (61,65, 68,136).

Once care of medical and nutritional problems has been initiated and is well in place, the assessment refocuses on the ongoing developmental needs of the child and the quality of interaction between family and child. Referral to early intervention or HeadStart programs is often indicated to enhance the child's level of cognitive development and to reduce the risk for developmental problems in later life (102). Under recent changes in regulations for Supplemental Social Security Income (SSI), children who fail to thrive may be eligible on the basis of their deficits in growth and development for SSI payments, which are frequently higher than those usually provided by Transitional Assistance to Needy Families (TANF). However, SSI standards for disability are strict and can be difficult to meet. Impoverished families should receive help in applying for these benefits. Moreover, whenever possible, services that supplement and struc-

ture the efforts of the primary caretaker, such as visiting nurses, trained homemakers, or respite day care, can be helpful and should be used. Various forms of mental health intervention, ranging from behavior modification of feeding problems to medication for a severely depressed parent to multigenerational family therapy, should be provided "as recommended" by the clinical assessment. Even after nutritional resuscitation has been achieved, families and children should be offered periodic reassessment as the child reaches school age to assure early identification of behavioral or psychoeducational problems, which may require specialized educational services.

Efficacy

Case reports have highlighted successful use of a range of specialized interventions for FTT infants and their families (62,67,203). Controlled studies of intervention in FTT are difficult to design and implement, given the substantial problems involved in engaging and maintaining families in treatment. Nevertheless, available follow-up studies have indicated that interventions are more likely to enhance children's physical growth and nutrition than they are to affect developmental outcomes (66,88–92,120,188).

Bithoney et al. (23) evaluated a multidisciplinary team-treatment approach including comprehensive assessment and treatment planning. This team included pediatricians, a pediatric nurse practitioner, a child development specialist, a pediatric gastroenterologist, and a social worker who delivered treatments including intensive case management and follow-up use of calorie-dense formulas and, when appropriate, referral for developmental stimulation, behavior modification (for eating disorders), visiting nurse, or homemaker services. Analysis of physical growth outcomes over a 6-month follow-up indicated that children with FTT who received the comprehensive, multidisciplinary team approach grew better than children with comparable physical growth deficits who received a typical management approach in a pediatric primary care clinic (23).

Controlled studies of interventions in the clinical setting for FTT are few and far between. The Black et al. (24) randomized trial of home intervention among 130 children with FTT recruited from pediatric primary care clinics is the most recent and comprehensive. Findings indicated more optimal cognitive development scores compared with infants of mothers who received clinic-based intervention. Home intervention was associated with better language development among infants and toddlers with FTT. At age 4 years, the children who received the home intervention also had better motor development. Children of less depressed mothers had better cognitive development and behavior during play (5,22).

The Infant Health and Development Project, a randomized clinical trial of home-and-center–based intervention among infants who were either born preterm or had low birth weight (less than 2,500 g), provided the opportunity for an assessment of the outcomes of 180 children with FTT. Casey et al. (36) found that children in the intervention and control groups were just as likely to experience FTT. Intervention was associated with better IQ scores and scores on the HOME inventory at 36 months. In addition, intensity of intervention appeared to make a difference. Children with FTT who attended the child development center for more than 250 days had more optimal cognitive development, behavior, and linear growth than did children who attended for fewer than 250 days.

Not all intervention studies have yielded positive findings. At least one study did not find significant differences in physical growth and/or development among three groups of children with FTT whose families received different, alternative models of home-based intervention (64).

Special Issues in Implementation

Parental Understanding of FTT and Acceptance of Clinical Management

To avoid overburdening families, practitioners must set treatment priorities in close collaboration with parents. Whenever possible, it is most useful to begin management with a problem that is salient to parents. In addition, goals for intervention should fit with the family's resources and understanding of the child's problem. Parents of FTT infants may have difficulty participating actively and productively in their child's clinical management for several reasons. The suspicion that they may have contributed, however unwittingly, to their child's growth deficiency is threatening to most parents. In addition, parents may be so preoccupied with personal, family, or financial stresses that they fail to comply with recommendations for treatment (63).

Another reason that parents may have difficulty participating is that their concepts of the etiology and appropriate treatment of their child's growth deficiency may differ substantially from those of professionals. For example, in contrast to professional concepts that FTT may relate to parental underfeeding or interactional problems, parents often focus on physical or biologic explanations of this problem (140). Sturm and Drotar (221) noted that maternal attributions of the FTT diagnosis included unspecified physical problems or illnesses (47%), specific physical problems (37%; e.g., colitis, family problems), constitutional (10%; e.g., "meant to be small"), and child behavior (7%; e.g., food refusal). Maternal perceptions of the physician's diagnosis most often included specific physical problems or growth difficulty rather than family or interactional problems. These findings suggested that mothers understood FTT predominantly as a physical or medical condition and had difficulty acknowledging the potential role of environmental factors. Parental perceptions that their child's FTT reflects physical rather than environmental problems may help to preserve their self-esteem. In addition, the co-occurrence of FTT with other physical symptoms and parental experiences with their child's hospitalization and extensive medical workup would be expected to reinforce their perceptions of the physical origins of FTT.

Differences in parent–practitioner concepts of the etiology and treatment of FTT may engender conflict and frustration and disrupt adherence to psychosocial treatment recommendations (221). For example, parents who believe strongly that their child's growth deficiency is a physical problem may expect a physical rather than psychosocial treatment for this problem, and may require more explanation and support than parents who are able or willing to acknowledge the relevant environmental factors. For this reason, practitioners should provide detailed explanations to parents concerning the psychological consequences of the child's FTT and malnutrition.

Enhancing Parental Participation in Assessment and Treatment Planning

To lessen parents' sense of threat and enhance their participation in the child's treatment planning and follow-up, parents should be informed in detail about the nature and purposes of all assessment procedures and helped to appreciate several basic facts: (a) their child's nutritional and physical problems present a significant hazard to his or her future psychological development and health; (b) these problems are correctable, but intervention is needed to reduce the risk to the child and prevent health and psychological problems in the future; and (c) intervention will be more likely to help their child if they participate actively (65).

Addressing parents' stated concerns about their child's problems may enhance their acceptance of assessment and eventually of an intervention plan. In addition, parents are more likely to accept a psychological or behavioral explanation of FTT if it is linked to their child's "special" temperament, behavior, or sensitivities. For example, management of meals, food selection, or caloric requirements can be interpreted as ways that parents can meet their child's special needs (65). Informing parents that their infant may be especially sensitive to stress or events in family life also provides a rationale to evaluate the impact of family routines or parental relationships on the child's growth and nutrition.

Our experience suggests that the Katon and Kleinman model of clinical negotiation is a useful framework in which to conduct clinical management with parents of children who fail to thrive (135). To establish a more informed basis of negotiation with parents, practitioners may find it helpful to assess parental beliefs about the etiology, consequences, and treatment of their child's condition. Specific questions that are useful in this assessment are listed in Table 12.7.

Other steps in this clinical negotiation process include the following: (a) carefully present the rationale and results of diagnostic procedures to parents and other family members; (b) openly acknowledge differences in viewpoints between the treatment team and parents concerning the child's condition and management; (c) if disagreements arise concerning diagnosis or treatment recommendations, try to develop a working compromise; (d) closely monitor the progress of communication with family members; and (e) engage in additional discussions as needed (65).

In our experience, open discussion of alternatives for the child's treatment has been more productive than engaging in debates about what may have caused FTT. Focusing on what parents can do to help the child in the future (rather than what they may have done in the past) also helps reduce parental guilt and emphasizes the positive opportunity parents now have to help their child (221). Parents are more

---

TABLE 12.7. *Questions to elicit parental attributions concerning failure to thrive*

1. How would you describe your child's condition?
2. When did you first know something was wrong?
3. How did you first know something was wrong with your child?
4. What did you do then?
5. What do you think is causing your child's condition?
6. Do you know other children with the same condition?
7. What do other people (family, friends) think about your child's condition?
8. What advice have they given you?
9. What do you think will help your child's condition?
10. What do you think might happen if nothing is done about your child's condition right now?
11. What questions do you have about your child's condition that you would like me to answer?

likely to accept recommendations for treatment if they feel that their opinions concerning their child's condition and treatment are respected and understood. For this reason, involving parents in the treatment process by asking their opinions and listening to their concerns and providing opportunity for expression of anger and frustration can be effective. Because many parents of FTT infants do not spontaneously volunteer their opinions about their child's condition, they often need considerable support to express their ideas and to participate in decisions concerning their child's care (61). In presenting recommendations to parents, the advantages and disadvantages of various treatment alternatives should be stated clearly. Discussion of treatment recommendations with other family members also can help to mobilize support within the family to help them accept their child's treatment or to identify resistant family members who might interfere with treatment.

Individualizing Intervention

Because children who fail to thrive and their families are such a heterogeneous group, effective intervention plans should be tailored to specific problems that are identified by clinical assessment. As shown in the following case example, dysfunctional parent–child relationship problems that result in FTT or are associated with FTT may benefit from interventions directed toward helping parents improve the frequency and quality of their feeding and stimulation.

Case Report

Ellen was hospitalized at age 5 months for FTT. She gained weight (0.4 kg) during 6 days of hospitalization on an age-appropriate diet. Comprehensive assessment revealed that Ellen had several strengths: she had age-appropriate interest in food, signaled the nursing staff when she was hungry, and had normal developmental status. Conversely, the assessment of Ellen's family indicated that her mother was a 22-year-old single parent who was overburdened by the care of three children. She did not have contact with Ellen's father or much support from her own family. Assessment of the mother–child interaction indicated several problems that became the focus of subsequent intervention. For example, Ellen's mother consistently ignored Ellen's cues that she was hungry and moved the bottle throughout the feeding to see how much Ellen was taking, which disrupted her feeding. Ellen's mother also reported that because Ellen did not seem to be hungry or responsive, she did not feed or stimulate her as much as she did her other children.

Intervention, which took place in the family home, helped the mother set up a feeding schedule in which Ellen was fed regularly and given a sufficient amount of calories to maintain age-appropriate weight gain. Increasing the frequency of interaction between Ellen and her mother, especially during feeding, was another goal of intervention. To support this goal, Ellen's mother was encouraged to hold her during feedings, strongly discouraged from propping the bottle, and was given education concerning her child's nutritional needs. To encourage Ellen's mother to provide age-appropriate stimulation for her needs, Ellen's mother was helped to make age-appropriate toys, such as a cradle gym, and to schedule specific times to play with her.

Ellen's progress was monitored by weighing her each week, charting her physical growth, and assessing her cognitive development and attachment. By age 12 months, 6 months after intervention had begun, she achieved age-appropriate physical growth and a secure attachment to her mother.

Dysfunctional Families

When the efficacy of parent-centered intervention is limited by chronic family problems, such as conflicts between parents, family-centered intervention may be necessary. Family-centered intervention involves multiple family members in achieving the following goals: (a) improvement in the organization and planning concerning allocation of family resources (attention and nutrition to the child);

(b) reduction of family conflict; (c) provision of emotional support to the child's primary caretaker to enhance the quality of nurturing and care-taking; and (d) management of acute family crises (64).

The way that family-centered intervention can improve the quality of the child's care is illustrated by Randy, who was first diagnosed with FTT at age 2 months. Randy's mother was highly stressed by the burden of his care and often asked the other adults, including his great-grandmother, two uncles, and an aunt, to feed him. This caretaking pattern reduced her level of involvement with Randy, however, and resulted in highly inconsistent care, which eventually culminated in decreased caloric intake and growth deficiency. After Randy's second hospitalization for FTT, his family was strongly encouraged to improve the organization of his care by increasing his mother's involvement in his care and decreasing the number of caretakers. In addition, his great-grandmother was encouraged to support his mother's primary involvement in his care by helping to feed his siblings. This intervention, which was reinforced in a series of home visits, eventually resulted in improved physical growth that was maintained for more than a year.

Indications for Protective Service Involvement

Practitioners inevitably encounter families of FTT infants who are both highly dysfunctional and resistant to recommended interventions. For this reason, the clinician must clearly and carefully document the family's response to intervention, as well as the child's physical, nutritional, and developmental progress.

Children with FTT who are referred to protective agencies fall into two broad categories: those whose safety, in the judgment of clinical personnel, requires placement away from their current caretakers, and those in less severe jeopardy, whose current caretakers require protective monitoring and support to obtain or comply with necessary services for the health and growth of the child.

Placement of a child with FTT outside of the home is the only safe intervention in certain situations, particularly when caretakers are out-of-control substance abusers, have inflicted injury on the child, have intentionally withheld available food from the child, or are profoundly psychiatrically or cognitively impaired, and when no other competent caretakers are available within the existing family system (32,98,138,150). School-age children with psychosocial dwarfism (more recently termed "hyperphagic short stature") are from such abusive situations and should be treated by removal from the home (95,143,179,211, 212).

Placement must be undertaken with great care because suboptimal foster care only worsens FTT (243). Because children who fail to thrive usually have multiple special needs requiring visits to many different professionals as well as specialized dietary, developmental, and medical management at home, foster parents must not be overburdened with the care of many other young or special needs children. Foster parents (whether professional or kinship) require the same intensive multidisciplinary support as biologic parents to provide adequate care for a child who is failing to thrive. To avoid deterioration of the child with FTT who is placed in foster care, clinicians should meet face to face with prospective alternate caregivers and educate them regarding the child's dietary and behavioral regimen, medical problems, and emotional needs. Foster parents and kinship caregivers should have a WIC referral, appropriate nutritional supplements, childcare equipment, and health insurance card before children are placed in their homes. The professional or kinship foster family must be willing to commit to close cooperation with clinic visits and home-based treatment for the child who fails to thrive. In general, having a protective services worker bring the child back and forth to medical care without the foster/kinship caregivers is ineffective because clinical change can be effected only when clinicians work directly and closely with the child's primary caregivers. Extra payment to the foster families of FTT children is warranted because of the child's increased dietary needs as well as frequent visits to health care and mental health/developmental professionals. Although expensive, well-supported foster care is far more cost effective in restoring normal growth and development in children from high-risk homes than is extended institutionalization, which is associated with a poor developmental prognosis (72,133,210).

Protective service intervention without placement out of the home may be useful when the family is seriously noncompliant with health and nutritional care of the child despite multiple efforts at voluntary outreach and the child continues to grow poorly. Close communication between the protective agency and the health care providers usually enhances parental compliance. In addition, in some jurisdictions, the only way to obtain needed services, such as home visits or developmentally appropriate day care, for a child who is failing to thrive, even from relatively compliant families, may be through protective service referral. Ideally, such services should be available through other community agencies without the stigma of protective service involvement, but in today's budget climate, this is often not the case. In our clinical experience in a municipal hospital with intensive multidisciplinary management, more than one half of all cases involving FTT in deprived urban families can be managed without any protective service involvement. For children from families with more material resources and greater access to private medical and mental health care, rates of required protective referral are probably lower.

CONCLUSION

FTT is a chronic condition that is the final common pathway of the interaction of diverse medical, nutritional, developmental, and social stresses. Effective care is multidisciplinary, respectful of parents, and sustained beyond the time of acute nutritional and medical crises. Ultimately, the goal of sustained interdisciplinary management is a thriving child in a thriving family.

REFERENCES

1. Acs G, Shulman R, Ng MW, et al. The effect of dental rehabilitation on the body weight of children with early childhood caries. *Pediatr Dent* 1999;21:109–113.
2. Agras S, Hammer L, McNicolas F. A prospective study of the influence of eating-disordered mothers on their children. *Int J Eat Disord* 1999;25:253–62.
3. Alfasi G. A failure to thrive infant at play: applications of microanalysis. *J Pediatr Psychol* 1082;7:111–123.
4. Als H, Tronic E, Adamson L, et al. The behavior of full-term but underweight infants. *Dev Med Child Neurol* 1976;18:590–602.
5. Altemeier WA III, O'Conner SM, Sherrod KB, et al. Prospective study of antecedents for non-organic failure to thrive. *J Pediatr* 1985;106:360–365.
6. American Academy of Pediatrics. *Report of the committee on infectious diseases.* 22nd ed. Elk Grove, IL: American Academy of Pediatrics, 1991.
7. Ashem B, Jones M. Deleterious effects of chronic undernutrition on cognitive abilities. *J Child Psychol Psychiatry* 1978;19:23–31.
8. Ashman L, et al. *Seeds of change: strategies for food security for the inner city.* Los Angeles: UCLA Urban Planning Department, 1993.
9. Atwood WJ, Berger JR, Kaderman R, et al. Human immunodeficiency virus type I infection of the brain. *Clin Microbiol Rev* 1993;6:339–366.
10. Barbour SD. Acquired immune deficiency syndrome of childhood. *Pediatr Clin North Am* 1987;34:247–268.
11. Barrett DE, Radke-Yarrow M, Klein RE. Chronic malnutrition and child behavior: effects of early caloric supplementation on social and emotional functioning at school age. *Dev Psychol* 1982;10:541–552.
12. Barrett DE, Frank DA. *The effects of undernutrition on children's behavior.* New York: Gordon Breach, 1987.
13. Bayley N. *Bayley Scales of Infant Development manual.* New York: Psychological Corporation, 1969.
14. Bayley N. *Bayley Scales of Infant Development manual.* San Antonio, TX: Psychological Corporation, 1993.
15. Belsky J. The determinants of parenting: a process model. *Child Dev* 1984;55:83–96.
16. Benoit D, Zeanah CH, Barton ML. Maternal attachment disturbance in failure to thrive. *Int Ment Health J* 1989;10:185–191.
17. Bergstrom WH. Twenty ways to get rickets in the 1990s. *Contemp Pediatr* 1991;December:88–93.
18. Berwick DM, Levy JD, Kleinerman R. Failure to thrive: diagnostic yield of hospitalization. *Arch Dis Child* 1982;57:347–351.
19. Bickel G, Carlson S, Nord M. *Household food security in the United States, 1995-1998 (Advance Report).* Washington, DC: USDA Food and Nutrition Service and Economic Research Service, 1999.
20. Bithoney WG, Rathbun JM. Failure to thrive. In: Levine M, et al., eds. *Developmental-behavioral Pediatrics.* Philadelphia: WB Saunders, 1983.
21. Bithoney WG. Elevated lead levels in children with nonorganic failure to thrive. *Pediatrics* 1986;78:891–895.
22. Bithoney WG, Newberger EH. Child and family attributes of failure to thrive. *J Dev Behav Pediatr* 1987;8:32–36.
23. Bithoney WG, McJunkin J, Michalek J, et al. Prospective evaluation of weight gain in both nonorganic and

organic failure to thrive children: an outpatient trial of a multidisciplinary team strategy. *J Dev Behav Pediatr* 1989;10:27–31.

24. Black MM, Dubowitz H, Hutchenson J, et al. A randomized clinical trial of home intervention for children with failure to thrive. *Pediatrics* 1995;95:807–814.

25. Black MM, Hutchenson JJ, Dubowitz H, et al. Parenting style and developmental status among children with nonorganic failure to thrive. *J Pediatr Psychol* 1994;19:689–707.

26. Black MM, Krishnakumar A. Predicting longitudinal growth curves of height and weight using ecological factors for children with and without early growth deficiency. *J Nutr* 1999;129(suppl 2):539S–543S.

27. Black MM. Zinc deficiency and child development. *Am J Clin Nutr* 1998;68:464S–4695.

28. Blumberg SJ, Bialostosky K, Hamilton WL, et al. The effectiveness of a short form of the Household Food Security Scale. *Am J Public Health* 1999;89:1231–1234.

29. Boyd LD, Palmer C, Dwyer JT. Managing oral health related nutrition issues of high risk infants and children. *J Clin Pediatr Dent* 1998;23:31–36.

30. Brandt I. Growth dynamics of low birthweight infants with emphasis on the prenatal period. In: Falkner F, Tanner J, eds. *Human growth, neurobiology and nutrition.* New York: Plenum Press, 1979.

31. Brown JL, Pizer HF. *Living hungry in America.* New York: Macmillan, 1987.

32. Bullard DM Jr., Glaser HH, Heagarty MC, et al. Failure to thrive in the "neglected" child. *Am J Orthopsychiatry* 1966;37:680–690.

33. Campbell JA. *Health insurance coverage, 1998.* Washington, DC: U.S. Bureau of Census, Consumer Income Series, 1999:60.

34. Casey PH. Failure to thrive: a reconceptualization. *J Dev Behav Pediatr* 1983;4:63–66.

35. Casey PH, Arnold WC. Compensatory growth in infants with severe failure to thrive. *South Med J* 1985; 78:1057–1060.

36. Casey PH, Kraemer HC, Bernbaum J, et al. Growth status and growth rates of a varied sample of low birth weight preterm infants: a longitudinal cohort from birth to three years of age. *J Pediatr* 1991;119:599–605.

37. Castner L, Anderson J. *Characteristics of food stamp households: fiscal year 1998 (Advance Report).* Alexandria, VA: 1999.

38. Center on Budget and Policy Priorities. *WIC Newsletter 1191* 1992;12:2–3.

39. Center on Budget and Policy Priorities. *Low unemployment, rising wages fuel poverty decline: concerns remain amidst the good news: analysis of the 1998 census poverty data.* Washington, DC: 1999.

40. Chase HP, Martin HP. Undernutrition and child development. *N Engl J Med* 1970;282:933–939.

41. Chasnoff IJ, Griffith DR, Friar C, et al. Cocaine/polydrug use in pregnancy: two year follow-up. *Pediatrics* 1992;89:284–289.

42. Chatoor I, Ganiban J, Colin V, et al. Attachment and feeding problems: a reexamination of nonorganic failure to thrive and attachment insecurity. *J Am Acad Child Adolesc Psychiatry* 1998;37:1217–1224.

43. Chavez A, Martinez C. Consequences of insufficient nutrition on child character and behavior. In: Levitsky DA, ed. *Malnutrition, environment, and behavior.* New York: Cornell University Press, 1979.

44. Chevalier P, Sevilla R, Sejas R, et al. Immune recovery of malnourished children takes longer than nutritional recovery: implications for treatment and discharge. *J Trop Pediatr* 1998;44:304.

45. Cole CR, et al. Should infants avoid apple and pear juices? *Arch Pediatr Adolesc Med* 1999;153:1098–1102.

46. Coleman RW, Provence S. Environmental retardation in infants living in families. *Pediatrics* 1957;19:285–291.

47. Coles CD, et al. Effects of prenatal alcohol exposure at school age: I. Physical and cognitive development. *Neurotoxicol Teratol* 1991;13:357–367.

48. Crittenden PM. Nonorganic failure to thrive: deprivation or distortion. *Int Ment Health J* 1987;8:51–55.

49. Dalaker J, Naifeh M. *Poverty in the United States: 1997.* Washington, DC: U.S. Bureau of Census, Current Population Reports, Series P60-201, U.S. GPO, 1998.

50. Dalaker J. *Poverty in the United States, 1998.* Washington, DC: U.S. Bureau of Center, Current Population Reports, Series P60-207, U.S. GPO, 1999.

51. Day N, Richardson G, Robles, N, et al. Effect of prenatal alcohol exposure on growth and morphology of offspring at 8 months of age. *Pediatrics* 1990;85:748–752.

52. Deren S. Children of substance abusers: a review of the literature. *J Subst Abuse Treat* 1986;3:77–94.

53. Dobbing J. Infant nutrition and later achievement. *Nutr Rev* 1984;42:1–7.

54. Doherty CP, et al. Zinc and rehabilitation from severe protein-energy malnutrition: higher-dose regimens are associated with increased mortality. *Am J Clin Nutr* 1998;68:742–748.

55. Dowdney L, Skuse D, Morris K, et al. Short normal children and environmental disadvantage: a longitudinal study of growth and cognitive development. *J Child Psychol Psychiatry* 1998;39:1017–1029.

56. Drewett RF, Corbett SS, Wright CM. Cognitive and educational attainments at school age of children who failed to thrive in infancy: a population-based study. *J Child Psychol Psychiatry* 1999;40:551–561.

57. Drotar D, Malone CA, Negray J. Environmentally based failure to thrive and children's intellectual development. *J Clin Child Psychol* 1980;10:236–247.

58. Drotar D, Malone CA, Negray J. Intellectual assessment of young children with environmentally based failure to thrive. *Child Abuse Negl* 1980;6:23–29.

59. Drotar D, Sturm LA. Paternal influences in nonorganic failure to thrive: implications for management. *Int Ment Health J* 1987;8:37–45.

60. Drotar D. Failure to thrive. In: Routh DK, ed. *Handbook of pediatric psychology.* New York: Guilford, 1988.

61. Drotar D, Sturm LA. The role of parent-practitioner communication in the management of non-organic failure to thrive. *Fam Syst Med* 1988;6:42–51.

62. Drotar D, Sturm LA. Prediction of intellectual development in young children with early histories of nonorganic failure to thrive. *J Pediatr Psychol* 1988; 13:281–296.

63. Drotar D. Behavioral diagnosis in nonorganic failure to thrive: a critique and suggested approach to psychological assessment. *J Dev Behav Pediatr* 1989;10:48–55.

64. Drotar D, Eckerle D. Family environment in nonorganic failure to thrive: a controlled study. *J Pediatr Psychol* 1989;14:245–257.

65. Drotar D, Wilson F, Sturm LA. Parent intervention in

failure to thrive. In: Schaefer CE, Briesmeister JM, eds. *Handbook of parent training: parents as cotherapists for children's behavioral problems.* New York: Wiley, 1989.

66. Drotar D, et al. Maternal interactional behavior with nonorganic failure to thrive infants: a case comparison study. *Child Abuse Negl* 1990;14:41–51.

67. Drotar D, Sturm LA. Behavioral symptoms, problem solving, and personality development of preschool children with early histories of nonorganic failure to thrive. *J Dev Behav Pediatr* 1992;13:226–273.

68. Drotar D, Sturm LA. Psychological assessment and intervention with failure to thrive infants and their families. In: Olson MR, Mullins LL, Gillman P, eds. *Sourcebook of pediatric psychology.* Baltimore: Johns Hopkins Press, 1994.

69. Evans SL, Reinhart JB, Succop RA. Failure to thrive: a study of 45 delayed cognitive development in infants at risk for later mental retardation. *Pediatrics* 1972;2: 440–457.

70. Fagan JF, Singer LT, Montie JE, et al. Selective screening device for the early detection of normal or delayed cognitive development in infants at risk for later mental retardation. *Pediatrics* 1986;78:1021–1026.

71. Faine MP, Oberg D. Snacking and oral health habits of Washington state WIC children and their caregivers. *ASDC J Dent Child* 1994;61:350–355.

72. Fitch MJ, et al. Cognitive development of abused and failure to thrive children. *J Pediatr Psychol* 1976;1: 32–37.

73. Fleisher DR. Comprehensive management of infants with gastroesophageal reflux and failure to thrive. *Curr Probl Pediatr* 1995;25:247–53.

74. Food Research and Action Center. *Community childhood hunger identification project, a survey of childhood hunger in the United States.* Washington, DC: 1995.

75. Fraiberg S, Adelson E, Shapiro B. Ghosts in the nursery. *J Am Acad Child Psychiatry* 1975;14:387–421.

76. Frank DA, Wong F. Effects of prenatal exposures to alcohol, tobacco, and other drugs. In: Kessler DB, Dawson P, eds. *Failure to thrive and pediatric undernutrition: a transdisciplinary approach.* Baltimore: Paul H. Brookes Publishing, 1999.

77. Frank DA, Zeisel SH. Failure to thrive. *Pediatr Clin North Am* 1988;35:1187–1206.

78. Frank DA. Malnutrition and child behavior: a view from the bedside. In: Brozek P, ed. *Malnutrition and behavior.* Lausanne, Switzerland: Nestle Foundation, 1984.

79. Frank DA, Allen D, Brown JL. Primary prevention of failure to thrive: social policy and implications. In: Drotar D, ed. *New directions in failure to thrive.* New York: Plenum Press, 1985.

80. Frank DA, Bauchner H, Parker S, et al. Neonatal body proportionality and body composition following in utero exposure to cocaine and marijuana. *J Pediatr* 1990;116:622–626.

81. Fried PA, O'Connell CM. A comparison of the effects of prenatal exposure to tobacco, alcohol, cannabis and caffeine on birth size and subsequent growth. *Neurotoxicol Teratol* 1987;9:79–85.

82. Fried PA, Watkinson B. 36- And 48-month neurobehavioral follow-up of children prenatally exposed to marijuana, cigarettes, and alcohol. *J Dev Behav Pediatr* 1990; 11:49-58.

83. Fried PA, Watkinson B, Gray R. Differential effects on cognitive functioning in 9- to 12-year olds prenatally exposed to cigarettes and marijuana. *Neurotoxicol Teratol* 1998;20:293–306.

84. Frisancho AR, Cole PE, Klayman JE. Greater contribution to secular trend among offspring of short parents. *Hum Biol* 1977;49:51–60.

85. Frommer E, Shea G. Antenatal identification of women liable to have problems in managing their infants. *Br J Psychiatry* 1973;123:149–156.

86. Fryer GE. The efficacy of hospitalization of nonorganic failure to thrive children: a meta-analysis. *Child Abuse Negl* 1988;12:375–381.

87. Gaensbauer TJ, Sands K. Distorted affective communications in abused/neglected infants and their potential impact on character. *J Am Acad Child Psychiatry* 1979;18:236–250.

88. Galler JR, Ramsey F, Solimano G. The influence of early malnutrition on subsequent behavior development. I. Degree of impairment in intellectual performance. *J Am Acad Child Psychiatry* 1983;22:8–15.

89. Galler JR, Ramsey F, Solimano G. The influence of early malnutrition on subsequent behavioral development. II. Classroom behavior. *J Am Acad Child Psychiatry* 1983;22:16–22.

90. Galler JR, Ramsey F, Solimano G. The influence of early malnutrition on subsequent behavioral development. III. Learning disabilities as a sequelae to malnutrition. *Pediatr Res* 1984;18:309–313.

91. Galler JR, Ramsey F, Solimano G. The influence of early malnutrition on subsequent behavioral development. V. Child's behavior at home. *J Am Acad Child Psychiatry* 1985;24:58–64.

92. Galler JR, Ramsey F, Solimano G. A follow-up study of the effects of early malnutrition on subsequent development. II. Fine motor skills in adolescence. *Pediatr Res* 1985;19:524–527.

93. Garbarino J, Sherman D. High risk neighborhoods and high risk families: the human ecology of child maltreatment. *Child Dev* 1990;51:188–198.

94. Georgieff MK, Mills MM, Zempel CE, et al. Catch-up growth, muscle and fat accretion and body proportionality of infants one year after neonatal intensive care. *J Pediatr* 1989;114:288–292.

95. Gilmour J, Skuse D. A case-comparison study of the characteristics of children with a short stature syndrome induced by stress (hyperphagic short stature) and a consecutive series of unaffected "stressed" children. *J Child Psychol Psychiatry* 1999;40:969–978.

96. Glaser HH, Heagarty MC, Bullard DM Jr, et al. Physical and psychological development of children with early failure to thrive. *J Pediatr* 1968;73:690-698.

97. Goldbloom RB. Failure to thrive. *Pediatr Clin North Am* 1982;29:151–166.

98. Goldson E, Cadol RV, Fitch MU, et al. Nonaccidental trauma and failure to thrive. *Am J Dis Child* 1976;130: 490–492.

99. Gomez F. Mortality in second and third degree malnutrition. *J Trop Pediatr* 1956;2:77–83.

100. Gordon AH, Jameson JC. Infant-mother attachment in parents with non-organic failure to thrive syndrome. *J Am Acad Child Psychiatry* 1979;18:251–259.

101. Graitcer PL, Gentry EM. Measuring children: one reference for all. *Lancet* 1981;2:297–299.

102. Grantham-McGregor S, Schofield W, Powell C. De-

velopment of severely malnourished children who received psychosocial stimulation: six year follow-up. *Pediatrics* 1987;79:247–254.

103. Grummer-Strawn L. Correspondence with Deborah A. Frank, MD. September 1999.
104. Guo S, Roche AF, Fomon SJ, et al. Reference data on gains in weight and length during the first two years of life. *J Pediatr* 1991;119:355–362.
105. Gupta MC, Urrutia JJ. Effect of periodic antiascaris and antigiardia treatment on nutritional status of preschool children. *Am J Clin Nutr* 1982;36:79–86.
106. Habicht JP, Matorell R, Yarbrough C, et al. Height and weight standards for preschool children: how relevant are ethnic differences to growth potential? *Lancet* 1974;1:611-614.
107. Weston JA, Colloton M, Halsey S, et al. A legacy of violence in nonorganic failure to thrive. *Child Abuse and Neglect* 1993;17:709–714.
108. Hamilton W, et al. *Household food security in the United States in 1995: summary report of the food security measurement study.* Alexandria, VA: USDA Food and Consumer Service, Office of Analysis and Evaluation, 1997.
109. Hanson J, Smith D. The fetal hydantoin syndrome. *J Pediatr* 1975;87:285–290.
110. Hanson J, Jones K, Smith D. Fetal alcohol syndrome. *JAMA* 1976;235:1458–1460.
111. Harsham J, Hayden Keller J, Disbrow D. Growth patterns of infants exposed to cocaine and other drugs in utero. *J Am Diet Assoc* 1994;94:999–1007.
112. Hattevig G, Sigurs N, Kiellman B. Effects of maternal dietary avoidance during lactation on allergy in children at 10 years of age. *Acta Paediatr* 1999;88:7–12.
113. Hawford JT. Growth problems in children: an approach to evaluation and therapy. In: Moss AJ, ed. *Pediatric update.* 1979.
114. Hediger M, Overpeck MD, Mauer KR, et al. Growth of infants and young children born small or large for gestational age: finding from the Third National Health and Nutrition Examination Survey. *Arch Pediatr Adolesc Med* 1998;152:1225–1231.
115. Heptinstall F, Puckering C, Skuss D, et al. Nutrition and meal-time behavior in families of growth retarded children. *Hum Nutr Appl Nutr* 1987;41A:390-402.
116. Herr T, Cook PR, Highfill G. In vitro testing in pediatric food allergy. *Otolaryngol Head Neck Surg* 1999;120:233–237.
117. Hillemeier AC. Gastroesophageal reflux: diagnostic and therapeutic approaches. *Pediatr Clin North Am* 1996;43:197–212.
118. Himes JH, Roche AF, Thissen D. Parent-specific adjustments for assessment of recumbent length and stature. *Monogr Pediatr* 1985;75:304–313.
119. Homer C, Ludwig S. Categorization of etiology of failure to thrive. *Am J Dis Child* 1980;133:848–851.
120. Horwood L, Mogridge N, Darlow BA. Cognitive, educational, and behavioral outcomes at 7 to 8 years in a national very low birthweight cohort. *Arch Dis Child* 1998;79:F12–F20.
121. Hufton IW, Oates RK. Nonorganic failure to thrive: a long-term follow-up. *Pediatrics* 1977;59:73–77.
122. Hurt H, Brodsky NL, Betancourt L, et al. Cocaine-exposed children: follow-up through 30 months. *J Dev Behav Pediatr* 1995;16:29–35.
123. Huston A, McLoyd V, Cull C. Children and poverty: issues in contemporary research. *Child Dev* 1991;65:275–282.
124. Jacobson JL, Jacobson SW, Sokol RJ. Effects of prenatal exposure to alcohol, smoking, and illicit drugs on postpartum somatic growth. *Alcohol Clin Exp Res* 1994;18:317–323.
125. James JM, Burks AW. Food hypersensitivity in children. *Curr Opin Pediatr* 1994;6:661–667.
126. James WP, Ferro-Luzzi A, Sette S, et al. The potential use of maternal size in priority setting when combating childhood malnutrition. *Eur J Clin Nutr* 1999;53:112–119.
127. Jarvinen K, Juntunen-Backman K, Suomalainen H. Relation between weak HLA-DR expression on human breast milk macrophages and cow milk allergy (CMA) in suckling infants. *Pediatr Res* 1999;45:76–81.
128. Jones YD, Nesheim MC, Habicht JP. Influence on child growth associated with poverty in the 1970s: an examination of HANES I and HANES II, cross-sectional US national surveys. *Am J Clin Nutr* 1985;42:714–724.
129. Kaila M, Salo MK, Isolauri E. Fatty acids in substitute formulas for cow's milk allergy. *Allergy* 1999;54:74.
130. Kanawati AA, McClaren DS. Failure to thrive in Lebanon. II. An investigation of the causes. *Acta Pediatr Scand* 1973;62:571.
131. Kapel N, Matarazzo P, Haouchine D, et al. Fecal tumor necrosis factor alpha, eosinophil cationic protein and IgE levels in infants with cow's milk allergy and gastrointestinal manifestations. *Clin Chem Lab Med* 1999;37:29–32.
132. Kaplowitz P, Webb J. Diagnostic evaluation of short children with height 3 SD or more below the mean. *Clin Pediatr* 1994;33:530–535.
133. Kapp MS. Regulation of growth in children with chronic illness: therapeutic implications for the year 2000. *Am J Dis Child* 1987;141:489–493.
134. Karniski W, Van Buren L, Cupoli J. A treatment program for failure to thrive: a cost/effectiveness analysis. *Child Abuse Negl* 1986;10:471–478.
135. Karniski W, Blair C, Vitucci J. The illusion of catch-up growth in premature infants. *Am J Dis Child* 1987;141:520–526.
136. Katon W, Kleinman A. Doctor-patient negotiation and other social science strategies in-patient care. In: Eisenberg L, Kleinman A, eds. *The relevance of social science for medicine.* Dordrecht, Holland: Reidel Press, 1981.
137. Kelly C, Ricciardelli LA, Clarke JD. Problem eating attitudes and behaviors in young children. *Int J Eat Disord* 1999;25:281–286.
138. Kielman A, McCord C. Weight-for-age as an index of risk of death in children. *Lancet* 1978;1:1247–1250.
139. Koel BS. Failure to thrive and fatal injury as a continuum. *Am J Dis Child* 1969;118:565–567.
140. Kotelchuck M. Nonorganic failure to thrive: the status of interactional and environmental theories. In: Camp BW, ed. *Advances in behavioral pediatrics.* Greenwich: Jai Press, 1980.
141. Kotelchuck M, Newberger EH. Failure to thrive: a controlled study of family characteristics. *J Am Acad Child Psychiatry* 1983;22:322–328.
142. Kramer V, Heinrich J, Wist M, et al. Age of entry to day nursery and allergy in later childhood. *Lancet* 1999;353:450–454.

143. Kramer-LeBlanc CS, Mardis A, Gerrior S, et al. *Review of the nutritional status of WIC participants.* Washington, DC: USDA Center for Nutrition Policy and Promotion, 1999.

144. Krieger I. Food restriction as a form of child abuse in ten cases of psychological deprivation dwarfism. *Clin Pediatr* 1974;13:127–133.

145. Kulig M, Bergmann R, Niggermann B, et al. Prediction of sensitization to inhalant allergens in childhood: evaluating family history, atopic dermatitis, and sensitization to food allergens. *Clin Exp Allergy* 1998;28: 1397–1403.

146. Lansky SB, Stephenson L, Weller E, et al. Failure to thrive during infancy in siblings of pediatric cancer patients. *Am J Pediatr Hematol Oncol* 1982;4:361–366.

147. Lassen K, Oei TPS. Effects of maternal cigarette smoking during pregnancy on long-term physical and cognitive parameters of child development. *Addict Behav* 1998;23:635–653.

148. Life Sciences Research Office. *Third report on nutrition monitoring in the United States.* Washington, DC: Federation of American Societies for Experimental Biology, 1995.

149. Linscheid TR. Disturbances of eating and feeding. In: Magrab P, ed. *Psychological management of pediatric problems.* Baltimore: University Park Press, 1978.

150. Linscheid TR, Rasnake LK. Behavioral approaches to the treatment of failure to thrive. In: Drotar D, ed. *New directions in failure to thrive: implications for research and practice.* New York: Plenum Press, 1985.

151. Mackner LM, Starr RH, Black MM. The cumulative effect of neglect and failure to thrive on cognitive functioning. *Child Abuse Negl* 1997;21:691–700.

152. MacLean WC. Protein-energy malnutrition. In: Grand RJ, Sutphen JL, Dietz WH, eds. *Pediatric nutrition.* Boston: Butterworth, 1987.

153. MacMahon KR, Kover MG, Felman J. *Infant mortality rate: socioeconomic factors.* Washington, DC: US Department of Health, Education, and Welfare, 1972.

154. Mahaffey KR, Amnest JL, Roberts J, et al. National estimates of blood lead levels: United States, 1976-1980: associated with selected demographic and socioeconomic factors. *N Engl J Med* 1982;307:573–579.

155. Maldonado J, Gil A, Narbona E, et al. Special formulas in infant nutrition: a review. *Early Hum Dev* 1998; 53(suppl):S23–S32.

156. Mathisen B, Skuse D, Wolke D, et al. Oral-motor dysfunction and failure to thrive among inner-city infants. *Dev Med Child Neurol* 1989;31:293–302.

157. McJunkin JE, Bithoney WG, McCormick C. Errors in formula concentration in an outpatient population. *J Pediatr* 1987;111:848–850.

158. McKay H, Sinisterra L, McKay A, et al. Improving cognitive ability in chronically deprived children. *Science* 1978;200:270–278.

159. McLaren DS. Vitamin A and the immune response. *J Indian Med Assoc* 1999;97:320–323.

160. Mendez MA, Adair LS. Severity and timing of stunting in the first two years of life affect performance on cognitive tests in late childhood. *J Nutr* 1999;129: 1555–1562.

161. Mitchell WG, Gorrell RW, Greenberg RA. Failure to thrive: a study in a primary care setting: epidemiology and follow-up. *Pediatrics* 1980;65:971–977.

162. Morales E, Craig LD, MacLean WC. Dietary management of malnourished children with a new enteral feeding. *J Am Diet Assoc* 1991;91:1233–1238.

163. National Research Council. *National research council recommended dietary allowances.* Washington, DC: National Academy Press, 1989.

164. Neuspiel DR, Hamel C, Hochberg E, et al. Maternal cocaine use and infant behavior. *Neurotoxicol Teratol* 1991;13:229–233.

165. Niggemann B, Sielaff B, Beyer K, et al. Outcome of double-blind, placebo controlled food challenge tests in 107 children with atopic dermatitis. *Clin Exp Allergy* 1999;29:91–96.

166. Nord M, Bickel G. *Estimating the prevalence of children's hunger from the current population survey food security supplement.* Washington, DC: USDA Economic Research Service and Food and Nutrition Service, 1999.

167. Nutrition and Consumer Services. *Women, infants and children: frequently asked questions.* USDA Internet Web Site.

168. Nutrition and Consumer Services. *School breakfast program facts.* USDA/FNS Internet Web Site.

169. Oates RK, Yu JS. Children with non-organic failure to thrive: a community problem. *Med J Aust* 1971;2: 199–203.

170. Orbak Z, Akin Y, Varo-glu E, et al. Serum thyroid hormone and thyroid gland weight measurements in protein-energy malnutrition. *J Pediatr Endocrinol Metab* 1998;11:719–724.

171. Ounstead M, Moar V, Scott A. Growth in the first four years. II. Diversity with groups of small-for-dates and large-for-dates babies. *Early Hum Dev* 1982;7:29–39.

172. Palmer S, Thompson RJ, Linscheid TR. Applied behavior analysis in the treatment of childhood feeding problems. *Dev Med Child Neurol* 1975;17:333–339.

173. Pearce DM. *When wages aren't enough: using the self-sufficiency standard to model the impact of child care subsidies on wage adequacy.* A report prepared for the Pennsylvania Family Economic Self-Sufficiency Project and the Women's Association for Women's Alternatives, Inc. (WAWA), 1998.

174. Peterson KE, Washington J, Rathbun JM. Team management of failure to thrive. *J Am Diet Assoc* 1984; 84:810–815.

175. Phillip M, Hershkovitz E, Rosenblum H, et al. Serum insulin-like growth factors I and II are not affected by undernutrition in children with nonorganic failure to thrive. *Horm Res* 1998;49:76–79.

176. Polan HJ. Disturbances of affect expression in failure to thrive. *J Am Acad Child Adolesc Psychiatry* 1991; 30:897–903.

177. Pollitt E. Failure to thrive: socioeconomic, dietary intake and mother-child interaction. *Fed Proc* 1975;34: 1593–1597.

178. Pollitt E, Eichler A, Chan CK. Psychosocial development and behavior of mothers of failure to thrive children. *Am J Orthop* 1975;45:525–537.

179. Pollitt E, Leibel R. Biological and social correlates of failure to thrive. In: Greene LS, Johnson E, eds. *Social and biological predictions of nutritional status, physical growth, and neurological development.* New York: Academic Press, 1980.

180. Powell GF, Brasel JA, Blizzard RM, et al. Emotional deprivation and growth retardation simulating idio-

pathic hypopituitarism: clinical evaluation of the syndrome. *N Engl J Med* 1967;276:1271-1283.

181. Powell GF, Low JL. Behavior in non-organic failure to thrive. *J Dev Behav Pediatr* 1983;4:26–31.

182. Powell GF, Low J, Speers MA. Behavior as a diagnostic aid in failure to thrive. *J Dev Behav Pediatr* 1987; 8:18–24.

183. Primus W, Rawlings L, Larin K, et al. *The initial impacts of welfare reform on the incomes of single-mother families.* Washington, DC: Center on Budget and Policy Priorities, 1999.

184. Pugliese MT, Weyman-Daum M, Moses N, et al. Parental health beliefs as a cause of nonorganic failure to thrive. *Pediatrics* 1987;80:175-182.

185. Ramey CT, Hieger L, Klisz D. Synchronous reinforcement of vocal responses in failure to thrive infants. *Child Dev* 1972;43:1449–1455.

186. Ramey CT, et al. Nutrition, response-contingent stimulation and the maternal deprivation syndrome: results of an early intervention program. *Mer Palm Q* 1975;21:45–53.

187. Ramey CT, Yeates KO, Short EJ. The plasticity of intellectual development: insights from preventive intervention. *Child Dev* 1985;55:1913–1925.

188. Rathbun JM, Peterson KE. Nutrition in failure to thrive. In: Grand RJ, ed. *Pediatric nutrition.* Boston: Butterworth, 1987.

189. Raynor P, Rudolf MC, Cooper K, et al. A randomized controlled trial of specialist health visitor intervention for failure to thrive. *Arch Dis Child* 1999;80:500–506.

190. Reilly S, Skuse DH, Wolke D, et al. Oral-motor dysfunction in children who fail to thrive: organic or nonorganic? *Dev Med Child Neurol* 1999;41:115–122.

191. Richards CA, Andrews PL, Spitz L, et al. Role of the mother's touch in failure to thrive: a preliminary investigation. *J Am Acad Child Adolesc Psychiatry* 1994;33:1098–1105.

192. Richardson GA, Conroy ML, Day NL. Prenatal cocaine exposure: effects on the development of school-age children. *Neurotoxicol Teratol* 1996;18:627–634.

193. Riordan MM, Iwata BA, Wohl MK, et al. Behavioral treatment of food refusal and selectivity in developmentally disabled children. *Appl Res Ment Retard* 1980;1:95–112.

194. Roesler TA, Barry P, Bock SA. Factitious food allergy and failure to thrive. *Arch Pediatr Adolesc Med* 1994; 148:1150–1155.

195. Rush D, Callahan KR. Exposure to passive cigarette smoking and child development. *Ann N Y Acad Sci* 1989;562:74–100.

196. Russell GF, Treasure J, Eisler I. Mothers with anorexia nervosa who underfeed their children: their recognition and management. *Psychol Med* 1998;28:93–108.

197. Salt P, Galler JR, Ramsey FC. The influences of early malnutrition on subsequent behavioral development. VII. The effects of maternal depressive symptoms. *J Dev Behav Pediatr* 1988;9:1–5.

198. Salvioli G, Faldella G, Alessandroni R, et al. Prevention of allergies of infants: breast-feeding and special formulas: influence on the response to immunization. *Acta Biomed Ateneo Parmense* 1997;68(suppl 1):21–27.

199. Scanlon KS. *Pediatric nutrition surveillance, 1997 full report.* Atlanta: Centers for Disease Control and Prevention, US Department of of Health and Human Services, 1998.

200. Schiffman R, Faber J, Eidelman AI. Obstructive hyper-

trophic adenoids and tonsils as a cause of infantile failure to thrive: reversed by tonsillectomy and adenoidectomy. *Int J Pediatr Otorhinolaryngol* 1985;9:183–187.

201. Schwartz J, Angle C, Pitcher H. Relationship between childhood blood levels and stature. *Pediatrics* 1986; 77:281–288.

202. Schwartz R. A practical approach to the otitis-prone child. *Contemp Pediatr* 1987;4:30–37.

203. Shaheen E, Alexaner D,Truskowsky M, et al. Failure to thrive: a retrospective profile. *Clin Pediatr* 1968;7:255-261.

204. Shapiro V, Fraiberg S, Adelson E. Infant-parent psychotherapy on behalf of a child in a critical nutritional state. *Psychoanal Study Child* 1976;31:461–491.

205. Shaywitz S, Cohen D, Shaywitz B. Behavior and learning difficulties in children of normal intelligence born to alcoholic mothers. *J Pediatr* 1980;96:978–985.

206. Sherman A. *Extreme child poverty rises sharply in 1997.* Washington, DC: Children's Defense Fund, 1999.

207. Siener K, Rothman D, Farrar J. Soft drink logos on baby bottles: do they influence what is fed to children? *ASDC J Dent Child* 1997;64:55–60.

208. Sills RH. Failure to thrive. *Am J Dis Child* 1978;132: 967–969.

209. Silver J, DiLorenzo P, Zukoski M, et al. Starting young: improving the health and developmental outcomes of infants and toddlers in the child welfare system. *Child Welfare* 1999;78:148–165.

210. Singer LT, Fagan JF. Cognitive development in the failure to thrive infant: a three year longitudinal study. *J Pediatr Psychol* 1984;9:363–383.

211. Singer LT. Extended hospitalization of failure to thrive infants: patterns of care and developmental outcome. In: Drotar D, ed. *New directions in failure to thrive.* New York: Plenum Press, 1985.

212. Skuse DH, Gilmour JA. Case-comparison study of the characteristics of children with a short stature syndrome induced by stress (hyperphagic short stature) and a consecutive series of unaffected "stressed" children. *J Child Psychol Psychiatry* 1999;40:969–978.

213. Skuse DH, Gill D, Reilly S, et al. Failure to thrive and the risk of child abuse: a prospective population survey. *J Med Screen* 1995;2:145–149.

214. Skuse DH. Non-organic failure to thrive: a reappraisal. *Arch Dis Child* 1985;60:173–178.

215. Skuse DH, Pickles A, Wolke D, et al. Postnatal growth and mental development evidence for a "sensitive period." *J Child Psychol Psychiatry* 1994;35:521–545.

216. Skuse DH, Reilly S, Wolke D. Psychosocial adversity and growth during infancy. *Am J Clin Nutr* 1994;48: S113–S130.

217. Smith MM, Lifshitz F. Excess fruit juice consumption as a contributing factor in nonorganic failure to thrive. *Pediatrics* 1994;93:438–443.

218. Smolak L, Levine MP, Schermer F. Parental input and weight concerns among elementary school children. *Int J Eat Disord* 1999;25:263–271.

219. Solomons NW. Assessment of nutritional status: functional indicators of pediatric nutriture. *Pediatr Clin North Am* 1985;32:319–234.

220. Stavrianos M. *Food stamp program participation rates: January 1994.* Alexandria, VA: USDA/FCS, 1997.

221. Sturm L, Drotar D. Maternal perceptions of the etiology of nonorganic failure to thrive. *Fam Syst Med* 1991;9: 53–59.

222. Sullivan PB. Nutritional management of acute diarrhea. *Nutrition* 1998;14:758–762.
223. Suskind RM. Malnutrition and the immune response. In: Suskind RM, ed. *Textbook of pediatric nutrition.* New York: Raven Press, 1981.
224. Trowbridge RI. Prevalence of growth stunting and obesity: pediatric nutrition surveillance system. *MMWR* 1984;32:23SS–26SS.
225. Niafeh M. *Trap door? revolving door? or both? Dynamics of economic well being: poverty. 1993-1994. Washington DC:* U.S. Census Bureau.
226. U.S. Centers for Disease Control. *Preventing lead poisoning in young children: a statement by the Centers for Disease Control.* Atlanta: U.S. Department of Health & Human Services, 1991.
227. Valenzuela M. Attachment in chronically underweight young children. *Child Dev* 1990;61:1984–1996.
228. Van Dyke DC, Mackay L, Ziaylek E. Management of severe feeding dysfunction in children with fetal alcohol syndrome. *Clin Pediatr* 1981;21:336–339.
229. Vande Veer B, Schweid W. Infant assessment: stability of mental functioning in young retarded children. *Am J Ment Retard* 1979;79:1–4.
230. Villar J, Smeriglio V, Martorell R, et al. Heterogenous growth and mental development in intrauterine growth-retarded infants during the first 3 years of life. *Pediatrics* 1984;74:783–791.
231. Viteri F. Primary protein-calorie malnutrition. In: Suskind RM, ed. *Textbook of pediatric nutrition.* New York: Raven Press, 1981.
232. Walravens P, Hambidge M, Koepfer D. Zinc supplementation in infants with a nutritional pattern of failure to thrive: a double-blind, controlled study. *Pediatrics* 1989;83:532–538.
233. Waterlow JC. Classification and definition of protein-calorie malnutrition. *Br Med J* 1972;3:530–555.
234. Weathers WT, Crane MM, Sauvain KJ, et al. Cocaine use in women from a defined population: prevalence at delivery and effects on growth in infants. *Pediatrics* 1993;91:350–354.
235. Wehler C, et al. *Community childhood hunger identification project: a survey of childhood hunger in the United States.* Washington, DC: Food Research Action Center, 1991.
236. Weston JA, Colloton M, Halsey S, et al. A legacy of violence in nonorganic failure to thrive. *Child Abuse Negl* 1993;17:709–714.
237. Whitten CF, Pettit MG, Fischoff J. Evidence that growth failure from maternal deprivation is secondary to under-eating. *JAMA* 1969;209:1675–1682.
238. Wiecha J, Palombo R. Multiple program participation: comparison of nutrition and food assistance program benefits with food costs in Boston, Massachusetts. *Am J Public Health* 1989;9:591–594.
239. Wilson GS, McCreary R, Kean J, et al. The development of preschool children of heroin-addicted mothers: a controlled study. *Pediatrics* 1979;63:135–141.
240. Wolf AW, Lozoff B. A clinically interpretable method for analyzing the Bayley Infant Behavior Record. *J Pediatr Psychol* 1985;10:199–214.
241. Wolke D, Skuse D, Mathisen B. Behavioral style in failure to thrive infants: a preliminary communication. *J Pediatr Psychol* 1990;15:237–254.
242. World Health Organization. *Measuring changes in nutritional status.* Geneva: WHO, 1983.
243. Wright CM, Matthews JNS, Waterston A, et al. What is a normal rate of weight gain in infancy? *Acta Paediatr* 1994;83:351–356.
244. Wyatt DT, Simms MD, Horwitz SM. Widespread growth retardation and variable growth recovery in foster children in the first year after initial placement. *Arch Pediatr Adolesc Med* 1997;151:814–816.
245. Zeiger RS, Sampson HA, Bock SA, et al. Soy allergy in infants and children with IgE-associated cow's milk allergy. *J Pediatr* 1999;134:614–622.
246. Zeskind PS, Ramey CT. Fetal malnutrition: an experimental study of its consequences on infant development in the caregiving environments. *Child Dev* 1978;49:1155–1162.
247. Zmora E, Gorodicher R, Bar-Ziv J. Multiple nutritional deficiencies in infants from a strict vegetarian community. *Am J Dis Child* 1979;133:141–144.
248. Zuckerman B, Frank DA, Hingson R, et al. Effects of maternal marijuana and cocaine use on fetal growth. *N Engl J Med* 1989;320:762–768.

13

Child Neglect

*Howard Dubowitz and †Maureen M. Black

*†Department of Pediatrics, University of Maryland School of Medicine;
*Division of Child Protection, University of Maryland Hospital; and
†Growth and Nutrition, University of Maryland Medical System, Baltimore, Maryland

The neglect of neglect has been well documented (16,17,133). Public and professional attention has focused largely on physical and sexual abuse, with little emphasis on the area of child neglect, yet neglect is the most prevalent form of child maltreatment, and is associated with substantial morbidity and mortality. Our goal in this chapter is to integrate the literature on child neglect to provide information that will be useful to practitioners, particularly health care providers.

DEFINITION

Child neglect has been difficult to define (16,58). Definitions have varied across disciplines, agencies, and states, in accordance with differing goals and thresholds (138). For example, although health care providers might view repeated nonadherence with medications as neglectful, such nonadherence would generally not meet the more stringent criteria of child-protective services (CPS), unless serious harm resulted. A district attorney, concerned with successfully prosecuting cases, would be even less likely to pursue medical noncompliance as a case of child neglect. Different definitions of neglect are needed to suit varying purposes; for example, child advocates might influence public policy by focusing on broad issues (e.g., lead in the environment), whereas prosecutors are concerned with criminal negligence (1).

Some authors have proposed broad definitions that incorporate not only caregiver acts and omissions, but also societal and institutional conditions (e.g., hunger, lack of health insurance) that adversely affect children (39, 63,80). More commonly, neglect has been narrowly defined as parental or caregiver acts of omission, such as inadequate supervision of a child (98). Although the child welfare system and many professionals focus primarily on parental omissions in care, this perspective is limited and may not afford adequate protection to children. Societal factors (e.g., poverty) that compromise the abilities of parents to care for their children also impair children's health and development. In this way, societal conditions influence how families nurture and protect their children. In addition, societal factors may directly affect the health and well-being of children. For example, environmental toxins, such as lead, can undermine children's health and well-being. Thus neglect must be evaluated within a societal context.

All disciplines and professionals concerned with children share a core common purpose in defining child neglect: to ensure the adequate care and well-being of children (58). This purpose may be best served by a single, broad definition of neglect including all instances in which the basic needs of children are not met, regardless of cause (39). Basic needs include adequate food, supervision, and protection; clothing; health care; education; a stable home; and the emotional needs for love and nurturance. In this view of neglect, the focus is on the child's needs, rather than on parental behavior. Parents remain primarily responsible for the care of their children, but the contributory roles of professionals, the community, and society also are acknowledged (39,80). This conceptual definition of neglect draws attention to the many factors, in addition to parental omissions in care, that may harm or endanger the well-being of children. By focusing more broadly, the array of potential contributory factors should be considered. A comprehensive understanding of what is underpinning the neglect helps guide appropriate interventions to address the basic needs of children and the conditions that compromise their well-being. A comprehensive appreciation of a child's and family's situation should also enhance professionals' abilities to develop and utilize interventions, regardless of CPS involvement.

Any definition of child neglect must take into account the heterogeneity within the phenomenon. Different forms of neglect, of varying severity and chronicity, and within differing contexts, require a range of responses tailored to the individual situation. For example, a parent's ignorance of a child's nutritional needs requires a very different response from protecting children from lead in the environment.

The degree to which children's needs are met can be viewed along a spectrum ranging from optimal to inadequate. At what threshold is a condition (e.g., lack of health care) endangering or harmful, or care (e.g., parental nonadherence to a medical recommendation) inadequate? It is often difficult to determine, for example, whether being a "latch-key child" is harming or endangering a child. Extreme situations might be clear, but the gray zone is vast, in part because of the paucity of information on how certain conditions affect children. A reasonable approach is to limit the definition of neglect to those conditions that are likely to harm children, and not those where our knowledge is quite uncertain. There is considerable agreement regarding what conditions jeopardize children's health and safety. Research has found that professionals and laypersons, people from different socioeconomic groups, and those in urban and rural settings hold similar views concerning adequate child care and child neglect (42,104,106).

It also is important to recognize the variability among children and their response to specific situations. Being a latch-key child might be appropriate for a mature child with adequate neighborhood supports, but endangering for another (15). In clinical practice, it is necessary to consider each child's specific situation to determine whether basic needs are being met.

In considering the impact of a situation on a child and the possibility of neglect, several factors should be evaluated: whether actual or potential harm occurred, the severity of harm involved, and the frequency/chronicity of the behavior/event(s).

Actual or Potential Harm

In current practice, neglect is often considered only when actual harm has occurred. However, in some situations, the potential for moderate to serious harm also is construed as neglect, such as when a young child is left unattended. Laws in most states, following federal regulations, do include the risk of harm in their definitions of child neglect (98). Some authorities argue, however, that "clear and identifiable harm or injury" is central to a definition of neglect (127), and professionals have been reluctant to judge a situation as neglect unless actual harm was evident (57).

The potential for harm is an important consideration in child neglect. Many forms of neglect have no immediate physical consequences, although there may be substantial and long-term psychological harm (71). For example, Zuravin (139) found that only 25% of children classified by a CPS agency as neglected had immediate physical harm.

Admittedly, the potential for harm can be difficult to predict. How does one estimate the risks of not keeping follow-up appointments? For most medical conditions, little information is available to estimate the risks; in the realm of mental health, predicting outcomes is even more difficult. Epidemiologic data can be helpful (for example, in estimating the risk of not wearing a seatbelt). Knowledge of a child's specific condition also can be informative, such as an asthmatic who has been repeatedly admitted to hospital after running out of medications.

It also is difficult to consider what degree of risk constitutes neglect. For example, an 80% risk is usually more worrisome that a 10% risk, but the specific nature of the risk must be considered. Some risks entail only minor harm; others might be life-threatening. In addition, taking risks and experiencing mishaps are important learning and developmental processes. Nevertheless, helping families minimize the likelihood of moderate to serious harm to their children is an important concern of pediatric primary care (e.g., anticipatory guidance on injury prevention).

Severity

The severity of neglect is typically based on the degree of harm involved. A serious injury is apt to be seen as more severe neglect than a minor injury; any injury is likely to be seen as more severe than a potential injury. Such thinking may sometimes be simplistic, however. For example, a young child left alone overnight might sleep soundly without incurring any harm. Nevertheless, such an incident representing inadequate supervision would be very worrisome.

The sequelae from neglect can be very serious. Approximately one half of the estimated 2,000 fatalities per year attributed to child maltreatment have involved neglect (32). The psychological sequelae of child neglect may be serious and should be considered in assessing the severity of a neglectful situation (56).

Frequency/Chronicity

A pattern of omissions in care has been an important criterion of neglect. Although single or occasional lapses in care are often considered "only human" and are not regarded as neglect, even a single omission in care can have devastating results, such as an unat-

tended toddler drowning in a swimming pool. In contrast, some omissions in care are unlikely to be harmful unless they are recurrent. For example, for a child to miss asthma medications occasionally may involve little risk, but that risk is far greater if medications are missed repeatedly. Only in the latter circumstance when the child's health is clearly in jeopardy is neglect an issue. Focusing on children's basic needs and the risks when these needs are not met is the key in assessing possible neglect. Therefore any dangerous or harmful omission in care constitutes neglect, whether it occurs once or many times.

In summary, we suggest that child neglect be defined as a condition in which a child's basic needs are not met, regardless of cause. Child neglect is a heterogeneous phenomenon, varying in type, severity, and chronicity. Both actual and potential harm are of concern, and the more serious the harm or risk, the more severe the neglect. A pattern of omissions in a child's care characterizes neglect, but single, momentary lapses in care or exposure to harm may also constitute neglect, particularly when serious risks are involved. Finally, the context in which the neglect occurs must be understood to tailor interventions to the specific needs of individual children and families.

INCIDENCE

Many cases of child abuse and neglect are not observed, detected, or reported to CPS (125), making it difficult to estimate the incidence or prevalence of child abuse and neglect. The best attempt was made in 1993 in the Third National Incidence Study (NIS-3), using a combination of CPS agencies and professionals in the community (e.g., physicians, teachers, childcare centers, and police). NIS-3 was conducted on a national probability sample of 42 counties throughout the United States. Community professionals, trained in advance of the study period, served as "sentinels" by noting those cases meeting the study's definitions of child maltreatment. Information on reported cases accepted for investigation was obtained from CPS.

The NIS-3 method included both strengths and shortcomings. By extending the definitions beyond those cases reported to CPS, the sampling strategy better reflects the true incidence of maltreatment. Establishing clear definitions of each form of maltreatment and verifying that each case met set criteria allow a clear understanding of what specifically was being counted. The definitions of abuse and neglect included the risk of harm or endangerment, in addition to actual harm. One study limitation was the absence of laypersons from the community group of sentinels; more than half of all reports to CPS are made by laypersons.

The incidence of different types of maltreatment in 1993 is shown in Table 13.1. It is noteworthy that 70% of cases involved neglect, with physical neglect being by far the most frequent type of neglect. Seven forms of physical neglect were examined, including (a) refusal of health care; (b) delay in health care; (c) abandonment; (d) expulsion of a child from the home; (e) other custody issues, such as repeatedly leaving a child with others for days or weeks at a time; (f) inadequate supervision, such as leaving a young child unsupervised for extended periods; and (g) other physical neglect, which included inadequate nutrition, clothing, or hygiene. Delay in health care was defined as "failure to seek timely and appropriate medical care for a serious health problem which any reasonable layman would have recognized as needing professional medical attention."

TABLE 13.1. *Incidence of child abuse and neglect in the United States in 1993*

Category	Number of children[a]	Rate per 1,000 children
Physical abuse	311,500	4.9
Sexual abuse	133,600	2.1
Emotional abuse	188,100	3.0
TOTAL ABUSE	590,800	9.4
Physical neglect	507,700	8.1
Emotional neglect	203,000	3.2
Educational neglect	285,900	4.5
TOTAL NEGLECT	917,200	14.6

[a]Children were classified in each category that applied, so the rows are not additive.

Educational neglect included three forms: (a) permitted chronic truancy (if the parent had been informed of the problem and had not tried to intervene); (b) failure to enroll/other truancy, such as causing a child to miss at least 1 month of school; and (c) inattention to special educational need. The special educational need criterion was defined as "refusal to allow or failure to obtain recommended remedial educational services, or neglect in obtaining or following through with treatment for a child's diagnosed learning disorder or other special education need without reasonable cause."

Seven forms of emotional neglect were examined, including (a) inadequate nurturance/affection; (b) chronic/extreme spouse abuse; (c) permitted drug/alcohol abuse (if the parent had been informed of the problem and had not attempted to intervene): (d) permitted other maladaptive behavior, such as chronic delinquency; (e) refusal of psychological care: (f) delay in psychological care; and (g) other emotional neglect, such as chronically applying expectations clearly inappropriate in relation to the child's age or developmental level.

Many forms of neglect are not identified as such and are not reported to CPS. For example, health care professionals usually consider neglect as very serious omissions in care, and they are unlikely to apply a highly stigmatizing label to less serious cases. Data from a variety of sources offer additional insight into the prevalence of neglect, mostly unsupervised children drowning or dying in house fires (20). Asser and Swan (6) reviewed 172 known deaths from 1975 to 1995 in which medical care was withheld because of religious beliefs. In most cases, the authors determined there was a high likelihood of excellent outcomes had the children received medical care.

Children's mental health needs are often not met. One study of youth between ages 9 and 17 years found that between 38% and 44% of children meeting stringent criteria for a psychiatric diagnosis in the prior 6 months had had a mental health contact in the previous year (84). Neglected dental care is widespread. For example, a study of preschoolers found that 49% of 4-year-olds had cavities, and fewer than 10% were fully treated (122). Neglected health care is not rare, and if access to health care and health insurance is a basic need in the U.S. today, more than 10 million children experience this form of neglect (4).

ETIOLOGY

Belsky (11) has provided a theoretic framework for understanding the etiology of child maltreatment, including neglect. There is no single cause of child neglect. Rather, multiple and interacting factors at the individual (parent and child), familial, community, and societal levels contribute to child maltreatment. For example, although maternal depression is often associated with child neglect, maternal depression does not necessarily lead to neglect. However, when maternal depression occurs together with other risks, such as poverty and few social supports, the likelihood of neglect increases.

Individual Level

Parental Characteristics

Maternal problems in emotional health, intellectual abilities, and substance abuse have been associated with child neglect. Emotional disturbances, including depression, have been a major finding among mothers of neglected children (108,132,139). Polansky et al. (108) described the apathy–futility syndrome in mothers of neglected children, characterized by an emotional numbness, loneliness, interpersonal relationships that involve desperate clinging, a lack of competence in many areas of living, a reluctance to talk about feelings, the expression of anger through passive aggression and hostile compliance, poor problem-solving skills, a pervasive conviction that nothing is worth doing, and an ability to evoke a sense of futility in others. Mothers of neglected children have been described as more bored, depressed, restless, lonely, and less satisfied with life than mothers of nonneglected children (134) and more hostile, impulsive, stressed, and less so-

cialized than either abusive or nonmaltreating mothers (50). Intellectual impairment, including severe mental retardation and a lack of education, also have been associated with neglect (75,90,102,134).

Maternal drug use during pregnancy has become a pervasive problem; more than 10% of urine toxicology screens in newborns are positive in both urban and suburban areas (61). Although most illicit drugs pose definite risks to the fetus and child, the magnitude of these risks and the long-term sequelae of drug exposure are still unclear (137). In addition to the direct effects of drugs, the compromised caregiving abilities of drug-abusing parents are a major concern. It has been proposed, mostly unsuccessfully, in legislatures of several states that maternal drug use be considered a form of child, or fetal, neglect (or abuse), with grounds for CPS involvement and even criminal prosecution. Many professionals prefer a therapeutic approach, offering appropriate services to mothers and babies (83). Only when such a plan fails and the child remains at significant risk is neglect considered with possible CPS involvement (90). High rates of drug addiction (134) have been found among families of neglected children (7). Jones (73) reported rates of 28% and 25% for alcohol and drug abuse, respectively, in families of children who had been neglected.

Child Characteristics

Theories of child development and child maltreatment emphasize the importance of considering children's characteristics because caregivers respond differently to these characteristics. For example, parents of children who are temperamentally difficult report more stress in providing care. Situations that lead to parental stress may contribute to child maltreatment (94). This association is supported by research that has, for example, found increased depression and stress in parents of chronically disabled children (116).

Several studies have found low birth weight or prematurity to be significant risk factors for abuse and neglect (13,64). Because these babies usually receive close pediatric follow-up as well as other interventions, however, it is difficult to discern whether their increased rates of reported maltreatment reflect greater surveillance. In addition, medical neglect might be expected to occur more often among children who require frequent health care (71), because their increased needs place them at risk for these needs not being met.

Other studies have found increased rates of abuse and neglect among children with chronic disabilities. Diamond and Jaudes (33) found cerebral palsy to be a risk factor for neglect. Increased neglect, but not abuse, also was found among a group of disabled children who had been hospitalized (60). Conversely, Benedict et al. (14) found no increase in maltreatment among 500 moderately to profoundly retarded children, 82% of whom also had cerebral palsy.

In summary, although child factors should be considered in evaluations of child neglect, the preponderance of the evidence suggests that child factors do not cause neglect, but may place difficult demands on parents that, in turn, increase the likelihood of neglect. Families of children with chronic illness or behavior problems may benefit from services, such as support, education, and respite care, to enable them to meet their children's needs. Further research is needed to identify the characteristics and conditions that influence children's vulnerability to neglect.

Family Level

Problems in parent–child relationships have been found among families of neglected children. Research on dyadic interactions indicates less mutual engagement by both mother and child (34) and frequent disturbances in attachment between mother and infant (28,44). Several other studies revealed the poor nurturing qualities of mothers of neglected children. In comparison with parents of abused and nonmaltreated children, parents of neglected children had the most negative interactions with their children (24). These parents made more requests of their children,

while being least responsive to requests from them. One study noted the negative and controlling behavior of mothers of neglected children during child-directed play (5). Bousha and Twentyman (21) found that mothers of neglected children interacted least with their children compared with mothers of abused and nonmaltreated children.

Although mothers of neglected children may have unrealistic expectations of their young children compared with matched controls (7), a lack of knowledge concerning child developmental milestones (e.g., when should an infant be able to sit unsupported) has not been clearly associated with child neglect (124). Deficient parental problem-solving skills, poor parenting skills, and inadequate knowledge of children's developmental needs have been associated with child neglect (7,65,74).

In his work with neglected children, Kadushin (75) described chaotic families with impulsive mothers, who repeatedly demonstrated poor planning and judgment. He further described the negative relationships that many mothers of neglected children have with the fathers of their children, particularly because the fathers had often deserted the family or were incarcerated. Most of the research on child neglect and high-risk families focuses on mothers and ignores fathers. This bias probably reflects the greater accessibility of mothers, and suggests that the frequently modest involvement of fathers in these families might be an additional contributor to child neglect, and a type of neglect in and of itself. A recent investigation of families with 5-year-old children found that father involvement protected children against neglect (41).

Neglect has been associated with substantial social isolation (105,134). Single parenthood without support from a spouse, family members, or friends poses a risk for neglect. In one large controlled study, mothers of neglected children perceived themselves as isolated and as living in unfriendly neighborhoods (107). Indeed, their neighbors saw them as deviant and avoided social contact with them. Mothers of neglected children in another study had less help with child care and fewer enjoyable social contacts compared with mothers of children who had not been neglected (74).

Several other studies have found an association between social isolation and child neglect. Wolock and Horowitz (134) found that "participation in a social network offers a family entry into a system of interpersonal and emotional exchanges," something that was lacking for many families of neglected children. Giovannoni and Billingsley (59) described a pattern of estrangement from kin among mothers of neglected children that included a lack of supportive relationships. Summarizing the literature on social support and child maltreatment, Seagull (114) asked whether social isolation is a contributory factor to neglect or a symptom of underlying dysfunction. In any event, social isolation does appear to be strongly associated with child maltreatment, and particularly with neglect.

Stress also has been strongly associated with child maltreatment. In one study, the highest level of stress, reflecting concerns about unemployment, illness, eviction, and arrest, was noted among families of neglected children compared with abusive and control families (51). Lapp (82) found stress was frequent among parents reported to CPS for neglect, particularly regarding family, financial, and health problems.

Crittenden (29) has described how distortions in two types of information processing (cognition and affect) can lead to neglect. She described three types of neglect associated with deficits in cognitive processing, affective processing, or both: (a) disorganized, (b) emotionally neglecting, and (c) depressed. The first type, disorganized, is characterized by families who respond to the immediate affective demands of situations, with little regard for the cognitive demands. The families operate in crisis mode and appear chaotic and disorganized. Children may be caught in the midst of this crisis, and consequently, their needs are not met. The second type, emotionally neglecting, includes families in which there is minimal attention to affect or to the emotional needs of the child. Parents may handle the demands of daily living (e.g., ensure that children receive food and clothing), but pay little or no attention to how the child feels. The third type, depressed, represents the classic image of neglect. Parents are depressed and therefore unable to process either cognitive or affective information. Children may be left to fend for themselves emotionally and physically. Although the intervention for these three different family patterns differs, they all rely on a family systems approach in which parent and child behavior are considered in context.

Community/Neighborhood Level

The community context and its support systems and resources influence parent–child relationships and are strongly associated with child maltreatment (54). A community with a rich array of services, such as parenting groups, high-quality and affordable child care, and a good transportation system, enhances the ability of families to nurture and protect their children. Informal support networks, safety, and recreational facilities also are important in supporting healthy family functioning. Garbarino and Crouter (54) described the feedback process whereby neighbors may monitor each other's behavior, recognize difficulties, and intervene. This feedback can be supportive and diminish social isolation, and may help families obtain necessary services.

A comparison of neighborhoods with low and high rates for child maltreatment showed that families with the most needs tended to cluster together in areas, often with the least social services (55). In addition to the role of personal histories, the authors attribute the formation of high-risk neighborhoods to political and economic forces. Families in a high-risk environment are less able to give and share and might be mistrustful of neighborly exchanges. In this way, a family's problems seem to be compounded rather than ameliorated by the neighborhood context, dominated as it is by other needy families.

Socioeconomic factors (i.e., poverty) appear to be strongly associated with child maltreatment (32,54). In addition, Garbarino and Crouter (54) found that parents' negative perceptions of the quality of life in the neighborhood were related to increased child maltreatment. In summary, communities can serve as valuable sources of support to families, or they may add to the stresses that families are experiencing.

Societal Level

Many factors at the broader level of the community or society compromise the abilities of families to care adequately for their children. In addition, these societal or institutional problems can be directly neglectful of children. "More than a dozen blue-ribbon commissions and task forces over the past decade have warned of the inadequacy of America's educational system and urged reform" (97). About 4 million (12.6%) young people aged 16 to 24 years have not completed high school and are not enrolled in school. In a national study, 70% of children with learning disabilities received special education services, according to their parents; only 25% of those with serious emotional or behavior problems received special services (136).

The harmful effects of poverty on the health and development of children are pervasive (94). In addition to its influence on family functioning, poverty directly threatens and harms the well-being of children (78,103, 130). For many children, living in poverty means exposure to environmental hazards (e.g., lead, violence), hunger, few recreational opportunities, and inferior health and health care. With one in five American children living in poverty (95), it is a critical national concern. Of all the risk factors known to impair the health and well-being of children, poverty is clearly important.

Poverty has been directly associated with neglect (134): "these families are the poorest of the poor" (59). Although poverty has been associated with all forms of child maltreatment, the contribution to neglect is particularly striking (3). It should be noted, however, that most low-income families are not neglectful of their children.

The child welfare system, the very system intended to assist children in need of care and protection, is another example of societal neglect. "If the nation had deliberately designed a system that would frustrate the professionals who staff it, anger the public who finance it, and abandon the children who depend on it, it could not have done a better job than the present child welfare system" (97). Inadequately financed, with staff who are generally undertrained and overwhelmed, and with poorly coordinated services, CPS are often unable to fulfill their mandate of protecting children. Not surprisingly, reports by the National Commission on Child Welfare and Family Preservation (96), the National Advisory Board to the National Center on Child Abuse and Neglect (93), and the National Center for Children in Poverty (95) have called for a drastic overhaul of the child welfare system.

MANIFESTATIONS OF CHILD NEGLECT

Different types of neglect have been described, reflecting differing basic needs of children that are not adequately met. We focus on the main types likely to be encountered by health care providers (Table 13.2). Specific is-

TABLE 13.2. *Manifestations of possible neglect encountered by pediatricians*

- Noncompliance (nonadherence) with health care recommendations
- Delay or failure in getting health care
- Refusal of medical treatment
- Hunger, failure to thrive, and, perhaps, unmanaged morbid obesity
- Drug-exposed newborns, older children
- Ingestions; injuries; exposure to second-hand smoke, guns, domestic violence; failure to use car seats/belts (**may** reflect inadequate protection from environmental hazards)
- Emotional affect (e.g., excessive quietness or apathy in a toddler), behavior (e.g., repetitive movements) and learning problems, especially if not being addressed; extreme risk-taking behavior (**may** reflect inadequate nurturance, affection, or supervision)
- Inadequate hygiene, perhaps contributing to medical problems
- Inadequate clothing, perhaps contributing to medical problems
- Educational needs not being met
- Abandoned children
- Homelessness

Noncompliance (Nonadherence) with Health Care Recommendations

This form of neglect occurs when inadequate health care results in actual or potential harm, such as when a severe asthmatic does not get or take prescribed medications. The term "nonadherence" is preferred because it avoids the blaming connotation of "noncompliance," recognizing the many potential contributors to health care recommendations not being implemented (86). It is important to ascertain that the child's condition is clearly attributable to a lack of care. For example, a brittle diabetic might be out of control despite good care. It also is helpful to acknowledge that some recommended care may not be important (e.g., a follow-up appointment for an ear infection in a child who appears well), so that such lapses in care should not be labeled neglect. Instead, some guidance for future management seems more appropriate. Similarly, lapses in primary care in a healthy child are unlikely to result in harm and should probably not be considered neglect, although encouragement to adhere to the health maintenance schedule would be reasonable.

A few issues are specific to the assessment and management of this form of neglect (86). Assessing the possible barriers to care is the key, as well as careful consideration of the physician–family relationship and communication. Management strategies include making the treatment as practical as possible, ensuring clear communication, and offering follow-up to help ensure that the plan is being implemented.

Delay or Failure in Getting Health Care

Medical neglect occurs when a child's health care needs are not appropriately met, resulting in actual or potential harm (40). Parents (or primary caregivers) are considered responsible for recognizing health problems in their children and for seeking necessary health care. This form of neglect pertains to a delay or failure in getting health care that results in actual or probable significant harm, such as a child with serious mental health problems not receiving help. There is a need to consider whether the delay in care was significant. For example, an infant may have severe gastroenteritis for days but appear quite well, before abruptly decompensating with dehydration. Care is needed before judging "if only the child was brought in earlier, this intensive care unit admission would have been avoided." As with other types of neglect, there may be multiple and interacting reasons that care is not sought or received; understanding these factors is the guide to appropriate intervention.

Current child welfare practice typically considers neglect when a child clearly has a health problem that a parent (or "average layperson") can reasonably be expected to recognize, but fails to do so, or fails to seek necessary health care in a timely manner. For example, severe respiratory distress in an asthmatic child should be obvious; in contrast, asymptomatic lead poisoning is rarely apparent. Failure or delay to seek care may be related to maternal factors such as depression, to family factors such as a lack of transportation, and to community factors such as limited access to health care.

From the child's standpoint, not receiving necessary health care constitutes neglect, regardless of the cause(s); however, identifying the contributory factors is crucial for planning an appropriate intervention. If a parent does not know how to mix infant formula, parent education is recommended. When a child is exposed to lead in the environment, in addition to the individual and family measures, a public health strategy is needed to remove the lead from the environment. When a lack of health insurance causes families to avoid health care expenses, social policies are needed to remove this obstacle.

Physicians may unknowingly contribute to medical neglect (86). In many instances, parents depend on health care providers to explain a child's condition and to plan for treatment. If the explanation is rushed or explained in "medicalese," parents may not understand the recommendations, and noncompliance, errors, and omissions in care may result. Health care providers share in the responsibility to ensure that children receive adequate health care.

A different scenario occurs when different cultural practices are followed, such as the Southeast Asian folkloric remedy. Used for a wide variety of symptoms, a hard object is vigorously rubbed up and down the body, producing substantial bruising. Aside from questions of abuse, concerns of neglect arise when alternative (to mainstream medicine) remedies are used, and complications ensue, in the context of clearly effective medical treatment (e.g., for bacterial meningitis). The threshold for intervention is guided by the level of certainty that a given treatment is harmful or not helpful, and where a distinctly preferable alternative exists (40). Sensitivity and humility are essential in broaching cultural differences, and often a satisfactory compromise can be found. It is important to avoid an ethnocentric approach (i.e., believing one's own way is best), and cultural relativism, a view that all cultures/cultural practices are equal and to be respected (79). This latter approach fails to recognize that there are cultural practices that are damaging (e.g., female genital mutilation). It is often best to also intervene with leaders of the group, minimizing the risk of the individual family being ostracized from their cultural group.

Refusal of Medical Treatment

A different manifestation of medical neglect may occur when parents actively refuse medical treatment, based on their belief that an alternative treatment is preferable and/or because the prescribed approach is prohibited by their religion. At one end of this spectrum are the cases in which a child is thought to be in need of treatment for a serious condition and the parents refuse permission to treat the child. Jehovah's Witnesses, for example, with their pro-

hibition of blood transfusions, routinely refuse surgery when the need for blood transfusions is anticipated. Another example is the Christian Scientist Church, with its own faith healers and its rejection of western medicine. Less dramatic examples of differing values might be the rejection of mental health interventions, or of dietary recommendations for obesity.

Asser and Swan (6) reviewed information from 172 child deaths between 1975 and 1995, attributed to a lack of medical care due to religious reasons. Almost all these deaths were deemed preventable, judging from the general state of medical treatment for the specific condition at the time of death. Deaths represent the "tip of the iceberg"; the morbidity is likely far greater.

At what point should alternative approaches and beliefs be challenged? At what point does one declare that a child's crucial health care needs are not being met and that a neglectful situation exists? How do we balance our concern with civil liberties and respect for varying beliefs in a pluralistic society with an interest in protecting children? The principle of *parens patria* establishes the state's duty to protect the rights of its younger citizens. Forty-six states, however, have religious exemptions from their child abuse statutes, stating for example "that a child is not to be deemed abused or neglected merely because he or she is receiving treatment by spiritual means, through prayer according to the tenets of a recognized religion" (2). These exemptions have largely been based on the arguments of various religious groups that the U.S. Constitution guarantees the protection of religious practice. This interpretation of the Constitution is contradicted by court rulings prohibiting parents from martyring their children based on parental beliefs (109) and from denying them essential medical care (72). The American Academy of Pediatrics strongly opposes the religious exemptions, advocating that "the opportunity to grow and develop safe from physical harm with the protection of our society is a fundamental right of every child," and "the basic moral principles of justice and of protection of children as vulnerable citizens require that all parents and caretakers must be treated equally by the laws and regulations that have been enacted by state and federal governments to protect children" (2).

As with cultural differences, assessment of these situations requires respect and humility, as well as some knowledge of the religion. Working with religious leaders and seeking compromise are important. Sometimes a satisfactory compromise cannot be reached, and the child is harmed or at risk of harm. Bross (23) presented criteria for legal involvement in this form of medical neglect. First, the treatment refused by the parents should have definite and substantial benefits over the alternative. Therefore, if the treatment has only a modest chance of success or if it carries a risk of major complications, the basis for advocating legal intervention is questionable, and neglect is probably not an issue. Second, not receiving the recommended treatment should result in serious harm. Most cases that have been settled in court have involved the risk of death or severe impairment, although some court decisions have mandated treatment for less serious conditions. Third, with treatment, the child is likely to enjoy a "high quality" or "normal" life. This criterion reflects the court's reluctance to mandate treatment for severely handicapped and terminally ill children. Of note, the Baby Doe laws concerning treatment of severely impaired newborns appear to have had little impact on how these cases are managed. Fourth, in the case of older children (e.g., teenagers), the youth consents to treatment. When these conditions are met, there is a legal basis for intervening. If efforts to provide treatment and reach a satisfactory compromise are not successful, legal intervention on behalf of the child may be necessary.

Hunger, Failure to Thrive, and, Perhaps, Unmanaged Morbid Obesity

Physicians are familiar with failure to thrive (FTT) or inadequate growth, in which psychosocial problems may contribute. Failure to thrive is addressed in Chapter 12; only a few points will be raised here. Care is needed in identifying children who are proportional and growing at an expected rate,

even if their growth parameters (weight-for-age and height-for-age) are low. Growth parameters are a crude reflection of nutritional status. The classic dichotomy of "organic and nonorganic" is no longer used because most growth problems involve both nutritional and psychosocial factors (19). Although neglect plays an important role in many cases of FTT, there are many other reasons for a child's growth to falter. Thus inferences of neglect should be based on a firm understanding of contributors to the child's condition and not automatically assumed in cases of FTT.

Poor growth is a relatively late result of inadequate nutrition, particularly in older children. Cutts et al. (30) found that hunger was relatively prevalent in a midwestern town, but not associated with impaired growth. Although pediatricians should continue to focus on growth, there is a need also to inquire about hunger and food shortages.

Obesity is a serious pediatric problem that has increased in prevalence over the past 30 years (67,123). Morbidity associated with adult obesity includes cardiovascular problems, hypertension, diabetes, psychosocial problems, and premature mortality. Recent analyses have shown the continuity of obesity from preschool years through adulthood (115), particularly when parents also are obese (129), emphasizing the importance of early prevention. In a recent 10-year follow-up investigation of 1,258 students (originally aged 9 to 10 years) in Copenhagen, Lissau and Sorensen (87) reported that after controlling for age, demographics, and childhood body mass index (BMI), children who were neglected (received little parent support) were sevenfold more likely to become obese as young adults than were children who were not neglected. Children who experienced multiple forms of neglect (lack of support and lack of hygiene) were 9.8 times more likely to become obese adults. The mechanisms linking neglect and obesity were not examined, but one possibility is that the children who experienced neglect looked to food for gratification.

Analogous to FTT, there should be a thorough assessment to understand the basis for obesity. Again, multiple and interacting factors may be involved. Whatever the causes, obesity that is not being addressed may be a form of neglect, deserving intervention.

Drug-Exposed Newborns and Older Children

Use of illegal drugs during pregnancy has been identified as a pervasive problem (61). Overall, there appear to be substantial risks to the developing fetus as well as to young children (25). Some of the risks may be attributable to associated risk factors (e.g., poor nutrition, legal drug use, cigarettes, alcohol, family problems) that frequently coexist with substance abuse. In any event, exposure *in utero* or later to illegal drugs is a form of neglect, requiring identification and intervention.

The very pervasive use of legal drugs (i.e., tobacco, alcohol) during pregnancy raises an important issue, given our knowledge of the risks involved. It is probably not helpful to label any use of these drugs as neglect; however, their use should be discouraged during pregnancy. Regarding older children, the risks of second-hand smoke, especially to vulnerable children with underlying lung disease, is clear. The same principle applies: behaviors that counter children's basic needs and harm them are forms of neglect. Approaches to prenatal substance exposure have varied greatly. Chasnoff and Lowder (25) offer an algorithm beginning with inducements to engage in drug treatment but leading to CPS and court involvement if therapeutic efforts fail.

Inadequate Protection from Environmental Hazards

A basic need of children is to be protected from environmental hazards, inside and outside of the home. Ingestions, injuries, exposure to guns, domestic violence, and failure to use car seats/belts may represent inadequate protection that threatens children's health. Consequently, health care professionals must be concerned to help prevent problems in these areas, and to identify these forms of possible neglect. Again, identifying neglect should not be a blaming response; rather it serves as a call to assess, understand, and intervene. It is beyond the scope of this chapter to discuss each of these issues; practical guidance on their assessment and management is offered elsewhere (41).

Inadequate Nurturance and Affection

Emotional (e.g., excessive quietness or apathy in a toddler), behavior (e.g., repetitive movements), and learning problems, especially if not being addressed, as well as extreme risk-taking behavior, may reflect inadequate nurturance and affection. Emotional, behavior, and learning problems occur for many reasons. In assessing such problems, health care providers need to consider an array of potential contributors, as described under Etiology. Another concern may be the nature of the family's response to an identified problem, or the lack of any response. Of all forms of neglect, inadequate nurturance and affection may be especially harmful (22).

Inadequate Supervision, Abandonment

Neglect occurs when children are not supervised in accordance with their developmental needs, resulting in clear risks to their health and well-being (e.g., an infant left unattended in a bathtub, a preschooler left home alone, a teenager out overnight without parental approval). Abandonment is the extreme form and has been defined as occurring when children are not "claimed" within 2 days. Another form of abandonment occurs when teenagers are forced to leave the home.

Inadequate Hygiene

This form of neglect occurs when a child repeatedly does not meet basic standards of hygiene (e.g., child obviously smelly or filthy, not just scruffy). Poor hygiene can contribute to medical problems (e.g., wound infection), as well as psychological concerns, if the child is teased or ostracized by peers.

The assessment should establish whether there has been a pattern of poor hygiene, what family members think about hygiene, what barriers they may face, and what consequences there may have been. In particular, are they amenable to improving their hygiene? Management includes kindly but forthrightly conveying one's concern and, with a social worker if possible, exploring ways to remedy the situation.

Inadequate Clothing

This form of neglect also involves a pattern in which a child repeatedly wears clothing that is obviously unsuitable for the weather or poorly fitting (e.g., lack of jacket in very cold weather, painfully small shoes). In extreme situations, inadequate clothing may contribute to health problems; more often it causes discomfort and possible ridicule. The approach is similar to that for inadequate hygiene.

Educational Needs Not Being Met

A child's educational needs are neglected when the child is not enrolled in school, when a child fails to attend without a satisfactory reason (>2 days/month), and when a child's special educational needs are not adequately met. "Home schooling" that is appropriately regulated appears to be an acceptable alternative. Health care providers are in a position to know about school attendance and possible barriers, especially those pertaining to the child's health. For children with learning and other disabilities, pediatric providers often play a valuable role in helping to ensure that children's special educational needs are met. School problems may result from abuse or neglect (43); these children are especially vulnerable to school failure if their families are not advocating on their behalf.

IMPACT OF NEGLECT ON CHILDREN

Two factors have hindered the research on the consequences of child neglect. First, children who are abused often also experience ne-

glect, and many investigators consider the two forms of maltreatment together, making it difficult to determine if there are specific consequences associated with neglect. However, investigators who have differentiated the effects of neglect from abuse have reported that children who have been neglected experience worse academic performance than do non-neglected children, especially when neglect occurs in combination with other forms of maltreatment (43). Second, neglect often occurs in the context of poverty, making it difficult to differentiate from the consequences of poverty. Elmer's classic work (47) among children from very low income families found that maltreatment had little impact because the detrimental effects of poverty were so devastating. However, her research involved relatively small sample sizes. Recent investigators have found that although poverty correlates with neglect, most children in low-income families are not neglected, and neglect exacerbates the negative aspects of poverty (66).

Much of the research on the impact of neglect has focused on infants, yet neglect can occur throughout childhood and adolescence. Children's needs change as they develop, beginning in infancy with total dependence and extending into adolescence and young adulthood with a continued, albeit lesser need for physical, emotional, and financial support. The sequelae of neglect may be viewed in terms of children's physical and psychosocial needs.

Physical Outcomes

Physical needs involve health, including the basic needs of food, shelter, and medical care, as well as protection from threats (e.g., poisons, environmental hazards). The risks of neglect of physical needs are significant and, in the most severe form, may lead to long-term morbidity or death.

Less severe forms of physical neglect may serve as warning signs to health care providers that a child is in need of protection and intervention. Inadequate growth may be a marker of family dysfunction (8). Children who do not grow adequately may experience permanent deficits in growth, school performance, and work capacity (36,52,91). Risk factors accumulate, such that children who are challenged by multiple forms of neglect may be at greater risk for negative sequelae than are children challenged in only one area (112). The negative consequences of neglect may be exacerbated when neglect occurs with other risks, such as failure to thrive (FTT). In a cross-sectional evaluation of infants and toddlers, the cognitive performance of children with both FTT and neglect was significantly below that of children with neither risk factor, neglect only, or FTT only (89). A longitudinal investigation of the same children at age 6 years examined the impact of early FTT and/or maltreatment on children's well-being reported by mothers, teachers, and standardized testing (77). The children who experienced both neglect and FTT as infants had more behavior problems at home and school, fewer cognitive skills, and less success at school than their peers with neither risk. Children who experienced only one risk had intermediate scores, supporting the accumulation of risk model (111,113). These results are consistent with findings from other investigators who have examined the accumulation of risk and found that multiple risks are much more detrimental than a single risk (34,112, 113). Thus neglect is a particularly serious threat when it occurs along with other risk factors such as FTT.

Psychosocial Outcomes

The impact of neglect on children's psychological development is best understood when evaluated with respect to general theories of child development. Children proceed through a series of developmental tasks from infancy through adolescence (9). These stages begin with attachment during the first year of life, the enduring and predictable relationship infants form with their caregivers. Autonomy and self-regulation are the primary tasks of the second and third years as toddlers acquire skills that contribute to their independence in both functional areas (eating, toileting) and interpersonal relationships (language). Peer

relationships, the tasks of early childhood, become increasingly important as children attend preschool and elementary school. Finally, during middle childhood, the child has to integrate the earlier tasks to develop the interpersonal skills necessary for satisfying relationships during adolescence (26,117). Although each task is associated with a specific age range, the tasks are not limited to that age range and extend throughout childhood from infancy through adolescence.

Infancy

Most of the maltreatment that occurs during infancy is neglect, given the dependency needs of infants. The interdependence between infants and their primary caregivers is well documented (12). As infants and caregivers look to one another for affective cues, they develop a synchrony in which responses stimulate expectations for subsequent interactions (12). Under ideal conditions, infants and caregivers develop a mutually satisfying pattern of interactions that facilitates healthy physical and psychological development in the infant. Infants learn that their needs will be met according to predictable cues, and they learn to trust their caregivers. When caregivers are not consistent in their responses, infants may be denied models to imitate and contingent feedback. Without satisfying interactions, infants may have difficulty developing trust and a secure attachment with their primary caregivers, and are at risk for subsequent emotional and relational problems.

In a recent application of developmental–ecologic theory among very low income, inner-city families of infants and toddlers, the relationships between neglect and child and family functioning differed by the type of neglect (62). Emotional neglect was associated with a path from family functioning through perceptions of child temperament. There were no direct links from family functioning, support, or life events to emotional neglect, but mothers who were involved in well-functioning families were more likely to regard their child as having an easy temperament, and children who were perceived as being relatively easy were less likely to experience emotional neglect. These findings illustrate the importance of conceptualizing neglect from a developmental–ecologic perspective that incorporates the family and the child's contribution through their temperament. The link between mothers' perceptions of their children's temperament and child neglect suggests that maternal perceptions of children's temperament is an important component of neglect that should be incorporated into intervention strategies. In contrast, when physical neglect was considered, there were no associations with child temperament and family context. Thus different factors may be associated with physical and emotional neglect.

School-Aged Children

Several investigators have shown that neglected children are more likely to exhibit developmental, emotional, and behavioral problems than are nonneglected children (5,34,37, 45). However, there is variation in the specific behavior problems shown by neglected children. Several investigators have noted that at times neglected children are passive and withdrawn, and at other times, they are aggressive (21,48). Thus children who have been neglected may have dysfunctional working models of social interactions, and in response to routine peer play, may display both withdrawn and aggressive behavior.

Egeland et al. (45,46) followed four groups of mother–child pairs (abusive, neglectful, psychologically unavailable, and nonmaltreating controls) and reported that children of neglectful and psychologically unavailable mothers were more likely to be anxiously attached when compared with nonmaltreated children. Without a secure attachment relationship with the primary caregiver, the tasks of autonomy and self-development and the ability to form trusting relationships with peers are threatened (118). Neglected children have fewer positive social interactions with peers than do nonneglected peers and are often less self-assured (68).

The vulnerability of neglected children has been well described in a longitudinal follow-up study (48). By early school age, neglected children had deficits in cognitive performance, academic achievement, classroom behavior, and personal social interactions with peers and adults. The neglected children rarely expressed positive affect and demonstrated more developmental problems than any other subgroup of maltreated children. Several authors have found that children with a history of neglect have more school absences (131), more retentions, and lower grades than do nonneglected children (43).

Risk and compensatory factors also influence children's adjustment to neglect. For example, a child who is intelligent, attractive, or talented may be more able to withstand neglectful situations than one who is not intelligent, not attractive, and has low self-esteem (49). Although protective factors may militate against some of the negative sequelae associated with neglect, Farber and Egeland (49) argued that the environmental challenges associated with maltreatment, and particularly with neglect or psychological unavailability, tend to overpower these protective factors, thereby increasing children's vulnerability.

Adolescence

The adolescent period is marked by transition as the dependency of childhood evolves into the independence (or interdependence) of adulthood. The primary tasks of adolescence are the ability to form multiple attachment relationships, to internalize standards of morality, and to assume responsibility for personal actions (81,119). Adolescents who have experienced prior neglect are at risk for emotional and behavioral problems if they have not mastered earlier developmental tasks successfully.

Neglect during adolescence can be particularly difficult to define, because the boundaries between adolescent independence and parental responsibility are unclear. As children age, the influence of parents is supplemented and sometimes replaced by the influence of peers and other forces in the community. Although adolescents do not require the close supervision required by younger children, they continue to require parental guidance and monitoring (81). Adolescents benefit from parents who adopt a democratic and respectful approach, and at the same time establish clear demands and are warm and accepting (119). Without access to parents who provide both supervision and nurturance, adolescents may be at increased risk for behavioral and emotional problems, such as engaging in high-risk behaviors (e.g., early initiation of sexual activity, substance abuse).

PRINCIPLES OF EVALUATION

The following section offers some generic principles for evaluating child neglect. They are based on ecologic theory in which children are evaluated in the context of their family and community.

1. The first step is to determine *whether a child is experiencing neglect*. This diagnosis or formulation should be based on whether a child's basic needs are being met. Also needed is a clear understanding of the family and community context, including the specific harm or risks involved in a particular situation.

    Related issues are the *immediacy of future harm or endangerment* and the *severity of the neglect*, because the safety and well-being of a child are paramount concerns. The issue of immediacy hinges on the particular circumstances: an abandoned infant faces immediate harm, whereas an inadequate diet in an older child usually entails longer term risks.

    The assessment of severity is based on the frequency and nature of prior and current incidents and their effect on a child, in addition to possible future harm. For example, a child with mild asthma might experience little harm if medications are frequently unavailable: a child with severe disease might be seriously harmed without necessary medications. In some instances, the harm or risks to a child are reasonably inferred from what is gener-

ally known of the effects of certain conditions, such as high lead levels.

2. Develop a *comprehensive understanding* of what is contributing to the neglectful situation. An accurate understanding of factors contributing to the neglectful situation is needed to help tailor the intervention to the specific needs of a child and family. The contributory family and community factors discussed in the section concerning etiology offer a useful guide to the issues that must be evaluated. Individual parent and child, familial, community, and societal factors all need to be considered.

3. An *interdisciplinary approach* is optimal because it is difficult for a single professional to evaluate adequately and to manage child neglect. A social work assessment addresses resources within the family and the community. For hospitalized children, a primary nurse might have helpful observations of the family and their relationships. Psychological evaluations can assess a child's developmental and emotional status and parents' abilities to nurture and protect their children. Teachers can provide valuable information on children's school behavior and performance. Health care providers can review the medical record for conditions and observations as well as compliance with appointments and recommendations. In summary, professionals must share information and work collaboratively to reach a comprehensive understanding of the situation and to plan accordingly.

PRINCIPLES OF PREVENTION AND INTERVENTION

Mrazek and Haggerty (92) have categorized prevention programs along three dimensions: universal, selected, and indicated. *Universal* or population-based interventions are designed to prevent child neglect for the entire population of children and are mass distributed. Examples include child-protection policies, mass media campaigns, and public service announcements to draw public attention to the importance of protecting children and promoting their optimal development. *Selected* interventions are directed toward families who are at high risk for child neglect. Their goal is to reduce the incidence of child neglect, often by reducing the risk factors that are associated with child neglect. Thus selected interventions are often targeted to families experiencing social isolation, high stress, few resources, poverty, and alcohol and/or substance abuse. *Indicated* interventions are directed toward families in which child neglect has already occurred. The goal of this type of intervention is to minimize the negative effects of neglect on the child and to break the cycle of child neglect by preventing further neglect.

In a recent review of prevention strategies for neglect, Holden and Nabors (69) noted the paucity of prevention programs and recommended the need for theory-driven, longitudinal programs that extend beyond the prevention of neglect to the promotion of healthy care-giving practices. Although the lack of specificity in the determinants of child neglect may be disheartening, as Belsky (10) pointed out, it provides multiple avenues for intervention. Home intervention has attracted national attention as an effective strategy in promoting the health and development of young children. The long-term successes noted by David Olds (100,101) in a home-visitation program among high-risk families in Elmira, New York, many of whom were adolescent mothers, are encouraging. In our own work among low-income children who were born healthy but experienced FTT in their first 2 years of life, we have found that early home intervention is effective in preventing neglect by promoting a nurturant home environment and reducing the developmental delays often experienced by low-income, urban children (18).

1. Interventions should be *based on existing knowledge and theory*. Interventions proven to be effective should be favored whenever possible. For example, because neglectful families often need basic parenting skills, a behavioral approach is usually preferable to insight-oriented psychotherapy (35).

2. Maternal mental health problems, particularly *depression*, occur commonly among families of neglected children. The publication of effective treatments for depressive symptoms (76,85), often based on cognitive-behavioral therapy, offers hope for the reduction of maternal depression among mothers of neglected children. Given the sensitivity of brief screening methods administered through paper-and-pencil tests (110), procedures for screening and referral could be introduced into health care practices for women and children.

3. *Ecologic theory* provides a conceptualization to understand child neglect and to guide prevention and intervention. Interventions should be targeted to many of the underlying contributory factors to neglect, including parenting limitations and environmental stresses, while using available strengths and resources. Project 12 Ways (88) is an example of a multimodal program providing an array of services tailored to the needs of individual families. Serving mainly neglectful families in rural Illinois, this program includes training in parenting skills, stress reduction, self (impulse) control, money management, job-finding services, weight reduction and smoking cessation, marital counseling, and teaching parents how to play with their children. Of note, the weight-control program has been very popular with parents and has served as an inducement to become involved with other aspects of the program. The importance of help with transportation has been noted and can make the difference in whether pediatric appointments are kept. Evaluations of Project 12 Ways have found short-term improvements in family functioning and diminished rates of child maltreatment (88).

4. Encourage the use of the *family's natural and informal supports*. Professionals must keep in mind the availability of support

from family and friends, and encourage their involvement. For example, by inviting fathers to participate in pediatric visits, pediatricians can convey to families the importance of fathers, and can facilitate fathers' involvement in child care, either directly or through support for the mother (41). If a mother needs time for herself, she might request help with babysitting from extended family members. A variety of other community resources, such as church or peer support groups (e.g., Family Support Centers, Parents Anonymous), can address the social isolation that is often associated with child neglect.

5. Begin with the *least intrusive approach*, and advance to more intrusive approaches if necessary. Successful intervention requires working with a family, and good rapport between professionals and the family is critical to effective help. Therefore intrusive approaches, or interventions that are perceived as punitive, should not be the first- or second-line strategies, unless the risk to the child is sufficiently serious to justify drastic measures. For example, if an infant has not been fed and is found alone and filthy, a report to CPS is clearly indicated.

   A useful first approach is to enhance the parents' child-rearing skills through anticipatory guidance. For example, noninflicted injuries may be prevented by discussing a toddler's emerging mobility and curiosity and the need to clear the home of potential hazards. Specific advice (e.g., remove small, hard objects that could cause a baby to choke) is more likely to be remembered than is more general guidance (e.g., safety-proof your house). Helping parents resolve a problem they identify as important can help establish rapport and trust.

6. Every state has an agency of *Child Protective Services (CPS)*, charged with the responsibility of ensuring that children are adequately protected. When clinicians suspect child abuse or neglect, they are obligated to contact CPS to investigate and to determine what services the family may need to ensure that the child is adequately protected. CPS should not be regarded as a punitive agency or a threat to families; the CPS report should be presented as an effort to clarify the situation and to obtain help if needed. The professionals who work for CPS often have expertise and resources to help families protect and nurture their children. Although they have the power to petition the courts to remove children from the care of their parents, they are guided by principles of family preservation, seeking to keep families together if possible.

7. The need for *structured interventions*. Videka-Sherman (128) emphasized the importance of structure in an intervention. This structure pertains to clear guidelines as to which families receive what services, how exactly interventions should be implemented, and the development of proximal, intermediate, and distal goals. Parents should participate in establishing goals, and goals should be reasonable and clearly identified, in writing.

8. *Home visitors.* Home-based intervention enables an appreciation of the family's circumstances, facilitates a rapport and connectedness between the interventionist and the family, and allows direct guidance in the setting in which recommendations need to be implemented. A randomized trial of nurse home visitors for high-risk mothers (low income, single, or adolescent) having their first babies improved the functioning of these families and reduced the incidence of child maltreatment (99). The most comprehensive package of services (i.e., prenatal and postnatal nurse home visitor, transportation to health care visits, and developmental screening of the children) yielded significant improvements, but only among the highest risk families (i.e., mothers who were low income, single, and adolescent). Although several evaluations of parent-aid or home-visitor programs suggest that home inter-

vention might be a particularly effective strategy, additional research is needed to refine our understanding of home visiting (126). For example, uncertainty persists regarding the optimal professional background of the home visitor, and the content, frequency, and duration of the intervention. Home visiting might be most effective when combined with other services in a comprehensive program. Despite limitations in our current knowledge, home visiting appears to be a promising strategy for families at risk for child maltreatment. One recommended approach is to make home visitors universally available, but optional, for all families with a new baby (93).

9. Interventions often must be *long term*. Brief crisis services, such as respite care, are cost-effective means of decreasing parent stress and providing immediate support to families, thereby reducing the likelihood of neglect. However, these types of services do not necessarily change underlying conditions that may lead to neglect. Comprehensive, long-term prevention programs, including center-based and home-visiting programs, have demonstrated effects on children's cognitive, academic, behavioral, and emotional adjustment, as well as parents' IQ and responsiveness with their children. Long-term programs are necessary to alter maladaptive patterns of family interaction, enhance problem solving and coping abilities, and address the broader conditions that may lead to poverty (e.g., poor educational attainment and unemployment) and possibly to neglect. The problems in many families of neglected children are often multiple, deeply rooted, and chronic; seldom are there quick fixes. It is helpful at the outset for both professionals and families to recognize that long-term intervention is probably necessary; in most instances, perhaps 12 to 18 months, and for some families, years. This time commitment raises the

dilemma for public policy of how best to allocate limited resources. Some have suggested that if good efforts are made for 18 months, yet little progress is achieved and the family remains at high risk, an alternative long-term plan for the child should be made (31).

10. The specific type of program most appropriate for the prevention of child neglect depends on families' specific needs (e.g., parents with severe emotional difficulties are better served by mental health services). Programs with a narrow focus (e.g., targeting individual family members without attention to the broader context) tend to be less effective than multilevel programs because parent, child, family, community, and societal factors are associated with child neglect. Because neglect takes several forms, it is difficult to define a specific set of program components that characterizes an effective prevention program; programs with the flexibility to tailor services to the specific needs of families (e.g., child's gender, age, developmental level) have been found to be most effective. Finally, effective programs build on family competencies and use these strengths to improve families' functioning.

Promising Interventions

Specific therapeutic interventions have been helpful to families of neglected children. For example, several programs have documented the effectiveness of behavioral management techniques (such as alternatives to hitting) with maltreating parents (27,121). The most effective programs focus on basic problem-solving skills and concrete family needs (31,120), provide positive behavior-management strategies, and address environmental factors (53).

Parents may benefit from a therapeutic relationship that includes nurturance, support, empathy, encouragement to express feelings, and motivation to change behavior. Parents of neglected children often require attention to their own emotional or interpersonal needs to nurture their children adequately. Insight-oriented therapy that is abstract, verbal, time consuming, and expensive, however, is often thought to be inappropriate for most parents of neglected children (5). An evaluation of 19 demonstration programs for maltreating families concluded that individual therapy was less effective than family or group therapy (31).

Although a family-level approach is generally needed, neglected children may require individual attention. The focus of CPS has largely been on parents, and few maltreated children have received direct services (31). Treatment of neglected children is needed to reduce the likelihood of psychological harm and of the possible intergenerational transmission of neglectful parenting. Preschool programs, for example, can provide stimulation and nurturance, while offering parents respite. It is important, however, that parents be included in any treatment of their children so that the therapeutic approach also can be implemented at home.

Few treatment programs are available specifically for neglected or maltreated children, and little evaluation research has been done in this area. Nevertheless, some specific interventions appear to be useful, including therapeutic day care programs for younger children and group therapy for older children and adolescents (70).

In a review of the empiric knowledge base for intervening in child neglect, Videka-Sherman (128) described the need to focus on building positive family experiences, "not just controlling or decreasing negative interaction." For example, parents of neglected children need to learn how to play with their children. One approach involves teaching mothers how to teach their children in a cognitive stimulation program (135). Children who had gone through the program had a higher IQ at age 6 years and were more likely to be in the appropriate grade at age 8 years compared with controls. Videka-Sherman also noted the need to be innovative and to look for resources in the homes of families of neglected children. Pots and pans can be used for play, and basic play materials, such as paper and crayons, might need to be provided.

Prevention by Pediatric Primary Care Providers

There is a need for early efforts to screen for risk factors for neglect and also to screen for neglect that may not be apparent. For example, without direct questioning, a mother's depression or a child's hunger may go undetected. Many of these problems are sufficiently prevalent to justify universal and systematic screening during health maintenance visits. Safety and injury prevention have long been concerns in pediatrics. We can build on this work, broadening our interest to consider additional hazards in children's environment, such as family violence.

One challenge is to educate and support health care providers who may have received little training in these areas and who feel understandably uncomfortable broaching such topics. Another challenge involves the time constraints in practice. There is a need to set priorities, to identify ways to screen briefly for these problems, and then briefly to assess and intervene. In many situations, the provider may be the important gatekeeper to needed services. In addition to screening, health care providers must be astute observers of risk factors or actual problems they may confront. For example, a parent may appear high on drugs, or a cold, angry disposition toward the child may be evident. These serve as "red flags" for providers to clarify the situation sensitively and to intervene as appropriate. Aside from problems, it is as important to identify strengths (35); these are valuable in directing the intervention. For example, a parent's wish to be a good parent might be the impetus to seek drug treatment. A teen's wish to play sports may motivate him to adhere to his asthma treatment plan. An understanding of both the risks and strengths in the family is critical for estimating risks, for the likelihood of successfully intervening, and for intervening optimally.

For children with chronic diseases, targeted health education and support help ensure adequate care. For other children, anticipatory guidance (38), whether it be about wearing a bike helmet or having a smoke alarm, is an effort to prevent harm and to ensure children's basic need to be protected from environmental hazards. Physicians' support, monitoring, and counseling are useful ways of helping families take adequate care of their children. At times, referrals to other professionals and agencies are necessary for services such as developmental evaluations, Women, Infants, and Children (WIC), Head Start, or psychotherapy. Helping a family obtain appropriate services is another valuable role that health care providers can play.

PRINCIPLES OF ADVOCACY

The ecologic model suggests that family and community factors contribute to child neglect. Health care providers can be effective advocates on behalf of children and families in a variety of ways. Explaining to a parent the safety needs of an increasingly mobile and curious toddler is one form of advocacy. Helping a family obtain services in the community is another form of advocacy, as is remaining involved with a family after a report to CPS is made. Finally, efforts to develop programs in a community and to improve social policies and institutional practices concerning children and families also are important forms of advocacy.

If poverty is a major contributor to child neglect (and other forms of child maltreatment), part of the treatment plan may be to help the family access services to reduce the negative consequences of poverty (e.g., emergency food, housing subsidies). From a broad perspective, a clinician may encourage parents to consider opportunities such as job training or further education.

From an advocacy perspective, clinicians may work in their communities to ensure that such programs exist and are accessible. Improving the care and well-being of children is a great challenge. It is impossible for any one person to carry out all the necessary measures. Much is known about children's needs, however, and together with colleagues and families, we should strive to meet those needs for all children.

REFERENCES

1. Aber JL, Zigler E. Developmental considerations in the definition of child maltreatment. In: Cicchetti D, Rizley R, eds. *New directions for child development.* San Francisco: Jossey-Bass, 1981.
2. American Academy of Pediatrics, Committee on Bioethics. Religious exemptions from child abuse statutes. *Pediatrics* 1988;81:169.
3. American Humane Association. *Highlights of official child abuse and neglect reporting, 1983.* Denver: American Humane Association. 1985.
4. Annie E. *Casey Foundation: kids count data book.* Baltimore: Annie E. Casey Foundation, 1999.
5. Aragona JA, Eyberg SM. Neglected children: mothers' report of child behavior problems and observed verbal behavior. *Child Dev* 1981;52:596.
6. Asser S, Swan R. Child fatalities from religion-motivated medical neglect. *Pediatrics* 1998;101:625.
7. Azar S, Robinson DR, Hekimian E, et al. Unrealistic expectations and problem solving ability in maltreating and comparison mothers. *J Consult Clin Psychol* 1984;52:687.
8. Barnett TJ. Baby Doe: nothing to fear but fear itself. *J Prenatal* 1990;10:307.
9. Barrett DE. Nutrition and social behavior. In: Fitzgerald HE, Lester BM, Yogman MW, eds. *Theory and research in behavioral pediatrics.* New York: Plenum Press, 1986.
10. Belsky J. Etiology of child maltreatment: a developmental-ecological analysis. *Psychol Bull* 1993;114:413.
11. Belsky J. Child maltreatment: an ecological integration. *Ant Psychol* 1980;35:320.
12. Belsky J, Rovine M, Taylor D. The Pennsylvania Infant and Family Development Project: the origins of individual differences in infant-mother attachment: maternal and infant contributions. *Child Dev* 1984;55:718.
13. Benedict M. White K. Selected perinatal factors and child abuse. *Am J Public Health* 1985;75:780.
14. Benedict MI, White RB, Wulff LM, et al. Reported maltreatment in children with multiple disabilities. *Child Abuse Negl* 1990;14:207.
15. Berman BD, Winkleby M, Chesterman E, et al. After-school child care and self-esteem in school-age children. *Pediatrics* 1992;89:654.
16. Black MM. The roots of child neglect. In: Reese RM, ed. *The treatment of child abuse.* Baltimore: Johns Hopkins University Press, 2000.
17. Black MM. Long-term psychosocial management of neglect. In: Reese RM, ed. *The treatment of child abuse.* Baltimore: Johns Hopkins University Press, 2000.
18. Black MM, Dubowitz H, Hutcheson J, et al. A randomized clinical trial of home intervention among children with failure to thrive. *Pediatrics* 1995;95:807.
19. Black MM, Feigelman S, Cureton P. Evaluation and treatment of children with failure to thrive: an interdisciplinary perspective. *J Clin Outcomes Manage* 1999; 6:60.

20. Bonner BL, Crow SM, Logue MB. Fatal child neglect. In: Dubowitz H, ed. *Neglected children.* Thousand Oaks, CA: Sage Publications, 1999:156–173.
21. Bousha DM, Twentyman CT. Mother-child interactional style in abuse, neglect, and control groups: naturalistic observations in the home. *J Abnorm Psychol* 1984;93:106.
22. Brassard MR, Hart SN, Hardy DB. The Psychological Maltreatment Rating Scales. *Child Abuse Negl* 1993; 17:715.
23. Bross DC. Medical care neglect. *Child Abuse Negl* 1982;6:375.
24. Burgess R, Conger R. Family interaction in abusive, neglectful, and normal families. *Child Dev* 1978;49:1163.
25. Chasnoff IJ, Lowder LA. Prenatal alcohol and drug use and risk for child maltreatment: a timely approach to intervention. In: Dubowitz H, ed. *Neglected children.* Thousand Oaks, CA: Sage Publications, 1999:132–155.
26. Cicchetti D. How research or child maltreatment has informed the study of child development: perspectives from developmental psychopathology. In: Cicchetti D, Carlson V, eds. *Child maltreatment.* New York: Cambridge University Press, 1984.
27. Crimmins DB, Bradlyn AS, Lawrence JS, et al. A training technique for improving the parent-child interaction skills of an abusive neglectful mother. *Child Abuse Negl* 1984;8:533.
28. Crittenden PM. Maltreated infants: vulnerability and resilience. *J Child Psychol Psychiatry* 1985;26:85.
29. Crittenden PM. Child neglect: causes and contributors. In: Dubowitz H, ed. *Neglected children.* Thousand Oaks, CA: Sage Publications, 1999:47–68.
30. Cutts DB, Pheley AM, Geppert JS. Hunger in midwestern inner-city young children. *Arch Pediatr Adolesc Med* 1998;152:489.
31. Daro D. *Confronting child abuse: research official child abuse and neglect reporting, 1983, Denver: American Humane Association, Neglect for Effective Program Design.* New York: The Free Press, 1988.
32. Daro D, McCurdy K. *Current trends in child abuse fatalities and reporting: the results of the 1991 50-State survey.* Chicago: National Center for the Prevention of Child Abuse, 1992.
33. Diamond LJ, Jaudes PK. Child abuse and the cerebral palsied patient. *Dev Med Child Neurol* 1983;25:169.
34. Dietrich KN, Starr RH, Weisfeld OE. In infant maltreatment: caretaker-infant interaction and developmental consequences at different levels of parenting failure. *Pediatrics* 1983;72:332.
35. DePanfilis D. Intervening with families when children are neglected. In: Dubowitz H, ed. *Neglected children.* Thousand Oaks, CA: Sage Publications, 1999:211–236.
36. Drotar D. The family context of nonorganic failure to thrive. *Am J Orthopsychiatry* 1991;61:23.
37. Drotar D, et al. Early psychological outcomes in failure to thrive: predictions from an interactional model. *J Clin Child Psychol* 1985;14:105.
38. Dubowitz H. Pediatrician's role in preventing child maltreatment. *Pediatr Clin North Am* 1990;37:989.
39. Dubowitz H, Black MM, Starr RH, et al. A conceptual definition of child neglect. *Criminal Justice Psych* 1993;20:8.
40. Dubowitz H. Neglect of children's health care. In: Dubowitz H, ed. *Neglected children.* Thousand Oaks, CA: Sage Publications, 1999:109–131.
41. Dubowitz H, Black MM, Kerr M, et al. Fathers and child neglect. *Arch Pediatr Adolesc Med* 2000;154: 135.
42. Dubowitz H, Klockner A, Starr RH, et al. Community and professional definitions of neglect. *Child Maltreat* 1998;3:235.
43. Eckenrode J, Laird M, Doris J. School performance and disciplinary problems among abused and neglected children. *Dev Psychol* 1998;29:53.
44. Egeland B, Brunquell D. An at-risk approach to the studies of child abuse and neglect. *J Am Acad Child Adolesc Psychiatry* 1979;18:219.
45. Egeland B, Sroufe A. Developmental sequelae of maltreatment in infancy. In: Rizley K, Cicchetti D, eds. *New directions for child development: developmental perspectives in child maltreatment.* San Francisco: Jossey Bass, 1981.
46. Egeland B, Stroule LA, Erickson M. The developmental consequences of different patterns of maltreatment. *Child Abuse Negl* 1984;7:459.
47. Elmer E. A follow-up study of traumatized children. *Pediatrics* 1977;59:273.
48. Erikson MF, Egeland B, Pianta R. The effects of maltreatment on the development of young children. In: Cicchetti D, Carlson V, eds. *Child maltreatment.* Cambridge: Cambridge University Press, 1989;579–619.
49. Farber FA, Egeland B. Invulnerability among abused and neglected children. In: Anthony EJ, Cohler BJ, eds. *The invulnerable child.* New York: Guilford, 1987.
50. Friedrich WN, Tyler JA, Clark JA. Personality and psychophysiological variables: its abusive, neglectful, and low-income control mothers. *J Nerv Ment Disord* 1985;173:449.
51. Gaines R, Sangrund A, Green AH, et al. Etiological factors in child maltreatment: a multivariate study of abusing, neglecting, and normal mothers. *J Abnorm Psychol* 1978;87:531.
52. Galler JR. The behavioral consequences of malnutrition in early life. In: *Nutrition and behavior.* New York: Plenum Press, 1984.
53. Gambrill ED. Behavioral interventions with child abuse and neglect. *Prog Behav Modif* 1983;15:1.
54. Garbarino J, Crouter A. Defining the community context of parent-child relations. *Child Dev* 1978;49:604.
55. Garbarino J, Sherman D. High-risk neighborhoods and high-risk families: the human ecology of child maltreatment. *Child Dev* 1980;51:188.
56. Gaudin JM. Child neglect: short-term and long-term outcomes. In: Dubowitz H, ed. *Neglected children.* Thousand Oaks, CA: Sage Publications, 1999:89–108.
57. Gelles R. Problems in the defining and labeling of child abuse. In: Starr RH, ed. *Child abuse prediction: policy implications.* Cambridge: Ballenger Publishing, 1982.
58. Giovannoni JM, Becerra RM. *Defining child abuse.* New York: The Free Press, 1979.
59. Giovannoni JM, Billingsley A. Child neglect among the poor: a study of parental adequacy in families of three ethnic groups. *Child Welfare* 1970;49.
60. Glaser D, Bentovim A. Abuse and risk to handicapped and chronically ill children. *Child Abuse Negl* 1979; 3:565.
61. Gomby DS, Shiono PH. Estimating the number of substance-exposed infants. In: *Future of children: drug*

exposed infants. Los Altos, Ca: Center for the Future of Children, 1991.

62. Harrington D, Black MM, Dubowitz H, et al. Child neglect: a model of temperament and family context. *Am J Orthopsychiatry* 1998;68:108.

63. Helfer RE. The neglect of our children. *Pediatric Clin North Am* 1990;37:923.

64. Herrenkohl EC, Herrenkohl RC. Some antecedents and developmental consequences of child maltreatment. In: Rizley R, Cicchetti D, eds. *Developmental perspectives on child maltreatment.* San Francisco: Jossey-Bass, 1981.

65. Herrenkohl R, Herrenkohl E, Egolf B. Circumstances surrounding the occurrence of child maltreatment. *J Consult Clin Psychol* 1983;51:424.

66. Herrenkohl RC, Herrenkohl EC, Egolf BP, et al. The developmental consequences of abuse: the Lehigh Longitudinal Study. In: Starr RL, Wolfe DA, eds. *The effects of child abuse and neglect: issues and research.* New York: Guilford Press, 1991:57–85.

67. Hill JO, Trowbridge FL. Childhood obesity: future directions and research priorities. *Pediatrics* 1998;101:570.

68. Hoffman-Plotkin D, Twentyman CT. A multimode assessment of behavioral and cognitive deficits in abused and neglected preschoolers. *Child Dev* 1984;55:794.

69. Holden EW, Nabors L. The prevention of child neglect. In: Dubowitz H, ed. *Neglected children.* Thousand Oaks, CA: Sage Publications, 1999:174–190.

70. Howing P, et al. Effective interventions to ameliorate the incidence of child maltreatment: the empirical base. *Social Work* 1989;34:330.

71. Jaudes PK, Diamond LJ. Neglect of chronically ill children. *Am J Dis Child* 1986;140:655.

72. Jehovah's Witnesses of Washington v King County Hospital. 278F Suppl. 488. (Washington, DC, 1967). Affirmed per curiam, 390 US 598, 1968.

73. Jones MA. *Parental lack of supervision: nature and consequence of a major child neglect problem.* Washington, DC: Child Welfare League of America, 1987.

74. Jones JM, McNeely RL. Mothers who neglect and those who do not: a comparative study. *Social Casework* 1980;61:559.

75. Kadushin A. Neglect in families. In: Nunnally EW, Chilman CS, Cox FM, eds. *Mental illness, delinquency, addictions, and neglect.* Newbury Park: Sage, 1988.

76. Kaslow NJ, Thompson MP. Applying the criteria for empirically supported treatments to studies of psychosocial intervention for child and adolescent depression. *J Clin Child Psychol* 1998;27:146.

77. Kerr M, Black MM, Krishnakumar A. Failure-to-thrive, maltreatment and the behavior and development of 6-year-old children from low-income urban families: a cumulative risk model. *J Child Abuse Neglect* 2000;24:587.

78. Klerman LV. The health of poor children: problems and programs. In: Huston AC, ed. *Children in poverty: child development and public policy.* New York: Cambridge University Press, 1991.

79. Korbin JE, Spilsbury JC. Cultural competence and child neglect. In: Dubowitz H, ed. *Neglected children.* Thousand Oaks, CA: Sage Publications, 1999:69–88.

80. Lally JR. Three views of child neglect: expanding visions of preventive intervention. *Child Abuse Negl* 1984;8:243.

81. Lamborn SD, Mounts NS, Steinberg L, et al. Patterns of competence and adjustment among adolescents from authoritative, authoritarian, indulgent and neglectful families. *Child Dev* 1991;62:1049.

82. Lapp J. A profile of officially reported child neglect. In: Trainer CNI, ed. *The dilemma of child neglect: identification and treatment.* Denver: The American Humane Association, 1983.

83. Larson CS. Overview of state legislative and judicial responses. In: *The future of children: drug exposed infants.* Los Altos, CA: Center for the Future of Children, 1991.

84. Leaf P, Alegria M, Cohen P, et al. Mental health service use in the community and schools: results from thr four-community MACA study. *J Am Acad Child Adolesc Psychiatry* 1996;35:889.

85. Lewinsohn PM, Clarke GN, Rhode P, et al. A course in coping: a cognitive-behavioral approach to the treatment of adolescent depression. In: Hibbs ED, Jensen PS, eds. *Psychosocial treatments for child and adolescent disorders: empirically based strategies for clinical practice.* Washington, DC: American Psychological Association, 1996:109–135.

86. Liptak GS. Enhancing patient compliance in pediatrics. *Pediatr Rev* 1996;17:128.

87. Lissau I, Sorensen TIA. Parental neglect during childhood and increased risk of obesity in young adulthood. *Lancet* 1994;343:324.

88. Lutzker JR, Rice JN. Project 12-Ways: measuring outcome of a large in-home service for treatment and prevention of child abuse. *Child Abuse Negl* 1984;8:519.

89. Mackner LM, Starr RH, Black MM. The cumulative effect of neglect and failure to thrive on cognitive functioning. *Child Abuse Negl* 1997;21:691.

90. Martin M, Walters S. Familial correlates of selected types of child abuse and neglect. *J Marriage Family* 1982;44:267.

91. Martorell R, Rivera J, Kaplowitz H. Consequences of stunting in early childhood for adult body size in rural Guatemala. *Ann Nestle* 1990;48:85.

92. Mrazek PJ, Haggerty RJ. *Reducing risks for mental disorders: frontiers for preventive intervention research.* Washington, DC: National Academy Press, 1994.

93. National Advisory Board on Child Abuse and Neglect. *Creating caring communities: blueprint for effective federal policy on child abuse and neglect.* Washington, DC: U.S. Department of Health and Human Services, 1991.

94. National Center for Children in Poverty. *Alive and well? A research and policy review of health programs for poor young children.* New York: Columbia University School of Public Health, 1991.

95. National Center for Children in Poverty. *Child welfare reform.* New York: Columbia University School of Public Health, 1991.

96. National Commission on Child Welfare and Family Preservation. *A commitment to change.* Washington, DC: American Public Welfare Association, 1990.

97. National Commission on Children. *Beyond rhetoric: a new American agenda for children and families: final report of the National Commission on Children.* Washington DC: Government Printing Office, 1991.

98. Office of Human Development Services. *CFR S1340.2 definitions.* Washington, DC: U.S. Department of Health Human Services, 1987.

99. Olds DL, Henderson CR Jr, Chamberlin R, et al. Preventing child abuse and neglect: a randomized trial of nurse home visitation. *Pediatrics* 1986;78:65.

100. Olds D, Eckenrode J, Henderson CR, et al. Long-term effects of home visitation on maternal life course and child abuse and neglect. *JAMA* 1997;278:637.

101. Olds D, Henderson CR Jr, Cole R, et al. Long-term effects of nurse home visitation on children's criminal and antisocial behavior: 15-year follow-up of a randomized controlled trial. *JAMA* 1998;280:1238.

102. Ory N, Earp J. Child maltreatment and the use of social services. *Public Health Rep* 1981;96:238.

103. Parker S, Greer S, Zuckerman B. Double jeopardy: the impact of poverty on early child development. *Pediatr Clin North Am* 1988;35:1227.

104. Polansky NA, Williams DP. Class orientation to child neglect. *Child Welfare* 1978;57:439.

105. Polansky NA, Ammons PW, Gaudin JM Jr. Loneliness and isolation in child neglect. *Social Casework* 1985;66:38.

106. Polansky NA, Chalmers MA, Williams DP. Assessing adequacy of child rearing: an urban scale. *Child Welfare* 1987;57:439.

107. Polansky NA, Gaudin JM Jr, Ammons PW, et al. The psychological ecology of the neglectful mother. *Child Abuse Negl* 1985;9:265.

108. Polansky N, et al. *Damaged parents:* an anatomy of child neglect. Chicago: University of Chicago, 1981.

109. Prince v Massachusetts, 3/21 U.S. 1944;158.

110. Roberts RE, Lewinsohn PM, Seeley JR. Screening for adolescent depression: a comparison of depression scales. *J Am Acad Child Adolesc Psychiatry* 1991;30:58.

111. Rutter M. Psychosocial resilience and protective mechanisms. *Am J Orthopsychiatry* 1987;57:316.

112. Sameroff AJ, Seifer R. Familial risk and child competence. *Child Dev* 1983;54:1254.

113. Sameroff AJ, Seifer R, Barocas R, et al. Intelligence quotient scores of 4-year-old children: social-environmental risk factors. *Pediatrics* 1987;79:343.

114. Seagull E. Social support and child maltreatment: a review of the evidence. *Child Abuse Negl* 1987;11:41.

115. Serdula MK, Ivery D, Coates RJ, et al. Do obese children become obese adults? A review of the literature. *Prev Med* 1993;22:167.

116. Shapiro J. Family reactions and coping strategies in response to the physically ill or handicapped child. *Soc Sci Med* 1983;17:913.

117. Sroufe LA. The coherence of individual development: early care, attachment and subsequent developmental issues. *Am Psychol* 1979;34:834.

118. Sroufe A, Waters 0. Attachment as an organizational construct. *Child Dev* 1977;48:1184.

119. Steinberg L, Dornbusch S, Brown BB. Ethnic differences in adolescent achievement: an ecological perspective. *Am Psychol* 1992;47:723.

120. Sudia C. What services do abusive families need? In: Pelton L, ed. *The social context of child abuse and neglect.* New York: Human Sciences Press, 1981.

121. Szykula SPA, Fleischman MJ. Reducing out-of-home placements of abused children: two controlled field studies. *Child Abuse Negl* 1985;9:277.

122. Tang J, Altman D, Robertson D, et al. Dental caries: prevalence and treatment levels in Arizona preschool children. *Public Health Rep* 1997;112:319-31.

123. Troiano RP, Flegal KM. Overweight children and adolescents: description, epidemiology, and demographics. *Pediatrics* 1998;101:497.

124. Twentyman C, Plotkin R. Unrealistic expectations of parents who maltreat their children: an educational deficit that pertains to child development. *J Clin Psychol* 1982;38:497.

125. U.S. Department of Health and Human Services. *Study findings: study of national incidence and prevalence of child abuse and neglect-1988.* Washington, DC: U.S. Government Printing Office, 1988.

126. U.S. General Accounting Office. *Home visiting: a promising early intervention strategy for at risk families.* Washington DC: U.S. Government Printing Office, 1990.

127. Valentine DP, Acuff DS, Freeman ML, et al. Defining child maltreatment: a multidisciplinary overview. *Child Welfare* 1984;58:497.

128. Videka-Sherman L. Intervention for child neglect: the empirical knowledge base. In: Cowan A, ed. *Current research on child neglect.* Rockville, MD: Aspen Systems Corporation, 1988.

129. Whitaker RC, Wright JA, Pepe MS, et al. Predicting obesity in young adulthood from childhood and parental obesity. *N Engl J Med* 1997;337:869.

130. Wise PH, Meyers A. Poverty and child health. *Pediatr Clin North Am* 1988;35:1169.

131. Wodarski JS, Kurtz PD, Gaudin JM, et al. Maltreatment and the school-age child: major academic, socioemotional, and adaptive outcomes. *Social Work* 1990;35:460.

132. Wolock I. Child developmental problems and child maltreatment among AFDC families. *J Sociol Soc Welfare* 1981;8:83.

133. Wolock I, Horowitz B. Child maltreatment as a social problem: the neglect of neglect. *Am J Orthopsychiatry* 1984;54:530.

134. Wolock I, Horowitz H. Child maltreatment and maternal deprivation among AFDC recipient families. *Soc Serv Res* 1979;53:175.

135. Yahraes H. Teaching mother's mothering. Rockville: NIMH, 1977. In: Videka-Sherman L, ed. *Intervention for child neglect: perinatal knowledge base: child neglect monograph: proceedings from a symposium.* Washington, DC: U.S. Department of Health and Human Services, 1988.

136. Zill M, Schoenborn CA. *Developmental, learning and emotional problems: health of our nation's children, United States, 1988. Advance data from Vital and Health Statistics, No. 190.* Hyattsville, MD: National Center for Health Statistics, 1990.

137. Zuckerman B. Drug-exposed infants: understanding the medical risk. In: *Future of children: drug exposed infants.* Los Altos, CA: Center for the Future of Children, 1991.

138. Zuravin SJ. Child neglect: a review of definitions and measurement research. In: Dubowitz H, ed. *Neglected children.* Thousand Oaks, CA: Sage Publications, 1999:24–46.

139. Zuravin S. *Child abuse, child neglect and maternal depression: is there a connection?* National Center on Child Abuse and Neglect: child neglect monograph: proceedings from a symposium. Washington DC: Clearinghouse on Child Abuse and Neglect Information, 1988.

14

Munchausen Syndrome By Proxy

Donna Andrea Rosenberg

Department of Pediatrics, University of Colorado Medical Center, Denver, Colorado

Munchausen syndrome by proxy (MSBP) is a somewhat bizarre form of abuse involving the persistent fabrication of illness in a child by an adult. It was first described in 1977 by Meadow (38), an English pediatrician, and the name is derived from Munchausen syndrome, the condition of self-inflicted illness in adults. In the decades since its initial description, and compared with other forms of child abuse, MSBP has proven to be a form of child maltreatment fraught with rather different diagnostic and legal problems. The perpetrator of MSBP, usually the child's mother, often evades the early detection of her noxious ministrations because the symptoms and signs she reports appear plausible and because she appears attentive and concerned. The perpetrator's history often sounds cogent to the physician, bespeaking a serious illness. Although doctors are educated to evaluate critically the reliability of an historian, pediatricians do not expect that a history is but an elaborate lie. Once the diagnosis has been considered, definitive inclusion or exclusion may be technically problematic. In consequence, ensuring civil court–ordered protection of the victim and any siblings also may prove difficult, and is uneven from location to location. Evaluation of the family, the information from which is intended to shape therapy and which is useful only when the perpetrator is forthcoming, is often stymied by the mother's refusal to participate or her indignant denial of her malfeasance, however compelling the evidence (21). Awareness of MSBP also varies significantly among mental health professionals (41), and the mother may be very persuasive, even to experienced evaluators (57). Criminal court proceedings undertaken against the perpetrator are still relatively rare, even in homicidal MSBP. Medical professionals continue to struggle with this form of child abuse.

DEFINITION

In MSBP, illness in a child is persistently and secretly simulated (lied about or faked) and/or produced by a parent or someone who is *in loco parentis,* and the child repeatedly presented for medical assessment and care. This often results in multiple medical procedures, both diagnostic and therapeutic. The definition specifically excludes physical abuse only, sexual abuse only, and nonorganic failure to thrive that is solely the result of nutritional/emotional deprivation.

By "simulated," one means that lies are told by the mother about the child's symptoms. For example, the mother may repeatedly report that her child has episodes of stiffening, shaking, or decreased level of consciousness, when in fact these never occurred, or she may tell the pediatrician that the child has hematuria, and bring in a urine sample that she has contaminated with her own menstrual blood. By "produced," one means that the mother secretly interferes with the child's body to produce symptoms or signs in the child, for example, by surreptitious suffocation, or by the administration of unprescribed and unnecessary medicines or substances, the fact or the extent of which are not proffered on history.

DEMOGRAPHICS

Hundreds of cases of MSBP have been reported worldwide, although it is likely that most cases of MSBP go unreported in the literature. Most of the literature concerning this form of maltreatment is published in English and originates in the United Kingdom and the United States. Cases of MSBP also have been reported from Canada; Australia; New Zealand; Western, Central, and Eastern Europe; the Middle East; South America; the Indian subcontinent; Central America; Africa; Ceylon; Japan; and Singapore. Clearly, MSBP is not a culture-specific disorder, nor is it confined to either a socialized or privatized medical system. It also appears that the perpetration of MSBP is not so uncommon as originally thought (52). One study in the U.K. estimated the combined annual incidence of MSBP, nonaccidental poisoning, and nonaccidental suffocation as at least 2.8/100,000 in children younger than 1 year (29).

Currently, statistics pertaining to MSBP rely on series from a single authorship or on meta-analysis. Meta-analysis is the quantitative repooling of data that have been acquired in like fashion, for the purpose of looking at a summary result. As with all statistical methods, meta-analysis has limitations, and no statistic based on sample population studies is entirely applicable to an individual patient.

In the overwhelming majority of cases of MSBP, the perpetrator is the mother, although fathers (27,33), other relatives (2), babysitters (45), and nurses (12) occasionally are implicated.

Boys and girls are victimized almost equally, and no special trend is noted as to birth order (48). Curiously, however, although several children in a family may be victimized sequentially, it is unusual for more than one child to be victimized within any given period (1), except during relatively brief transition periods. Typically, if the original victim survives, that child's medical troubles melt away when another child comes along and develops unusual and inexplicable troubles.

Most victims of MSBP are infants and toddlers (29,48). Presumably, the younger children are more commonly affected because they are pre- or semiverbal and relatively helpless physically. They are therefore easier to manipulate and assault. Although victimization of the children commonly begins in infancy or toddlerhood, there is usually a delay in making the correct diagnosis. In one series, the average time from onset of symptoms and signs to diagnosis was 15 months, but it might be as long as 20 years (48) or never (31). Older child victims of MSBP, whose abuse has generally begun years earlier, may adopt the false symptoms and signs as their own (16,23). Some evidence suggests that these children may go on to develop Munchausen syndrome themselves (13) or some type of personality disorder (44,49). There is at least one report of an elementary school–age victim whose mother desisted from the longstanding, painful, and disfiguring abuse after the child's threat to expose her (10).

In one series, 25% of cases of MSBP involved simulation only, 25% involved production only, and 50% involved both simulation and production of illness. As much as 95% of the time, the perpetrator continues victimizing the child in the hospital (48), often in the most egregious ways (55).

Short-term morbidity for the children, by definition, is 100%, much of it related to the diagnostic and therapeutic procedures ordered by the doctor. Long-term morbidity, defined as pain and/or illness that causes permanent disfigurement or impairment, is harder to assess statistically. At least 8% of the surviving victims of MSBP have some kind of long-term morbidity as a result of complications of the attack or, rarely, complications from medical procedures (35,48). This figure is probably an underestimate, however, and does not include long-term psychological morbidity, which may be considerable (30,48).

Although it is currently impossible, for methodologic reasons, to assess the mortality rate from MSBP, it is important to state that some children do die because of an ultimate fatal attack. Perhaps the perpetrator accidentally goes too far, having meant to make the child ill but not to kill the child. Perhaps it is a final act of unbridled hostility toward the child. Whatever the intent, within this syndrome, children are at some risk of death. In one series, 33% of the children died (35). In another, 9% of the children died (48). All were infants and toddlers, and the causes of death notably featured suffocation and poisoning. Other causes of death have been described (48), and still others, as yet undescribed, are possible. Furthermore, siblings of victims of MSBP tended to die in alarming numbers, often with the misdiagnosis of sudden infant death syndrome (SIDS), and there is every reason to believe that they died in a homicidal manner (4,9,35,36). Child fatality review teams are springing up throughout the country, and, with the availability to these teams of multidisciplinary records and expertise, they are discovering cases of MSBP that had previously but incorrectly been designated as accidental, natural, or undetermined manner of death.

A few cases of adult victims of adult perpetrators of MSBP have been reported (5,53, 54). The methods of assault included repeated injection of gasoline or turpentine under the skin, and injection of insulin.

CLINICAL AND LABORATORY FINDINGS

Symptoms and signs and laboratory findings in MSBP cover an enormous spectrum, but the most common presentation is apnea. Seizures, bleeding, central nervous system depression, diarrhea, vomiting, fever (with or without sepsis or other localized infection), and rash also are quite common (48). At no time, however, should any list be considered inclusive, as we continually expand our understanding of the breadth of presentations of this syndrome. Table 14.1 lists some of the presentations of MSBP.

Nissen fundoplications are unnecessarily performed with distressing frequency in victims of MSBP, as are operations for the installation of a central venous catheter. Both procedures result in direct-line access to the child and therefore the possibility of further intraluminal assaults on the child, with feces, saliva, contaminated water, drugs, salt, and many other substances (19). Some child victims of MSBP are developmentally delayed as a result of the damage done by the inflicted illness or as a result of chronic hospitalization or lack of stimulation. Malnutrition may be the result of the chronically inflicted illness, surreptitious withholding of food, prolonged emetic, laxative, or other drug assault, or other causes. MSBP also may present in the context of a bona fide chronic disease, when the caretaking parent has intentionally and surreptitiously withheld treatment to exacerbate the child's illness significantly (28,34).

The perpetration of MSBP may terminate with the homicide of the child. Probably the most common cause of death in homicidal MSBP is suffocation, but there are many causes of death, among which are poisoning with various drugs, inflicted bacterial or fungal sepsis, hypoglycemia, and salt or potassium poisoning. Too frequently, both suffocation and other homicidal deaths are signed out incorrectly as to cause and manner. Either the significantly positive clinical history is undiscovered or ignored, or a scene investigation is delayed or inadequate, or the autopsy, if performed, has not included all necessary dissections or tests.

A significantly positive clinical history would feature one or more items listed in Table 14.2. If any of these factors figure in the clinical history, MSBP should be suspected in the differential diagnosis, along with possible genetic, metabolic, toxicologic, or environmental causes of death. These factors are not diagnostic criteria for MSBP. They are historical flags that should spur further investigation, and in particular an exhaustive autopsy.

TABLE 14.1. *Some clinical presentations of Munchausen syndrome by proxy*[a]

	Symptom, sign, or laboratory finding
Head, eyes, ears, nose, throat, mouth	Bleeding from ears nose, throat,
	Epistaxis
	External otitis
	Hearing impairment
	Nasal excoriation
	Nystagmus
	Otorrhea
	Tooth loss
Respiratory	Apnea
	Asthma
	Bleeding from upper respiratory tract
	Cyanosis (and other color changes including pallor)
	Cystic fibrosis
	Hemoptysis
	Respiratory arrest
	Sleep apnea
Cardiovascular	Bradycardia
	Cardiomyopathy
	Cardiopulmonary arrest
	Hypertension
	Rhythm abnormalities (including bradycardia, tachycardia, ventricular tachycardia, and others)
	Shock
Gastrointestinal	Abdominal pain
	Anorexia
	Bleeding from nasogastric tube/ileostomy
	Crohn's disease
	Diarrhea
	Esophageal burns
	Esophageal perforation
	Feculent vomiting
	Feeding problems
	Gastrointestinal ulceration
	Hematemesis
	Hematochezia or melena
	Hemorrhagic colitis
	Intestinal pseudo-obstruction
	Malabsorption syndromes
	Polyphagia
	Pseudomelanosis coli
	Retrograde intussusception
	Vomiting (cyclic or otherwise)
Genitourinary	Bacteriuria
	Hematuria
	Menorrhagia
	Nocturia
	Polydipsia
	Polyuria and/or impaired urinary concentrating ability
	Pyuria
	Renal failure
	Urination from umbilical micropenis
	Urethral stones
	Urine gravel

TABLE 14.1. *(Continued)*

	Symptom, sign, or laboratory finding
Neurologic, musculoskeletal, developmental, psychiatric	Arthralgia
	Arthritis
	Ataxia
	Behavioral/personality change (including anxiety, panic reactions, rage, disorientation, and others)
	Developmental delay (failure to attain and/or loss of milestones)
	Headache
	Hyperactivity
	Irritability
	Lethargy
	Morning stiffness
	Psychotic symptoms
	Sleep disturbances: prolonged sleep/other
	Seizures
	Sexual abuse
	Syncope
	Unconsciousness
	Weakness
Skin	Abscesses
	Burns
	Eczema
	Excoriation
	Rash
Infectious, immune, allergic	Allergies (to food and others)
	Bacteremia (uni- and/or polymicrobial)
	Fevers
	Immunodeficiency
	Osteomyelitis
	Septic arthritis
	Urinary tract infection
Abnormalities of growth	Failure to gain weight or weight loss
Hematologic	Anemia
	Bleeding diathesis
	Bleeding from specific sites (see system)
	Easy bruising
	Leukopenia
Metabolic, endocrine, fluid and electrolyte	Acidosis
	Alkalosis
	Biochemical chaos
	Creatine kinase and aldolase increase
	Dehydration
	Diabetes
	Glycosuria
	Hyperglycemia
	Hyperkalemia
	Hypernatremia
	Hypochloremia
	Hypoglycemia
	Hypokalemia
	Hyponatremia
Other	Abuse (sexual, physical, other)
	Diaphoresis
	Foreign-body ingestions
	Hypothermia
	Peripheral edema
	Poisonings
	Premature birth

[a]Including items reportedly observed by mother or actually observed by medical staff.

TABLE 14.2. *Review of clinical history in a dead child: circumstances suggestive of Munchausen syndrome by proxy*

A history of repeated medical visits for unusual, poorly defined, unpredictable or unresponsive illness, especially apnea and seizures, which had never been confirmed to be witnessed at their starting moment by anyone other than the mother; *and* a full medical evaluation of the child that revealed no organic abnormality that could *fully* account for the child's reported illness, *or* a partial medical evaluation of the child that excluded major causes for the child's reported illness, *or* any medical evaluation that came to a conclusion about the child's diagnosis but whose accuracy, on review, is seriously questioned; OR

Ill sibling of decedent, especially if was or is ill with chronic, poorly defined medical problems; OR

Dead sibling of decedent, or dead unrelated child in the same home as decedent, especially if any of the following is found: (a) if other child's death was signed out as SIDS; (b) if death followed a poorly defined or chronic illness; (c) if the cause of death was allegedly an illness that overwhelmingly is nonfatal in childhood; (d) if the cause of death was related to poisoning/intoxication; (e) if the cause of death was the result of an unusual accident; (f) if the death followed a presumed illness that was either unsubstantiated or excluded at autopsy; *or* (g) if the explanation for the death was inadequate; OR

Mother with chronic, poorly defined medical problems

SIDS, sudden infant death syndrome.

The usefulness of the autopsy as an investigative tool for determining cause and manner of death is obviously enhanced when it is done in the most thorough manner. Specifically, evidence of poisoning should be diligently searched for, with the necessary toxicologic studies done from vitreous, blood, urine, gastric contents, tissues, or other sources. A "routine toxicology study" may be inadequate and, in any case, includes somewhat different studies, depending on the laboratory. Specific requests may be necessary to have specific tests done. Consultation with the laboratory director is often useful. If thin-layer chromatography is positive, the nature of the substance may be more specifically delineated with gas chromatography/mass spectrophotometry. The laboratory should be requested to preserve the samples securely, as they may be needed later for repeated studies or other studies not originally considered. If both serum sodium and urine sodium are elevated and the child is not dehydrated, salt poisoning should be suspected. The premortem blood sodium or the postmortem vitreous sodium is useful. Postmortem vitreous urea nitrogen is a reliable study, and may be useful as a reflection of hydration status. It is interpreted in the context of other renal function studies, in the same way as is blood urea nitrogen. As with all children suspected of having been maltreated, a skeletal survey should be done to look for fractures. Microbiology studies may be central to determining whether the child was the victim of inflicted microbial assault. When postmortem blood samples are positive, care must be taken to discriminate between those that reflect infection in the child and those that are the result of postmortem blood contamination with bowel organisms. The condition and contents of any lines into the child (central venous catheter, gastrostomy, endotracheal tube, shunt, pacemaker, etc.) should be examined closely, and it may be prudent to preserve them. As in a clinical situation, there should be careful attention to chain of evidence for laboratory specimens and biomedical appliances.

Homicidal suffocation deaths (32) deserve further comment because they are still too commonly misdiagnosed as SIDS. It is reemphasized here that if any significant history precedes death, then SIDS, by definition, is excluded. The current definition of SIDS is "the unexpected death of an infant younger than 1 year of age that remains unexplained after a complete review of the clinical history, death scene investigation, and autopsy." What this really means is that, after a thorough evaluation, although certain causes and manners have been definitively excluded, the cause and manner of death remain undetermined. Despite this, and for reasons having more to do with a combination of well-meaningness and/or politicking than with scientific durability, it is still acceptable to use the term SIDS as a cause of death on a death certificate. SIDS deaths are considered deaths of a natural manner. Always be concerned when sudden death occurs in a child who had apnea before death, especially apnea that featured attacks beginning only in the mother's presence, and when the mother called someone to see the baby, the child was hypoxic (i.e., cyanotic, grey, gasping, and limp) (46). The physical findings of suffocation more commonly seen in adult victims (head and neck petechiae and/or bruising, defensive marks, etc.) are almost always absent in young children (15). Intraalveolar hemosiderin found at autopsy may be a marker of past smothering (39).

PERPETRATORS

What are the characteristics of the perpetrator of MSBP, and why does she do this? First, it is important to mention that no psychologic test can include or exclude perpetration of MSBP. Second, there is no classic profile for a perpetrator, meaning that possessing certain characteristics does not entirely implicate a suspect, and lacking certain characteristics does not entirely exclude a suspect.

The perpetrator of MSBP is usually the mother. She sometimes has had nursing, medical, or paramedical training, perhaps never completed. She may be married or single or divorced, but if married, the relationship with her husband, although perhaps seemingly satisfactory, is usually shallow. Although she was described originally as generally affable with medical and nursing staff, broader experience shows that she may have a hostile, difficult, and demanding personality. Some mothers, in their roles as champions of their ill children, have had good success at enlisting the admiration of their communities, or in making useful, powerful, or lucrative contacts, or in obtaining benefits consequent on the child's illness, including wish-fulfillment

trips. Features of Munchausen syndrome and a history of problems related to her reproductive system (including spontaneous abortions during motor vehicle accidents), unsubstantiated by her medical records, are not uncommon in these mothers, but they may lack a documented psychiatric history, or it may be unavailable (it is often difficult to find out if psychiatric records exist, much less what they contain.) Forty-one percent of adult patients with Munchausen syndrome develop symptoms by age 18 years and have a characteristic background of abuse and neglect coupled with an illness (44).

Mothers have been variably diagnosed psychiatrically as normal, depressed, borderline personality disorder, hysterical personality disorder, narcissistic personality disorder, or unspecified personality disorder (8). It is not to be understood from this that the mother has some kind of disease that renders her incapable of discerning right from wrong, that makes her compulsively perform acts outside her consciousness, or that makes her either the unwilling or unwitting captive of an irresistible impulse. Only very, very rarely does the mother carry the diagnosis of psychosis (48). Some reports cite a history of significant childhood maltreatment in these mothers (26), including physical and sexual abuse (30), with the generational legacy of abuse in some way "medicalized," from the mother's exposure to the medical field, either as a patient or a close party to a sick person. The mother may become suicidal when her duplicity is uncovered or when she becomes aware of professional suspicions. Psychiatric interventions should be offered and available. Why MSBP is overwhelmingly a female-perpetrated form of child abuse is not clear, although female patterns of learned behavior and expression of hostility have been proposed. It certainly stands in contrast to almost every other form of child abuse and neglect (except sexual abuse), in which male and female perpetrators figure in approximately equal numbers.

No evidence whatsoever suggests that the perpetrator of MSBP is unaware of her actions. On the contrary, the planning and organization often involved, the minute attention to secrecy, the fact that the assaults are committed without witnesses, and the carefully woven fabric of lies presented to the doctor all suggest great awareness. The perpetration of MSBP is volitional. It is also violent. The fact that the violence is encased in duplicity only hides, but does not diminish, its violence.

Most mothers do not have a criminal history, but occasionally one does. They may break into their own homes to stage thefts, or set fires, sometimes collecting insurance settlements. They also may be dangerous to others in their midst, with the homicide of relatives or children in their charge, for example, having occasionally been proven or highly suspected.

Perpetrators also may be dangerous to medical professionals. They have been known to undertake criminal behavior such as stalking, breaking and entering, theft, fraud, destruction of property, and death threats. It is no longer uncommon for the perpetrator of MSBP to make false allegations of malpractice by the doctor to professional or licensing bodies, or to sue the doctor and/or hospital on one or several of a number of pretexts: defamation of character, malicious reporting, malpractice, wrongful detention of the child, or wrongful death.

DIAGNOSTIC STRATEGIES

Failure to diagnose MSBP means that a fundamentally healthy child and his siblings could be killed or irreversibly damaged. Conversely, the failure to exclude MSBP may mean that necessary treatment is withheld from an ill child, or that a family is not offered prognostic information or genetic counseling. The single largest impediment to making a diagnosis of MSBP is the failure to include it in the differential diagnosis. Once the diagnosis is entertained and a diagnostic strategy designed, the diagnosis is usually included or excluded relatively quickly.

Once MSBP is considered, the difficulties in pursuing the diagnosis generally revolve around the dilemma of not wishing to expose the child to any more potential risk and yet needing reasonably definitive proof. This clinical judgment call is best made with the assistance of the director of medical services, the head nurse, the primary care nurse, the hospital child-protection team, and, if necessary, the hospital lawyer. It is at this point that social services and their representative lawyer should be notified of a possible child abuse case. The diagnostic strategy (or often, strategies) must maximize diagnostic capability while minimizing risk to the child, and must obviously take into account access to, and condition of, the child.

When MSBP is suspected, confirmation or elimination of the diagnosis may be undertaken through one or several of a number of strategies: the search for evidence of illness fabrication, the search for evidence of an explanation other than MSBP, the separation of the child from the suspected perpetrator, and records review.

The first diagnostic strategy, the search for evidence of illness fabrication, includes such tests as toxicology studies if poisoning is suspected, blood group typing or subtyping if contamination with exogenous blood is suspected, or hidden video monitoring if surreptitious suffocation is suspected. The medical literature contains some fascinating accounts in which evidence of commission has been thus captured: ipecac poisoning is uncovered by finding the bottles in the child's hospital room, by finding a postmortem blood sample positive for the alkaloids in ipecac (51), and by toxicologic studies in a living child (20); factitious bleeding is exposed by minor blood group typing of erythrocytes in urine (42) and by injecting radiolabeled erythrocytes as comparisons to the child's "bleeding sites" (25); factitious diabetes mellitus is confirmed by using ascorbic acid as a marker for the child's own urine (40); mothers are covertly videotaped while suffocating the children they claim had intractable apnea (47,55,56).

To a great extent, one must choose, or even design, the test depending on the fabrication that is suspected. The search for evidence of illness fabrication must be very carefully planned and executed. Depending on the situation, this involves proper chain of evidence, preservation of laboratory specimens, continuous monitoring and recording of video units with plans to intervene immediately and decisively if assault is seen, and precise coordination with law enforcement and/or social services. The advantage of this diagnostic strategy is that, if positive evidence is uncovered and is reliable, it is more likely to be accepted as definitive, both medically and legally. The disadvantage is that the child is, potentially, exposed to at least one more assault. If the test is negative, then it is often not possible to distinguish between absence of assault, failure to capture the assault, or a false-negative test.

One diagnostic strategy in the search for evidence of illness fabrication is covert videomonitoring. It is a highly useful, if somewhat controversial, strategy. A video camera with its lens in, for example, what appears to be a sprinkler head or smoke alarm, may be purchased and then hard wired into a monitoring and recording unit in a nearby room. At the time of this writing, such a system involves an expenditure of approximately $10,000.00 (U.S. currency), which, on the scale of things, is a rather small investment. Tertiary care hospitals should seriously consider the diagnostic benefits of such a system, especially when undertaking remodeling. Obviously, this type of system must be in place before the child's admission. If the hospital room has a private bathroom, it is wise to close it off to avoid the possibility of an assault to the child outside the range of the video.

Useful clinical data may be accrued with videotaping (11,17,47,55,56,58). One investigator who videotaped mothers smothering their children noted,

Smothering has been labelled "gentle" battering. We reject this. The video and physiological recordings showed that both children struggled violently until they lost consciousness. Considerable force was used to obstruct their

airways, and this force was needed for at least 70 seconds before electroencephalographic changes, probably associated with loss of consciousness, occurred. Interestingly, in both cases a soft garment was used to smother the children and no marks were seen on the lips or around the nose.

The authors further delineated features of the multichannel recordings, "a combination of which may in future prove to be pathognomonic of this type (smothering) of apnea . . ." The features included the sudden onset of large body movements during a relatively regular breathing pattern (from struggling induced by airway obstruction); a series of large breaths at about 1 minute after the onset of the episode, with a characteristically prolonged expiratory phase, at a relatively slow rate (a response to severe arterial hypoxia); a severe degree of sinus tachycardia; and last, at about 1 minute after the onset of the episode, large slow waves and a subsequent isoelectric baseline on the electroencephalogram typical of hypoxia (56).

If videotaping is planned, the multidisciplinary team may want to consult with the hospital attorney. Continuous observation of the videotape by closed circuit television is essential, and it is wise to notify hospital security and the local police department, because one may need their participation.

The subject of diagnostic, covert videotaping in the hospital has engendered some animated debate, with authors addressing the legal, ethical, and logistic aspects of videotaping (18,22,24,37,50,59,60). Some are concerned with the rights of privacy of parents in the hospital. Other authors pointed out that the parental rights to privacy are abrogated when that parent is the agent of the child's possible destruction. In this pediatrician's opinion, the videotape may be considered the equivalent of other tests undertaken in the usual diagnostic process that do not individually require consent; the general medical consent form signed on behalf of the child at the time of admission to the hospital covers most procedures. Furthermore, child abuse statutes in every state permit the taking of pictures without parental consent if child abuse is suspected. To date, no medical person or institution has been successfully sued for using covert videomonitoring as a diagnostic strategy. At the time of this writing, the Department of Health in the U.K., acknowledging that there was "little doubt that children suffer ill health and are sometimes left severely disabled or die as a consequence of their carers either inducing or fabricating their illnesses," was about to convene an expert multidisciplinary panel to "review the identification of situations where children have had illnesses induced or fabricated by their carer . . . and issue guidelines which should include the use of covert video surveillance" (14).

The second diagnostic strategy, the search for an explanation other than MSBP, has often been extensive by the time that MSBP is suspected, but it has not necessarily been exhaustive. There are certain situations in which an exhaustive search for an explanation other than MSBP is the best diagnostic strategy: when there exists neither the opportunity nor the diagnostic test that could capture evidence of commission, or when the search for evidence of illness fabrication would expose the child to grave risk. The contending diagnoses on the differential should be those that are subject to definitive inclusion or exclusion. For example, if a child is repeatedly presented to the hospital with apnea that begins only in the presence of the mother, the disorders that might be causing the child's apnea (however unlikely, for example, a cerebral space-occupying lesion or gastroesophageal reflux) can be searched for, and can therefore be definitively included or excluded. Positive test results must be carefully scrutinized to ensure that they are positive neither as a result of maternal contamination/ intervention, nor as a result of being "overcalled" (i.e., the range of normal for the test is not reliably delineated). Certain gastrointestinal tests seem to be especially vulnerable to this problem, in particular gastrointestinal motility studies (3) and esophageal pH probe studies. The advantage of this diagnostic strategy is that the gathering of diagnostic evidence does not involve exposing the child to the possibility of another assault. The disadvantage is that it can

be time consuming and expensive, and there may be risks to the patient of various diagnostic procedures or prolonged hospitalization.

The third diagnostic strategy, the separation of the child from the parent, may be a very useful diagnostic strategy, and in certain circumstances, it carries the most diagnostic weight and is the least malignant. It is important to have a baseline against which to compare the child's subsequent course during separation, whether that separation occurs in hospital or in a foster home. The baseline is the well-documented history of the child's symptoms and signs as provided by the mother. Therefore it is important that the only major change that is made in the child's care during the separation is the presence of the caretaker. It is sometimes the case that the fabrication of illness causes irreversible medical problems, or that the fabrication of illness is piled onto already existing illness. Only reversible conditions of the child can be expected to improve, and these only to the degree and at a rate that is consonant with the condition itself. The advantage of this diagnostic strategy is that it can be definitive without exposing the child to further risk. The disadvantage is that, if it turns out that it is not MSBP, then an ill child has been separated unnecessarily and perhaps harmfully from his or her mother, and correct diagnosis has been delayed. One way to minimize the possible disadvantages is to have supervised visits with the mother. The supervision must be constant and scrupulous, with no foods or medicines or candy permitted.

The fourth diagnostic strategy is records review. This diagnostic strategy involves the reformulation of a differential diagnosis—one that is comprehensive without being promiscuous—and the critical reevaluation of this differential. This strategy, which one would suppose to have been implicit in the medical care already provided, follows from the observation that the pivotal facts, although present in the medical record, are frequently obscured by the sheer volume of information. In other words, the crucial data are there, but are buried. Furthermore, the importance of a comprehensive survey of the child's medical presentation has been repeatedly overshadowed by the immediacy of the crises. Curiously, the more chronic and intractable the child's problem, the less likely it may be that it is given a fresh, comprehensive look. Finally, a sort of colonial system of medical care sometimes evolves, with fragments of the child's condition being parceled off to subspecialists, whose purview extends only to the shoreline of their organ systems of interest. How, or even whether, these fragments converge to form some cohesive empire of illness may be unexplored.

Records review may be the preferred diagnostic strategy, because it is low risk and often definitive. Records review may be the only diagnostic strategy available when, for example, the child is alive but unavailable for some reason, when the symptoms and signs of fabrication are long gone, or when the child is dead.

For most pediatric patients, a thorough records review is straightforward: we read, we remember. Records are relatively brief and come from a small number of medical facilities. That a substantially different approach to records review is in order when MSBP is suspected is a consequence of three typical features: the record is mammoth, the legal implications are broad, and the stakes are high. Records often run to thousands of pages, sometimes from dozens of medical facilities. The doctor may be called to testify in civil and/or criminal proceedings, where the medical facts—perhaps hundreds of thousands of them—may be minutely tracked and challenged, as may the process by which the diagnosis was distilled from the facts. A computerized system for data entry, storage, organization, and retrieval is often indispensable, and any of a number of commercially available database-management systems can be adapted for this purpose.

Because the medical and nursing records are often complicated, it is best if someone (or several people) experienced in both inpatient and outpatient pediatrics reviews the records. There are advantages and disadvantages to working with original medical records. The advantages are that poor quality or missed duplication of records is not an issue, and that vital information on oversized pages (e.g., nursing records from the pediatric intensive care unit) is accessible. The disadvantages are considerable: pages cannot be numbered; accessibility, space, and the simultaneous availability of the record and the necessary computer equipment are generally problematic.

In reality, it is commonly impossible to review original records, because of geographic or logistic problems. In these usual circumstances, care must be taken to ensure, as far as possible, that photocopied records, or records scanned onto a CD-ROM, are complete. In the process of the records review, it is often helpful to compile a cumulative list of prescribed medications, operations, consultations, hospitalizations, diagnoses explored, diagnostic tests performed and their results, interventions attempted, school days missed, and outside consultations.

When records are voluminous, it is optimal to have a small team of people reviewing the records and making notes in a similar way. Sometimes, elective medical students and residents can be enlisted. A system using index cards or computer database-management software is recommended. Records should be page-numbered immediately, so that data can be noted with their corresponding page numbers and later found again.

The diagnostic strategies used to detect MSBP in its most common presentations are outlined in Table 14.3. Obviously, these diagnostic strategies will not fit every type of suspected event, and one must tailor the diagnostic strategy to the type of perpetration suspected. This effort may involve contacting colleagues in related fields for information or to seek help.

Occasionally, the distinction between MSBP and pathologic doctor-shopping, or magnification of a child's real but minimal illness for the parent's own psychologic or fiscal gain may not be clear. For those cases that seem to fall at the edges of the definition of MSBP, it is worth remembering that the name applied to the child's circumstances is not so material as a careful assessment of the threatened harm to the child.

TABLE 14.3. *Some methods of fabrication and corresponding diagnostic strategies in Munchausen syndrome by proxy*

Presentation	Method of simulation and/or production	Method of diagnosis
Apnea	Manual suffocation	• Videomonitoring • Implantable ECG recorder • Diagnosis by exclusion • Patient with pinch marks on nose • Mother caught

	Poisoning
	  Tricyclic antidepressants
	  Hydrocarbon
		• Toxicology (gastric/blood)
		• Toxicology of i.v. fluid

Seizures	Lying	• Diagnosis by exclusion

	Poisoning
	  Phenothiazines
	  Hydrocarbons
	  Salt
	  Tricyclic antidepressants
		• Toxicology of blood, urine, i.v. fluid, milk
		• Serum and urine sodium concentrations

	Suffocation/carotid sinus pressure	• Witnessed • Forensic photos of pressure points
Diarrhea	Phenolphthalein/other laxative poisoning	• Stool/diaper positive
	Salt poisoning	• Assay of formula/gastric contents
Vomiting	Emetic poisoning	• Assay for drug
	Lying	• Hospital observation

CNS depression	Drugs
	  Diphenoxylate and atropine (Lomotil)
	  Insulin
	  Chloral hydrate
	  Barbiturates/narcotics
	  Aspirin
	  Diphenhydramine
	  Tricyclic antidepressants
	  Acetaminophen
	  Hydrocarbons
	  Chlordiazepoxide
	  Phenytoin
	  Carbamazepine
		• Assays of blood, gastric contents, urine, i.v. fluid; analysis of insulin type

	Suffocation	• See "apnea" and "seizures"
Bleeding	Rodenticide (warfarin) poisoning	• Toxicology
	Phenolphthalein poisoning	• Diapers positive
	Exogenous blood applied	• Blood group typing (major and minor) • ^{51}Cr labeling of erythrocytes
	Exsanguination of child	• Single-blind study • Mother caught in the act
	Addition of other substances (paint, cocoa, dyes)	• Testing; washing
Rash	Drug poisoning	• Assay
	Scratching	• Diagnosis of exclusion
	Caustics applied/painting skin	• Assay/wash off

TABLE 14.3. *(Continued.)*

Presentation	Method of simulation and/or production	Method of diagnosis

Fever	Contamination with infected material
	• Materials
	  Saliva
	  Feces
	  Dirt
	  Contaminated water
	  Coffee grounds
	  Vaginal secretions
	  Others
	• Target tissues
	  Blood
	  Skin
	  Bones
	  Bladder
	  Others
		• Caught in the act
		• Improper taping of line discovered
		• Type of organism growing from infected sites
		• Trial separation
		• Epidemiology (relative-risk assessment)
		• Diagnosis by exclusion

	Falsifying temperature	• Careful charting, rechecking (esp. urine for core body temp)
	Falsifying chart	• Careful charting, rechecking • Duplication (ghost record) of temperature chart in nursing station

CNS, central nervous system; ECG, electrocardiographic. Adapted from Rosenberg DA. Web of deceit: a literature review of Munchausen syndrome by proxy. *Child Abuse Negl* 1987;11:547–563, with permission.

DIAGNOSTIC CRITERIA

When Munchausen syndrome by proxy is suspected, the strength of the known facts may extend from weak to definitive. Thus there may be different degrees of diagnostic conviction, not only from case to case, but also within a case, depending on the stage of the assessment. Here, therefore, diagnostic criteria for a definitive diagnosis, a provisional diagnosis, and a possible diagnosis of MSBP are provided. Because the gathering of evidence in a case may, ultimately, diminish the likelihood or altogether exclude MSBP, diagnostic criteria for the uncertain diagnosis and the definitely excluded diagnosis also are enunciated.

Diagnostic criteria serve to discriminate efficiently between one particular diagnosis and all others. Collectively, the diagnostic criteria for a disorder are the smallest set of findings that must be present to make a diagnosis.

Each diagnostic criterion must be present to make a diagnosis. Each criterion must be pivotal, meaning that its presence is required for, and its absence excludes, the diagnosis. Each finding must be credibly observable by human senses. Other competent observers, using the same method, would observe the finding the same way. Thus the observation would be replicable.

To summarize, then, each criterion is necessary, and collectively the criteria are sufficient, for diagnosis.

Definitive Diagnosis

The definitive diagnosis of MSBP is the clear diagnosis. One can make a definitive diagnosis in one of two ways: by inclusion or by exclusion.

A diagnosis by inclusion is one supported by incontrovertible evidence of commission. For example, if a mother smothers the child she had previously and repeatedly presented for apnea, and if her act were captured with covert videotaping in hospital, then the definitive diagnosis of MSBP would be one by inclusion. Table 14.4 lists the criteria for the definitive diagnosis by inclusion of MSBP.

A diagnosis by exclusion is one in which all other possible explanations for the child's condition have been considered and excluded. A diagnosis by exclusion is the only diagnosis left standing after an exhaustive investigation. For example, if a child presents with recurrent apnea that begins exclusively in one person's

TABLE 14.4. *Munchausen syndrome by proxy: Criteria for a definitive diagnosis by inclusion*

1. Test/event is positive for tampering with child or with child's medical situation,
   AND
2. Positivity of test/event is not credibly the result of miscommunication, misunderstanding, or test error,
   AND
3. No other explanation for positive test/event is medically possible

presence and results in observable clinical compromise, if the child is conclusively shown to not otherwise exhibit apnea, and if all possible medical conditions that could account for the apnea are properly investigated and definitively excluded, then the definitive diagnosis of MSBP would be one by exclusion. Table 14.5 lists the criteria for the definitive diagnosis by exclusion of MSBP.

Provisional Diagnosis

The provisional diagnosis of MSBP is the diagnosis that, among contending diagnoses, is more likely than any other. Table 14.6 lists the criteria for provisional diagnosis of MSBP.

Possible Diagnosis

A possible diagnosis of MSBP is one among several likely diagnoses. Table 14.7 lists the criteria for the possible diagnosis of MSBP. Medical professionals are legally mandated to

TABLE 14.5. *Munchausen syndrome by proxy: Criteria for a definitive diagnosis by exclusion*

1. All competing diagnoses have been credibly eliminated, so that
   a. if the child is alive, the competing diagnoses are those that took into account the child's major medical findings and that account for the entirety of the child's presentation. [A major medical finding is one that is objectively observed, sufficiently specific as to help formulate the range of diagnoses, and verifiable in the record],
      OR
   b. if the child is alive, separation of the child from the alleged perpetrator results in resolution of the child's reversible medical problems, in accordance with their degree and speed of reversibility. No variable other than the separation can logically and fully account for the child's improvement,
      OR
   c. if the child is dead, autopsy examination does not reveal a cause of death that is credibly of accidental, natural, or suicidal manner,
      AND
2. No findings exclude the diagnosis of MSBP

TABLE 14.6. *Munchausen syndrome by proxy: Criteria for provisional diagnosis*

1. Test/event is presumptively positive for tampering with the child or the child's medical situation. No other explanation is medically probable. No findings exclude the diagnosis of MSBP
   OR
2. Child has, or had, a condition that cannot be fully explained medically, despite thorough evaluation. Cogent hypothesis suggests a faked medical condition. No findings exclude the diagnosis of MSBP
   OR
3. Child has, or had, a condition that cannot be fully explained medically. Evaluation has been extensive but not exhaustive. Cogent hypothesis suggests medical condition is faked. Further tests to include/exclude an uncommon organic diagnosis are impossible to do (if, for example, child is deceased), would be highly invasive, present a large medical risk to the child, or are unlikely to yield a definitive answer. No findings exclude the diagnosis of MSBP

TABLE 14.7. *Munchausen syndrome by proxy: Criteria for possible diagnosis*

1. Test/event is presumptively positive for tampering with child, or with child's medical situation. No other explanation is readily apparent. No findings exclude the diagnosis of MSBP

    OR

2. Child has a condition that cannot be fully explained medically, despite a respectable initial evaluation, at least. Cogent hypothesis suggests a faked medical condition. No findings exclude the diagnosis of MSBP

report child abuse to the local authority when they have a reasonable suspicion of it. Reasonable suspicion is not a term of art in medicine, but roughly translates into the set of diagnostic criteria here noted as possible diagnosis.

Inconclusive Determination: Can't Know

It is obvious that, rather than increasing the weight of medical evidence in support of a diagnosis of MSBP, accumulating data may instead diminish its likelihood. Medical criteria for inconclusive findings—that is, for MSBP's being indeterminate—are therefore articulated here. I cannot know means that, although the collection of data is complete, the data are insufficient to determine the diagnosis. One can neither confidently eliminate nor establish MSBP as the diagnosis. Can't know differs from possible diagnosis because implicit in a can't know determination is the assertion that all relevant and available records have been reviewed. This is in contrast to a possible diagnosis, in which there is an ex-

TABLE 14.8. *Munchausen syndrome by proxy: Criteria for inconclusive determination*

1. The relevant and available information has been reviewed

    AND

2. One is left with a differential diagnosis, rather than a diagnosis

    AND

3. It is not possible to affirm one diagnosis conclusively

    AND

4. It is not possible to exclude all but one diagnosis conclusively on the differential

    AND

5. It is not possible to prioritize reliably the likelihood of the competing diagnoses remaining on the differential

pectation of further diagnostic strategy. Table 14.8 lists the criteria for an inconclusive determination (can't know).

Definitely Not

Definitely not MSBP means that the diagnosis can be absolutely eliminated. This means that a wholly credible alternative explanation is at hand. To allow degrees of certainty within this diagnostic option, the physician might want to use some kind of qualifier, for example, probably not MSBP. Probably not MSBP is about the same as saying that, in all likelihood, an alternative explanation is at hand. The fact that diagnostic criteria for the exclusion of MSBP are included means that it is inevitable, as with other pediatric disorders, that there will be more suspected than actual cases. Recognizing this means also recognizing the need for the swiftest and most decisive diagnostic test, but one whose risk to the child does not appear to be excessive. Extreme care must be taken not to overdiagnose MSBP, or to marry oneself to the diagnosis in the absence of sufficient evidence, simply because one has considered it. Cases of misdiagnosed MSBP (43) are a real tragedy for the family and child. Table 14.9 lists the criteria for excluding the diagnosis of MSBP.

TABLE 14.9. *Munchausen syndrome by proxy: Criteria for excluding the diagnosis*

1. An alternative diagnosis has been credibly proven

    OR

2. What had appeared to be possible falsification of illness has been wholly and credibly accounted for in some other way

INTERVENTION

It would be folly to give a list of directives to take in all cases in which MSBP is suspected. The reader, however, may find the following considerations useful.

1. Optimally, the child can be protected and the data either definitely to include or exclude the diagnosis can be simultaneously collected. Realistically, this is often not the case. Professionals find themselves poised between weighing the eventual usefulness of these data against the possibility of a mishap occurring to the child during the data-collection process. When further diagnostic procedures place the child in a situation of untenable risk, the protection of the child is always the paramount consideration. Because child protection is a civil matter, the legal burden of proof is preponderance of the evidence. Thus absolute diagnostic proof is not necessary, and in its absence, epidemiologic evidence pertaining to the case may be sufficiently compelling (see later discussion).

2. Involve a multidisciplinary team early on. The team should include not only the usual members of the existing team, but also some individuals who are not customarily members of a hospital child-protection team. The social worker from the county to which the case has been reported is a pivotal person. Much will depend on this person's communication with the medical staff and understanding of the case. Given the volume and complexity of the data to digest and the generally high rate of staff turnover among county social workers, it is preferable for the social workers to work in pairs. Any way to circumvent the widespread and inefficient practice of having an "intake worker" start the case and then an "ongoing worker" continue it should be pursued. The supervisor of the social workers and the county attorney should similarly be included in the multidisciplinary team from the start.

Two psychiatrists and/or psychologists should be engaged to participate. Optimally, one is assigned to the family and the other to the medical and nursing staff. The family needs not only extended evaluation but also support. After confrontation of the family with the suspected diagnosis, the mother, who is generally the alleged perpetrator, as well as the father, are at increased risk for suicide. The child also needs to be at least developmentally and, if of sufficient age, psychologically evaluated. Interactional assessments by an experienced developmental psychologist may be fruitful.

Assigning a psychiatrist for the medical and nursing staff is not superfluous. Multidisciplinary teams break down over these cases. It is axiomatic that cases of MSBP cause polarization of opinions and emotions among the hospital staff, who have often worked with the family for years. The sense of betrayal experienced by some staff members is enormous and painful. One nurse commented, "On an intellectual level, the diagnosis was sensible, but on an emotional level, the suspicion was almost impossible to accept" (7). Others simply cannot fathom that this situation is possible; unfortunate and unnecessary rifts occur among the staff. Anticipating the need for a mental health professional to help all the staff with their feelings is good primary prevention.

Police and other law-enforcement personnel also should be involved early, especially if videotaping in the hospital is anticipated. Should an episode of intentional infliction of harm come to light during the videotaping, the police generally prefer to have prior knowledge of the case and may want to be prepared with an arrest warrant.

The primary care nurse and the head nurse should be included in the multidisciplinary child-protection team. The primary care nurse is often the person who has spent the most time with the child and the family over an extended period and multiple hospitalizations. He or she often has valuable information about a case that may not be known to the others on the team, and this individual certainly must be included in any plans that involve diagnostic procedures for MSBP. The primary care nurse often becomes responsible for such important items as documentation and chain of evidence of specimens.

Finally, it is often advisable to have a good clinical epidemiologist participating with the multidisciplinary team from the beginning, because data of commission (e.g., a videotape showing the mother suffocating the baby; a definitive blood test showing exogenous insulin in the child's body) often are unobtainable. The diagnostic alternative to these data is the calculation of the relative risk to the child of being in the maternal care. For example, if the child has an unspecified illness characterized by vomiting, failure to thrive, and multiple hospitalizations, an epidemiologist can review the child's records and calculate the relative risk to the child of losing weight at home compared with that of losing weight in the hospital. In the absence of data of commission, relative-risk data may be the most compelling evidence to present to the court. It is helpful if the data can be interpreted to the court in lay language by the epidemiologist or by the attending clinician.

The multidisciplinary child-protection team is under no obligation to include the mother's attorney (if she has engaged one) or any other professionals who may divulge either the diagnostic strategies planned or the content of the proceedings to the family. Be careful.

3. Because medical records in cases of suspected MSBP are often voluminous, efficient review must be organized prospectively. Otherwise, the result of the records review is a mass of detail from which no trends can be elicited and therefore no conclusions drawn. Therefore in beginning the review of the records, one shortly recognizes certain patterns and then formalizes these preliminary obser-

vations into questions one asks of the data: In a child with a chief complaint of intractable vomiting, did the child have any documented episodes of vomiting while in the presence of a doctor or nurse? In a child with repeated episodes of apnea, how many episodes, if any, actually began in the presence of someone other than the mother? In a child with recurrent fevers in the hospital, who actually took and charted the temperatures when the child was febrile?

4. All medical records of all siblings must be reviewed, including autopsy reports and death certificates. It often requires some vigor to obtain these records, but they are vital. Neither police summaries nor social work records are sufficient.

5. Review the parents' medical, educational, and work history, as far as possible from documents, especially if the parent claims various illnesses or some medical education.

6. Several methods may be used, singly or in combination, to gain access to records. Sometimes it is possible to have signed parental consent to obtain the records. Otherwise, the lawyers on the multidisciplinary team may advise canvassing the area with subpoenas or requesting court-ordered discovery of records.

7. Presentation of the review of records to the multidisciplinary team should include as brief as possible a chronologic review, followed by a review of discrepancies, if any. How does the mother's history compare with the observed clinical findings in the child? How do the laboratory test results compare with the given histories (e.g., are drug levels continually subtherapeutic with a history of absolute compliance?) It is impossible to list all of the possible questions, but the data will tell the reviewer which questions are important. In reviewing a case of suspected MSBP, it is essential to consider and explore all possible organic explanations.

Genuine illness and MSBP may coexist. The discovery of a real illness does not exclude MSBP; the question then becomes, Does the type and severity of this illness reasonably explain the child's symptoms and signs?

8. When presenting a case of MSBP to the civil or juvenile court, some strategies of presentation may assist the trier of fact in coming to a conclusion.

   Despite the many hours spent in reviewing records and making an extensive chronologic compilation of the child's medical history, presentation of the information to the court in long, narrative form often only confuses, rather than elucidates the material. A short summary is often better. Questions may then be asked to clarify or expand on particular events.

   Graphs and charts, clearly readable and with a single issue to illuminate, often better illustrate a complex issue than a long, verbal narrative. For example, a growth chart may show that the child consistently gains weight in the hospital but loses weight at home. A histogram may show the number of apnea episodes that originated in the presence of the mother compared with the number that originated in the presence of the nursing staff or grandmother.

   Cases typically involve conflicting medical opinions, and the parents usually have medical experts testify in their behalf. These experts may be one's colleagues. A clear grasp of the medical and epidemiologic evidence and a professional, nonadversarial attitude is always best.

   The perpetrator only rarely admits to MSBP, but curiously, she will more often agree to voluntary services as long as the court is not involved and a dependency petition is not filed. No success with this approach has been reported. Experience has shown that court-ordered intervention is necessary if there is any hope of successful protection of the child.

9. It is prudent to recommend out-of-home placement for the child (30,48). This measure ensures protection of the child and a diagnostic period of separation to see how the child's health fares. The fact that a mother has hitherto only simulated but not produced illness is no guarantee that she will not do something more nefarious to the child in the future. Simulators may become producers of illness. Confrontation of the parent with the news of the suspected diagnosis does not, in and of itself, ensure safety for the child (6,30,48).

   The reader is warned in particular about the dangers of placing the child with a family member or friend. The perpetrator may have access to the child, despite that relative's or friend's promises to the contrary. This places the child at potential dire risk.

10. If the child is to remain in the hospital for a time, all visits with all family members must be supervised by a medically experienced person to ensure that no one is tampering with the child's medical care. Sometimes the best course of action is to ask the court for a short (i.e., 10-day to 2-week) period of hospitalization with only supervised parental visits as a diagnostic trial to determine if the child's symptoms floridly persist. If they do not, concern about MSBP is heightened. If they do, ask the court to vacate the order and turn attention to a fresh look for an organic diagnosis. This approach is useful only if the child's symptoms and signs, if induced, would reasonably be expected to abate rather quickly in the absence of ongoing assault.

11. It is prudent to recommend out-of-home placement of siblings, because they may become the next victims if they remain in the home. At least, all siblings must have court-ordered medical evaluations and review of records.

12. Once the child is in foster care, his or her health status must be monitored and documented closely by the same physicians. Although often it is optimal to have the original doctor or set of doctors involved in the child's ongoing care, this arrangement sometimes is not practical for reasons of geography or temperament.

13. A troublesome issue is, When is it safe to send the child home? If the diagnosis is indeed MSBP, it seems sensible that the same guidelines that apply to other forms of child abuse and neglect apply in consideration of when to send the child home (i.e., the perpetrator must acknowledge that she committed these acts, she must have some insight into the reasons for it, and she must provide reasonable assurance that not only insight but also sufficient change has occurred to ensure the safety of the child). Very little information is available on family reunification after psychiatric intervention. In one study, family reunification was thought to be feasible in certain cases, but the authors cautioned that long-term follow-up is necessary to monitor the safety of the child and to assess whether the perpetrator's mental health has deteriorated (6). The mother's therapist will discuss with the court and the child-protection team those issues that concern the safety of the child. If the mother and the psychiatrist insist that all the information is privileged, the court has no way to determine that the children will be safe at home, and other permanent arrangements must be made for them.

14. Even if the children are removed permanently and parental rights are terminated, subsequent children born to the mother are at high risk of being victims of MSBP. Sometimes, no formal method is available by which to keep track of the mother's pregnancies and peregrinations, but every effort must be made to protect future children.

LEGAL CONSIDERATIONS

Because a diagnosis of MSBP can lead to various legal proceedings in which the physician's testimony is requested, it is well to keep a few guideposts within view.

In a courtroom or out, you are not required to translate your degree of diagnostic conviction into a legal equivalent. Terms such as probable cause, reasonable suspicion, preponderance of the evidence, clear and convincing evidence, and evidence beyond a reasonable doubt have a specific meaning in the law. If asked if the evidence conforms to any of these burdens, or if you have a reasonable degree of medical certainty about the diagnosis (a popular question), use the medical language that is meaningful to you and distill it to lay terms that best embody your meaning. You are cautioned against using legal terminology unless definitions have been precisely rendered for you and are in the court record.

Be alert to attempted manipulation by lawyers. The disputatious lawyer is no more a threat, in this regard, than the pleasingly respectful lawyer. Do not let yourself be badgered. Equally, do not let yourself be flattered or lulled into a small, but medically unjustifiable, resizing of your opinion, or into being persuaded that you are a standard-bearer for a good and righteous cause. Remind the lawyer that you are in court only to provide as balanced, thorough, and comprehensible an interpretation of the medical data as is possible. Remember: all practicing attorneys have jobs that are different from those of all doctors.

A diagnosis of MSBP may have been based, at least in part, on the information you have reviewed. You may be asked if your opinion would change, given different or additional information. In reality, there are few instances in which you can be absolutely sure that you have reviewed all existing records. If you are asked if you might change your diagnosis, or your degree of conviction about it, should you be given new information, often the most accurate answer is that it is possible but, absent the information and the time to think it over, you have no way of gauging the likelihood of that possibility.

It is the job of the trier of fact (i.e., the judge or jury), not yours, to determine if your conclusion and the reasons for it contribute to a finding that the burden of proof has been met.

CONCLUSION

A child who is a victim of MSBP is at high risk of harm. The fact that the perpetrator abruptly desists from the assault does not ensure that the situation is even minimally adequate for the child. The impetus to attack the child repeatedly, the ability to objectify the child in the first place and use the child as a tool, generally reflect a lack of empathy so profound as to likely hobble the overall capacity for mothering. Regrettably, cases involving MSBP may first be identified by a multidisciplinary child-fatality review board, but even though it is too late to help the child who died, other children in the family may be protected as a result. The dangerousness of perpetrators of MSBP should never be underestimated.

REFERENCES

1. Alexander R, Smith W, Stevenson R. Serial Munchausen syndrome by proxy. *Pediatrics* 1990;86:581–585.
2. Atoynatan TH, O'Reilly E, Loin L. Munchausen syndrome by proxy. *Child Psychiatry Hum Dev* 1988; 19:3–13.
3. Baron HI, Beck DC, Vargas JH, et al. Overinterpretation of gastroduodenal motility studies: two cases involving Munchausen syndrome by proxy. *J Pediatr* 1995;126: 397–400.
4. Beal SM, Blundell HK. Recurrence incidence of sudden infant death syndrome. *Arch Dis Child* 1988;63: 924–930.
5. Ben-Chetrit E, Melmed RN. Recurrent hypoglycaemia in multiple myeloma: a case of Munchausen syndrome by proxy in an elderly patient. *J Intern Med* 1998;244: 175–178.
6. Berg B, Jones DP. Outcome of psychiatric intervention in factitious illness by proxy (Munchausen's syndrome by proxy). *Arch Dis Child* 1999;81:465–472.
7. Blix S, Brack G. The effects of a suspected case of Munchausen's syndrome by proxy on a pediatric nursing staff. *Gen Hosp Psychiatry* 1988;10:402–409.
8. Bools C, Neale B, Meadow R. Munchausen syndrome by proxy: a study of psychopathology. *Child Abuse Negl* 1994;18:773–788.
9. Bools CN, Neale BA, Meadow SR. Co-morbidity associated with fabricated illness (Munchausen syndrome by proxy). *Arch Dis Child* 1992;67:77–79.
10. Bryk M, Siegel PT. My mother caused my illness: the story of a survivor of Munchausen by proxy syndrome. *Pediatrics* 1997;100:1–7.
11. Byard RW, Burnell RH. Covert video surveillance in Munchausen syndrome by proxy: ethical compromise or essential technique? *Med J Aust* 1994;160:352–356.
12. Carrell S. Texas nurse found guilty of killing child. *Am Med News* 1984;1–27.
13. Conway SP, Pond MN. Munchausen syndrome by proxy abuse: a foundation for adult Munchausen. *Aust N Z J Psychiatry* 1995;29:504–507.
14. Department of Health, United Kingdom. Report of a review of the research framework in north Staffordshire hospital NHS trust: executive summary of the report and recommendations. 8 May 2000; http://www.doh.gov.uk/wmro/northstaff.htm
15. DiMaio DJ, DiMaio VJM. *Forensic pathology.* New York: Elsevier, 1989.
16. Douchain F. Lithiase urinaire "factice": syndrome de Munchausen par procuration? *Presse Med* 1987;16:179.
17. Epstein MA, Markowitz RL, Gallo DM, et al. Munchausen syndrome by proxy: considerations in diagnosis and confirmation by video surveillance. *Pediatrics* 1987;80:220–224.
18. Evans D. The investigation of life-threatening child abuse and Munchausen syndrome by proxy. *J Med Ethics* 1995;21:9–13.
19. Feldman KW, Hickman RO. The central venous catheter as a source of medical chaos in Munchausen syndrome by proxy. *J Pediatr Surg* 1998;33:623–627.
20. Feldman KW, Christopher DM, Opheim KB. Munchausen syndrome-bulimia by proxy: ipecac as a toxin in child abuse. *Child Abuse Negl* 1989;13:257–261.
21. Feldman MD. Denial in Munchausen syndrome by proxy: the consulting psychiatrist's dilemma. *Int J Psychiatry Med* 1994;24:121–128.
22. Feldman MD. Spying on mothers [Letter]. *Lancet* 1994;344:132.
23. Janofsky JS. Munchausen syndrome in a mother and daughter: an unusual presentation of folie á deux. *J Nerv Ment Dis* 1986;174:368–370.
24. Johnson P, Morley C. Spying on mothers. *Lancet* 1994; 344:132–133.
25. Kurlandsky L, Lukoff JY, Zinkham WH, et al. Munchausen syndrome by proxy: definition of factitious bleeding in an infant by ^{51}Cr labeling of erythrocytes. *Pediatrics* 1979;63:228–231.
26. Lesnik-Oberstein M. Munchausen syndrome by proxy [Letter]. *Child Abuse Negl* 1986;10:133.
27. Makar AF, Squier PJ. Munchausen syndrome by proxy: father as perpetrator. *Pediatrics* 1990;85:370–373.
28. Masterson J, Dunworth R, Williams N. Extreme illness exaggeration in pediatric patients: a variant of Munchausen's by proxy? *Am J Orthopsychiatry* 1988;58:188–195.
29. McClure RJ, Davis PM, Meadow SR, et al. Epidemiology of Munchausen syndrome by proxy, non-accidental poisoning, and non-accidental suffocation. *Arch Dis Child* 1996;75:57–61.
30. McGuire TL, Feldman KW. Psychologic morbidity of children subjected to Munchausen syndrome by proxy. *Pediatrics* 1989;83:289–292.
31. Meadow R. Mothering to death. *Arch Dis Child* 1999; 80:359–362.
32. Meadow R. Unnatural sudden infant death. *Arch Dis Child* 1999;80:7–14.
33. Meadow R. Munchausen syndrome by proxy abuse perpetrated by men. *Arch Dis Child* 1998;78:210–216.
34. Meadow R. Neurological and developmental variants of Munchausen syndrome by proxy. *Dev Med Child Neurol* 1991;33:270–272.
35. Meadow R. Suffocation, recurrent apnea, and sudden infant death. *J Pediatr* 1990;117:351–357.
36. Meadow R. Recurrent cot death and suffocation [Letter]. *Arch Dis Child* 1989;64:179–180.
37. Meadow R. Video recording and child abuse [Editorial]. *Br Med J* 1987;294:1629–1630.
38. Meadow R. Munchausen syndrome by proxy: the hinterland of child abuse. *Lancet* 1977;2:343–345.

39. Milroy CM. Munchausen syndrome by proxy and intra-alveolar haemosiderin. *Int J Legal Med* 1999;112:309–312.

40. Nading JH, Duval-Arnould B. Factitious diabetes mellitus confirmed by ascorbic acid. *Arch Dis Child* 1984;59:166–167.

41. Ostfeld BM, Feldman MD. Factitious disorder by proxy: awareness among mental health practitioners. *Gen Hosp Psychiatry* 1996;18:113–116.

42. Outwater KM, Lipnick RN, Luban NLC, et al. Factitious hematuria: diagnosis by minor blood group typing. *J Pediatr* 1981;98:95–97.

43. Rand DC, Feldman MD. Misdiagnosis of Munchausen syndrome by proxy: a literature review and four new cases. *Harv Rev Psychiatry* 1999;7:94–101.

44. Raymond CA. Munchausen's may occur in younger persons. *JAMA* 1987;257:3332.

45. Richardson GF. Munchausen syndrome by proxy. *Am Fam Physician* 1987;36:119–123.

46. Rosen CL, Frost JD, Glaze DG. Child abuse and recurrent infant apnea. *J Pediatr* 1986;109:1065–1067.

47. Rosen CL, Frost JD Jr, Bricker T, et al. Two siblings with cardiorespiratory arrest: Munchausen syndrome by proxy or child abuse? *Pediatrics* 1983;71:715–720.

48. Rosenberg D. Web of deceit: a literature review of Munchausen syndrome by proxy. *Child Abuse Negl* 1987;11:547–563.

49. Roth D. How "mild" is mild Munchausen syndrome by proxy? *Isr J Psychiatry Rel Sci* 1990;27:160–167.

50. Samuels MP, Southall D. Covert surveillance in Munchausen's syndrome by proxy: welfare of the child must come first [Letter]. *BMJ* 1994;308:1101–1102.

51. Schneider DJ, Perez A, Knilans TE, et al. Clinical and pathological aspects of cardiomyopathy from ipecac administration in Munchausen's syndrome by proxy. *Pediatrics* 1996;97:902–906.

52. Schreier HA, Libow JA. Munchausen syndrome by proxy: diagnosis and prevalence. *Am J Orthopsychiatry* 1993;63:318–321.

53. Sigal M, Altmark D, Gelkopf M. Munchausen syndrome by adult proxy revisited. *Isr J Psychiatry Rel Sci* 1991;1:33–36.

54. Sigal MD, Altmark D, Carmel I. Munchausen syndrome by adult proxy: a perpetrator abusing two adults. *J Nerv Ment Dis* 1986;174:696–698.

55. Southall DP, Plunkett BM, Banks MW, et al. Covert video recordings of life-threatening child abuse: lessons for child protection. *Pediatrics* 1997;100:735–760.

56. Southall DP, Stebben VA, Rees SV, et al. Apnoeic episodes induced by smothering: two cases identified by covert video surveillance. *Br Med J (Clin Res Ed)* 1987;294:1637–1641.

57. Szajnberg NM, Moilanen I, Kanerva A, et al. Munchausen-by-proxy syndrome: countertransference as a diagnostic tool. *Bull Menninger Clin* 1996;60:229–237.

58. Thomas T. Covert video surveillance: an assessment of the Staffordshire protocol. *J Med Ethics* 1996;22:22–25.

59. Wade R. Video tape and patients' rights [Letter]. *Aust N Z J Psychiatry* 1994;28:525–526.

60. Williams C, Bevan VT. The secret observation of children in hospital. *Lancet* 1988;1:780–781.

15

Photodocumentation of the Abused Child

Lawrence R. Ricci

The Spurwick Child Abuse Program, Portland, Maine; Department of Pediatrics,
University of New England College of Osteopathic Medicine, Biddeford, Maine;
Department of Pediatrics, University of Vermont College of Medicine, Burlington, Vermont

Photographic documentation of visual findings is an important component of any child abuse evaluation. High-quality photographs of physical findings may be valuable in influencing courts to adjudicate that child abuse has taken place (13). Photographs may be used for consultation, peer review, and teaching of such concepts as cutaneous injury pattern recognition and hymen anatomy and trauma.

Although some institutions have access to professional photographic staff, either inside the institution through a media department or outside through law enforcement, many do not (9). It is incumbent on the medical providers evaluating abused children to assure adequate photographic documentation of visible lesions, either by taking the photographs themselves or by arranging for someone to take them. Even when photographs are taken by professional photographers, law-enforcement officials, or child-protective workers, the medical provider is still responsible for seeing that all areas of importance are documented adequately. Indeed, many states require reporting medical professionals to make reasonable efforts "to take or cause to be taken" color photographs of any areas of visible trauma (9).

Medical providers who care for abused children should be familiar with the basic principles and techniques of clinical photography. These principles include good equipment, adequate lighting, and planned composition. The key equipment concerns are camera, lens, lighting, and film. A quality lens, adequate flash, and proper technique are of far greater importance than brand or features of camera (22). No particular system is best. Decisions should be based on the needs of the photographer and the cost of the system. The ideal system not only produces consistent, reliable results but also is comfortable and easy to use.

CAMERAS

Camera systems for photographing the physically abused child range from expensive and sophisticated 35-mm close-up systems (5, 20,24,28,29) to less expensive and simpler, instant or self-developing cameras (3). Systems recommended for photographing the sexually abused victim range from expensive colposcopic cameras (24,28,29) to 35-mm close-up systems (5,20) and most recently video. Despite new technologic advances, such as videotape, digital still and video cameras, and computer-based digital image manipulation, 35-mm slide, and print photography remains the standard for patient documentation (11). However, analog and digital video and the newer megapixel digital still cameras provide adequate, and in some cases such as video, if not superior documentation.

Specific camera types include instant-processing cameras, fixed-focus lens or variable-focus point and shoot 35-mm cameras, and traditional 35-mm single-lens reflex (SLR) cameras. Newer 35-mm autofocus point-and-shoot cameras offer the simplicity of a compact camera and the versatility of a 35-mm SLR.

Instant-processing cameras have the advantage of simple operation and low cost. Their disadvantages include poor resolution and poor color rendition when compared with 35-mm film (9). This deficiency is particularly problematic when photographing faint bruises or small lesions. Because of their limited close-up capability, instant-processing cameras are unsuitable for photography of the genitorectal area. Additionally, they require expensive film that is difficult to reproduce and store. The only argument for using an instant-processing camera is that the print develops just after the photograph is taken, thus guaranteeing at least some form of documentation. One compromise, particularly when immediate documentation is needed, is to take both instant and 35-mm photographs (19).

Fixed-focus lens point-and-shoot or compact 35-mm cameras are inexpensive and easy to use, yet much like instant-processing cameras, offer limited close-up capability and expandability. Typically, the viewfinder does not view the same image as the lens. This feature, coupled with fixed-focus that can get no closer than 6 to 7 feet, often creates blurred images when the photographer attempts to magnify the image by moving in closer than the close-focusing limit of the lens. These cameras often have fixed aperture and shutter speed, limiting their range in varying photographic situations. Compact cameras, much like instant-processing cameras, have little to recommend them in the clinical setting (19).

Serious medical photography requires a camera that offers control over aperture, focusing, and shutter speed. As well, the camera should be able to accept a variety of lenses and other attachments. The 35-mm format offers unrivaled choice of cameras, lenses, and accessories, and hence excellent resolution and close-up capability. The most widely used 35-mm camera is the 35-mm SLR. A reflex camera is one in which the viewing systems use a mirror to reflect the image directly from the lens onto the viewing screen. The mirror flips out of the way to expose the film when the

shutter is released. A 35-mm SLR uses 35-mm film and a single lens for both viewing and recording the image. The photographer then sees the same image as the lens and the film, important when using close-up or zoom lenses.

The most versatile system for the relatively skilled photographer combines a 35-mm SLR camera body with a series of lenses (e.g., 50 mm, 105 mm, 35- to 105-mm zoom, macro lens) and both hotshoe and ring flash (20). The accessories are used in various combinations depending on the particular clinical circumstances. Attached to a 35-mm camera, a macro lens allows photographs of fine anatomic detail not otherwise visualized (Fig. 15.1).

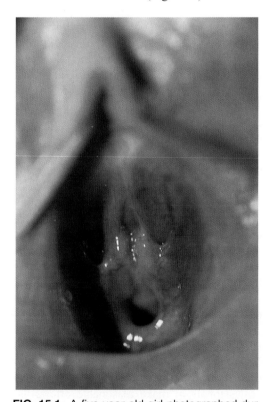

FIG. 15.1. A five-year-old girl photographed during a sexual abuse examination using the camera in Figure 15.2. Magnification is 1× (1:1). Lighting and resolution are excellent. The chief complaint was vaginal bleeding reportedly after a self-inflicted fingernail scratch while bathing. A vertical linear abrasion located to the left of the urethra is consistent with the history. Note how depth of field is limited both in front of and behind the lesion. Also note the vertical format or orientation of the image to best show neighboring anatomy.

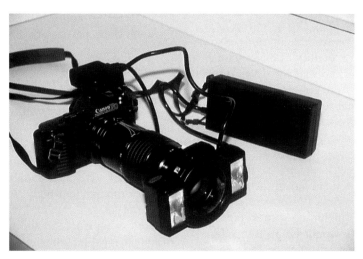

FIG. 15.2. Example of a true macro (1:1) 35-mm camera system, a Canon T50 camera body with databack and motor drive, Kiron 105-mm 1× (1:1) manual-focus macro lens, and Canon ML-1 ring flash. This kind of system with magnification range of 0.1× (1:10) to 1× (1:1) is unexcelled in versatility and photographic quality.

Prepackaged 35-mm camera systems that allow true macro reproduction (1×) include the Canon EF EOS Auto-focus 100/f-2.8 Macro lens with ML-3 Macro Ring Lite (camera body separate) or the Yashica/Contax Dental Eye II.

These systems offer totally integrated (dedicated) flash that self-adjusts during shooting. Their versatility and expandability make them unexcelled (Fig. 15.2). They compare favorably with and are significantly less expensive than colposcopic cameras for photographing the sexually abused child. Unfortunately, their technical requirements are prohibitive for the occasional user.

The simplest system for a multiuser environment or for those unable to master a 35-mm SLR is one of the newer 35-mm cameras, once called "bridge" cameras because they bridged the gap between easy-to-use compact cameras and more versatile 35-mm cameras. They are now called point-and-shoot cameras (Fig. 15.3). These cameras combine the simplicity and ease of use of a point-and-shoot camera with the versatility, expandability, and close-up capability of a 35-mm SLR. They are relatively inexpensive, fully automatic, and incorporate tele-

photo and limited macro (up to 0.25×) capability, built-in flash, autofocus, motor drive, and optional databack. They ensure nearly foolproof film loading and shooting with electronic fail-safes. An example of an auto-focus point-and-shoot camera is the Olympus IS-3 with 35–180 mm zoom lens, built-in flash, and databack.

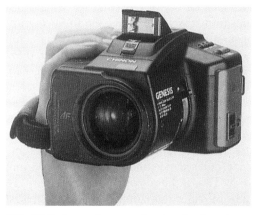

FIG. 15.3. An early example of a simple yet versatile point-and-shoot 35-mm camera with a single noninterchangeable 35- to 80-mm lens, small built-in flash, autofocus, and limited macro capability to 0.25× (1:4). Addition of accessory close-up lenses can increase magnification to 0.5× (1:2).

LENSES

Lens quality more than anything else determines picture quality. Lenses come in three basic types: normal focal length, wide angle, and long or telephoto. The labeling of a particular focal length is dictated by the format (negative or transparency image size) of the camera. A normal lens is one in which the focal length approximately equals the diagonal measurement of the camera film format (the diagonal of 24 × 36 mm). For a 35-mm camera (35 mm refers to the total film width including sprockets), a normal focal length would be 50 to 55 mm. A wide-angle lens would then be 28 to 35 mm, whereas a long lens would be 80 mm or greater.

The ideal lens for medical photography should have good optics, medium telephoto focal length to minimize distortion (85 to 105 mm), and macro or close-up capability up to 1× (the image on the negative or transparency is magnified to life size).

Magnification is the ratio of image size on the negative or transparency to actual object size (image size/object size). It can be expressed as a ratio (1:2), a fraction (1/2), a decimal (0.5×), or a percentage (50%). Close-up is 0.1 to 0.5×, extreme close-up is 0.5 to 1×, and true macro is 1 to 35×. Photographing, for example, an 8-year-old child by using a 35-mm format would produce the following images at different magnifications: 0.05×, full body; 0.1×, half body; 0.2×, face, hand; 0.5×, ear, lips, eye, genitorectal area; 1×, fingernail, introitus; 2×, hymen.

The maximal magnification of a lens can be checked by focusing the camera on a metric ruler at the closest focusing distance of the lens (19). With a 35-mm SLR, the viewfinder screen and film are both 36 mm wide. Thus if the screen or the film "sees" 36 mm of ruler horizontally (at the closest working distance of the lens), the magnification is 1×. If the screen sees 72 mm, the magnification is 0.5× (m = 36 mm/number of millimeters "seen" horizontally on the viewfinder screen).

A 90- to 110-mm lens is recommended for close-up work, particularly facial, when using a 35-mm camera (16). Long lenses compress or flatten perspective. This flattening is advantageous in face shots, in that features such as the nose are less distorted. For torso or full-length photography, a 50- or 55-mm lens is adequate (11). In general, a medium telephoto lens, such as a 105-mm lens, is best for everything from 0.2 to 1× (head and neck down to fingernails), whereas a 55-mm lens should be used for full and half-body lengths only (0.05 to 0.1×) (9,27).

In close-up work, an additional advantage of longer focal length is greater working distance. A typical 50-mm lens at 0.1× has a close working distance of 25 cm. A 100-mm lens doubles this working distance. Children may be less fearful if the camera is farther away (i.e., the subject-to-lens distance is increased). In addition, flash illumination becomes more uniform as the distance increases (5).

Zoom lenses offer variable focal length, which allows one lens to be used for both close-up and distant work. By changing the focal length to bring the subject closer, they allow the photographer to remain stationary while changing the magnification. Some zoom lenses provide macro capability up to 0.25×.

MACROPHOTOGRAPHY

For close work greater than 0.5×, a macro lens offers the best solution (20). A macro lens is capable of providing 1× or greater magnification, although the term is often used to describe any close-focusing lens. Lenses sold as "zoom with macro focusing" are not true macro lenses and often magnify only up to 0.25×. True macro lenses have their barrels embossed with magnification, especially from 0.5 to 1×. Examples of true macro lenses include the Canon 100-mm f-2.8 1:1 Macro AF and the Nikon 105-mm f-2.8 1:1 Micro AF (Fig. 15.2). As used here, the "f" rating signifies the widest aperture or lens diaphragm opening (the lower the number, the larger the opening and hence the more light that can enter through the lens).

An f-number (or f-stop) is a numeric representation of the diameter of the diaphragm opening or aperture of the lens. A sequence of f-numbers on the lens dial calibrates the aperture in regular steps or stops. The f-numbers generally follow a standard sequence such that the interval between one stop and the next represents a halving or doubling in image brightness. As the number become higher, the aperture is reduced.

A relatively inexpensive alternative to a macro lens is a set of close-up or supplementary lenses placed over the normal lens to magnify the image (19). These auxiliary lenses may provide reasonable magnification up to 0.5× (Fig. 15.4); however, using close-up lens attachments to achieve magnification greater than 0.5× significantly reduces image quality. Beyond 0.5×, a macro lens offers the best option. Bellows and extension tubes, although cumbersome and difficult to use, are another option. Colposcopic camera attachments use the extension-tube principle to achieve 1× or greater magnification.

A problem particular to close-up work is narrow depth of field (19). Depth of field is the zone of sharpness extending in front of and behind the center of focus. It is determined by aperture, lens focal length, and subject-to-lens distance. The larger the aperture (the smaller the f-number), the narrower the depth of field. In the close-up range, depth of field can be quite narrow (a typical 105-mm macro lens at 1× magnification and f-22 has a maximal depth of field of 6 mm). This limitation can be a significant problem when photographing cavities, such as the rectum, that may have a greater depth than the depth of field of the lens (Fig. 15.5A and B). This problem may necessitate a series of photographs, each focused at different points near and far, none of which captures the entire area. When depth of field is a problem, it is important not only to focus carefully but also to try to position the subject and/or the camera so that all of the important parts to be photographed fall in a plane parallel to the film. A powerful flash can improve depth of field by allowing a smaller aperture.

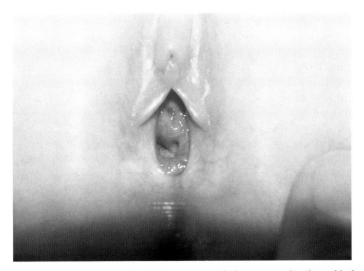

FIG. 15.4. A four-year-old girl photographed during a sexual abuse examination with the camera in Figure 15.3. Magnification of 0.5× (1:2) is achieved by adding a supplementary close-up lens (+6 diopter). Resolution is fair and the image is a bit overexposed, although the hymen is visualized adequately at least for major trauma. Shadow at bottom is from the top-mounted flash blocked by the lens.

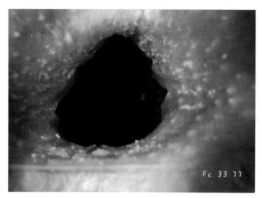
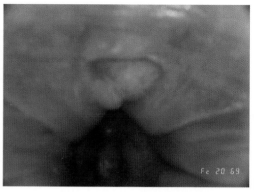

A   B

FIG. 15.5. Examples of anal-rectal photography. **A.** A 15-year-old girl in the prone knee-chest position with gentle buttock traction is photographed with the camera in Figure 15.2. Magnification is 1× (1:1). Viewing magnification would have been 8× had this photograph been obtained through a variable magnification colposcope. Entire dilated anal-rectal area with adequate angle of view and adequate depth of field are shown. **B.** A subacute fissure is evident at 12 o'clock position in a 4-year-old boy using the camera in Figure 15.6. Photographic magnification is 2× (2:1), whereas viewing magnification through the binoculars is 16 power. The lesion is well delineated but depth of field is limited as is the angle of view. Variable magnification particularly from 4 to 16 power is a useful option in colposcope photography.

COLPOPHOTOGRAPHY

The colposcope is a binocular viewing device (often with varying magnification) and attached light source. A camera can be added by an extension tube for photographic documentation (Fig. 15.6). Typically, a standard 35-mm camera body is used. Many examiners now attach a video camera for teaching and documentation (15).

A drawback to colposcopic photography, basically macrophotography through an extension tube rather than a macro lens, is limited depth of field (4 mm or less) compared with better macro lenses (6 to 8 mm) and at magnifications above 1× limited viewing angle (see Fig. 15.5). The singular advantage of the colposcope, however, is that the same instrument provides illuminated and magnified viewing along with photographic capability so that examination and documentation can occur simultaneously.

Although the primary use of colposcopic photography is documenting abnormalities, some examiners routinely photograph all sexual abuse examinations, even those with normal findings. Besides providing educational material, this practice may have comparative value if the same child is later reexamined.

Colposcopes can differ significantly from one manufacturer to another in quality, accessories, and cost. Ease of use, quality of

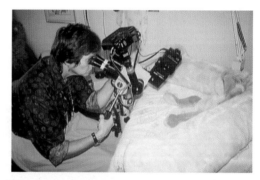

FIG. 15.6. Example of a colposcope with T-mounted camera allowing 2× (2:1) photographic magnification and simultaneous 16-power viewing, a Frigitronics colposcope with Canon T90 camera body (databack, motor drive, and remote shutter release), and Vivitar hotshoe mounted flash. This system only allows viewing at 16 power and photography at 2× (2:1), although quality of photography at 2× (2:1), although quality of photographic image is excellent. Quantum Turbo battery attached to the flash allows 2 seconds recycle time.

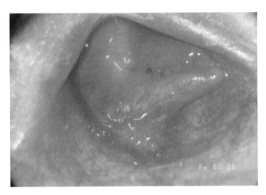

FIG. 15.7. A two-year-old girl photographed during a sexual abuse examination with the colposcope in Figure 15.6. Magnification is 2× (2:1). Lighting and resolution are excellent. Three punctate submucosal hemorrhages are located on the vaginal surface of the hymen at 5 o'clock position consistent with penetrating trauma. These subtle findings would not have been as well documented using less magnification. Note the databack identification code in the lower right hand corner.

optics and light source, magnification, and photographic capabilities are important features. The most useful magnification range is between 4 and 16 power. Four power, which refers to the magnification in the eyepiece, is equal to 0.5× or 1:2 reproduction on the slide. Eight power equals 1× or 1:1, whereas 16 power creates an image on the slide that is 2 times life size, 2× or 2:1. Features to consider for photographing through a colposcope include a beam splitter rather than a mirror, a high-quality ring flash with rapid recycle time (less than 5 seconds is good; less than 2 seconds is ideal), a motor drive, and databack for the camera. A remote shutter release, either hand or foot controlled, allows both of the examiner's hands to be free for picture taking by an assistant or even the child.

Photographing genitorectal findings may be difficult through the colposcope because of rapid changes in genitorectal shape, excessive magnification (narrow angle of view), and narrow depth of field (Fig. 15.5) (1). A good lighting source for the camera is critical. The colposcope must provide adequate resolution, exposure, and depth of field (Figs. 15.7 and 15.8A and B). Any system chosen must be tested thoroughly by the examiner before clinical use.

A less expensive and quite adequate alternative to colposcopic photography is the use of a 35-mm camera equipped with macrofocusing lens and ring flash (Figs. 15.1 and 15.5) (19). Even less expensive, although with limited magnification and resolution, is a bridge camera with close-up lenses (Fig. 15.4).

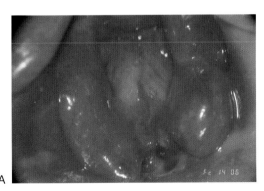
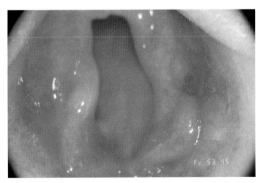

A   B

FIG. 15.8. A two-year-old girl with extensive penetrating trauma to the hymen and vagina at 6 o'clock position photographed using the colposcope in Figure 15.6. **A:** 3 days after the trauma; **B:** months later. Magnification is 2× (2:1). Detail and lighting are excellent, although had trauma been most extensive, such a narrow angle view would have been adequate. **A** was useful legally in demonstrating that the injury required significant penetration. Note the databack identification code in the lower right hand corner.

LIGHTING

No single aspect affects the quality and usefulness of a medical/legal photograph more directly than lighting. Proper lighting can show texture, color, depth, and contour. Improper lighting can hide detail in shadow, wash out bruises, and even misrepresent evidence (9,25,27).

Short of three-source studio lighting, electronic flash offers the best light for indoor color medical photography (11,25). The two basic types of electronic flash units are a traditional point source flash mounted to the side or top of the camera and a ring flash encircling the camera lens (Figs. 15.2 and 15.3).

A ring flash provides the best overall lighting in the form of shadowless, uniform illumination (19). It is particularly useful when photographing cavities and recesses such as the mouth, vagina, and rectum. Shadowing for detail, important in black-and-white photography, is less important when using color film, which uses varying colors and hues to separate detail. Controlled shadowing, however, may still be effectively used to demonstrate texture in bites and abrasions.

With modern through-the-lens (TTL) metering systems, flash use has become simple (19). Dedicated flashes are designed to work best with a particular camera. Connection of the flash to the shutter for synchronization may be through a coaxial cable or direct through a shoe fitting on the camera (hotshoe). Many electronic flash guns have automatic exposure control. Light from the flash is reflected from the subject back to a sensing cell. When sufficient light has been reflected, the cell cuts off the current, and the light is switched off. The light-producing power of a flash is measured by its guide number: guide number = the distance in feet × f-stop. A higher guide number represents a more powerful flash. A more powerful flash allows a smaller aperture and hence greater depth of field.

Limitations of an electronic flash include reflections, particularly from mucous membranes and dark skin; loss of three-dimensional quality of textured areas, such as abrasions; washout of subtle colors by overexposure; and inadequate lighting, especially if a hotshoe-mounted flash is blocked by a long lens (Fig. 15.3) (9,27). Reflections and loss of texture can be minimized by taking photographs from differing perspectives or angles. The lens-shadowing problem can be obviated by using a ring flash. When using electronic flash, it is important to remove or neutralize other point light sources prone to create exposure imbalance, such as shadow-producing operative lights or partially illuminating sunlight.

Flash-recycle time, the time it takes the flash capacitor to recharge and be ready to fire again, is especially important when photographing children (19). The difference between 2 to 5 seconds and 10 to 15 seconds may be the difference between a good photograph and none at all with a child who is unwilling to sit still for the several seconds it takes a slow flash to recycle. As batteries discharge, recycle time lengthens; thus fresh alkaline batteries should always be used. Spare batteries should be readily available. Lithium ion or rechargeable nickel metal hydride batteries, although more expensive, shorten recycle time and last significantly longer. A remote rechargeable battery pack, such as the Quantum Turbo, can improve flash recycle time considerably.

FILM

Thirty-five millimeter color slide film, sometimes called color transparency or color reversal film, remains the standard for medical use (11,25). Color film offers a distinct advantage over black-and-white in that color film uses the various hues of the subject to separate details more effectively than do shades of gray (9). Color also portrays the findings more realistically and can be used to age bruises. Color slides are relatively inexpensive, quickly developed, and easy to file, and they can be converted into satisfactory color prints if necessary (11,25). Although color negative or print film offers greater exposure and contrast latitude and hence is more forgiving of exposure mistakes, color slide film provides a first-generation image that can be projected. Color negative film necessitates a second-generation conversion into a print, sometimes resulting in color-balance distortion. Conversion of color negatives to slides or color slides to prints results in loss of sharpness and color balance.

Duplicating slides or prints may alter color and resolution (9). Two sets of slides should be shot initially (i.e., each view should be photographed twice). One set can be used in court, and the other set is retained with the child's record. Magnification should be accomplished in the original photograph by varying camera distance and/or lens focal length, and not in the print- or slide-making process (Figs. 15.9 and 15.10A–D; see also Figs. 15.1, 15.7, and 15.8). As a rule, only one patient should be photographed on each roll of film. Even if a roll has only a few exposures, it should be developed rather than kept in the camera, thus avoiding accidental

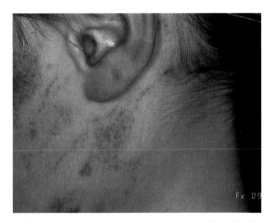

FIG. 15.9. A three-year-old boy with classic hand imprint pattern injury to the face photographed with the camera in Figure 15.2. Magnification is 0.25× (1:4). This magnification clearly reveals not only the thin linear markings characteristic of a handprint, but also the bruising extending behind the ear. This photograph alone demonstrates that the injury could not have occurred as alleged from a fall. Note the databack identification code in the lower right hand corner.

exposure of the film or confusion of subjects. Images of more than one child may be included in one roll if a strict segregation and identification system is in place and if the film is never left partially exposed in the camera.

Film speed is the sensitivity of the film emulsion to light, as measured by its ISO (International Standards Organization) rating. A film rated at 400 ISO is twice as light sensitive or "fast" as one rated at 200 ISO. Slower film (lower ISO rating) offers finer grain, which in turn means greater sharpness and definition. Slower film, however, requires more light and/or a larger aperture. A larger aperture results in narrower depth of field. Film should be fast enough to provide an aperture of f-11 or f-16. Medium-speed (100 to 200 ISO) daylight film allows a smaller aperture for greater depth of field yet minimal grain (25).

A flash should always be used when shooting indoors with daylight film (19). Daylight film is color balanced to give accurate color rendition in average daylight. The color temperature of daylight is 5,000° Kelvin. Normal indoor lighting has a color temperature of 3,000° Kelvin and will create significant color distortion if daylight film is used without a flash. Electronic flash is standardized to the same color temperature as average daylight (10).

Film may be refrigerated or frozen to prolong its effective shelf life. Film that is refrigerated, however, requires 3 hours at room temperature to reach a usable temperature; 24 hours is needed if the film is frozen (10).

Differences in image processing may be noted between film laboratories as well as at the same laboratory with development of successive roles of film if quality control of the development process is not maintained (25). Using Kodak processing laboratories assures quality control and standardization (4).

After the film is developed, each image should be reviewed for both technique and content. No photographs, even poor ones, should be discarded. This action could be misconstrued as destruction of evidence (11,23).

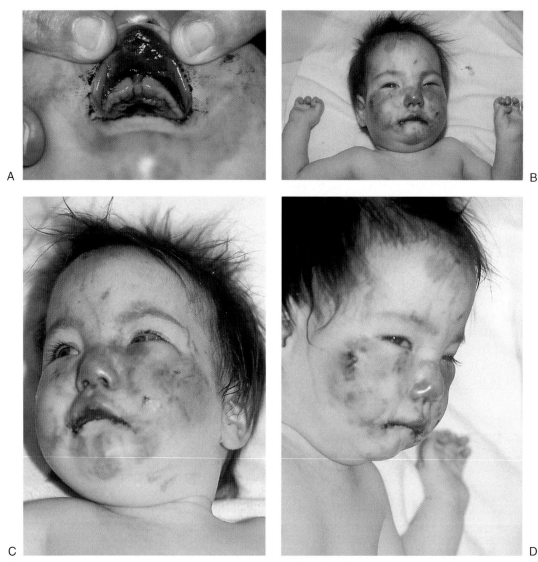

FIG. 15.10. A one-year-old girl with extensive injury to the face and upper lip photographed with the camera in Figure 15.2. Magnification in **A** is 0.5× (1:2). This view at this magnification dramatically illustrates the force required to produce such an injury and was instrumental in convincing the court judge that an adult caretaker, not a 3-year-old sibling, had inflicted this and the other facial trauma. **B-D:** Varying perspective facial views at 0.25× (1:4) magnification. **C** best shows the left scleral hemorrhage, whereas **D** best shows the dramatic edema of the left periorbital region.

A storage/filing system should be established in a cool, dry, and low-light location. Each slide should be stored in a clear plastic sheet to minimize handling of the slide and to allow viewing and easy storage. Stored slides last many years with proper use, care, and storage (10). A slide used for lectures or left out in the light, however, will fade after only a few years (6).

PHOTOGRAPHIC COMPOSITION

Composition is the proper arrangement of the elements in a photograph. The compositional goal of medical photography is accurate documentation of the patient's condition. Artistic composition is less important than consistency of technique and reproducibility of results. A technically excellent photograph or series of photographs may not be admissible as evidence if they do not establish both the scale and the anatomic location of the trauma (9). Perspective (viewpoint), scale, and background must be carefully considered.

Medical photography must show injuries as realistically as possible and should not be used to enhance or exaggerate trauma. It is useful to photograph burns, dirty abrasions, and even unkempt children both before and after cleaning. Lesions, as they change over time, should be rephotographed (9). Just as varying perspective can add a three-dimensional quality, photographs of the same child over time can add a fourth dimension (Fig. 15.8).

Perspective or viewpoint refers to the relation between objects at different distances from the camera as well as the angle from which the objects are viewed. Proper perspective is important in accurately depicting a scene. Perspective can be altered by subject-to-lens distance, lens focal length, magnification, point of view, and size of the final photograph (23).

The following compositional principles should be kept in mind when photographing abused children (Table 15.1):

1. At least one, if not several, pictures should contain an anatomic landmark (Figs. 15.11 and 15.12A and B). The inclusion of an elbow or knee allows the viewer to identify the location of a wound. Anatomic or background material unnecessary to the photograph, however, should be left out. By adhering to this principle, the main subject will occupy a larger part of the picture and will be easier to study. As well, unneeded and possibly confusing visual information will be omitted (22,25,26).

2. At least two photographs should be taken of each finding, one including identifying landmarks and one close-up with the lesion filling the frame. Magnification should be

TABLE 15.1 *Photography shooting tips*

Before	Establish a protocol or checklist for operation.
	Decide in advance who will use the camera.
	Always shoot a test roll before using a new system.
During	Compose the picture the way you usually look at the area.
	Keep the photographer and subject at the same level.
	Arrange the subject so that the surface of interest is parallel to the film plane.
	Take several shots from different angles and distances.
	Take one photograph with landmarks and one, as close as possible, of the lesion alone.
	Magnify in an original, not in a blow-up.
	Bracket shots if correct exposure is uncertain.
	Take a photograph of patient's name.
	Take a photograph of the face to identify the patient.
	Shoot more slides rather than plan to duplicate.
	Never leave partially exposed film in the camera.
After	Review pictures after development.
	Keep notebook of photographs and technique.
	Label prints or slides.

obtained in the original and not achieved in a blow-up (Figs. 15.1 and 15.7 to 15.10). The finding of interest should occupy as much of the frame as the camera allows.

3. The subject should be arranged so that the surface of interest is parallel to the film surface or plane. Likewise, the camera and the subject should be at the same level (22,25,26). An exception to this rule applies to colposcopic photography, in which the upward-tilting genitalia of a child requires that the camera be tilted down from above (15).

4. Varying perspective—taking a number of exposures from different angles and distances—is useful, particularly because electronic flash may produce unpredictable reflections (4,25). Likewise, because the skin is a curved surface, some lesions may require several photographs to reveal the pathologic findings fully (Figs.

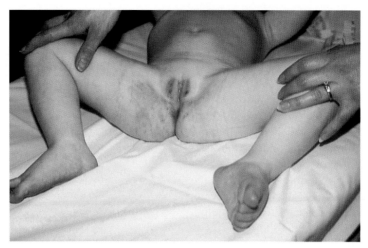

FIG. 15.11. A two-year-old girl with extensive bruising of the labia and perianal region photographed with the camera in Figure 15.3 at the 55-mm setting on the zoom (equivalent to a standard 55-mm lens). Magnification is 0.1× (1:10). View demonstrates extent of trauma in relation to surrounding anatomy but is limited in detail. Close-up views would help particularly in assessing trauma to the vagina and rectum. Nevertheless, this view showing the bruising into the rectal area was particularly useful in convincing the trial judge that sexual assault had occurred.

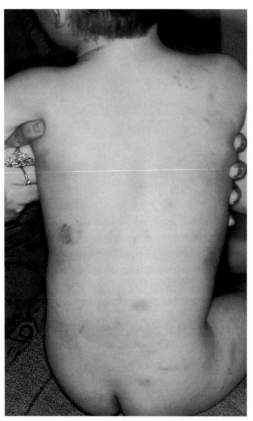
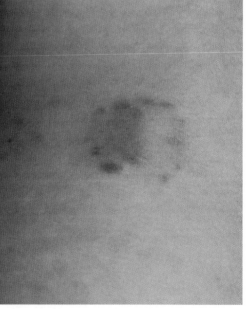

A   B

FIG. 15.12. A three-year-old boy with bites on his back photographed with the camera in Figure 15.2. Magnifications are 0.1× (1:10) **(A)** and 0.5× (1:2) **(B)**, respectively. Full back view **(A)** demonstrates two bites (right shoulder and left flank) in relation to neighboring anatomy. Close-up view of the flank bite **(B)** demonstrates detail of teeth imprint. Size of teeth and arch suggest the bite came from another child as alleged. A measuring tape in the viewing field would have been helpful even though precise measurements were documented in the record.

15.10 and 15.13A–C). Areas of trauma that have texture or are swollen (contusions, lacerations, abrasions, and blisters) may lose their three-dimensional quality when light strikes them directly. Offsetting the camera-to-subject axis by 15 degrees allows the light source to glance off the lesion and create contour shadowing.

5. The picture should be composed in the way the examiner would normally look at the anatomic area. The horizontal format is standard. When necessary, however, such as for full-body images, the vertical format is used (Fig. 15.1).

6. The size of lesions may be documented on the photograph by positioning a measuring device, such as an adhesive metric scale, directly above or below the injury (9,23). Photographs are no substitute, however, for clearly written and detailed descriptions of the dimension, shape, color, size, and location of lesions. Size along with color may be distorted in the photograph.

A standardized color bar, although awkward to use, may be placed in the photographic plane for comparison with the color of the lesion. This step assures that if color is distorted in the developing process, adequate comparisons can still be made. If color is a significant concern, however, as when trying to age a bruise, it is more useful to document the color carefully in writing than to rely on the photograph.

7. It is desirable but not always possible to have a standard set of views for each area photographed (27). The four cardinal

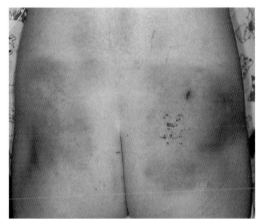

A

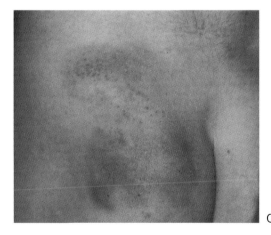

C

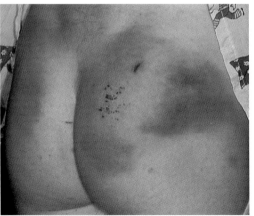

B

FIG. 15.13. A five-year-old girl hit with a paddle and photographed with the camera in Figure 15.2. Magnification is 0.2× (1:5). Three views were required to illustrate the extent of the buttock pattern injury. Multiple views **(A-C)** showing a curving multiplanar injury are useful in illustrating how such an injury could not have resulted from an accidental fall.

anatomic positions, anteroposterior (AP), posteroanterior (PA), and right and left lateral, should be kept in mind when photographing children. Young children may not cooperate with such positioning plans, however, again reinforcing the usefulness of multiple views from varying perspectives (Fig. 15.13).

8. Forensic bite-mark photography is a specialized branch of medical photography and is best performed by or interpreted by a forensic dentist or pathologist. The basic objective of photographing bites is the accurate recording of all aspects of the mark. Size, shape, color, depth of indentations, and three-dimensional contours must be preserved. No one medium is suitable for all these functions. Photographs, both black-and-white and color, can record the first three features, whereas dental impressions show the last two. Ultimately, the photographs may be enlarged to life size and compared with a representation of the suspect's teeth (4).

   Frequently the clinical practitioner takes the initial photographs. The same principles as described throughout this chapter apply to photographing bite marks. Multiple views from multiple perspectives are particularly important in delineating texture and shape. Parallel views best depict shape and size, whereas obliquely directed views and lighting highlight texture. Some views should show neighboring anatomy; others should magnify the bite as much as the camera and lens will allow (Fig. 15.12).

9. Keeping a record or log of photographic data (date, time, location, case number, camera, lens, aperture, shutter speed, film, light source, subject distance, and macro lens magnification) helps reconstruct cases, particularly for courtroom verification; aids in learning and teaching; and encourages consistent technique if the child requires more photographs later.

10. Background is important (11,26,27). The background wall should be nonreflective,

TABLE 15.2. *Sample checklist for camera operation*

1. Secure lens to cameral body.
2. Remove lens cap.
3. Secure flash to camera hotshoe.
4. Load film.
5. Set film speed on camera and flash.
6. Set lens aperture (usually to automatic).
7. Check flash setting and turn on flash.
8. Focus and compose the picture.
9. Shoot.
10. Check to be sure flash has fired.
11. Advance film.
12. Check to be sure the film is advancing.
13. Rewind film when done shooting.
14. Only then open back to remove film.

ideally a matte-finish neutral gray, green, or blue. Glossy background surfaces can produce a glare. A cluttered room makes a poor background for medical photographs. Materials unnecessary for the photo should be deleted. A backdrop may be useful.

11. Before photographing children, it is important to establish both a protocol and a checklist for operation (Table 15.2). Who will take the photographs and how the film will be handled after picture taking should be identified. The photographer should always shoot a test roll first when using a new camera setup.

COMMON PHOTOGRAPHIC ERRORS

Despite the advent of simple and sophisticated electronic cameras, traditional camera-operation errors continue to occur.

1. The subject is blurred. This problem is usually caused by improper focusing, often because the photographer was trying to get closer than the minimal focusing distance of the lens in an attempt to magnify the image. This problem is particularly common with viewfinder fixed-focus compact cameras. Sometimes movement of subject or camera will cause blurring. Shutter speeds less than 1/90 second for normal lens and less than 1/125 second for telephoto lens

should not be used. If the camera is autofocus, a problem will occur if the subject of interest is outside the center focusing ring. For example, if the subject is in the foreground and off to the side, the camera may focus on a centered background object, throwing the foreground out of focus.

2. The negative is clear or the transparency is black. Most likely, the film was never exposed because it did not advance in the camera. The most common cause of this problem is failure to load the film properly (the film sprocket holes never caught properly in the film-transport sprockets). It is important to load film correctly and to ensure that the film is being transported through the camera by checking that the rewind knob turns as the film is advanced. Because of this problem, some centers recommend shooting a backup set of instant prints with a Polaroid camera. Newer, nearly foolproof electronic cameras either fail to shoot at all or show on the data screen that the film is not advancing.

3. The film is over- or underexposed. Incorrect exposure continues to be a problem in photography despite advances in automatic exposure control. Exposure depends on the brightness of the image, the camera aperture, the length of time the photographic material is exposed (shutter speed), and film speed. The usual cause of incorrect exposure is incorrect setting of either the aperture, film speed, shutter speed, or flash. Camera and flash settings should be checked carefully.

   An exposure technique some professionals use to avoid over- or underexposure is bracketing. If the final combination of film and flash indicates an aperture of f-16, three frames are exposed, one at a setting of f-16, one overexposed at f-11, and the third underexposed at f-22. One of the three should be perfectly exposed (4,25).

4. The print or slide has distorted color, often yellow or green. This error occurs

most commonly because color daylight film is used indoors without a flash. Always use a flash indoors, even if the room is bright.

PHOTOGRAPHING CHILDREN

When photographing children, it is important to explain to the child what is going to happen in language the child will understand (19). Allowing the child to try out the camera and flash often aids in gaining trust. Most cameras, particularly those mounted on a colposcope, can be provided with a remote switch that the child may control. Children should be allowed to assume a position of comfort. It is better to have a cooperative child, somewhat out of optimal photographic position yet not moving, than an uncooperative, moving child. The photographer can compensate for incorrect anatomic position with multiple views. If the child will not move, the photographer should.

It is often useful to involve a trusted support person in the photographic session. Infants and toddlers may be photographed more easily if they are held in the lap of a guardian or assistant. Apart from being a comfort to the child in unfamiliar surroundings, such a person provides an extra pair of hands (18).

Film-advancing motor drives are almost mandatory when photographing children, as is a fast recycling flash. Because an unexpected flash may be alarming, children should be allowed to preview and even try out the flash.

The photographer must at all times be cognizant of the potential traumatic effect of photographs on the abused child, with regard to both the photographic process itself and the use of these photographs in court. Some children may refuse photographic documentation, despite the photographer's best efforts. This refusal should, as much as possible, be respected. Similarly, the adverse effects of photographing children, particularly sexually abused children, should not be underestimated. These issues should be addressed openly and sympathetically both before and after the evaluation.

LEGAL ISSUES

In child abuse litigation, photographs of the injured child may be important in proving nonaccidental injury. For photographs to be used as court evidence, they must be properly verified and relevant to the issue (8).

Verification requires that the photographer or physician testify that the pictures accurately portray the findings (9). A physician who examined the child, even though not the photographer, may verify that they accurately represent the findings. The photographer/physician should be able to state how the photograph was taken. Practitioners should not, however, portray themselves as photography experts. Such a portrayal might lead to questions on obscure optical and film concepts and potentially discredit the medical witness.

From a medicolegal perspective, photographs of abused children should convey a fair and accurate representation of the scene. Pictures that are inadmissible because of technical error (out of focus, distorted, unidentifiable, too dark, etc.) must be avoided (21). Seeking a second opinion from a photograph requires that the image reasonably reflect the original findings. To help verify that the photographs are actually of a particular child, two pictures can be taken: one of the child's name and one of the child's face. Likewise, an identifying sign may be placed in front of the patient for each picture. The inclusion of such signs or labels in the photograph, however, is time consuming and distracting (22). An alternative for identification is the use of a camera databack. Many 35-mm cameras have available databack attachments that imprint the time, date, and an identifying code on each frame. Another advantage of a databack is that, because the imprint is always located in the bottom right of the transparency or negative right/left, top-to-bottom orientation is simpler (Figs. 15.5 and 15.7 to 15.9).

Once processed, the slides or prints should be labeled. At a minimum, the slide should be labeled with a medical record number and the date the photographs were taken. Each print or slide may optionally contain the name of the child, age, date of birth, date and time of photograph, hospital number, name of photographer, and name of practitioner.

Relevance is a judicial decision (17). Photographs may have evidentiary value yet be deemed prejudicial to the defendant. Whether the probative value outweighs the prejudicial danger remains a decision for the trial judge. Photographs are generally considered admissible, however, if they shed light on the issue, enable a witness to describe better the objects portrayed, permit the jury to understand the testimony better, or corroborate testimony (Figs. 15.8 to 15.11). Courts generally permit physicians to explain and illustrate their testimony with a photograph. Some states require that reasonable efforts be made by the reporting hospital or physician "to take or cause to be taken" color photographs of any areas of visible trauma on the child (9). Many provide for immunity from civil or criminal prosecution for the person arranging for or taking photographs if done in good faith.

Consent forms should always be completed when even remotely identifying features are included in the picture. Conversely, it is not necessary to obtain consent when no identifiable features are evident. Likewise, many child abuse laws state that permission is not needed for the taking of photographs as a part of a child abuse evaluation. Going through the process of obtaining consent, however, can establish an alliance with the family. A variety of consent forms is available including a model form drafted by the American Medical Association (5,22,25).

Each institution should have a policy for the handling and the release of photographs (9). For an unbroken chain of evidence, film should change hands as infrequently as possible. With each transfer, the signature of an authorized recipient should be affixed to a list of the materials received and include date, time, and place. Outside laboratory processing may be acceptable, even if the laboratory staff does not sign for the film because sending film out is the normal business procedure for the institution (23). Courts usually accept films sent to Kodak for processing by first-class mail as an unbroken chain of custody (14). Kodak will, on request, enclose an affidavit ensuring the receipt, correct processing, and return of the film. The use of Kodak processing laboratories for color film assures quality control, standardization, and legal acceptability.

An particular legal concern about digital photographs is that such photographs are easily manipulated. Although concerns have been expressed that digital images will not be accepted in court, to date (late 1999) there is no case law excluding digitally obtained images. Of course, changing 35-mm slides and negatives by color or contrast or brightness manipulation has always been possible. The new concern over digital image alteration appears to be based both on the ease with which such changes can be made and on the possibility of drastic, substantive change such as selectively enhancing one element of the image over another. Original images for courtroom use should of course never be altered. If a copy is altered to improve viewing such as by enlargement or by brightening, such changes should be clearly noted. Ultimately, however, photographs are useful only as demonstration aids for the examiner to explain the findings. As such, they should be as fair and accurate a representation of the findings as possible. Capturing and recording a digital image on a disk is really no different from capturing and recording a chemical image on silver-based film (7).

EMERGING TECHNOLOGIES

Obtaining a photograph that adequately represents the findings of an abused child can be challenging, given both the inherent plasticity of some of these structures and general motion by the child (15). This problem has led some authorities to work with video photographic techniques for both documentation and teaching (15).

Video cameras combined with high-resolution printers make examination and documentation easier and more precise for both sexual and physical abuse. Modern video technology uses optical sensing semiconductor devices (charged coupled device, CCD) to transfer light to digital electronic information, which is then stored on videotape. Traditional analog VHS or S-VHS cameras record an analog signal, whereas newer digital video cameras record a digital signal on the tape. Video cameras are easy to use and satisfactory for most uses. The image produced can be reviewed immediately, eliminating the wait for film development. Video offers a three-dimensional quality to documentation, can capture the movement of the subject itself, and can offer a near infinite number of perspectives (7).

The standard consumer format for videotape is VHS. The 8-mm format allows use of a smaller audiocassette-size tape and hence a smaller camera. The 8 mm is comparable in quality to standard VHS and is easier to store. Hi-8 and Super VHS (S-VHS) video cameras offer a significant improvement in image quality or resolution over 8 mm and VHS. Digital video cameras are better still (VHS and 8-mm video record 200 lines of resolution; S-VHS and Hi-8 can record 400 lines; digital video, 500 plus lines) (7).

One of the drawbacks of video documentation is the inability to produce 35-mm–quality still photographs. Some examiners record both video and 35-mm images. Video can be converted to digital stills for printing by using a video capture card or transferred directly to a usable Polaroid size, still using a video printer. The use of a video camera either colposcopically mounted or stand alone to document findings combined with a video printer for immediate still-image production is a versatile combination.

Digitized images—whether digitized primarily by using a digital still or digital video camera or secondarily by scanning a slide, negative, or print, or by grabbing a frame from a video—can be transmitted via the Internet or direct computer-to-computer connection to colleagues for discussion. The use of such telemedicine communication techniques has emerged as a powerful tool in child abuse consultation and education (7).

An example of a digital video camera is the Sony Mini DV Handycam DCR-TRV9. An example of a 2-megapixel (1,600 × 1,200 pixel image) digital still camera is the Nikon Coolpix 9500 with 3× zoom. Digital still cam-

eras that produce megabyte images require a large flash memory card and superior batteries such as lithium or nickel metal hydride. Such megapixel cameras can produce an 8 × 10-inch photograph that rivals 35 mm (Figs. 15.14A–D and 15.15A and B).

Ultraviolet (UV) photography has an established role in clinical forensic medicine and is beginning to see use in child abuse assessments (2). Reflected UV photographs can reveal long-healed bite marks, belt imprints, and wound remnants. A drawback of UV 35-mm photography is that the image cannot be seen until after development. Recently a hand-held, image-intensifier UV viewer has been developed by Hamamatsu that allows di-

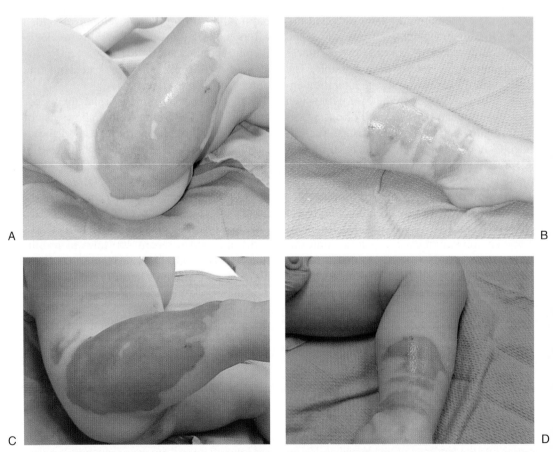

FIG. 15.14. A, B: Digital still images using a Nikon Coolpix 9500 with attached flash of the hot-liquid spill burns sustained by a 6-month-old child. **C, D:** The same child photographed with a Sony digital video camera. These images are frames grabbed from the video. Ambient fluorescent lighting was used.

A

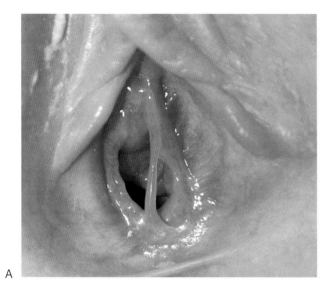

B

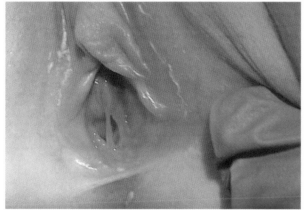

FIG. 15.15. A: Digital still image using a Nikon Coolpix 9500 with attached flash of a hymenal examination of a 14-year-old girl, showing hymenal band. **B:** The same child photographed with a Sony digital video camera. The frame was grabbed from the video. Ambient fluorescent lighting was used.

rect and immediate viewing and recording of UV images from skin (12).

CONCLUSION

Because photographs offer the only certain method of preserving perishable visual findings, they may serve several useful purposes. Photographs can be reviewed after the examination to double-check findings or perhaps even to discover previously unnoticed findings. If the magnification is precisely known, measurements can be obtained directly from the photograph. Photographic findings can be discussed among colleagues and consultants or can be compared with recent published

data. The development of regional peer review groups to enhance technical and interpretive skills is to be encouraged. Photographs taken during an initial examination can provide a standard for subsequent comparison. Likewise, if a second opinion is required, photographs may save the child from the trauma of reexamination. In court, photographs can provide a powerful and convincing statement, whereas a simple verbal description might fail (Figs. 15.8, 15.10, and 15.11). Even when not used directly in court, photographs may enhance testimony by jogging the examiner's memory of specific findings (19). In those circumstances in which photographs cannot be obtained, a clear and complete narrative, accompanied by detailed drawings at a minimum, should be obtained.

Whether child abuse has occurred and who is responsible is a legal issue for the courts to decide. Corroborative physical evidence photographically documented can be an important adjunct to the legal process. A normal examination, particularly of the sexually abused child, does not exclude the possibility of abuse, however, as many children present without current physical evidence. The need for a sensitive medicolegal history continues to be paramount.

The guiding principles of medical photography are good equipment, adequate lighting, and planned composition. Equally important is a working knowledge of camera equipment, film procedure, and medicolegal implications. Physicians who provide medicolegal examinations of abused children must have access to adequate photographic equipment and a working knowledge of photographic techniques.

REFERENCES

1. Adams JA, Phillips P, Ahmad M. The usefulness of colposcopic photographs in the evaluation of suspected child sexual abuse. *Adolesc Pediatr Gynecol* 1990;3:75–82.
2. Barsley RE, West MH, Fair JA. Forensic photography: ultraviolet imaging of wounds on skin. *Am J Forensic Med Pathol* 1990;11:300–308.
3. Baum E, Grodin MA, Alpert JJ, et al. Child sexual abuse, criminal justice, and the pediatrician. *Pediatrics* 1987;79:437–439.
4. Bernstein ML. The application of photography in forensic dentistry. *Dent Clin North Am* 1983;27:151–170.
5. Cordell W, Zollman W, Karlson H. A photographic system for the emergency department. *Ann Emerg Med* 1980;9:210–214.
6. Eaton GT. Proper storage of photographic images. *J Audiov Media Med* 1985;8:94–98.
7. Finkel MA, Ricci LR. Documentation and preservation of visual evidence in child abuse. *Child Maltreatment* 1997;2:322–330.
8. Flower MS. Photographs in the courtroom "Getting it straight between you and your professional photographer." *North Kentucky State Law Forum* 1974;2: 184–211.
9. Ford RJ, Smistek BS. Photography of the maltreated child. In: Ellerstein NS, ed. *Child abuse and neglect: a medical reference.* New York: John Wiley and Sons, 1981.
10. Freehe CL. Photography in dentistry: equipment and technique. *Dent Clin North Am* 1983;27:3–73.
11. Gilmore J, Miller W. Clinical photography utilizing office staff: methods to achieve consistency and reproducibility. *J Dermatol Surg Oncol* 1988;14:281–286.
12. Hubbard SB. Ultraviolet photography. *Photo Electronic Imaging* 1992:40–42.
13. Ladson S, Johnson CF, Doyt RE. Do physicians recognize sexual abuse? *Am J Dis Child* 1987;141:411–415.
14. Luntz LL, Luntz P. *Handbook for dental identification: techniques in forensic dentistry.* Philadelphia: JB Lippincott, 1973.
15. McCann J. Use of the colposcope in childhood sexual abuse examinations. *Pediatr Clin North Am* 1990;37: 863–880.
16. Morello D, Converse J, Allen D. Making uniform photographic records in plastic surgery. *Plast Reconstr Surg* 1977;59:366–373.
17. Myers JEB, Carter LE. Proof of physical child abuse. *Mo Law Rev* 1988;53:189–224.
18. Reeves C. Pediatric photography. *J Audiov Media Med* 1986;9:131–134.
19. Ricci LR. Photographing the physically abused child: principles and practice. *Am J Dis Child* 1991;145: 275–281.
20. Ricci LR. Medical forensic photography of the sexually abused child. *Child Abuse Negl* 1988;12:305–310.
21. Scott CC. *Photographic evidence.* 2nd ed. St Paul: West Publishing, 1969.
22. Sebben JE. Office photography from the surgical viewpoint. *J Dermatol Surg Oncol* 1983;9:763–768.
23. Spring GE. Evidence photography: an overview. *J Biol Photogr* 1987;55:129–132.
24. Teixeira WRG. Hymenal colposcopic examination in sexual offenses. *Am J Forensic Med Pathol* 1981;2:209–215.
25. Weiss CH. Dermatologic photography of nail pathologies. *Dermatol Clin* 1985;3:543–556.
26. Whitesell J. The basics of medical photography in plastic surgery. *J Plast Reconstr Surg Nurs* 1981;1:89–92.
27. Williams AR. Positioning and lighting for patient photography. *J Biol Photogr* 1985;53:131–143.
28. Woodling BA, Heger A. The use of the colposcope in the diagnosis of sexual abuse in the pediatric age group. *Child Abuse Negl* 1986;10:111–114.
29. Woodling BA, Kossoris P. Sexual misuse: rape, molestation and incest. *Pediatr Clin North Am* 1981;28:481–499.

General Photography References

Hedgcoe J. *John Hedgecoe's complete photography course.* New York: Simon and Schuster, 1979.
Hedgcoe J. *The book of photography.* New York: Alfred A Knopf, 1987.
Langford M. *Michael Langford's 35 mm handbook.* New York: Alfred A Knopf, 1988.
Shipman C. *How to select and use canon SLR cameras.* Los Angeles: HP Books, Price Stern Sloan, 1987.
White W. *The Kodak Workshop Series close-up photography.* New York: Eastman Kodak Company, 1984.

16

Child Abuse by Poisoning

Jan Bays and *Kenneth W. Feldman

*Child Abuse Response and Evaluation Services, Emanuel Children's Hospital and Healthcare Center;
and Department of Pediatrics, Oregon Health Sciences University, Portland, Oregon; *Department of
Pediatrics, University of Washington School of Medicine; *Child Protection Team, Children's Hospital
and Regional Medical Center; and *Odessa Brown Children's Clinic, Seattle, Washington*

The Poison Prevention Packaging Act of 1970 dramatically reduced the morbidity and mortality from unintentional poisoning in children (78). As the child's access to toxins was reduced by child-resistant containers, increasing concern has arisen that some cases of childhood poisoning result from child abuse. Although Kempe (75) first mentioned child abuse by poisoning 30 years ago, intentional poisoning remains an underrecognized and underreported type of abuse. In 1965, Dine (36) suggested the term child abuse by chemical or drug administration. In 1990, the Index Medicus first added the subheading "chemically induced" under the larger heading for child abuse.

INCIDENCE

Accidental poisoning of children is common. Children younger than 3 years account for 42%, and those younger than 6 years, 56% (978,000) of the 1.8 million toxin exposures reported to the American Association of Poison Control Centers' surveillance system during 1993 (87). Fortunately childhood poisonings have a much lower case fatality rate than do those in older people; only 4.3% of poisoning deaths affect children younger than 6 years. Intentional suicidal ingestions and adult exposure to drugs of abuse are much more likely to be fatal. Intentional poisoning is less common than is accidental poisoning. The Poison Centers' surveillance system

listed "malicious intent" in 5,400 toxin exposures (0.5% of all exposures) (87). However, among the tabulated poisoning deaths, none is listed as having malicious intent. The American Humane Association reported 222 cases of child abuse by poisoning in the United States in 1981 (51). Thirty-one cases of intentional, inflicted, nonsuicidal poisoning were reported in more than 10,000 cases of toxic exposure in Honolulu. Eleven (0.1%) of these cases occurred in children of 15 years and younger. No fatalities were reported (175).

Child Abuse by Poisoning

Dine and McGovern (37) reviewed 48 cases of child abuse by poisoning in 1982, and Tenebein (158) compiled 27 additional cases in 1986. In this chapter, an additional 91 reports of poisoning by substances other than alcohol and illicit drugs are compiled in Table 16.1. This table does not reflect aggregate reports of the interface between intentional poisoning and Munchausen syndrome by proxy (MSBP) (Table 16.2). Case reports of more than 100 children poisoned by alcohol and drugs of abuse are listed in Tables 16.3 and 16.4. Only the more severe or unusual cases reach the literature. Thus the literature is likely to underestimate vastly the number of intentional poisonings.

Intentional poisoning is more lethal than accidental childhood poisoning (101). Deaths

TABLE 16.1. *Child abuse by poisoning*

Reference	Agent	Age	Sex	Clinical features	Abuser	Admit*	In hospital*	Other types of abuse	Survival	Comments
46	Barbiturate	4 days	M	None	Mother	–	+	–	Survival	MSBP*
57	Barbiturate	2 yr	M	↓LOC, *coma	Mother	–	–	–	Death	Died 3 days after hospital discharge
90	Barbiturate	2 yr	M	LOC, cardiac arrest, foot pain	Mother	–	+	–	Survival	Mom Munchausen
113	Barbiturate	14 yr	F	↓LOC, ataxia, diplopia nystagmus	Father	a*	–	–	Survival	Father poisoned two other sibs at puberty
177	Barbiturate	20 mo	M	↓LOC, ataxia, seizures	Mother	o	–	–	Survival	Pill fragments found by lavage
70	Barbiturates	4 yr	M	Ataxia	Mother	–	+	+	Survival	Arthralgia, hematuria, fever, phenothiazines, phentermine, methaqualone
96	Phenytoin	4 yr	M	"Seizures," weight loss, extreme lethargy	Mother	a	+	–	Survival	No seizures once off medication in foster care
113	Phenytoin	8 yr	M	Vomiting, ataxia ↓LOC, nystagmus	Stepfather	–	–	–	Survival	Stepfather taking antiepileptics
158	Codeine	2 mo	M	↓LOC, apnea, miosis	Mother	–	+	–	Survival	
65	Benzodiazepine	12 days	M	Apnea, cyanosis, ↓LOC, jittery	Mother	–	–	–	Survival	
65	Benzodiazepine, codeine, phenobarbital	27 days	M	Apnea, cyanosis, hypotonia	?	–	–	–	Survival	Four episodes ALTE*, poisoned again after return home
65	Meperidine, phenothiazine	24 days	F	Apnea, cyanosis, hypertonia	Father	a	–	–	Survival	Father sedated child to help mother rest
65	Meperidine, promethazine hydrochloride	33 days	M	Apnea, cyanosis, hypertonia	Mother	a	–	–	Survival	Mother "sedated" child
158	Phenothiazines	24 mo	F	↓LOC, ataxia	Stepfather	–	–	–	Survival	Prior aspirin poisoning
114	Amitriptyline	2 mo	F	Unresponsive	Mother	a	–	–	Death	16-year-old mother, pills found on endotrachial tube at autopsy
118	Amitriptyline	10 mo	F	Recurrent loss of consciousness	Mother	o	+	–	Survival	Sibling died of PxAb*
155	Imipramine	4 yr	M	Drowsy, ataxia	Mother	–	+	–	Survival	Mother tried homicide/suicide previously with drugs
177	Tricyclic	5 mo	F	Seizures, respiratory arrest	Mother	–	–	–	Survival	
65	Acetaminophen	20 days	M	Lethargy, icterus	Mother	–	–	–	Death	Survived initial poisoning but died of "SIDS" at 26 wk; no autopsy
28	Glibenclamide	11 yr	F	Seizures, unconscious, hypoglycemia	Mother	–	+	–	Survival	Many medical procedures, including subtotal pancreatectomy. Cured by foster placement
104	Insulin, phenothiazines, laxative	17 mo	F	↓LOC, hypoglycemia	Mother	a	–	–	Survival	MSBP, siblings also probably victims
177	Insulin	2.5 mo	M	Seizures, hypoglycemia	Mother	–	–	–	Impaired	Sibling died of diet-pill overdose
5	Arsenic	9 yr	M	Vomiting, abdominal pain	Mother	c	–	–	Death	MSBP, mother attempted suicide twice

Ref	Agent	Age	Sex	Symptoms	Perpetrator				Outcome	Comments
5	Arsenic	8 yr	M	Vomiting, abdominal pain	Mother	c	–	–	Death	MSBP, mother attempted suicide twice
86	Arsenic	u	F	Nausea, coldness	Mother	–	–	–	Survival	Sib also similar abuse
17	Ipecac	1.5 mo	F	Hypotonia, poor sucking reflex, weak cry, dehydration	Mother	a	+	–	Survival	MSBP, mother added ipecac to expressed breast milk in hospital
37	Ipecac	4 yr	F	Vomiting & diarrhea, dehydration, heart failure	Mother	a	+	–	Death	
46	Ipecac, ephedrine	9 mo	F	Recurrent vomiting & diarrhea, hypotonia, FTT*	Mother	–	+	–	Survival	Diagnosed at eleventh hospitalization, bulimic mother
81	Ipecac	12 mo	U	V & D, FTT	Mother	–	+	–	Survival	
94 or 95	Ipecac	1 mo	F	V & D, FTT	Mother	+	+	–	Survival	3 older sibs laxative poisoning
138	Ipecac	5 yr	M	V & D, cardiac dysfn	Mother	+	+	–	Death	Cardiac dysfunction. On cath
164	Detergent	3 yr	?	Vomiting & diarrhea, burning in throat & anus	Parents	–	–	+	Survival	Physical abuse
28	Black pepper	5 mo	M	Death of pepper aspiration	Mother	a	–	–	Death	Punishment for putting fingers in mouth
		2 yr	F	Death of pepper aspiration	Godfather	a	–	–	Death	Punishment for eating pepper
		2.5 yr	F	Death of pepper aspiration	Mother	a	–	+	Death	Punishment for taking sibling's bottle, PxAb
		2.5 yr	M	Death of pepper aspiration	Mother, boyfriend	c	–	+	Death	Punishment for unknown offense. PxAb
		3.5 yr	F	Death of pepper aspiration	Mother	a	–	+	Death	Punishment for taking sibling's bottle, PxAb
		4 yr	M	Death of pepper aspiration	Self	–	–	–	Death	Pica
		5 yr	M	Death of pepper aspiration	Foster mother	a	–	–	Death	Punishment for lying
		10 yr	M	Death of pepper aspiration	Adult friend	a	–	+	Death	Punishment for not eating breakfast, PxAb forced to eat Worcestershire & Tabasco sauce by "big brother"
56	Metallic foreign bodies	6 mo	F	Esophageal symptoms	?	–	–	–	Survival	Thumbtack, screw, & carpet tack among multiple foreign bodies in stomach
83	Chloral hydrate	3 yr	F	Coma	Mother	–	+	+	Survival	Prior NA caustic injestion
25	Lasix	5 yr	M	V & D Barter's?	Mother	?	+	–	Survival	
42	Castor oil	18 mo	M	Diarrhea	Mother	+	–	–	Survival	Mother Munchausen, phenobarbital
52	Phenolphthalein	17 mo	M	Diarrhea	Mother	+	+	–	Survival	2 sibs hosps diazepam
52	Phenolphthalein	26 mo	M	Fever, V & D, rash, ataxia	Mother	+	+	–	Death	Death unexplained resp
59	Muriatic acid	21 mo	F	Stridor, respiratory distress	Baby sit	+	–	+	Survival	Prior forced FB ingest
59	Muriatic acid	3 yr	F	Croup	Baby sit	–	–	–	Survival	
70	Warfarin	7 yr	F	Hemorrhage	Mother	–	+	+	Survival	Multiple unexplained symptoms, sib of ref 70, folic didscfic
80	Bisacodyl	11 yr	M	Diarrhea, hyper NA	Mother	+	+	–	Survival	
81	Cold med.	6 mo	u	Coma, FTT	Mother	–	+	–	Survival	
81	Cooking oil	10 yr	u	Vomit, pneumonia	Mother	–	+	–	Survival	
86	Phenobarbital		{F	Seizures, FTT	Mother	–	–	–	Survival	Sugar/corn syrup OD
86	Caustics			Skin burns	Mother	–	–	–	Survival	

407

continued

TABLE 16.1. *(Continued.)*

Reference	Agent	Age	Sex	Clinical features	Abuser	Admit*	In hospital*	Other types of abuse	Survival	Comments
103	Paracetamol	3 mo	M	Hepatic failure	Father	–	–	+	unknown	Also warfarin & caffeine
147	Chlorpromazine	18 mo	F	Prolonged sleep	Mother	–	+	–	Survival	History of seizures
167	Phenothiazine	5 yr	M	Stupor, fever	Mother	–	+	+	Survival	Blood gravel in urine, vomiting
167	Sugar	22 mo	F	Diabetic seizure	Mother	–	+	–	Survival	MSBP
169	Imipramine	7 yr	M	Unconscious	Mother	+	+	–	Survival	
174	Ethylene glycol	6 mo	F	Lethargy, acidosis	Baby sit	–	–	–	Survival	
138	Ipecac	4 yr	M	V & D	Mother	–	+	–	Survival	
92	Ipecac	8 mo	M	Recurrent V & D, hypotonia	Mother	a	+	–	Survival	Diagnosed at fourth hospitalization
92	Ipecac	10 mo	F	Recurrent V & D	Mother	o	+	–	Survival	Diagnosed after multiple hospitalizations. Mother had bottles of ipecac in purse
92	Ipecac	21 mo	M	Recurrent V & D, dehydration	Mother	–	+	–	Survival	Diagnosed after multiple hospitalizations
154	Ipecac	16 mo	M	Recurrent V & D, muscle weakness, ↑CPK, FTT	Mother	–	–	–	Survival	Diagnosed after three hospitalizations
170	Laxatives	?	?	?	Mother	–	–	–	Survival	Three siblings of child poisoned with ipecac
81	Laxatives	6 yr	u	Seizures, apnea, vomit, abd pain	Mother	–	+	–	Survival	
50	Epsom salts	4 mo	F	Diarrhea, dehydration, weight loss, poor	Mother	a	+	–	Survival	
5	Mineral oil	10 mo	M	?	Mother	a	+	–	Survival	MSBP, sibling died of "SIDS" after mother placed him in freezer until he suffocated
158	Toluene	13 mo	M	↓LOC, seizures, hydrocarbon odor to breath	Parents	o	–	–	Survival	Parents inhaling toluene & drinking alcohol
45	Isopropyl alcohol	2 yr	M	Coma, hypothermia (33°C) shock	Father	–	–	+	Survival	Contusion, scald burns, ingestion of 100 mL isopropyl alcohol
134	Isopropyl alcohol	4 yr	F	Found dead	Mother, boyfriend	a	–	+	Death	Alcohol applied to immersion burns left alone in room for 27 h
135	Ethylene glycol	8 mo	F	Intoxicated, vomiting, lethargy, acidotic	Parents	–	–	–	Survival	
132	Caustic	11 yr	F	Progressive upper gastrointestinal ulceration, esophageal stricture, recurrent sepsis	Mother?	c	+	–	Survival	MSBP, many procedures, & hospitalizations near death from induced sepsis. Cured by foster placement
65	Air freshener	28 days	M	Recurrent apnea, cyanosis, choking	Mother	o	+	–	Survival	Air freshener added to infant's bottle
124	Caffeine	5 wks	M	Agitated/irritable	Father	+	–	+	Death	Died of inflicted head injury
107	Caffeine	14 mo	F	V & D, dehydration ↓LOC	Mother, boyfriend	–	–	+	Death	Lacerated spleen, rib fractures, caffeine diet pills abused by mother & sold by mother's boyfriend

408

Ref	Poison	Age	Sex	Presentation	Perpetrator	Key admit	In hospital	Outcome	Comments
3	Salt (NaCl & KCl)	6 yr	M	Abdominal pain, collapse	Stepfather	a	–	Death	Salt substitute added to food as punishment for child using too much salt
33	Salt	3 yr	F	Somnolence, dehydration, FTT, hypernatremia	Mother?	–	–	Survival	Trichotillomania, water deprivation
56	Salt	1 yr	M	Vomiting, FTT, lethargy, cardiac arrest, hypernatremia	Mother	c	–	Death	
103	Salt	5 mo	F	Hyper Na	Father	–	–	Death	FTT, bizarre eating
38	Salt	5 yr	F	Seizures, hyper Na	Mother	–	+	Survival	
74	Water	8 yr	F	Unconscious, hypothermia, hyponatremia	Foster parents	a	–	Survival	Water drinking chosen as humane punishment after "much counseling"
162	Water	4 yr	F	Collapse, status epilepticus, hyponatremia, FTT*	Mother	a	–	Survival	Physical abuse, gained 5.5 lb in 7 days in hospital
37	Peppers	33 mo	M	Coma after beating	Mother, boyfriend	a	+	Death	Twenty small peppers found in esophagus; subdural & retro-peritoneal bleeds at autopsy
164	Jalapeno peppers	7 yr	?	V & D, burning in throat & anus	Parents	–	+	Survival	Physical abuse
	Tabasco sauce	5 yr	?	V & D, burning in throat & anus	Parents	–	+	Survival	Physical abuse

*Key admit, admission of guilt by perpetrator; in hospital, poisoning continued in hospital. M, male; F, female; LOC, level of consciousness; MSBP, Munchausen syndrome by proxy; SIDS, sudden infant death syndrome; FTT, failure to thrive; ALTE, apparent life-threatening event; CPK, creatine phosokinase; a, admitted guilt; o, observed or evidence found; c, convicted; V & D, vomiting and diarrhea; PxAb, physical abuse.

TABLE 16.2. *Case series of Munchausen syndrome by proxy and poisoning*

Ref.	Author	Study years	MSBP victims (n)	Poisoned (n)	Poison fatality (n)
130	Rosenberg	1966–1987	117	NR	5
19	Bools	1976–1986	56	15	2
93	McClure	1992–1994	97[a]	44	5
49	Feldman	1974–1998	104	18	0

NR, not reported.
[a]From a series of 128 victims of MSBP, intentional poisoning, intentional suffocation, or a combination of the three.

TABLE 16.3. Child abuse by poisoning: substance abuse

Reference	Agent	Age	Sex	Clinical features	Abuser	Survival	Comments
9	Cocaine	Not born	F	Death	Mother	Death	Fetal demise due to maternal cocaine use
11	Cocaine	3 mo	F	Seizures	?	Survival	Heavy crack smoking in home
11	Cocaine	9 mo	M	Drowsiness	Uncles	Survival	Uncles smoked crack in apartment
11	Cocaine	2 yr	M	Seizures, lethargy	Baby sit	Survival	Babysitter smoked crack
11	Cocaine	3 yr	M	Nausea, too wobbly to stand	Adult male	Survival	Adult male smoked crack all night
26	Cocaine	11 days	M	Seizures, apnea	Mother	Survival	Topical cocaine powder used on nipples to relieve pain
27	Cocaine	2 wk	F	↓LOC, ataxia, seizures	Mother	Survival	Breast-feeding by cocaine-using mother
29	Cocaine	8 wk	F	Found dead	Parents	Death	Parents didn't ask cause of death, arrested in another city for sale & use of cocaine
29	Cocaine	10 wk	F	Found dead, babysitter	Parents?	Death	Parents used & sold cocaine
43	Cocaine	4 mo	F	Seizure	Mother?	Survival	Mother may have used cocaine to sedate child
43	Cocaine	9 mo	F	Seizures, in stasis for 90 min	Baby sit	Survival	Drugs accessible at home of babysitter; cocaine found in gastric lavage
43	Cocaine	14 mo	M	Seizures	?	Survival	Use of cocaine in home night before
43	Cocaine	3 yr	F	Seizures	?	Survival	Claimed child found cocaine on street and ate it
63	Cocaine	6 wk	M	LOC, hypothermia 31°C, diarrhea, dehydration FTT*	?	Survival	Mother admitted infant frequently exposed to crack cocaine smoke
63	Cocaine	3 mo	F	Vomiting and diarrhea, seizures, cerebral infarcts, sagittal vein, thrombosis, dehydration	Parents?	Death	Parents smoked cocaine daily; said they would not "waste" cocaine on the baby
63	Cocaine	12 mo	M	Epistaxis, H flu sepsis, pericardial effusion	Mother?	Survival	Mother entered drug treatment, denied all but passive exposure to infant
63	Cocaine	14 mo	M	Fever, ear pain, Sz	Aunt?	Survival	Aunt smoked crack while caring for infant, denied feeding him cocaine
77	Cocaine	20 mo	F	Drooling, vomiting, lethargy, esophagitis, epiglottitis	Mother?	Impaired	Ingested lye used in crack preparation; esophageal stricture; required hyperalimentation and gastrostomy
121	Cocaine	4 yr	F	Anal fissure, anal laxity	Parents	Survival	Parents accused each other of hiding rock cocaine in the child's rectum
123	Cocaine	4 yr	F	LOC, vomiting, bloody diarrhea, cardiovascular collapse	?	Survival	Rock cocaine lying on kitchen table at house where cocaine was used
125	Cocaine	9 mo	F	Sz, apnea, hyperthermia, hypertension	?	Survival	Infant found playing in remnants of party where cocaine was used
152	Cocaine	Birth	F	Intrauterine death	Mother	Death	Intrauterine cocaine toxicity
152	Cocaine	6 wk	M	Found dead	Stepbro.	Death	Homicide from cocaine-laced formula
9	Opiate	5 days	M	Death	?	Death	Accidental "overdose" with opiates
32	Heroin	10 mo	M	Found dead, presumpt-	Mothers	Death	Multiple injections of heroin by mother's boyfriend to stop baby crying
65	Methadone	5 days	M	Apnea, cyanosis, LOC, hypotonia	Mother	Survival	Mother admitted giving her own methadone to treat the baby's withdrawal
140	LSD*	22 mo	M	Crying, agitation, hallucinations	?	Survival	Mother admitted child may have ingested LSD left in house by friend
141	PCP*	2 mo	F	7 children w/symptoms	?	Survival	Deliberate poisoning of formula vs. passive
141	PCP*	10 mo		100% LOC, lethargy–coma			
141	PCP*		F	100% blunted/absent pain response	?	Survival	Passive inhalation at a party
141	PCP*	13 mo	F	86% hypotonia			Passive inhalation at a party
141	PCP*			71% ataxia			Passive inhalation at a party
141	PCP*	14 mo	F	57% blank stare, 57% miosis	?	Survival	Passive inhalation at a party

141	PCP*			57% nystagmus	?	Survival	Passive inhalation at a party
141	PCP*	18 mo	F	27% seizure, 27% opisthotonos	?	Survival	Passive inhalation at a party
141	PCP*	5 yr	M	27% disconjugate gaze	?	Survival	Passive inhalation at a party
141	PCP*				?	Survival	Passive inhalation at a party
171	PCP*	11 days	M	6 children with symptoms	?	Survival	Passive inhalation vs. deliberate intoxication
171	PCP*			100% lethargy		Survival	Passive inhalation vs. deliberate intoxication
171	PCP*	8 mo	F	67% nystagmus, 67% ataxia	?	Survival	Passive inhalation vs. deliberate intoxication
171	PCP*			50% opisthotonos, 50% staring			Passive inhalation vs. deliberate intoxication
171	PCP*	13 mo	F	33% irritability, 33% coma	?	Survival	passive inhalation vs. deliberate intoxication
171	PCP*			33% hypertonic, 33% miosis			passive inhalation vs. deliberate intoxication
171	PCP*	13 mo	M		?	Survival	passive inhalation vs. deliberate intoxication
171	PCP*	18 mo	F		?	Survival	passive inhalation vs. deliberate intoxication
171	PCP*	5 yr	F		?	Survival	passive inhalation vs. deliberate intoxication
82	THC*	?	?	3 children in coma	—	Survival	Apparently accidental ingestion of 1 g of hashish by 3 children
97	THC*	1 yr	F	5 children with symptoms	—	Survival	Apparently accidental ingestion
97	THC	2 yr	M	Stupor; sluggish pupils; one patient required atropine and a ventilator for respiratory depression	—	Survival	Apparently accidental ingestion
97	THC			" "	—	Survival	Apparently accidental ingestion
97	THC			" "	—	Survival	Apparently accidental ingestion
142	THC	?	?	25 children, aged 5 mo to 10 yr, w/symptoms including sleepiness, giggling, ataxia, hyperactivity, and crying	Babysitter	Survival	Nine girls admitted intoxicating a total of 25 children with marijuana while babysitting from 1 to 15 times for each child
157	THC	2 yr	F	Ataxia, hand tremor	Babysitter	Survival	Neighbor gave marijuana-laced cookies to babysitter
157	THC	3 yr	F	Ataxia, voracious appetite, LOC, labile affect, tremor, conjunctival hyperemia	Babysitter	Survival	Neighbor gave marijuana-laced cookies to babysitter
157	THC	4 yr	M	Ataxia, voracious appetite, LOC, labile affect, tremor, conjunctival hyperemia	Babysitter	Survival	Neighbor gave marijuana-laced cookies to babysitter
15	Alcohol			15 intoxicated toddlers	—	Survival	"Morning after" ingestion of alcohol left out after party the night before
15	Alcohol			4 intoxicated toddlers	—	Survival	Intoxicated while attending family celebration
15	Alcohol			2 intoxicated toddlers	Prnt/Bbysit	Survival	Given alcohol by parent or babysitter
15	Alcohol			5 boys, aged 7 to 14 yr	Friends	Survival	Forced to drink under duress
15	Alcohol			4 boys, aged 7 to 14 yr	Adult men	Survival	Forced to drink as part of sexual abuse
24	Alcohol	5 yr	M	Found dead	Mother, boyfriend	Death	Infant died of ingestion of cologne (70% ethanol) and salicylates. Mother and boyfriend pled guilty
37	Alcohol	4 yr	M	Vomiting and drowsiness	Dad's friend	Survival	Prior poisoning with propoxyphane (Darvon)
61	Alcohol	6 yr	F	Coma, shock, hypothermia (34°C)	Father	Survival	Father forced child to drink a cup of brandy. Peritoneal dialysis required. Physical abuse also
122	Alcohol	1 yr	M	Found moribund	Mother's boyfriend	Death	Mother's boyfriend fed baby rum and Coke to quiet him. Physical abuse

PCP, phencyclidine; LSD, lysergic acid diethylamide; THC, tetahydrocannabinol; alcohol, ethyl alcohol; M, male; F, female; LOC, level of consciousness; SIDS, sudden infant death syndrome; Sz, seizures.

TABLE 16.4. *Child abuse by poisoning: occult cocaine exposure*

Reference	Agent	Age	Clinical features	Comments
76	Cocaine	2 wk to 5 yr	Urine drug screens of 250 children at Boston City Hospital ER, informed consent, anonymous. 18 parents refused	2.4% positive for cocaine metabolite: 1-mo-old w/pneumonia; 4-mo with reactive airway disease, 5-mo with otitis media, 9-mo with bronchiolitis, 19-mo with laceration, 22-mo with fever, rule-out sepsis
79	Cocaine	<16 yr	Urine drug screens of 36 children at Case Western ER w/unexplained seizure in the past 12 hr (excluding trauma, metabolic, infection, febrile and epilepsy)	11% positive for cocaine; 14-mo "accidental ingestion," 32-mo "accidental ingestion," 14-yr intentional ingestion; 15-yr intentional ingestion
106	Cocaine	1 wk–24 mo	Retrospective review of toxicology results on about 600 infant autopsies. Scene investigation	2.7% positive for cocaine or cocaine metabolites. Passive inhalation thought to be the cause
126	Cocaine	<2 days	Toxicology screens on 43 infants dying at less than 2 days of age with no cause of death at gross or microscopic autopsy	40% positive for cocaine and/or cocaine metabolites; 23% positive for opiates
131	Cocaine	1 mo–5 yr	Urine drug screens of 460 children at Michigan Children's ER who required urine testing for fever, vomiting, or other symptoms. Anonymous, no consent	5.4% positive for cocaine and/or cocaine metabolites. No positive patients were breast-fed
144	Cocaine	<30 yr	1,680 consecutive urine and serum toxicology screens at Boston Children's Hospital	4.6% positive for cocaine and/or cocaine metabolites; 4 neonates, 11 adolescents, 3 infants, 7-mo with symptoms whose parents and babysitter were cocaine users; 2-mo with apnea whose mother used cocaine in pregnancy; 6-week-old whose mother admitted breast-feeding while using cocaine

of accidental poisonings have declined from more than 600 per year before 1971 to fewer than 150 per year in 1981, for a mortality rate of less than 0.04% (110). In 1992 there were 39 poisoning deaths among children younger than 15 years in the U.S., for a mortality rate of 0.06/100,000 children (111). In contrast, among the 48 cases of inflicted poisoning reported by Dine and McGovern (37), the mortality rate was 17%. In the 75 cases of Tenebein (158), mortality was 18.7%, with two additional suspicious deaths occurring later. The mortality rate for the cases in Table 16.1 was 26%. Rosenberg (130) reported 10

child fatalities attributed to MSBP, of which five (50%) involved poisoning. McClure et al. (93) observed that five of eight fatalities in a series of 128 MSBP, suffocation, and poisoning victims had been poisoned.

Data on fatalities that result from abusive poisoning are scanty. Several studies offer regional information. Of 3,972 poisoning fatalities investigated by the Cuyahoga County Coroner's Office in Cleveland, Ohio, between 1951 and 1985, 14 were homicidal poisonings (3). Six of these occurred in children younger than 16 years. Five of the six children died of carbon monoxide inhalation. The sixth was poisoned with potassium chloride. In Vermont, between 1971 and 1985, the total number of homicides was 264. Three were homicidal poisonings, all in children 3 years old or younger (3). In Oregon, four of 117 child fatalities related to abuse between January 1985 and March 1992 involved inflicted poisoning. A 4-year-old girl died after her mother gave amitriptyline to quiet her. Two children died when their mother gave herself and her children organophosphate insecticide, apparently to escape domestic violence and child abuse inflicted by her husband. The mother lived. A 2-year-old child was asphyxiated when the mother's boyfriend poured red chili pepper in his mouth as punishment for crying. Another 4-year-old child was the victim of carbon monoxide poisoning in a suicide–homicide by the father (State of Oregon, Department of Human Resources, unpublished data).

The paucity of case reports of morbidity and mortality from abuse by poisoning may relate to clinicians' failure to entertain the diagnosis. Miller (105) reviewed the charts of 228 children evaluated at the Mayo Clinic hospital for toxic ingestion. He found that in no case were suspicions of child abuse or neglect documented. He emphasized that professionals should consider at least lack of supervision, if not intentional administration, in the differential diagnosis of these patients.

Not only must the diagnosis be considered, but appropriate toxicology screens also must be done. Hickson et al. (65) attempted to estimate the incidence of poisoning as a cause of apparent life-threatening events. Of 216 patients admitted to Vanderbilt University Hospital in a 6-year period, at least nine (4%) were poisoned by parents. Because drug screens were ordered in only about 20% of cases, this is a minimal estimate of frequency.

The true incidence of child abuse by poisoning is unknown. Most cases are probably undetected. In fatal poisoning, detection occurs only in those cases in which autopsy is performed. Those are identified only if the pathologist does the appropriate toxicology or electrolyte screens. In nonfatal poisoning, detection occurs in only those children in whom symptoms are sufficiently bizarre or severe to cause physicians to test for toxic agents.

It is naive to think that when a child is discovered to be the victim of intentional poisoning on one occasion that this has been or will be the only episode. Many children who are intentionally poisoned probably never present for medical care, recover at home, or are never diagnosed. To paraphrase statements by Kempe, child abuse by poisoning will be detected only in proportion to the physician's willingness to entertain the diagnosis and to test for it.

PATTERNS OF UNINTENTIONAL POISONING

It is helpful to know the characteristics of unintentional poisoning to be able to distinguish it from possible intentional poisoning (58,71,78,85,173,175). The peak age group sustaining accidental poisoning is 2- to 3-year-old toddlers. Two-year-old children account for about one half of all cases. Accidental poisoning is rare in infants younger than 1 year (0.1% to 8%).

Unintentional ingestion also is uncommon in children between ages 6 and 10 years (2% to 4%). After age 10 years, the incidence of intentional ingestion and suicide attempts increases. Suicide attempts in children should not escape the notice of child welfare workers. The Oregon State Child Fatality Committee Report for 1985 revealed that of seven children, ages 5 to 14 years, who committed suicide, Children's Services Division had prior contacts with all but one (86%) (44).

The child's home is the most common site of accidental ingestion. It typically occurs during daylight hours, with peak times around 10 a.m. and 4 to 7 p.m. An adult is usually present in the home. According to one report, 78% of accidental ingestions occurred while the children were being watched or were within earshot of the parent (56). Drugs are the most common poisons ingested by 2- to 3-year-old children, whereas household products are most common in the 1- to 2-year-old age groups (173). Often the substance ingested was recently moved, used, or placed in a location likely to be more accessible and to attract the attention of the child (58). Household products sold or temporarily stored in containers similar to those normally used for foods increase the risk that a child will mistake the chemicals for a foodstuff. Less than 2 hours typically elapses between the time of ingestion and the time when medical advice is sought (175).

CLINICAL PRESENTATION IN DELIBERATE INTOXICATION

Children who have been deliberately poisoned may present in several ways (101).

1. The child is brought to a medical facility with a history of accidental ingestion. The history will be accepted at face value, particularly if the child is an active toddler. Only if the child or another observer is able to give an alternate history will the true cause be discovered.

2. The child is seen with signs of poisoning and no history to explain the symptoms. If toxicology screens are not performed, the child may recover with symptomatic treatment and be discharged without a diagnosis. If toxins are found, the parents may deny knowledge of the cause or invent implausible explanations.

   Differential diagnoses considered in those cases later proven to be intentional poisoning include sepsis, meningitis, seizures, intracranial hemorrhage, head trauma, gastroenteritis, apnea, an apparent life-threatening event, sudden infant death syndrome (SIDS), bleeding diathesis, and metabolic derangement (130,171).

3. The child has recurrent unexplained illness such as seizures, vomiting and diarrhea, or apneic spells. Repeated medical workup is negative until administered toxins are discovered. The parents also may create factitious symptoms by means other than poisoning. These cases overlap with MSBP (see Chapter 14).

4. The child dies unexpectedly. Autopsy may or may not reveal the cause of death.

HISTORICAL FACTORS THAT AROUSE CONCERN

Many factors that arouse suspicion of intentional intoxication are the same as those listed 15 years ago by Schmitt and Kempe (137). Clinical indicators of possible intentional poisoning are listed in Table 16.5.

Taking the History: Toxin Availability

The history-taker should make a complete list of drugs in the child's environment, including medications or remedies being used by parents, siblings, grandparents, baby-sitters, or anyone else in recent contact with the child.

Dine (36) described a 19-month-old child with eight hospital admissions for symptoms finally attributed to poisoning by perphenazine. The mother continued to deny any possible access to or ingestion of drugs. Finally, the pediatrician contacted the mother's physician and learned that the mother had been hospitalized for postpartum depression after two suicide attempts. She had been supplied with perphenazine during her ongoing outpatient treatment.

TABLE 16.5. *Clinical indicators of abuse by poisoning*

Age
  Younger than 1 yr or between 5 and 10 yr
History
  Nonexistent, discrepant, or changing
  Does not fit child's development
  Previous poisoning in this child
  Previous poisoning in siblings
  Does not fit circumstances or scene
  Third party, often a sibling, is blamed
  Delay in seeking medical care
Toxin
  Multiple toxins
  Substances of abuse
  Bizarre substances
Presentation
  Unexplained seizures
  Life-threatening events
  Apparent sudden infant death syndrome
  Death without obvious cause
  Chronic unexplained symptoms that resolve
    when the child is protected
  Other evidence of abuse or neglect

When making a list of drugs given to the child, vitamins, antipyretics, cold and cough medicines, herbs, teas, tonics, and natural or ethnic remedies should be included. Ask if anyone in the house has a substance-abuse problem. Was this child born drug or alcohol exposed? Are there indications that this child lives in a house where illegal drug activity is common?

Toxin Accessibility

The physician should determine where and in what type of container this substance was stored at the time of the ingestion. Information from accidental ingestion of drugs shows that often the drug was used or moved to a location where the child could see and obtain it within a few hours of the ingestion. Tenenbein (158) described a 24-month-old child brought to the emergency department by her stepfather with decreased level of consciousness and ataxia. Results of toxicologic studies were positive for chlorpromazine and phenothiazine metabolites. The child had been admitted at age 10 months with salicylate poisoning, also incurred while in her stepfather's care. The stepfather was being treated with chlorpromazine for chronic schizophrenia. A home visit confirmed that this medication was kept on a high shelf inaccessible to the child.

Home investigation might include a public health nurse visit to evaluate toxin accessibility and the plausibility of the scenario before deciding whether protective service referral is appropriate.

Developmental Abilities

A developmental history should be taken to discover if the child can crawl, walk, climb up to cabinets, feed him- or herself, and open pill containers, medicine cabinets, or refrigerators. To ingest a toxin accidentally, a child must be capable of crawling, cruising, or walking to the location of the poison, extracting it from a container, if any, and getting the substance into his or her mouth. Children begin crawling at around age 7 to 9 months, cruising and holding onto furniture at around 9 months, and walking at about 12 months. They can messily feed themselves a large object, such as a cracker or leaf of a household plant, at about age 7 months, but do not have the "neat pincher grasp" required to pick up a small pill, capsule, or rock of crack cocaine and successfully get it into the mouth until about age 10 to 12 months. If the family gives a developmental history that seems unlikely, test the child in the hospital. Some 9-month-olds do walk and put small objects into their mouths; others sit like placid lumps, cannot feed themselves, and show no interest in exploration.

Of the 75 cases of child abuse by poisoning reviewed by Dine and McGovern (37) and Tenenbein (158), 31% involved children aged 1 year or younger. Of the additional cases reviewed in this chapter, approximately 40% of those involving substances of abuse (Tables 16.3 and 16.4) and 24% of those involving other substances (Table 16.1) occurred in children aged 1 year or younger. Friedman (56) described a 6-month-old girl brought into the emergency department with esophageal symptoms. Barium contrast radiography during swallowing revealed a linear metallic foreign body in the esophagus. An abdominal radiograph showed multiple foreign bodies, including a thumbtack, a screw, and a carpet tack. A 6-month-old child is not capable of obtaining and ingesting such an array of objects. Either a determined older sibling or, more likely, an adult is responsible. Barnett (10) described another 6-month-old child who was hospitalized because of toxic effects apparently from swallowing a centipede (later excreted in the diaper). No bites on the skin or in the mouth were found. As is typical of many reports of ingestions in infants, the question of how a centipede got into this small infant's mouth was not addressed.

When a sibling is blamed for injury to a child, child abuse or at least neglect should be suspected. Dogruyol and Gurpinar (39) reported the case of a 4-day-old infant with pneumonia. When a nasogastric tube could not be inserted, investigation revealed that a bean was obstructing the esophagus. The infant's 4-year-old sister had spent a great deal of time playing with him using playthings such as beans. The authors considered that "since self-introduction of a foreign body is impossible at this age," the accident represented a form of neglect.

Stresses in the Home

Inquiries should be made as to whether there is an adult in the family with a history of mental illness, abuse in childhood, drug or alcohol abuse, or frequent or unusual illnesses. One theory links marital discord with child abuse poisonings. It hypothesizes that the parent attacks a child seen as favored by the spouse. The created illness, at the child's expense, helps to restore a balance in the marital relationship (56). Swann and Glascow (155) described a 4-year-old boy who had four hospital admissions in 8 days. The first two admissions were for falls and epistaxis. The last two were for seizures with shock. Toxicologic tests of the urine obtained at the earlier admissions revealed imipramine (45 µg/L). Toxicologic analysis of the urine from 4 days into the fourth hospital admission revealed desipramine at even higher levels (770 µg/L). Further inquiry indicated that the father was a paraplegic as the result of a motorcycle accident. The mother was depressed and drank heavily. One year previously, the family had moved from England to Northern Ireland. The mother had attempted to commit suicide and to kill the patient and his older sister with medication prescribed for the father.

Prior Similar History

It is important to take a history of prior poisonings or unusual illnesses in the child and its extended family, and of unexplained deaths of siblings. Telephone consultation with the physician or medical examiner involved is advised. Prior medical records should be obtained. It is best to not take the family's history at face value, particularly if they say that

records are unavailable because a doctor moved or a hospital lost them (130).

Recurrent Poisoning

Recurrent poisoning presents a diagnostic problem. Is the household unsafe? Is the child unsupervised or neglected, making a bid for attention, or being poisoned? In one study (88), 41% of children between ages 3 and 5 years who had been accidentally poisoned were "repeaters." Of 585 repeaters younger than age 5 years, 18% had two prior ingestions, and 4.4% had three prior ingestions. One child had nine prior ingestions; one, 12; and one had 15! Disturbingly, 34 (12%) of 585 repeaters were younger than 1 year.

Repeated ingestions are not correlated with safety hazards in the home. They occur more often in families with increased stress, poor emotional support, low coping abilities on the part of the mother, and higher levels of physical and mental illness (56,88). Wright (unpublished data) has developed a profile of a child who is likely to ingest poison repeatedly. The child is younger than other victims at first poisoning; is more impulsive, aggressive, and destructive; and frequently makes caretakers angry. The child is likely engaged in a variety of autonomy struggles with the parents. He or she has had many opportunities to watch others take medicine and is more likely to have penetrated a fastened container. Wright has characterized repeated poisonings as an indirect form of child abuse. The family creates a stress-ridden environment, producing a stress-ridden, reactive child. The child, who has minimal help or protection from the environment, poisons himself. When a child is repeatedly poisoned, family intervention is indicated to discover if neglect or abuse is occurring and to remedy unsafe conditions.

LABORATORY TESTING

Clinicians rely on toxicology screens to detect poisoning. Several factors can affect whether a positive result of toxicologic tests is obtained on an intoxicated child. These include the time since ingestion, amount ingested, whether it was a single or repeated exposure, rate of absorption and excretion, the type of specimen obtained, and the screening methods used.

Clinicians must be aware that routine toxicology screens are limited. Some common poisons are not detected and must be requested specifically. Wiley (172) reviewed this problem and listed common drugs that cause coma and circulatory depression, but are not detected on routine drug screening (Table 16.6). The clinician should make an intelligent guess as to the type of poison involved and then confer with the toxicologist. Different test selection and methods will be appropriate, depending on the suspected toxins.

TABLE 16.6. *Poisons undetected by drug screening*

Poisons causing coma	
Miosis present	*Mydriasis present*
Clonidine	Carbon monoxide
Chloral hydrate	Cyanide
Organophosphates	Methemoglobinemia
Tetrahydrozoline	LSD
(OTC eye drops)	
Bromide	

Poisons Causing Circulatory Depression

Hypotension with bradycardia	*Hypotension with tachycardia*
Calcium channel blockers	β-adrenergic agonists
β-adrenergic blockers	Iron
Bretylium	Amatoxin-containing
Clonidine	mushrooms
Digitalis	Colchicine

Poisons that must be specifically requested
Antiepileptics
Benzodiazepines (some)
Caffeine
Emetine
Ethylene glycol
Fentanyl (and other "designer drugs")
Insulin
Laxatives
Oral hypoglycemic agents
PCP

LSD, lysergic acid diethylamide; OTC, over the counter; PCP, phencyclidine.
Reprinted from Wiley JF. Difficult diagnosis in toxicology. *Pediatr Clin North Am* 1991;38:725, with permission.

Clinicians should know the limitations of their toxicology laboratory. When 13 reference laboratories received blind samples containing known concentrations of drugs, more than 90% had unacceptable false-negative rates for barbiturates, amphetamines, cocaine, and morphine. In a study of children admitted for poisoning, 14% had overdosed with a substance not detected by testing available at their toxicology laboratory (172). Belson et al. (16) spoke to the other side of this issue. Of 234 childhood intoxications, 227 were either clinically suspected or detected by an enzyme immunoassay screen (EMIT) for a limited number of toxins. Seven required further high-pressure liquid chromatography (HPLC) for identification. The authors suggested that the added expense of the comprehensive HPLC testing was usually not warranted. However, no instances of intentional poisoning were included. These might involve more exotic toxins than those commonly ingested or detected by the limited screen. This recommendation also ignores the evidentiary value of specific and reliable toxin identification in abuse. Samples of all body fluids should be analyzed, including urine, blood, and vomitus/gastric aspirate. "Chain of custody" procedures are often indicated for toxicology samples.

Feldman et al. (46) described a child poisoned repeatedly with ipecac whose urine tested negative. Finally, a sample of vomitus from the child was positive on a thin-layer chromatography (TLC) toxicology screen, but was negative by mass spectrophotometric (mass spec) screening. A control, undiluted sample of syrup of ipecac also was negative by mass spec. The time elapsed since ingestion also affects results. When seven poisoned children were treated at the emergency department with ipecac, TLC toxicology screens of urine from all seven patients were negative. Five had positive and two had negative TLC screens of gastric contents for ipecac. The five children with positive gastric screens had vomited within 20 to 90 minutes of ingesting ipecac. The two children with negative TLC results had vomited 70 minutes after ingestion. Although specific for ipecac, TLC is not sensitive. HPLC is more sensitive and reliable in detecting ipecac, including in urine.

Clinicians may have to resort to unusual methods to confirm the diagnosis of inflicted poisoning. Proesmans et al. (120) described poisoning that produced recurrent renal failure in a 7-year-old boy. The boy's urine and stains on his underwear were fluorescent yellow. Subsequent TLC showed a band not present in control urine, identified as glafenin, an analgesic. The child was able to pick glafenin out of a "line-up" of similar-appearing tablets. He identified it as the "vitamins" he had been given by his mother. The author then ingested glafenin herself. Two hours later, her urine was fluorescent yellow and had chromatographic characteristics that matched the urine of her young patient. Confronted with this evidence, the mother confessed.

COMMONLY USED POISONS AND THEIR PRESENTATIONS

Ipecac

Intentional ipecac poisoning is relatively common (17,31,46,81,92,95,138,154). Syrup of ipecac is widely available without prescription and is often dispensed to families by physicians concerned about accidental poisoning in toddlers. Although ipecac is widely known to induce emesis immediately, prolonged administration or intoxication also causes colitis (92) and evidence of cardiac and skeletal muscle weakness (138). Creatine phosphokinase (CPK) and aldolase levels, as well as serum and urine levels of emetine, should be measured. Electrocardiogram and cardiac ultrasound may be helpful. Standard toxicology screens may not include emetine; it must be requested specifically. Even if ipecac is detected, laboratories may fail to report it because of its widespread use to treat ingestions.

Laxatives

Laxative abuse manifests with chronic or recurrent diarrhea, sometimes leading to fail-

ure to thrive. When a reasonable medical workup is unproductive, laxative administration should be suspected. Stimulant laxatives cause secretory diarrhea. Stools are voluminous and watery, even if the patient is not eating. Stools do not contain blood, pus, or abnormal concentrations of carbohydrates or fat. Further analysis reveals an increase in stool sodium and chloride concentrations and narrowing of the osmotic gap (53).

Ex-Lax contained phenolphthalein, but was recently reformulated to replace the phenolphthalein with sennasides. It is sold in a form that appears and tastes like a small bar of chocolate. Phenolphthalein may cause a pink tinge of the stool or the diaper, which sometimes is mistaken for blood. The presence of phenolphthalein or aloes can be detected by the pink color that appears when stool water or urine is alkalinized to a pH of 8.5 by adding drops of dilute potassium hydroxide. When dilute acid is added, the pink disappears.

Other laxatives are suspected if stool water contains elevated levels of sulfate, magnesium, or anthracines (2), or the child is hyperphosphatemic (149). Long-term abuse of anthracene, including senna, cascara, and aloes, causes deposition of brown pigment in the bowel mucosa, which is visible at sigmoidoscopy (168). Kudo et al. (80) described the identification of bisacodyl by gas chromatography/mass spec in an 11-year-old child with induced diarrhea.

Volk (168) described an 8-month-old child whose mother induced chronic diarrhea by feeding apple juice concentrate, which has a high osmotic load. Measurement of osmolarity and electrolyte concentration in fecal fluid also can help to diagnose laxative-induced diarrhea. If the osmolarity is less than twice the sum of the sodium and potassium concentrations in stool (no osmotic gap), then hyponatremia and high fecal electrolyte concentrations indicate secretory diarrhea. A low fecal urea content eliminates urine contamination. If the osmotic gap is more than 100 mmol/L and osmolarity is normal, it is reasonable to suspect administration of laxatives containing magnesium salts, such as Epsom salts (50,176).

Black and Red Pepper

A common form of punishment is putting soap or other noxious or irritating substances in the child's mouth. Sometimes the consequences can be disastrous. Cohle (28) described eight children who died after aspiration of pepper. In only one case was accidental ingestion considered. In the other cases, pepper was administered as punishment, and the perpetrators were charged with homicide. In four patients, the initial history was incorrect. The mother of a 5-month-old infant said the dead child had ingested the pepper herself. The estimated volume of pepper in the larynx and bronchi was 12 mL. The mother later confessed that she had given the pepper to prevent the baby from putting his fingers in his mouth.

Four of the eight children in the series had been abused previously, and all but one child were younger than 6 years. The one older child, aged 10 years, had been punished by his "Big Brother" for not eating breakfast. The man pinched the boy's nose closed and forced pepper and Worcestershire sauce in his mouth. The assailant had previously forced the child to ingest horseradish and Tabasco sauce, beaten the child, and held his head in the toilet. The authors emphasized the importance of a good history and a thorough scene investigation, including examination of the pepper container. A careful physical examination or autopsy to document mucosal injuries and evidence of physical abuse is needed. Estimate the amount of pepper ingested. They concluded, "Nearly all cases of pepper aspiration are a manifestation of child abuse."

Tominack and Spyker (164) described three children, ages 3, 5, and 7 years, who were disciplined repeatedly for minor offenses by administration of Tabasco sauce or hot peppers. "A split jalapeño pepper was placed in the child's mouth and a timer set for 15 to 20 minutes. If the child spit the pepper out, swallowed it or vomited before the time expired, he was given a fresh pepper and the timer was reset. Liquid dishwasher detergent or Tabasco sauce was given in a similar manner." The children complained of burning in their mouth, throat, and sometimes the anus with passage of stools. They told of crying at night from residual pain. They also had been disciplined by being beaten with a metal ruler. Authorities were alerted when one child appeared at school with the mouth taped shut with wide duct tape "wrapped securely around the head so that the neck was fixed in flexion and only the nostrils were exposed."

A 10-year-old boy who was seen at our hospital described being punished by having hot peppers placed in his mouth and a belt fastened around his feet. If he moved, the belt would be jerked, causing him to fall over backward and choke on the pepper. If he vomited, he was forced to eat another pepper. The child also had been physically assaulted. He had a BB gun shot at him and was orally sodomized by the same perpetrator, the mother's boyfriend (L.H. Keltner, unpublished data).

Use of hot pepper is abusive because it is painful and has the potential to cause mucosal injury to eyes and the respiratory and gastrointestinal tracts. The resulting pharyngeal edema may cause death. Physicians and child welfare workers should ask about whether children have had anything put into their mouths or if they were made to eat anything as punishment.

Salt Poisoning and Water Deprivation

Thirty-three cases of child abuse by salt administration are cited in the literature. Seven (21%) of the 33 had evidence of physical abuse, and 10 (30%) died (3,12,33,38,47,56, 100,102,103,116,128). Children poisoned with salt present with vomiting, lethargy, dehydration, hypothermia, and seizures. Serum sodium concentration is typically greater than 180 mEq/L, and urine sodium levels also are elevated. Salt may be given to treat or punish enuresis, along with water restriction.

Feldman and Robertson (47) described two children abused by salt poisoning and probable forcible water restriction. Both had evidence of physical abuse. The parents of one child said they had used salty foods to treat the child's sudden onset of voracious appetite and remarkable thirst. These behaviors were not seen in 20 days of hospitalization or thereafter in foster care. The other child, a 3-year-old girl, was reportedly found with a cup of salt beside her crib.

Friedman (56) described a 1-year-old boy who, during admission for failure to thrive, had a cardiac arrest and died. His serum sodium level was greater than 200 mEq/L. The mother was tried and found guilty of adding salt to his formula.

A 5-year-old child who was given spoonfuls of salt for enuresis was admitted to William Beaumont Army Medical Center with diarrhea, lethargy, and dehydration. His serum sodium value was 184 mEq/L, with a urine sodium content of 360 mEq/L and urine osmolarity of 860 mOsm/L. He also had inflicted burns on the feet and ankles (12).

A 6-year-old boy died of hyperkalemia and hypernatremia after eating food his stepfather had seasoned heavily with Lite Salt, a salt-substitute mixture of potassium chloride and sodium chloride. The stepfather intended to "break" the child of the habit of adding too much salt to his food (3).

Large amounts of salt must be administered forcibly to produce symptoms in a child out of infancy. Meadow (100) tried to give a 14-month-old child enough salt to duplicate a serum sodium level of 165 to 170 mmol/L. The child's mother had been able to achieve this level, apparently by salt administration. He was able, with difficulty, to give 20 g of salt, which raised the serum sodium level to only 147 mmol/L.

Desprez et al. (33) diagnosed water deprivation and probable salt intoxication in a girl just younger than 3 years who was hospitalized with a serum sodium level of 186 mmol/L, a urine sodium level of 178 mmol/L, and a urine osmolarity of 710 mOsm/L. She complained constantly of thirst. At school she had been seen licking water from glass windows and drinking from puddles. She had been hospitalized previously for failure to thrive, trichotillomania, and encopresis.

Meadow (102) described the largest series of salt poisoning. Of 12 child victims, three had other fabricated illness; four, failure to thrive or neglect; one, other physical abuse; and two died. A median of 3 months of abuse preceded diagnosis. In most cases the abuse had been repetitive.

Bizarre eating and drinking habits have characterized psychosocial dwarfism. These include stealing or hoarding food, eating from garbage cans, and drinking urine and water from toilets or fishbowls (68). These symptoms appear to be caused not only by emotional deprivation but also by deliberate withholding of food and water from children by abusive caretakers. Salt, or other crystalline substances such as sugar, given in sufficient quantities to remain as undissolved crystals in the stomach, is radiopaque.

Water Intoxication

Water can be forcibly administered as punishment. Children may have apnea, seizures, and hypothermia. Serum sodium concentrations are 125 mmol/L or lower. Eight children who became ill after being forced to drink water as punishment were reported. Two children also had evidence of physical abuse (25%), and all survived (74,108,158,162).

Keating et al. (74) described one child in a series of 34 pediatric patients with water intoxication who had been the victim of "malicious forcing of water on a child." This 8-year-old girl had been physically abused as an infant. She had threatened to stab her foster parent to death. After "much counseling," the foster parents chose to punish the child by having her drink water. After being forced to drink 12 glasses, she lost consciousness. Her sodium concentration was 120 mmol/L.

Mortimer (108) reported the case of a 4.5-year-old boy who had generalized convulsions, hypothermia, and a serum sodium level of 117 mmol/L. He had a fracture of the arm and multiple bruises. The foster parents, who had cared for him for 7 months, said that the child craved fluid and drank from bizarre sources. These included flower pots and a water hose. The child said that the foster father had forced him to drink from the hose. After diuresis, the child was discharged to a new foster home and had no further fluid or electrolyte problems.

Chadwick (unpublished data) treated two critically ill hyponatremic children who had acute water intoxication. One had sustained anal lacerations, probably as a result of water enemas, and the other had a rupture of the stomach when water was administered with a garden hose. As Mortimer stated, "Presumably if water is forced into the oral cavity . . . the victim has only two options. Either he inhales the water with the probability of drowning or he swallows the water with the consequence of acute water intoxication" (108).

Tileli and Ophoven (162) described a case of water intoxication. They suggested that many, if not most, cases of apparent psychosocial dwarfism with bizarre eating/drinking habits are directly related to abusive behavior involving food and water.

A 4.9-year-old girl was admitted to the hospital after being found limp and unresponsive by her parents. They said that she had been drinking from a garden hose over the last 8 hours. At the time of hospitalization, she was unconscious. She had generalized hypertonic extensor posturing and responded only to deep pain. Her serum sodium concentration was 108 mEq/L. She had multiple ecchymoses and abrasions, including injuries around the mouth. The child's height and weight were less than the 5th percentile, and her bone age was 2.5 years. When her serum sodium content was corrected, the child regained consciousness. She stated that her parents had forced her to drink water as punishment. She would "be good if she didn't have to drink any more water." Her mother admitted forcing the child to drink large amounts of water as punishment for bed-wetting. She also admitted severe corporal punishment inflicted by herself and the child's siblings, whom she could not control. The child gained 2.58 kg (5.5 lb) during a 1-week stay in the hospital (162).

Water intoxication occurs for many reasons other than abuse. Of 34 water-intoxicated children described by Keating (74), only one had been forced to drink water as punishment. (One other infant was readmitted later with a nonaccidental fracture of the humerus.) Nonabusive causes of water intoxication include infant swimming lessons, iatrogenic administration of oral or parenteral water, drinking quantities of cold water for the pain of toothache, and ingestion of excessive water to dilute urine for drug testing or during athletic events, like marathon runs. Parents who run out of formula cause a growing problem of water intoxication in infants. They substitute either dilute formula or plain water. The daily allotment of formula provided by the Supplemental Food Program for Women, Infants, and Children (WIC) is indeed "supplemental." It is not sufficient to provide adequate calories for infants aged 4 months or older. If a family does not or cannot buy additional formula, and offers water instead, the infant may drink enough water to become hyponatremic.

Carbon Monoxide

Carbon monoxide poisoning of children can be either accidental or homicidal. Most intentional cases occur when a depressed parent attempts suicide by carbon monoxide poisoning and "takes the children with them." Adelson (3) described five children who died of carbon monoxide exposure when a parent (one father and two mothers) attempted suicide. Ironically, all the parents survived. If a child is poisoned by carbon monoxide and the parent has no signs or symptoms, further investigation is warranted. However, because carbon monoxide is heavier than oxygen, it concentrates near the floor. This places short or recumbent people at greater risk of intoxication.

Accidental carbon monoxide poisoning occurs when fuel is burned in inadequately ventilated spaces. Most exposures involve motor vehicles, home furnaces, water heaters, and indoor use of barbecues or portable gas and kerosene heaters. Paint stripper containing methylene chloride can be absorbed through the skin and be converted to carbon monox-ide. Cases are not always easy to unravel. Pi-att et al. (115) described a 2.5-month-old in-fant with recurrent neurologic deterioration that progressed to death. It was discovered in retrospect that the child's symptoms had worsened each time she was transported in the family car. These included 30-minute rides to the physician's office and the hospital. No carbon monoxide was measurable in the front seat, but toxic levels of carbon monoxide were found to be leaking through a small crack in the floor of the back seat where the infant always rode.

Acetaminophen and Aspirin

Acetaminophen and aspirin are inexpensive and readily available. Because they are used commonly, their presence on a toxicology screen may pass unnoticed. Greene et al. (60,66) described a 6-week-old child initially thought to have been accidentally poisoned with acetaminophen. The child was hospital-ized for 11 days and given 17 doses of acetyl-cysteine. The history included the admission that he had been given, in error, two forms of acetaminophen with different brand names (Tempra and Tylenol). However, 6 weeks after discharge, the child died at home. An autopsy was not performed. The death was attributed to SIDS. Several months later, a 3-week-old sib-ling was admitted for possible seizures. A urine drug screen was positive for phenothiazines and diazepam. The mother, who had ceased breast-feeding 1 week before, denied giving medication to the child or taking medication herself. The infant was placed in protective custody. The authors stated, "Cases of poorly explained overdosages in infancy should raise the question of intentional poisoning. Physi-cians must maintain a certain index of suspi-cion about these cases as they do with cases in-volving unexplained injuries . . . cases like this support the current trend to obtain autopsies in cases of suspected SIDS" (see also Chapter 20). Meadow (103) also described a 3-month-old boy who developed hepatic failure after poisoning with paracetamol by his father.

Insulin and Oral Hypoglycemics

Several case reports demonstrate child abuse by administration of insulin or oral hypoglycemic agents (13,23,37,99,104,128, 177). The clinical presentations included lethargy, coma, and unexplained hypo-glycemia. Ketosis is usually lacking; its presence suggests that the hypoglycemia did not result from a hyperinsulinemic state. In-vestigation ultimately reveals a probable source of insulin, needles, or oral hypo-glycemics, often of a family member who is diabetic. In one case, a 13-month-old boy had a 35-hour period of severe hypoglycemia in the hospital despite aggressive infusions of 10% and 20% glucose. He had a 3-year-old brother with "brittle" diabetes, whose glucose lability also may have been attribut-able to deliberate administration of inappro-priate doses of insulin (13).

Several methods have been used to deter-mine if child abuse is the cause of hypo-glycemia. C-peptide levels should be mea-sured. If the insulin is of endogenous pancreatic origin, C-peptide is released in an equimolar ratio. Human C-peptide does not crossreact with porcine or bovine C-peptide. "The triad of hyperinsulinism, hypoglycemia, and a low serum C-peptide level is considered to be diagnostic of exogenous hyperinsulin-ism" (99).

An early case was proved by adding a tracer to the suspected vial of insulin. Serial plasma samples can be used to determine the time of insulin administration and whether short- or long-acting insulin was used. Species-spe-cific antiserum also has been used to provide more certain evidence of exogenous bovine or porcine insulin poisoning (13).

Hyperglycemia, again without ketosis, can result from forced feeding of excess sugars. McGuire and Feldman (95) described a child with recurrent coma accompanying hyper-glycemic, nonketotic dehydration. Each time he had profuse watery, osmotic diarrhea and hypokalemia. He finally related that his mother was forcing him to drink honey. Ven-ter and Joubert (166) also reported a 22-

month-old child with diabetic symptoms due to sugar administration.

Household Substances

Caffeine

One case of death from intentional poisoning with caffeine has been reported. An ambulance was called to the home of a 14-month-old girl who was vomiting. It was sent away by the mother, who said the child was all right. Three hours later, the ambulance was called again. The now moribund child was brought to the hospital where she died. She had been admitted 11 days before with unexplained lethargy, irritability, and bruises. Autopsy revealed healing fractures of three ribs and a healing laceration and hematoma of the spleen. Injuries were thought, by microscopic findings, to be at least 10 to 14 days old. The blood caffeine level was 117 mg/L, and the blood theophylline level was 36 mg/L, evidence of prolonged toxicity. Investigation revealed abundant "amphetamine look-alike" caffeine capsules in the home. The mother was known to abuse these pills. The mother's boyfriend sold them on the street. Both caretakers denied knowledge of how the poisoning or injuries occurred (107).

Accidental caffeine poisoning has been reported in four children, two of whom died. A 15-month-old mistakenly given 90 mL of 20% caffeine solution (approximately 18 g) in the hospital died 5 hours later. A 5-year-old child died after ingesting 53 diuretic tablets containing about 3 g of caffeine. This case should have been investigated with an eye to possible abuse or neglect, unless the pills were small and tasted particularly good. A 1-year-old child who ingested 10 to 15 small No-Doz tablets recovered in 48 hours. Scene investigation revealed a shoebox containing 20 different bottled medications and dozens of loose pills, raising the issue of neglect (153). Another 1-year-old child was severely poisoned after taking eight to 10 caffeine diet pills. She developed serious respiratory failure and required two treatments with charcoal hemoperfusion. She was hospitalized for a total of 6 weeks (34). Rivenes (124) described caffeine poisoning presenting as unexplained tachycardia. The infant had been given it by his father 3 weeks before his death after inflicted head injury (124).

Nicotine

No cases of intentional poisoning with nicotine are reported, although accidental ingestions of nicotine are common. In one study of 51 children who ingested cigarettes, 45% developed signs or symptoms of toxicity. Of five children who ingested nicotine resin gum, four were adversely affected. Probably because unwrapping and chewing gum takes more dexterity, the children who chewed or swallowed nicotine gum were older, aged 20 months to 9 years. The children who ingested cigarettes were younger. All except one was younger than 18 months (and perhaps closer to the ground). Signs and symptoms included agitation, lethargy, tachycardia, hypotension, abdominal pain, vomiting, and seizures. Aspects of this study raise concerns about whether some of the children were victims of nonaccidental exposure. The authors reported that the youngest child in their study was 5 months old. Forty (78%) of the 51 children were between 7 and 12 months old. It would be an advanced 5-month-old child who could locomote to, pick up, and ingest cigarettes (151).

Industrial Compounds

Saulsbury et al. (136) described intentional poisoning of an 11-month-old boy with an intravenous injection of a hydrocarbon. The child had been hospitalized previously for episodes of apnea. During a second hospitalization for seizures, he had a sudden respiratory arrest. A strong odor of hydrocarbon was noted on his breath, and oily droplets were found in the intravenous line. Gas chromatography revealed naphtha, a hydrocarbon widely used as an industrial solvent and the major constituent of lighter fluid. The mother admitted injecting something into her son's intravenous line. She was found guilty of attempted manslaughter. One of the 10 cases of the surgical manifestations of MSBP reported by Lacey (81) presented after forced instillation of cooking oil in the child's nares. Aspiration pneumonia resulted.

Friedman (56) has warned fellow otolaryngologists to be aware that caustic ingestions may be an overlooked form of child abuse or neglect. Dine and McGovern (37) reported a case of a 10-year-old girl who was forced to ingest lye-contaminated toilet bowl cleaner by her mother. The mother tried unsuccessfully to commit suicide. The child died of complications of lye ingestion after 5 years. Another case of suspected purposeful administration of a caustic substance involved an 11-year-old girl who had recurrent gastrointestinal ulceration. She underwent esophageal dilation, gastrostomy, fundal plication, placement of eight central venous catheters, total parenteral nutrition, and several exploratory surgeries before foster placement "cured" her symptoms (132).

A 20-month-old girl had upper airway and esophageal burns as a result of exposure to a lye solution used in the production of crack cocaine. Esophageal strictures formed, requiring insertion of a gastrostomy tube and central hyperalimentation. The lye had been left in a cup on the kitchen table after a party the night before. The mother denied that cocaine had been used at the party, but the infant's urine drug screen was positive for cocaine metabolites (77). Gotschlich (59) described oropharyngeal and esophageal injury in a 21-month-old due to forced ingestion of muriatic acid pool cleaner. The child's 3-year-old sister had had similar, but milder, symptoms a month before after care by the same sitter. She had been hospitalized and treated with repeated doses of dexamethasone for presumed croup.

Ethylene glycol is an extremely toxic solvent used in automotive antifreeze and windshield de-icer solutions. Most glycol poisonings are accidental or suicidal. Because ethylene glycol is colorless, odorless, and sweet, accidental poisoning is not rare. This substance frequently poisons dogs. A typical presentation includes inebriation without the odor of alcohol on the breath, central nervous system depression, metabolic acidosis with a widened anion gap, and calcium oxalate crystalluria. Saladino and Shannon (135) described an 8-month-old child who was the victim of apparent intentional and probably repeated poisoning with ethylene glycol. Because ethylene glycol is not detected by routine toxicology screens or by the methods used to measure other alcohols, the diagnosis was made serendipitously during investigation for inborn errors of metabolism. Studies revealed elevated levels of breakdown products of ethylene glycol: glycine and glycolic acid. Serum from the first day of admission was reanalyzed and showed an ethylene glycol level of 85mg/dl. Woolf (174) also described a 6-month-old girl with recurrent hyperglycinemia and urinary glycolic aciduria, which was initially thought to have resulted from an inherited metabolic disorder. Ethylene glycol was finally identified in the infant's blood and bottle. The opposite situation occurred in a case of Shoemaker's (146) in which propionic acid was misidentified on gas chromatography as ethylene glycol. The infant was placed in protective custody, only to have recurrent symptoms 2 months later. A correct diagnosis of methylmalonic acidemia was then made.

An unusual case of child abuse involved a 9-year-old boy who came to the emergency department with his left eye glued shut with cyanoacrylate adhesive (18). The history, that an unknown child had thrown the glue, did not fit the injury. The lower lid was everted and had an even application of glue, consistent with forceful opening of the eye and reflex constriction of the lids. The child was living with an alcoholic, violent father. He had been treated for a fractured clavicle and rib at age 4 years. The mother had two black eyes. She said she could not guarantee the safety of the child if he was returned home. Conservative medical treatment was unsuccessful. The lids were separated with the child under anesthesia. The case was reported to child welfare authorities.

Prescription Drugs

Not surprisingly, the drugs involved in child abuse by poisoning are those most often prescribed for adults. Any drug available may be used. Case reports include poisoning with barbiturates, chloral hydrate, phenothiazines, diazepam, tricyclic antidepressants, diuretics, antiepileptics, anticoagulants, theophylline, and furosemide (Table 16.1) (25,70,95,93, 158). "Terrifying possibilities of child abuse therefore abound with the multiple drugs available with and without prescriptions" (2).

Alcohol and Illicit Drugs

Prenatal Exposure

Prenatal exposure to drugs and alcohol can cause damage to the developing fetus. The reader is referred to a recent review of the literature (14). Prenatal exposure to drugs or alcohol has been considered child neglect or abuse. It is argued that if a woman voluntarily becomes pregnant and intends to give birth and raise the child, then she has an obligation to that child. The Michigan Appeals Court has written (98), "Since a child has a legal right to begin life with a sound mind and body, . . . we believe it is within this best interest to examine all prenatal conduct bearing on that right . . . . We hold that a newborn suffering narcotics withdrawal symptoms as a consequence of maternal drug addiction may properly be considered a neglected child."

Children raised in addicted households are at risk of both accidental and intentional poisoning. This involves not only ordinary toxins but also substances of abuse. It is naive to think that parents who use drugs and alcohol to treat their own physical and emotional distress will not do the same with their children.

Howard (69) related that in his study of addicted infants, "A significant number of parents experienced their first exposure to drugs and alcohol through their own parent's encouragement. One mother . . . was introduced to heroin by her own father. Another mother told us that when she was upset as a child, her mother would mix her a drink and say, 'Drink this, it will make you feel better.' A third mother stated that her own father 'shot me up with heroin when I threatened to call the cops on him.' "

Schwartz and Einhorn (141) listed four methods by which children may become intoxicated with substances of abuse: accidental ingestion of drugs or alcohol (such as chewing on butts of drug-laced cigarettes), passive inhalation, deliberate poisoning, or accepting drugs offered by an older child. These methods cannot always be distinguished. In one report of a child intoxicated by cocaine, the authors seem to have accepted at face value statements by the parents that they had not given their child cocaine because they would not "waste" their cocaine on the infant (63). Almost all cases of intoxication of preadolescent children by alcohol or illegal drugs represent neglect. The caretakers had knowledge of the risk of exposure in the environment. Table 16.3 summarizes reported cases of children poisoned by alcohol and drugs of abuse.

Accidental Exposure

Drugs can pass through breast milk. The American Academy of Pediatrics' committee statement on drugs in breast milk should be seen for reference (6). They may produce apnea and convulsions in the nursing infant (27). In one case, a mother said she had used a topical cocaine powder on her sore nipples for pain relief (26). At our facility, we tell mothers who are abusing alcohol or drugs that they cannot breast-feed. We had one infant admitted with apnea after ingesting cocaine through breast milk. Another woman, when advised of the dangers of using cocaine while breast-feeding, said she had witnessed a friend's baby having convulsions after the mother used cocaine and then breast-fed. Another mother, when asked why she continued to breast-feed and use cocaine, said she hoped that breast-feeding would help her stop using (it did not).

The term "morning after syndrome" was coined in the 1960s to describe children who became intoxicated after ingesting the dregs of alcohol left in glasses after adult parties the night before. Recently the same phenomenon has been described with cocaine. The parents found a 9-month-old child in the living room playing with the uncleared remains of the food and drink. A party the night before involved alcohol and cocaine powder. Shortly thereafter, the child had seizures. On admission to the hospital, she was hyperthermic and hypertensive. Urine toxicologic analysis was positive for cocaine at the time of admission, and for cocaine and metabolites 36 hours later (125).

In homes in which adult addicts are in methadone maintenance programs, "take-home" doses of methadone mixed with fruit juice are attractive for ingestion by children. This may have lethal consequences. A few deaths of children occur this way each year in the New York City area (32).

Accidental poisoning by drugs is not a new problem. Among 2,000 child welfare cases reported by the Queensland Society for the Prevention of Cruelty to Children (160) between 1891 and 1897 were several cases of apparently accidental poisoning by drugs. Three infants younger than 2 years died of narcotics overdose. A toddler died after ingesting brandy while his mother was attending mass. In that era, some commonly used infant remedies contained toxic substances such as opium, bromide, and a mixture of opium and gin. Concerns of neglect were raised in 12.3% of 1,746 childhood ingestions admitted to three pediatric hospitals from 1988 to 1990 (161).

Passive Inhalation

Children have been intoxicated by passive inhalation of free-base cocaine or phencyclidine (PCP) smoked in poorly ventilated rooms or closed cars. Signs and symptoms include lethargy, vomiting, nausea, apnea, seizures, and coma (11,63,106,141).

Deliberate Poisoning

Sturner et al. (152) described a 6-week-old infant who was found unresponsive in his crib by his mother. On arrival in the emergency department, he was cold and stiff, and had a clump of hair clenched in his fist. The only findings at autopsy were cocaine in urine,

blood, gastric contents, cerebrospinal fluid, and the formula in the infant's bottle. Investigation revealed that a 15-year-old stepbrother, who had assaulted the mother the night before, might have poisoned the formula.

Deliberate poisoning may occur when caretakers wish to amuse themselves or to sedate a child. In a survey of middle-class adolescent girls enrolled in drug treatment, 11% said they and their friends had deliberately intoxicated children with whom they were baby-sitting (142). Nine girls admitted to intoxicating 25 children, aged 5 months to 10 years. The teenage baby-sitters, usually acting as a group, had blown several puffs of marijuana smoke into the noses, mouths, or faces of the children. They often repeatedly intoxicated the same child. The median was 4 times, with a range of 1 to 15 times per child. The children had exhibited signs of intoxication, including sleepiness, giggling, ataxia, hyperactivity, and crying. Older child victims were warned to keep the episodes a secret. None of the parents had discovered the abuse. Three teenage baby-sitters said they had also given beer to children as young as 5 months. Another study confirmed these findings. Of 25 teenagers who used marijuana daily, 20% convinced a younger sibling to try marijuana, 52% got a pet dog or cat "high," and 12% got an infant "high" while baby-sitting (21).

In an article concerning the forensic pathology of drug-related child abuse, Densen-Gerber (32) stated,

> Another type of child-abuse death uniquely seen only in drug-saturated environments occurs when the addicted mother or boyfriend injects heroin or methadone in the child's milk or juice. This deed is done to sedate the child so that the cries do not interfere with the parent's drug taking, prostitution or other activities. Occasionally, it arises out of pure sadism by the adult who, while high on drugs, feels it would be a great joke to see the reactions of a child or pet, usually a dog. Death has occurred from such activity.

She described a 10-month-old child who was found dead in bed. The infant was thought to be a victim of SIDS until autopsy revealed multiple injection sites on its thigh. Toxicology screens revealed heroin, morphine, and quinine (used to cut street drugs) in the baby's tissues. The mother admitted that her boyfriend had repeatedly injected heroin into the infant when annoyed by its crying. This time, the infant had "overdosed." The mother's chief concern was to prevent her boyfriend–pimp from going to jail.

Deliberate intoxication of children is not a new problem. In the 19th century, reports of the Queensland Society for the Prevention of Cruelty to Children (161) cited 37 cases involving "supplying intoxicants to children," as well as 13 cases of "sending children to hotels for drink," and 17 cases of "neglect through drunkenness."

Phencyclidine

Six children with symptomatic PCP poisoning were reported by pediatricians at the UCLA Medical Center (171). The youngest victim was 11 days old. The authors collected an additional 10 reported cases involving children aged 6 years and younger. Symptoms of PCP intoxication in children, which were somewhat different from those in adults, included bizarre behavior (such as lethargy, staring spells, and intermittent periods of unresponsiveness), ataxia (most apparent in the toddler group), and vertical and horizontal nystagmus. Pupil changes are inconsistent. The child gives an initial impression of extreme agitated attention, while actually being poorly responsive. Muscle tone is normal, decreased, or increased. In the latter case, prolonged isometric muscle contractions and opisthotonic posturing can occur with subsequent elevation of serum CPK levels. One child required resuscitation after a full cardiac arrest at home, and one infant had bloody spinal fluid on two taps, suggesting an intracerebral hemorrhage. In all cases, caretakers denied the possibility of exposure to PCP or any other drugs. When the hospital Child Abuse Team presented the toxicology data to the families, the majority admitted that PCP was available. However, they had no explanation how the exposure occurred. Accidental ingestion, purposeful administration, and passive inhalation were all considered possible.

The use of PCP in adult caretakers places children at risk. The drug induces symptoms of psychotic illness with aggression and unusual physical strength. A 30-year-old woman intoxicated with PCP attempted to drown and smother her 4-year-old son. She then pulled a knife on her husband, saying she wanted to see blood dripping. She was actively hallucinating. She had to be placed in four-point restraints and sedated heavily. After recovering, she had no memory of these happenings and no knowledge of how she had ingested the drug (54).

The use of PCP seems to be relatively localized to areas such as Los Angeles and Washington, DC (40). It is important to remember that PCP is not included on routine toxicology screens and must be requested specifically. TLC is not so sensitive as EMIT in detecting PCP and its analogues (115).

Marijuana

Both accidental and purposeful intoxication with marijuana has been reported (Table 16.3). In our experience, minor intoxication is relatively common and is likely to go undetected. In a review of 105 pediatric poisonings treated at Hospital Sainte Justine in Montreal (82), three children had become comatose after accidental ingestion of about 1 g of hashish. The authors of this study (personal communication) also have seen children who were sedated by adults intentionally blowing marijuana smoke in their faces. In one report, (97), five children between the ages of 1 and 4 years became intoxicated after ingesting 1/2 to one marijuana joint or reefer. The joints were estimated to contain 3.6 to 15 mg of tetrahydrocannabinol (THC) each. Symptoms developed within 20 minutes and included stupor and slow pupillary response. A 2-year-old child required atropine and positive-pressure ventilation for respiratory depression.

Cocaine

As cocaine use has become widespread among adults, cocaine exposure and intoxication has become common in children (Tables 16.3 and 16.4). Children may inhale crack cocaine fumes in cars or small rooms, accidentally ingest cocaine, or be given cocaine deliberately. The "body packer syndrome" is well described in adults who use body cavities to hide drugs. If the drugs are absorbed, death can occur. Children are not immune to this syndrome. In a brief report (121), the parents of a 4.5-year-old girl accused each other of inserting rock cocaine in the child's rectum to hide it. The child's examination revealed genital and anal erythema, anal laxity, and a small anal fissure. Toxicologic analysis was positive for a cocaine metabolite.

Cocaine has become a strikingly prevalent environmental contaminant (Table 16.4). Rogers et al. (126) found cocaine or its metabolites in 40% of 43 infants in Los Angeles who died at younger than 2 days without an obvious cause of death at autopsy. One infant, stillborn at 30 weeks with no evidence of malformation or placental abnormalities, had a level of cocaine in the range considered fatal for adults. Rogers (126) concluded that cocaine exposure is an important cause of unexpected fetal and perinatal death in Los Angeles County. He recommended, in areas where cocaine use is high, measuring cocaine and benzoylecgonine concentrations in infants younger than 2 days who died without an obvious cause identified at autopsy. Mirchandani et al. (106) reported toxicologic evidence of cocaine exposure in 16 (2.6%) of approximately 600 infants dying unexpectedly before age 2 years in the Philadelphia area.

Several surveys provide additional evidence of the prevalence of cocaine exposure in childhood and adolescence. If these studies, done at large urban hospitals, can be generalized, clinicians can expect that 2% to 6% of children seen in emergency departments with complaints unrelated to drug exposure and 11% of children presenting with unexplained seizures will have positive toxicologic results for cocaine or its metabolites (Table 16.3) (76,79,131,144).

A series of six cases representing the spectrum of infant deaths related to cocaine as seen by a medical examiner in Rhode Island was described in 1991 (152). These cases included one involving a 35-weeks-gestation fetus that died *in utero* with cocaine intoxication. A 7-week-old infant was found dead when his parents awakened from cocaine-induced sleep. Autopsy showed that the infant, who had tested positive for cocaine at birth, had died of severe dehydration and starvation, complicated by a necrotic, ulcerated diaper rash. A 6-week-old infant died of acute cocaine intoxication after ingesting formula that had been laced with cocaine by a 15-year-old stepbrother. The author recommended that "all fetuses, infants, and children should be tested for cocaine and other drugs at autopsy examination." Additionally, a scene investigation should be done, with consideration given to passive drug intoxication, active contamination of baby food and formula, or suffocation (152).

Signs and symptoms alerting clinicians to possible cocaine exposure include lethargy, unsteady gait, seizures, focal neurologic deficit, intracranial hemorrhage, hemorrhagic diarrhea (123), pharyngeal or esophageal inflammation, hyperthermia, tachycardia, cardiac arrhythmias, and death (11).

A positive toxicology screen for cocaine in a child almost always means abuse or neglect and should be reported. It is important to rule out legitimate medical or dental exposure to cocaine. TAC (tetracaine, adrenaline, and cocaine) has been used as a topical anesthetic when suturing lacerations in children. It is absorbed and can produce a positive toxicology result for cocaine or its metabolites within 15 minutes (159).

Alcohol

Alcohol intoxication in young children is a serious problem. Beattie et al. (15) reported that 1,000 children younger than 15 years are admitted to hospital each year in England and

Wales with acute alcohol intoxication. In their series of 143 acutely intoxicated children, 53 were younger than 7 years. Most episodes were related to "accidental access in the child's own home . . . often aggravated by domestic upset or an apparent general lack of surveillance." Several cases raised concern about abuse or neglect. Fifteen were classic "Sunday morning" scenarios. Toddlers drank alcohol left out from parties the night before while their parents were still asleep. Four toddlers became intoxicated at family parties. Two were given alcohol by a baby-sitter or parent. Five children were accompanied to the hospital by drunken parents.

Complications were common. Ten children younger than 7 years arrived at the hospital unconscious from hypoglycemia, and one child was seizing. Hypothermia was seen in children presumed to have been drinking out of doors. Physical trauma related to intoxication was seen in 14 cases. Ten children were unconscious after sustaining head trauma from falls while drunk; four required facial sutures, and one was treated for burns. Nine boys had been forced to drink to the point of drunkenness, one at gunpoint.

A 1980 report from Austria (61) details a case of child abuse by alcohol poisoning. A 6-year-old girl was forced by her father to drink about 100 g of plum brandy, several times the lethal dose. The father admitted punishing the child because she was "insolent and not educable." She was admitted to hospital deeply comatose, in shock, with a rectal temperature of 34°C. She had evidence of physical abuse. Her injuries included multiple hematomas and traumatic alopecia. Blood alcohol content was 4.98 g/L. She required mechanical ventilation and peritoneal dialysis.

Two reports concern fatalities from poisoning by alcohol. A 1-year-old infant died after the mother's boyfriend gave him rum and Coke to stop his crying. Autopsy revealed erosion of the fundus of the stomach and a blood alcohol content of 0.12% (122). In the second case, a 5-year-old child was found cold and stiff with cloudy corneas after his parents called police to report that he was "breathing funny." Au-topsy showed that he died of poisoning with Avon cologne (70% alcohol) and salicylates. Ethanol levels were 74 mg/dL in blood and 293 mg/dL in gastric contents. Multiple contusions were evident on the face, back, and extremities. The mother and her boyfriend pled guilty to manslaughter (24).

In years past, breast-feeding mothers were advised to drink alcohol to facilitate milk let-down. This practice may not be benign. Passive alcohol intoxication has been observed in breast-fed infants (163). Regular exposure to alcohol through breast milk also may have a detrimental effect on the motor development of breast-fed infants (89).

The differential diagnosis of alcohol poisoning includes ingestion of mouthwash, which comes in attractive colors and pleasant flavors. It is a common cause of accidental ethanol poisoning in children (84). The depressant effect of alcohols increases with the length of their carbon chain. Isopropyl or "rubbing" alcohol has twice the narcotic effect of ethyl ("drinking") alcohol. It is poorly absorbed through the skin, but well absorbed through inhalation. Accidental isopropyl alcohol intoxication has been described in infants who were sponged with rubbing alcohol to reduce fever or were dressed with a diaper or swaddled in a sheet wet with alcohol (94).

Not all cases of isopropanol poisoning are accidental. In one report (45), calculations indicated that a 2.5-year-old, deeply comatose boy had ingested almost 100 mL of rubbing alcohol. He had evidence of physical abuse. He had been admitted 3 weeks previously for scald burns to the lower extremities and genital area. The German physicians treating the child thought that the large amount of alcohol indicated a forced ingestion. The case could not be investigated further because the boy's father was an American soldier who was ordered back to the U.S.

DIFFERENTIAL DIAGNOSIS

Every effort should be made to exclude other causes of poisoning before making the diagnosis of intentional poisoning. Causes that might be missed without a thorough investigation include dispensing errors, substitution errors, use of natural remedies, and accidental poisoning with substances that are not detected on a toxicology screen and cause symptoms mimicking abuse.

In the last category is the decongestant imidazoline, an ingredient in many over-the-counter drugs for nasal and ophthalmic use. Two toddlers had significant toxicity after accidentally ingesting Visine and Murine Plus eye drops (67). Clinical signs of poisoning include periods of hyperactivity alternating with periods of depression of the cardiopulmonary and central nervous systems, tremor, hallucinations, seizures, apnea, and coma. The therapeutic index of this drug is low; "appropriate" administration of this drug in doses as small as one or two nose drops to an infant has caused respiratory depression. Routine toxicology screens rarely pick up imidazoline substances in blood or urine, so a thorough history is important. Further confusion can occur when accidental poisoning produces lesions usually associated with abuse. For example, overuse of imidazole decongestants has caused subarachnoid hemorrhage and cerebral infarction.

Accidental diphenoxylate-atropine (Lomotil) poisoning can be confusing because it can cause both early atropinic effects and/or later opiate effects. Recurrent symptoms of respiratory and central nervous system depression can occur 12 to 24 hours after the ingestion, leading to suspicion of ongoing poisoning. Cerebral edema causing death has occurred in three patients (91).

The differential diagnosis becomes particularly difficult when a child with physical signs of abuse (bruises, fractures, abnormal genital findings) also is poisoned. Suspicion of intentional poisoning is naturally higher, but accidental poisoning as well as suicide attempts are more likely to occur in an abusive household (1).

Alternative Medicine and Vitamins

Physicians evaluating children who appear to have been poisoned should ask about plants in and around the home, herbal remedies, and vitamin doses. Parents may poison their children intentionally or unintentionally through the use of herbal remedies or vitamins. In a patient population that is likely to use traditional medicines, these substances are a potential source of serious poisoning. Of 1,306 patients admitted to a South African hospital for acute poisoning, 15.8% had been poisoned by traditional medicines. Children between ages 1 and 5 years were affected most often (64%). Traditional medicines accounted for 52% of all deaths, carrying a three-fold higher risk of mortality than other poisons (166).

A 5-month-old Indian child, who was treated by a Native American "curer" with an unidentified rectal suppository, required admission to an intensive care unit for screaming, hematemesis, severe tachycardia, and seizures. A serum theophylline level 12 hours after the suppository was given was 141 µg/mL (165). Another infant died as a result of the mother's ingestion during pregnancy of a tea containing coltsfoot (*Tussilago farfara*) and butterbur (*Petasites officinalis*). Both plants contain pyrrolizidine alkaloids, which are potent liver toxins (157).

Two cases of severe hepatic disease caused by herbal teas have been described in Mexican-American children from Arizona. One child developed cirrhosis. The other child, aged 2 months, died of what appeared to be Reye syndrome after the parents gave an herbal tea supposedly containing an innocuous herb gnaphalium, folk-named *gordolobo*. On analysis, the tea actually contained *Senecio*, which is similar in appearance to harvesters but is highly toxic. The authors stated,

> The routine use of herbal teas may not be elicited in a drug history, nor would their use be considered as a cause of distress. Administration of herbs may be denied. Further, herbs may be known by several folk names, depending on the geographic location. Since nomenclature may be confusing, analysis of any ingested herb must be done in suspected cases (55).

The use of toxic herbal teas was once so common in Jamaica that an educational campaign against their use was successful in reducing the national incidence of venoocclusive liver disease in children (139). Adults have been poisoned by drinking herbal tea containing mistletoe (*Verbascum album*) and Chinese herbal medicine containing aconite (*Aconitum* sp) (157).

Lead-containing folk remedies such as azarcon, albayalde, and greta are commonly used by Mexican-American families and healers and have caused serious poisoning (8). An abdominal radiograph showing heavy metal densities can help make the diagnosis.

Hmong folk remedies can contain mixtures of vegetable medicines, opium, and Western drugs. These remedies have caused toxicity in infants. A Hmong backache remedy used by Southeast Asian immigrants in Wisconsin was found to contain a complex combination of aspirin, acetaminophen, caffeine, and opium (133,150).

Other sources of accidental poisoning to consider are contamination of water from wells or storage containers, home-canned foods, household or outdoor plants, and field mushrooms. Intentional mushroom poisoning has not been reported. However, we observed a 9-year-old boy whose 15-year-old, conduct-disordered sibling had brewed tea from mushrooms. He gave the neighbor children the tea. Only his sibling became symptomatic, with visual hallucinations, confusion, and agitation. His skin was red and dry, and his pupils widely dilated. Small-capped, brown mushrooms with long, thin stems were brought in the cheesecloth in which they had been brewed. The child recovered by the next morning. Methemoglobinemia has occurred in infants fed homemade baby food high in nitrates or well water into which fertilizer has leached.

Vitamin intoxication has occurred as part of megavitamin therapy for disorders such as learning disabilities or minimal brain dysfunction. A 7-year-old child was admitted to our hospital with symptoms of toxicity after large doses of vitamins A and D were prescribed by a chiropractor, and a naturopath gave additional doses. A case of vitamin administration requiring intervention by child welfare authorities was reported when a 4-year-old boy was admitted to Yale–New Haven Hospital with irritability, fever, hepatomegaly, diffuse bone pain, and abnormal liver enzymes (145). His grandmother, who owned a health food store, denied giving the child vitamins. However, the child had been seen at nursery school eating vitamins continually from a bottle he brought to school. He had been seen by a physician known to prescribe megavitamin therapy and had a vitamin A level 10 times normal. The child was placed in foster care after a 4-week hospitalization.

Labeling and dispensing errors should be in the differential diagnosis when a child is poisoned. An 18-month-old boy developed disorientation, vomiting, tachycardia, and lethargy after being given a rectal suppository prescribed by his pediatrician. Investigation revealed that the pharmacist had supplied medication containing aminophylline and phenobarbital instead of aspirin and phenobarbital (165). A 17-day-old infant presented with convulsions and opisthotonic posturing after being given regular doses for 1 week of a hexachlorophene solution that had been mislabeled sulfisoxazole (Gantrisin) (64).

Errors by caregivers also should be investigated. A 15-month-old boy presented with acute liver failure and encephalopathy after his mother ran out of 80-mg tablets of acetaminophen and instead gave him 500-mg tablets for 2 weeks (4). Problems also can occur when caregivers dose children simultaneously with different brand names of the same medication, such as acetaminophen, resulting in overdosage.

One infant developed extreme hypocalcemia, hyperphosphatemia, and hypernatremia after a foster sibling poured a greater than prescribed amount of phosphosoda laxative into the child's bottle. The sibling was helping because the foster mother had broken her leg (149).

Apparent accidental poisoning has occurred when formula was diluted with a solvent other than water. Saladino and Shannon (135) described a 3-month-old girl who was accidentally poisoned when her family's well broke down. They used water from a base-ment storage tank containing 29% ethylene glycol (which is odorless) to mix formula. More worrisome is the case of a 6-week-old infant who was fed Similac formula diluted with a methanol-containing windshield washer fluid. The odor of windshield washer fluid was detectable in 110 mL of gastric aspirate. The question of why the parents had not also detected the odor when preparing the formula was not addressed (20).

Errors because of language problems or communication should be evaluated. Hexa-chlorophene poisoning occurred in an 8-day-old infant fed pHisoHex by a Spanish-speak-ing mother. The container, provided at the time of discharge from the hospital nursery, was labeled in English to be used for bathing only (64).

Poisoning and Other Types of Abuse

Physical child abuse is a frequent accompa-niment of deliberate poisoning. Dine and Mc-Govern (37) found that 20% of poisoned chil-dren had evidence of physical abuse. Of the 91 cases in Table 16.1, 23% had other injuries related to abuse.

Pickering (117) reported the case of a 19-day-old infant with hypoglycemia and cardiac arrest resulting from salicylate poisoning. The author thought that the mother had given the aspirin overdose accidentally, intending to se-date the child. He acknowledged that "the borderline between deliberate and accidental poisoning is not always easy to define." The baby was discharged and went home with the mother after a month-long hospitalization. Eight years later, she was admitted after an as-sault. The mother beat the child's head against a wall and inflicted extensive bruises on her legs with a belt. The author then diagnosed the patient as a victim of battered child syn-drome manifest as poisoning, stating, "It would thus be reasonable to examine samples of the blood and urine of battered babies on admission for evidence of poisoning until the incidence of this manifestation is deter-mined."

A retrospective review (129) of the records of 147 consecutive children admitted to a children's medical center during 1 year with presumed accidental poison ingestions re-vealed that 37% had previous emergency de-partment visits or admissions for traumatic injuries, 7% for previous poisoning, 6% for both poisoning and trauma, and 1.4% for fail-ure to thrive. Seven percent had suspicion or proof of child abuse documented in the chart, and 2.7% were considered neglected. When county child abuse records were reviewed, 18% of the victims of ingestion also had been investigated as victims of possible abuse. These findings differed from those of a con-trol group. Three cases of intentional poison-ing outside the study population also were found. The authors concluded that there may be a strong association between childhood poisoning and more classic forms of child abuse. They warned clinicians to be alert to the possibility that intentional poisoning may be common.

A brief report from Wales (109,148) indi-cated that abused children are significantly more likely to have apparent accidental poi-soning than are control subjects. On retro-spective review of records, 10 of 80 abused children had prior poisoning episodes com-pared with two of 80 controls. The authors thought the episodes were accidental rather than deliberate and represented a symptom of family stress.

Parents who abuse children also may poi-son them in an attempt to cover up the abuse, to relieve the child's symptoms, or to avoid detection. A 4-year-old girl was found dead after the mother's boyfriend had inflicted hot-water immersion burns to "teach her a lesson" after she wet her pants. The child had second-degree burns to 30% of the lower extremities and a blood isopropyl alcohol level of 50 mg/dL. The mother had treated the burns by applying gauze soaked with isopropyl alco-hol. She left the child alone in her room with-out food or water for 27 hours until she died (134). In a current case of fatal abuse with head trauma, anal penetration, and a head-first immersion burn, the child had high postmortem heroin levels. The caretaker had been bingeing on both heroin and alcohol at the time of the abuse. He may have used the heroin as pain relief for the child after causing the other injuries.

Pedophiles sometimes use alcohol or marijuana to intoxicate their young victims (J. Bays and L. Bays, unpublished data). In the Beattie study discussed earlier, of 143 children admitted with acute alcohol intoxication to University Hospital in Nottingham and the Royal Hospital for Sick Children in Glasgow (15), four boys had been forced to drink alcohol in association with sexual abuse by adult men. One boy was forced to drink at knifepoint before being sexually assaulted. The authors recommended considering sexual abuse as a motive if adults give children alcohol.

In a study of 1,179 toxicology screens from cases of suspected sexual assault from 49 states, ElSohly (41) found 60% positive by immunoassay for at least one and 35% for multiple psychoactive drugs. Positives included 38% for alcohol, 18% for cannabinoids, 8% for cocaine metabolites, 8% for benzodiazepines, 4% for amphetamines, 4% for γ-hydroxybutyrate (GHB), 2% for opiates, and 1% each for propoxyphene and barbiturates. No cases positive for PCP or methaqualone were found. Although many victims may have ingested the drugs willingly, some are likely to have surreptitiously been given medications with the intent of reducing resistance to sexual advances. Although alcohol remains the standard, benzodiazepines [in particular, flunitrazepam (Rohypnol)] have a current reputation for sexual disinhibition and amnesia in "date rape" (143).

We evaluated an 8-year-old girl whose father injected cocaine into her vagina before raping her. She described her vagina feeling "numb." Her father told her he was doing it because he loved her. We are aware of other cases of child sexual abuse in which cocaine was used to numb the child's vagina.

Densen-Gerber (32) wrote graphically of her experiences in New York City where more than two thirds of all children dying of child abuse come from addicted families. She lists the many facets of child abuse related to parental substance abuse, including child battering, starvation, intentional administration of drugs, and accidental ingestion of methadone. She describes deaths in fires caused when parents high on drugs fall asleep with lighted cigarettes, or when small children are left alone while parents go out to obtain and use drugs. She stated that fatal falls result when "parents, especially prostitutes, will place the baby on a fire escape or windowsill during warm weather, in part for cool breezes but also so that the child will not interfere with the parent's occupation." She described drowning deaths of infants left alone in bathtubs by substance-abusing parents with impaired judgment.

Densen-Gerber also warned of death of suffocation when narcotized or intoxicated parents "lie over" a child. In one instance, a mother injected herself with heroin and then fell asleep on a mattress that she inadvertently had lowered on top of her infant. She awoke 6 hours later to find the child smothered. In another report (152), a baby exposed to cocaine *in utero* was found dead at age 4 months after being put down to sleep. The autopsy findings were consistent with SIDS, but scene investigation revealed the true cause of death to be traumatic asphyxia. She had been wedged between the back of a couch and her father's body as he slept. A third death of overlying associated with intoxication occurred in a 1-month-old infant who was found dead in bed by his mother. The infant was prone, with his father's arm draped over the base of his neck and upper shoulders. The father, upset over the loss of his only son, gave specimens for toxicologic analysis. They were positive for tetrahydrocannabinol and an extrapolated blood alcohol level of 0.12 mg/dL at the time of the infant's death (114).

Munchausen Syndrome and "Simple Poisoning"

Many cases of MSBP involve child abuse by poisoning (see also Chapter 14). Rosenberg (130) reviewed 117 cases of MSBP. Of the eight most common presentations of MSBP, only one, fever, was not at times produced by poisoning. Ten of the 117 children died, three of salt poisoning, and two of other poisons.

Criteria for MSBP include factitious illness, chronic or recurrent illness, and fraudulent medical histories presented by the parents. The American Society on the Abuse of Children MSBP task force has recommended separating the diagnosis of the child victim as Pediatric Condition Falsification (PCF) from the diagnosis of the perpetrator (7). To diagnose the perpetrator with Factitious Disorder by Proxy (FDP), the perpetrator's primary motivation for fabrication should be the attention the perpetrator obtains from the child's illness. The reader is referred to the original working draft for further discussion of the differential diagnosis of both the child and the perpetrator. Originally, Meadow (100) excluded child abuse by poisoning from MSBP unless the parents fabricated other acts. Zitelli et al. (177), however, recommended that poisoning be labeled MSBP "when the parents present a factitious history."

The largest single series of the interface between MSBP and intentional poisoning also includes intentional suffocation. It comes from the British Pediatric Association Surveillance Unit (93). For the 2 years from 1992 to 1994, members reported all evaluated cases with any of the three conditions. Reports of 128 cases were received for an incidence of 0.5 cases/100,000 children younger than 16 years and 2.8 cases/100,000 younger than 1 year. Fifteen children were victimized by poisoning alone, 26 by both poisoning and MSBP, one by poisoning and suffocation, and two by all three conditions. In all, 44 children were poisoning victims. All eight deaths resulted from either or both poisoning (five) or suffocation (four). The majority of poisonings (71%) were from medications. In particular these were anticonvulsants and sedative/pain relievers. Household products including salt, bleach, and carbon monoxide also were reported. Thirty-eight of the children had experienced multiple poisoning events. Thirty-four of the 83 families,

which had other children, contained sibs who had also been abused. These included five who had been poisoned. Fifteen of these families had prior sibling deaths involving 18 children in all. The authors emphasized the strong interrelationship of intentional poisoning with MSBP and intentional suffocation. In a follow-up study of these children, it was noted that only eight of the survivors of poisoning were eventually returned home after the abuse (30). Although none of these eight was re-abused, four of 22 poisoning families with sibs had a prior child death. Five other families had recognized abuse of prior sibs. In all, 40% of families had previously abused sibs. In a previous study of 56 MSBP victims from Leeds, England, from 1976 to 1988, the primary form of abuse had been poisoning in 15 (26%) (19). Ten of 26 sibs also were recognized to have been poisoned.

Feldman (49) reported 71 PCF victims with either asthma, allergy, drug sensitivities, or sinopulmonary infections from a larger group of 104 PCF victims from 68 families. Eighteen (25%) also had induced intoxications. Although not reported, seven (21%) of the 33 other PCF victims also had induced intoxications. Not only were children victimized by direct intoxication, but caretakers also reported false or exaggerated histories of intoxications and complications of medical treatment caused intoxications. In all, 34 (32%) of the entire group of PCF victims had actual or factitious intoxications (49). Six (38%) of a previously reported 16-child subgroup of these patients, who had central venous catheters placed, were among those with intoxications (48).

If a child is found on one occasion to be the victim of nonaccidental poisoning, it is likely that previous episodes of poisoning have occurred and/or that future episodes will occur if the child is left unprotected (93). Any child who is the victim of what appears to be a single episode of poisoning ought to be considered a potential victim of MSBP (5). A careful history should be taken on the child, siblings, and parents. Complete medical records should be obtained to verify the facts against the history given (22). A psychosocial evaluation on the apparent perpetrator (usually the mother) is warranted. A verbal child should be interviewed alone. Hospital records and discharge diagnoses should document child abuse and MSBP. Child abuse authorities should be notified so that the family is entered into a statewide registry, aiding detection if they present to another health-care facility. Zitelli et al. (130,177) suggested such a statewide medical registry of Munchausen syndrome and MSBP patients. If professionals fail to recognize MSBP, they risk become unwitting participants in the syndrome.

Poisoning and SIDS

A forensic text states, "A small percentage of infants who die of apparent SIDS may have been poisoned, either accidentally or intentionally. If routine toxicology testing is not done, or if the toxicology screen does not include the substance administered, such poisonings will not be detected" (35).

A series of 170 infants dying of apparent SIDS between 1983 and 1987 were studied at the University of Arkansas (114). With parental consent, autopsies, cultures, and a complete set of radiographs were performed on infants aged from 1 week to 12 months who died suddenly with no known medical illness. After autopsy, 101 infants were diagnosed as SIDS (59%). Eight infants (4.7%) were found to have died of child abuse or neglect. One died of asphyxia when overlain by his intoxicated father. The 16-year-old mother poisoned another. She crushed amitriptyline pills and gave them to the infant to stop crying. In this case, poisoning would not have been diagnosed because routine toxicology screens were not part of the study protocol. Although the postmortem examination was negative, the discovery of pink pill fragments on an endotracheal tube that had been sent with the body led to toxicology testing.

A potential relation between phenothiazine-containing medication (Phenergan) and sleep apnea, episodes of near-miss SIDS, and unexpected death in infants has been ob-

served (73). Another study of eight infants referred to the Southwest SIDS Research Institute (62) raises concerns that colic medications may contribute to apparent life-threatening events in infants. The medications implicated, dimenhydrinate (Dramamine) and atropine, scopolamine, hyoscyamine, and phenobarbital (Donnatal), contain central nervous system depressants including atropine, scopolamine, ethanolamines, alcohol, and phenobarbital. The authors concluded, "Because of the common use of CNS depressant agents and smooth muscle relaxants for the treatment of colic . . . the authors strongly recommend that all infants presenting with an apparent life-threatening event have serum and urine drug screens as part of their initial evaluation."

MOTIVE

Fischler (51) divided abuse by poisoning into four categories. The first is impulsive acts under stress. An example is a caretaker who uses alcohol or sedatives to quiet a fussy baby. The second is neglect or lack of supervision. An example would be the "morning after syndrome," in which children ingest drugs or alcohol left out after an adult party. The third is bizarre child-rearing practices. An example would be forcibly restricting water or feeding salt to control enuresis. The last is MSBP. The caretaker repeatedly feigns or creates factitious illness in the child.

Alternatively, motives for poisoning could include

1. Idiosyncratic or folk medical belief systems;
2. Punitive acts, such as administering oral pepper as punishment;
3. Aggressive acts: poisoning to dispose of an unwanted child;
4. Recreational intoxication: getting the child "high" for entertainment;
5. Unauthorized use of prescription or illicit medications to relieve symptoms: giving narcotics to mask the pain of physical abuse;

6. To obtain sexual advantage as in "date rape";
7. Consequences of child neglect: poor supervision and toxin storage; or
8. Falsifying disease, as in MSBP.

The authors of a forensic textbook (35) stated,

> Poisoning is very easy in children, because they are dependent upon adults for feeding. The perpetrators are generally not psychotic, but just wish to dispose of the child for some reason or another. Because of this, it is a very good idea to perform complete toxicological analysis on young children in which no anatomical cause of death is apparent. This is especially true of SIDS cases. The authors have had a number of apparent SIDS deaths in which toxicological analysis revealed the deaths to be due to drug overdose. In one two year span, there was an obvious homicide, an accident due to misinterpreting the dispensation of medication by the mother, and a third undetermined as to manner, but most probably a homicide. In a fourth case, where a child died of asphyxia when cotton was wedged down its throat, there was also a toxic level of propyl alcohol in the blood.

In a series of nine poisoned infants described by Hickson (65), seven of the perpetrators of poisoning were mothers. Five parents admitted administering the agents. Their reasons included, "an apparent attempt to harm an infant, the need to sedate a fussy infant, or a gross misunderstanding of the potential risk of various agents to infants." One mother gave her infant methadone as a home treatment for neonatal withdrawal. One teenaged mother denied the poisoning but admitted that her husband, who traveled often, paid more attention to the family when the infant was ill. As Hickson says, however,

> One cannot take all histories at face value because parents who physically abuse their children often invent plausible explanations for injuries . . . . The fact that multiple agents were used in four of the cases, that poisonings occurred twice in the same family and occurred more than once in the same patients, continuing even while they were still in the hospital, and that four of the nine parents denied knowledge of a drug ingestion even after the screen

results were positive demonstrates elements of child abuse by poisoning.

As evidence of deliberate intent, poisoning frequently continues while the child is in the hospital. In a series of 75 children reported by Tenenbein (158), 40% were victims of ongoing poisoning in the hospital. Of the 91 children listed in Table 16.1 who were alive at presentation, 37 (40%) were poisoned in the hospital.

TREATMENT AND PREVENTION

Rogers et al. (127) stated,

> Interest in the diagnostic problem of nonaccidental poisoning . . . may have diverted attention from the equal problem of subsequent management . . . . We think the psychiatric aspects of this tragic family disorder differ in many respects from classical child abuse and that at present they are a long way from being understood.

They recommended psychiatric inpatient treatment for parent and child rather than punitive legal action.

There are only a few accounts of psychotherapeutic treatment of a child victim of child abuse by poisoning. An 8-year-old, growth-retarded, boy was admitted to the hospital with the mother complaining that he was "in constant pain, only able to lie in a bed or a push-chair, eyes closed behind dark glasses." He was placed in foster care after diuretic poisoning was diagnosed. The therapist described the boy's state of "inner confusion . . . as if the differentiations between good and bad, health and sickness, being alive or dead had hardly been achieved." Therapeutic sessions were filled with "sadistic fantasies and morbid preoccupations" (156). Rosenberg (130) discussed psychiatric follow-up of a few child victims of MSBP. One was withdrawn and preoccupied with themes of being poisoned and attacked. Chronic invalidism also may occur. Liebow did a follow-up study of 10 adults who had been MSBP victims during childhood. Distress and dysfunction were common (86). The two older MSBP victims described by McGuire and Feldman (95) developed conversion disorders during adolescence. Thirty-two percent of the children described by Feldman (49) exhibited conduct or behavior disorders, and 25% were thought to have attention deficit disorder.

The literature concerning treatment of adults who poison children is not optimistic. Meadow (101) wrote of child abuse by poisoning as requiring more planning and deliberation than the usual forms of child abuse. Baugh et al. (12) wrote, "any form of intentional poisoning is probably a more pathologic form of abuse than more violent acts such as extreme corporal punishment . . . . Child abuse by intentional poisoning appears to reflect greater pathology than other forms of abuse." Davis (30) also expressed the concern that poisoning victims and their sibs remain at considerable risk if left with the perpetrator.

Saulsbury (136) stated,

> The psychological profile of parents who poison their children may differ from that of parents who engage in other forms of abuse or neglect. There is a higher incidence of mental disturbances and character disorders in parents who poison their children, in contrast to those who are physically abusive. These groups are not mutually exclusive, however, inasmuch as up to 20% of poisoned children have also been physically abused.

Jones (72) observed that parents who intentionally poison their children are resistant to change and difficult to treat. He lists other parental factors increasing the risk associated with untreatability. These include severe abuse of the caretaker during childhood, persistent denial of abusive behavior, alcohol or drug abuse, psychotic delusions involving the child, lack of empathic feeling for the child, violent behavior, and severe personality disorder, particularly if combined with a mental handicap.

If a child who has been poisoned is returned to an abusive home, frequent urine toxicologic screening should be considered in addition to other monitoring procedures. Once the diagnosis of child abuse by poisoning is made, psychiatric consultation for the perpetrator should be sought. Confrontation is associated with a significant risk of a maternal suicide attempt (2,130). Court protective orders may be required to get the perpetrator to accept this consultation.

Home nurse visitation programs can reduce the incidence of childhood emergency department visits, accidents, accidental poisonings, and also child abuse and neglect (112). These programs might be a method of preventing child abuse by poisoning, but are more likely to affect poisoning due to neglect or social chaos.

Intentional poisoning is a serious form of child abuse that occurs in families from all socioeconomic levels. Like its all too frequent companion, physical abuse, it passes undetected, is underreported, and is potentially lethal. To paraphrase findings by Kempe, no child ever died of a toxicology screen, but many may suffer and die if we do not obtain one.

REFERENCES

1. Child Protective Services Program. *A report of Oregon fatalities due to abuse or neglect 1985-1989.* Salem, OR: State of Oregon, Department of Human Resources, 1990.
2. Ackerman NB Jr, Strobel CT. Polle syndrome: chronic diarrhea in Munchausen's child. *Gastroenterology* 1981;81:1140–1142.
3. Adelson L. Homicidal poisoning: a dying modality of lethal violence? *Am J Forensic Med Pathol* 1987;8: 245.
4. Agran PF, Zenk KE, Romansky SG. Acute liver failure and encephalopathy in a 15-month-old infant. *Am J Dis Child* 1983;137:1107.
5. Alexander R, Smith W, Stevenson R. Serial Munchausen syndrome by proxy. *Pediatrics* 1990;86:581.
6. American Academy of Pediatrics Committee on Drugs. Transfer of drugs and other chemicals into human milk. *Pediatrics* 1994;93:137–150.
7. Definitional issues in Munchausen syndrome by proxy. American Professional Society on the Abuse of Children Munchausen by Proxy Task Force. *Am Professional Soc Abuse Child Advisor* 1998;11:7–10.
8. Baer RD, Garcia de Alba J, Cueto LM, et al. Lead-based remedies for empacho: patterns and consequences. *Soc Sci Med* 1989;29:1373–1379.
9. Bailey DN, Shaw RF. Cocaine- and methamphetamine-related deaths in San Diego County (1987): homicides and accidental overdoses. *J Forensic Sci* 1989;34:407.
10. Barnett PL. Centipede ingestion by a six-month-old infant: toxic side effects. *Pediatr Emerg Care* 1991;7: 229–230.

11. Bateman DA, Heagarty MC. Passive freebase cocaine ("crack") inhalation by infants and toddlers. *Am J Dis Child* 1989;143:25–27.

12. Baugh JR, Krug EF, Weir MR. Punishment by salt poisoning. *South Med J* 1983;76:540–541.

13. Bauman WA, Yalow RS. Child abuse: parenteral insulin administration. *J Pediatr* 1981;99:588–591.

14. Bays J. Substance abuse and child abuse: the impact of addiction on the child. *Pediatr Clin North Am* 1990;37:881–904.

15. Beattie JO, Hull D, Cockburn F. Children intoxicated by alcohol in Nottingham and Glascow, 1973-84. *Br Med J* 1986;292:519–521.

16. Belson MG, Simon HK. Utility of comprehensive toxicologic screens in children. *Am J Emerg Med* 1999;17:221–224.

17. Berkner P, Kastner T, Skolnick L. Chronic ipecac poisoning in infancy: a case report. *Pediatrics* 1988;82:384–385.

18. Blinder KJ, Scott W, Lange MP. Abuse of cyanoacrylate in child abuse. *Arch Ophthalmol* 1987;105:1632–1633.

19. Bools CN, Neale BA, Meadow SR. Co-morbidity associated with fabricated illness (Munchausen syndrome by proxy). *Arch Dis Child* 1992;67:77–79.

20. Brent J, Lucas M, Kulig K, et al. Methanol poisoning in a 6-week-old infant. *J Pediatr* 1991;118:644–646.

21. Buchta R. Deliberate intoxication of young children and pets with drugs: a survey of an adolescent population in a private practice. *Am J Dis Child* 1988;142:701–702.

22. Burman D, Stevens D. Munchausen family. *Lancet* 1977;2:546.

23. Caruso M, Bregani P, Natale B, et al. Ipoglicemia indotta: un insolito caso di maltrattamento infantile. *Minerva Pediatr* 1989;41:525–528.

24. Case MES, Short CD, Poklis A. Intoxication by aspirin and alcohol in a child: a case of child abuse by medical neglect. *Am J Forensic Med Pathol* 1983;4:149–151.

25. Chan DA, Salcedo JR, Atkins DM, et al. Munchausen syndrome by proxy: a review and case study. *J Pediatr Psychol* 1986;11:71–80.

26. Chaney NE, Franke J, Wadlington WB. Cocaine convulsions in a breast-feeding baby. *J Pediatr* 1988;112:134–135.

27. Chasnoff IA, Lewis DE, Squires L. Cocaine intoxication in a breast-fed infant. *Pediatrics* 1987;80:836–838.

28. Cohle SD, Trestrail JD, Graham MA, et al. Fatal pepper aspiration. *Am J Dis Child* 1988;142:633.

29. Cravey RH. Cocaine deaths in infants. *J Anal Toxicol* 1988;12:354–355.

30. Davis P, McClure RJ, Rolfe K, et al. Procedures, placement, and risks of further abuse after Munchausen syndrome by proxy, non-accidental poisoning, and non-accidental suffocation. *Arch Dis Child* 1998;78:217–221.

31. Day L, Kelly C, Reed G, et al. Fatal cardiomyopathy: suspected child abuse by chronic ipecac administration. *Vet Hum Toxicol* 1989;31:255–257.

32. Densen-Gerber J. The forensic pathology of drug-related child abuse. *Leg Med Annu* 1978;135–147.

33. Desprez PH, Vaudour G, Burquin C, et al. Privation d'eau: une forme inhabituelle de maltraitance. *Arch Francaises Pediatr* 1990;47:287–289.

34. Dietrich AM, Mortensen ME. Presentation and management of an acute caffeine overdose. *Pediatr Emerg Care* 1990;6:296–298.

35. Dimaio D, Dimaio VJM. *Forensic pathology.* New York: Elsevier, 1989.

36. Dine MS. Tranquilizer poisoning: an example of child abuse. *Pediatrics* 1965;36:782–785.

37. Dine MS, McGovern ME. Intentional poisoning of children: an overlooked category of child abuse: report of seven cases and review of the literature. *Pediatrics* 1982;70:32–35.

38. Dockery WK. Fatal intentional salt poisoning associated with a radiopaque mass. *Pediatrics* 1992;89:964–965.

39. Dogruyol H, Gurpinar AN. A foreign body in a four day old infant's esophagus: a case of negligence. *Turkish J Pediatr* 1989;31:163–166.

40. *Drug use forecasting* (DUF) *fourth quarter 1988.* Washington, DC: US Department of Justice, June 1989.

41. ElSohly MA, Salamone SJ. Prevalence of drugs used in cases of alleged sexual assault. *J Anal Toxicol* 1999;23:141–146.

42. Epstein MA, Markowitz RL, Gallo DM, et al. Munchausen syndrome by proxy: considerations in diagnosis and confirmation by video surveillance. *Pediatrics* 1987;80:220–224.

43. Ernst AA, Sanders WM. Unexpected cocaine intoxication presenting as seizures in children. *Ann Emerg Med* 1989;18:774–777.

44. Oregon Children's Services Division. *Fatal child abuse and neglect in Oregon 1985 and 1986.* Salem, OR: Oregon Children's Services Division, 1988.

45. Fechner VG, Kernbach-Wighton G, Bohn, G. Kindesmifshandlung oder akzidentelle Vergiftung mit Isopropanol? *Beitr Gerichtl Med* 1989;47:73–75.

46. Feldman KW, Christopher DM, Opheim KB. Munchausen syndrome/bulimia by proxy: ipecac as a toxin in child abuse. *Child Abuse Negl* 1989;13:257–261.

47. Feldman KW, Robertson WO. Salt poisoning: presenting symptom of child abuse. *Vet Hum Toxicol* 1979;21:341–342.

48. Feldman KW, Hickman RO. The central venous catheter as a source of medical chaos in Munchausen syndrome by proxy. *J Pediatr Surg* 1998;33:623–627.

49. Feldman KW, Stout JW, Inglis AF. Asthma, allergy and sinopulmonary disease in pediatric condition falsification. *Child Maltreat* (in press).

50. Fenton AC, Wailoo MP, Tanner MS. Severe failure to thrive and diarrhea caused by laxative abuse. *Arch Dis Child* 1988;63:978–979.

51. Fischler RS. Poisoning: a syndrome of child abuse. *Am Fam Physician* 1983;28:103–108.

52. Fleisher D, Ament ME. Diarrhea, red diapers, and child abuse. *Clin Pediatr* 1997;17:820–824.

53. Forbes DA, O'Laughlin EV, Scott RB, et al. Laxative abuse and secretory diarrhea. *Arch Dis Child* 1985;60:58–60.

54. Foster HM, Narasimhachari N. Phencyclidine in CSF and serum: a case of attempted filicide by a mother without a history of substance abuse. *J Clin Psychiatry* 1986;47:428–429.

55. Fox DW, Hart MC, Bergeson PS, et al. Pyrrolizidine

(*Senecio*) intoxication mimicking Reye syndrome. *J Pediatr* 1978;93:980–982.

56. Friedman EM. Caustic ingestions and foreign body aspirations: an overlooked form of child abuse. *Ann Otol Rhinol Laryngol* 1987;96:709–712.

57. Gairdner D. Commentary. *Arch Dis Child* 1980;55:646–647.

58. Garrettson LK, Bush LP, Gates RS, et al. Physical change, time of day and child characteristics as factors in poison injury. *Vet Hum Toxicol* 1990;32:139–141.

59. Gotschlich T, Beltran RS. Poisoning of a 21-month-old child by a baby-sitter. *Clin Pediatr* 1995;134:52–53.

60. Greene JW, Craft L, Ghishan F. Acetaminophen poisoning in infancy. *Am J Dis Child* 1983;137:386–387.

61. Grubbauer HM, Schwarz R. Peritoneal dialysis in alcohol intoxication in a child. *Arch Toxicol* 1980;43:317–320.

62. Hardoin RA, Henslee JA, Christenson CP, et al. Colic medication and apparent life-threatening events. *Clin Pediatr* 1991;30:281–285.

63. Heidemann SM, Goetting MG. Passive inhalation of cocaine by infants. *Henry Ford Hosp Med J* 1990;38:252–254.

64. Herskowitz J, Rosman NP. Acute hexachlorophene poisoning by mouth in a neonate. *J Pediatr* 1979;94:495–496.

65. Hickson GB, Altemeier W, Martin E, et al. Parental administration of chemical agents: a cause of apparent life-threatening events. *Pediatrics* 1989;83:772–776.

66. Hickson GB, Greene JW, Ghishan FK, et al. Apparent intentional poisoning of an infant with acetaminophen. *Am J Dis Child* 1983;137:917.

67. Higgins GL, Campbell B, Wallace K, et al. Pediatric poisoning from over-the-counter imidazoline-containing products. *Ann Emerg Med* 1991;20:655–658.

68. Hopwood NJ, Becker DJ. Psychosocial dwarfism: detection, evaluation and management. *Child Abuse Negl* 1979;3:439.

69. Howard J, et al. The development of young children of substance-abusing parents: insights from seven years of intervention and research. *Zero to Three* 1989;9:8.

70. Hvizdala EV, Gellady AM. Intentional poisoning of two siblings by prescription drugs. *Clin Pediatr* 1978;17:480–482.

71. Jacobson BJ, Rock AR, Cohen MJ, et al. Accidental ingestions of oral prescription drugs: a multicenter survey. *Am J Public Health* 1989;79:853–856.

72. Jones DPH. The untreatable family. *Child Abuse Negl* 1987;11:409.

73. Kahn A, Hasaerts D, Blum D. Phenothiazine-induced sleep apneas in normal infants. *Pediatrics* 1985;75:844–847.

74. Keating JP, Schears GJ, Dodge PR. Oral water intoxication in infants: an American epidemic. *Am J Dis Child* 1991;145:985–990.

75. Kempe CH, Silverman FN, Steele BF, et al. The battered-child syndrome. *JAMA* 1962;181:17–24.

76. Kharasch S, Vinci R, Glotzer D, et al. Unsuspected cocaine exposure in young children. *Am J Dis Child* 1990;144:441.

77. Kharasch S, Vinci R, Reece R. Esophagitis, epiglottitis, and cocaine alkaloid ("crack"): "accidental" poisoning or child abuse? *Pediatrics* 1990;86:117–119.

78. King WD, Palmisano PA. Ingestion of prescription drugs by children: an epidemiologic study. *South Med J* 1989;82:1468–1471.

79. Krug SE, Marble P, Lubitz DL, et al. Screening for cocaine intoxication in children with unexplained seizures in the emergency department. *Am J Dis Child* 1991;145:410.

80. Kudo K, Miyazaki C, Kadoya R, et al. Laxative poisoning: toxicological analysis of bisacodyl and its metabolites in the urine. *J Anal Toxicol* 1998;22:274–278.

81. Lacey SR, Cooper C, Runyon DK, et al. Munchausen syndrome by proxy: patterns of presentations to pediatric surgeons. *J Pediatr Surg* 1993;28:827–832.

82. Lacroix J, Gaudreault P, Gauthier M. Admission to a pediatric intensive care unit for poisoning: a review of 105 cases. *Crit Care Med* 1989;17:748–750.

83. Lansky LL. An unusual case of childhood chloral hydrate poisoning. *Am J Dis Child* 1974;127:275.

84. Leung AKC. Ethyl alcohol ingestion in children: a fifteen year review. *Clin Pediatr* 1986;25:617–619.

85. Lewis HH, Cronje RE, Naude SP, et al. Accidental poisoning in childhood. *S Afr Med J* 1989;76:429–431.

86. Liebow JA. Munchausen by proxy victims in adulthood: a first look. *Child Abuse Negl* 1995;19:1131–1142.

87. Litovitz TL, Clark LR, Soloway RA. The 1993 annual report of the American Association of Poison Control Centers toxic exposures surveillance system. *Am J Emerg Med* 1994;12:546–584.

88. Litovitz TL, Flagler SL, Maneguerra AS, et al. Recurrent poisonings among paediatric poisoning victims. *Med Toxicol Adverse Drug Exp* 1989;4:381–386.

89. Little RE, Anderson KW, Ervine H, et al. Maternal alcohol use during breast-feeding and infant mental and motor development at one year. *N Engl J Med* 1989;321:425–430.

90. Lorber J, Reckless JPD, Watson JBG. Nonaccidental poisoning: the elusive diagnosis. *Arch Dis Child* 1980;55:643–647.

91. McCarron MM, Challoner, KR, Thompson, GA. Diphenoxylate-atropine (Lomotil) overdose in children: an update (report of eight cases and review of the literature). *Pediatrics* 1991;87:694–700.

92. McClung HJ, Murray R, Braden NJ, et al. Intentional ipecac poisoning in children. *Am J Dis Child* 1988;142:637–639.

93. McClure RJ, Davis PM, Meadow SR, et al. Epidemiology of Munchausen syndrome by proxy, non-accidental poisoning, and non-accidental suffocation. *Arch Dis Child* 1996;75:57–61.

94. McFadden SW, Haddow JE. Coma produced by topical application of isopropanol. *Pediatrics* 1969;43:622–633.

95. McGuire TL, Feldman KW. Psychologic morbidity of children subjected to Munchausen syndrome by proxy. *Pediatrics* 1989;83:289–292.

96. Mahesh VK, Stern HP, Kearns GL, et al. Application of pharmacokinetics in the diagnosis of chemical abuse in Munchausen syndrome by proxy. *Clin Pediatr* 1988;27:243–246.

97. Malizia E, Andrucci G, Alfani F, et al. Acute intoxication with nicotine alkaloids and cannabinoids in children from ingestion of cigarettes. *Hum Toxicol* 1983;2:315–316.

98. Matter of baby X. 97 Mich App 111, 293 NW 2nd 736, 1980.

99. Mayefsky JH, Sarnaik AP, Postellon DC. Factitious hypoglycemia. *Pediatrics* 1982;69:804–805.

100. Meadow R. Munchausen syndrome by proxy: the hinterland of child abuse. *Lancet* 1977;2:343–345.

101. Meadow R. ABC of child abuse: poisoning. *Br Med J* 1989;298:1445–1446.

102. Meadow R. Non-accidental salt poisoning. *Arch Dis Child* 1993;68:448–452.

103. Meadow R. Munchausen syndrome by proxy abuse perpetrated by men. *Arch Dis Child* 1998;78:210–216.

104. Mehl AL, Coble L, Johnson S. Munchausen syndrome by proxy: a family affair. *Child Abuse Negl* 1990;14:577–585.

105. Miller KA. Suspected child abuse and neglect presenting as an ingestion of toxic substances. *Vet Hum Toxicol* 1981;23:32.

106. Mirchandani HG, Hellman F, English-Rider R, et al. Passive inhalation of free-base cocaine ("crack") smoke by infants. *Arch Pathol Lab Med* 1991;115:494–498.

107. Morrow PL. Caffeine toxicity: a case of child abuse by drug ingestion. *J Forensic Sci* 1987;32:1801–1805.

108. Mortimer JG. Acute water intoxication as another unusual manifestation of child abuse. *Arch Dis Child* 1980;55:401–403.

109. Murphy J, Sibert JR, Evans R, et al. Accidental poisoning preceding nonaccidental injury. *Arch Dis Child* 1981;56:78–79.

110. National Center for Health Statistics. *Vital statistics of the United States 1978. Vol 2: mortality.* Hyattsville, MD: U.S. Department of Health and Human Services, 1981.

111. National Center for Health Statistics. *Vital statistics of the United States 1978: Vol 2A: mortality.* Hyattsville, MD: U.S. Department of Health and Human Services, 1996.

112. Olds DL, Henderson CR, Chamberlin R, et al. Preventing child abuse and neglect: a randomized trial of nurse home visitation. *Pediatrics* 1986;78:65–78.

113. Osborne JP. Non-accidental poisoning and child abuse [Letter]. *Br Med J* 1976;1:1210.

114. Perrot LJ, Nawojczyk S. Nonnatural death masquerading as SIDS (sudden infant death syndrome). *Am J Forensic Med Pathol* 1988;9:105–111.

115. Piatt JP, Kaplan, Bond GR, et al. Occult carbon monoxide poisoning in an infant. *Pediatr Emerg Care* 1990;6:21–23.

116. Pickel S, Anderson C, Holliday MA. Thirsting and hypernatremic dehydration: a form of child abuse. *Pediatrics* 1970;45:54–59.

117. Pickering D. Salicylate poisoning as a manifestation of the battered child syndrome. *Am J Dis Child* 1976;130:675.

118. Pickering D, Moncrieff M, Etches PC. Non-accidental poisoning and child abuse [Letter]. *Br Med J* 1976;1:1210–1211.

119. Press S. Crack and fatal child abuse. *JAMA* 1988;260:3132.

120. Proesmans W, Sina JK, Debucquoy P, et al. Recurrent acute renal failure due to nonaccidental poisoning with glafenin in a child. *Clin Nephrol* 1981;16:207–210.

121. Reinhart MA. Child abuse: cocaine absorption by rectal administration. *Clin Pediatr* 1990;29:357.

122. Richards RG, Cravey RH. Infanticide due to ethanolism. *J Anal Toxicol* 1978;2:60.

123. Riggs D, Weibley RE. Acute hemorrhagic diarrhea and cardiovascular collapse in a young child owing to environmentally acquired cocaine. *Pediatr Emerg Care* 1991;7:154–155.

124. Rivenes SM, Bakerman PR, Miller MB. Intentional caffeine poisoning in an infant. *Pediatrics* 1997;99:736–738.

125. Rivkin M, Gilmore HE. Generalized seizures in an infant due to environmentally acquired cocaine. *Pediatrics* 1989;84:1100–1102.

126. Rogers C, Hall J, Muto J. Findings in newborns of cocaine-abusing mothers. *J Forensic Sci* 1991;36:1074–1078.

127. Rogers DW, Bentovim A, Tripp JH. Nonaccidental poisoning: the elusive diagnosis. *Arch Dis Child* 1981;56:156–157.

128. Rogers DW, Tripp J, Bentovim A, et al. Non-accidental poisoning: an extended syndrome of child abuse. *Br Med J* 1976;1:793–796.

129. Rogers GC, Baird J. Association between childhood poisoning and trauma and child abuse and neglect. Unpublished data.

130. Rosenberg DA. Web of deceit: a literature review of Munchausen syndrome by proxy. *Child Abuse Negl* 1987;11:547–563.

131. Rosenberg NM, Meert KL, Knazik SR, et al. Occult cocaine exposure in children. *Am J D Child* 1991;145:1430–1432.

132. Rubin LG, Amelides A, Davidson M, et al. Recurrent sepsis and gastrointestinal ulceration due to child abuse. *Arch Dis Child* 1986;61:903–905.

133. Rubio EL, Ekins BR, Singh PD, et al. Hmong opiate folk remedy toxicity in three infants. *Vet Hum Toxicol* 1987;29:323–325.

134. Russo S, Taff ML, Mirchandani HG, et al. Scald burns complicated by isopropyl alcohol intoxication: a case of fatal child abuse. *Am J Forensic Med Pathol* 1986;7:81–83.

135. Saladino R, Shannon M. Accidental and intentional poisonings with ethylene glycol in infancy: diagnostic clues and management. *Pediatr Emerg Care* 1991;7:93–96.

136. Saulsbury FT, Chobanian MC, Wilson WG. Child abuse: parenteral hydrocarbon administration. *Pediatrics* 1984;73:719–722.

137. Schmitt BD, Kempe CH. The pediatrician's role in child abuse and neglect. *Curr Probl Pediatr* 1975;5:3–47.

138. Schneider DJ, Perez A, Knilans TE, et al. Clinical and pathologic aspects of cardiomyopathy from ipecac administration in Munchausen's syndrome by proxy. *Pediatrics* 1996;97:902–906.

139. Schoental R. Herbal medicines to avoid. *Nature* 1972;238:106–107.

140. Schwartz JG, Hopkovitz AM. LSD intoxication. *J Fam Pract* 1988;27:550–551.

141. Schwartz RH, Einhorn A. PCP intoxication in seven young children. *Pediatr Emerg Care* 1986;2:238–241.

142. Schwartz RH, Peary P, Mistrett D. Intoxication of young children with marijuana: a form of amusement for "pot"-smoking teenage girls. *Am J Dis Child* 1986;140:326.

143. Schwartz RH, Weaver AB. Rohypnol: the date rape drug. *Clin Pediatr* 1998;37:321–322.

144. Shannon M, Lacouture PG, Roa J, et al. Cocaine exposure among children seen at a pediatric hospital. *Pediatrics* 1989;83:337–342.

145. Shaywitz BA, Sizel NJ, Pearson HA. Megavitamins for minimal brain dysfunction: a potentially dangerous therapy. *JAMA* 1977;238:1749–1750.

146. Shoemaker JD, Lynch RE, Hoffman JW, et al. Misidentification of propionic acid as ethylene glycol in a patient with methylmalonic acidemia. *J Pediatr* 1992;120:417–421.

147. Shnaps Y, Frand M, Rotem Y, et al. The chemically abused child. *Pediatr* 1981;68:119–121.

148. Sibert JR, Murphy JF. Child poisoning and child abuse. *Arch Dis Child* 1980;55:822.

149. Smith MS, Feldman KW, Furukawa CT. Coma in an infant due to hypertonic sodium phosphate medication. *J Pediatr* 1975;86:395–398.

150. Smith RM, Nelson LA. Hmong folk remedies: limited acetylation of opium by aspirin and acetaminophen. *J Forensic Sci* 1991;36:280–287.

151. Smolinski SC, Spoerke KG, Spiller SK, et al. Cigarette and nicotine chewing gum toxicity in children. *Hum Toxicol* 1988;7:27–31.

152. Sturner WQ, Sweeney KG, Callery RT, et al. Cocaine babies: the scourge of the 90's. *J Forensic Sci* 1991;36:34–39.

153. Sullivan JL. Caffeine poisoning in an infant. *J Pediatr* 1977;90:1022–1023.

154. Sutphen JL, Saulsbury FT. Intentional ipecac poisoning: Munchausen syndrome by proxy. *Pediatrics* 1988;82:453–456.

155. Swann A, Glascow J. Child abuse: we must increase our level of suspicion. *Ulster Med J* 1982;51:115–120.

156. Szur R. Psychotherapy with a child who has been poisoned. *Child Abuse Negl* 1979;3:505–508.

157. Talalaj S, Czechowitcz A. Hazardous herbal remedies are still on the market. *Med J Aust* 1990;153:302.

158. Tenenbein M. Pediatric toxicology: current controversies and recent advances. *Curr Probl Pediatr* 1986;16:198–233.

159. Terndrup TE, Walls HC, Mariani PS, et al. Plasma cocaine and tetracaine levels following application of topical anesthesia in children. *Ann Emerg Med* 1992;21:162–166.

160. Thearle MJ, Gregory H. Child abuse in nineteenth century Queensland. *Child Abuse Negl* 1988;12:91–101.

161. Thyen U, Leventhal JM, Yazdgerdi SR, et al. Concerns about child maltreatment in hospitalized children. *Child Abuse Negl* 1997;21:187–198.

162. Tileli JA, Ophoven JP. Hyponatremic seizures as a presenting symptom of child abuse. *Forensic Sci Int* 1986;30:213–217.

163. Tolis AD. Hypoglycemic convulsions in children after alcohol ingestion. *Pediatr Clin North Am* 1965;12:423–425.

164. Tominack RL, Spyker DA. Capsicum and capsaicin: a review: case report of the use of hot peppers in child abuse. *Clin Toxicol* 1987;25:591–601.

165. Vaucher Y, Lightner ES, Walson PD. Theophylline poisoning. *Pediatrics* 1977;90:827–830.

166. Venter CP, Joubert PH. Aspects of poisoning with traditional medicines in Southern Africa. *Biomed Environ Sci* 1988;1:388–391.

167. Verity CM, Winckworth C, Burman D, et al. Polle syndrome: children of Munchausen. *Br Med J* 1979;2:422–423.

168. Volk D. Factitious diarrhea in two children. *Am J Dis Child* 1982;136:1027–1028.

169. Watson JBG, Davies JM, Hunter JLP. Nonaccidental poisoning in childhood. *Arch Dis Child* 1979;54:143–144.

170. Weinberg D, Lande A, Hilton N, et al. Intoxication from accidental marijuana ingestion. *Pediatrics* 1983;71:848–850.

171. Welch MJ, Correa GA. PCP intoxication in young children and infants. *Clin Pediatr* 1980;19:510–514.

172. Wiley JF. Difficult diagnoses in toxicology. *Pediatr Clin North Am* 1991;38:725–737.

173. Wiseman HM, Guest K, Murray VS, et al. Accidental poisoning in childhood: a multicentre survey. 1. General epidemiology. *Hum Toxicol* 1987;6:293–301.

174. Woolf AD, Wynshaw-Boris A, Rinaldo P, et al. Intentional ethylene glycol poisoning presenting as an inherited metabolic disorder. *J Pediatr* 1992;120:421–424.

175. Yamamoto LG, Weibe RA, Matthews WJ. Toxic exposures and ingestions in Honolulu: I. a prospective pediatric ER cohort; II. A prospective poison center cohort. *Pediatr Emerg Care* 1991;7:141–148.

176. Zahavi I, Shaffer EA, Gall DG. Child abuse with laxatives. *Can Med Assoc J* 1982;127:512–513.

177. Zitelli BJ, Seltman MF, Shannon RM. Munchausen's syndrome by proxy and its professional participants. *Am J Dis Child* 1987;141:1099–1102.

17

Immersion Injury in Child Abuse and Neglect

Kenneth W. Feldman

*Department of Pediatrics, University of Washington School of Medicine; Child Protection Team,
Children's Hospital and Regional Medical Center; and Odessa Brown Children's Clinic,
Seattle, Washington*

Although drowning is the second leading cause of death from unintentional injury between ages 1 and 14 years and the fifth leading cause at younger than 1 year (31), it has received little attention in the child abuse literature. Early case series of abused children lack reference to drowning as a cause of child abuse (13,16,21,33,54). However, Adelson's 1961 description of 46 child homicides included 10 who would be considered to have died of abuse and three of neglect (2). Five of the entire series died of drowning, including four bathtub immersions. It is unclear how many of the drownings fit the child abuse pattern. Subsequent studies of child homicide (6,9,15,30) and series of childhood immersion injury (36,44) have begun to recognize instances of inflicted immersion injury. Abuse and neglect should be considered in a variety of drownings. Events thought to be unintentional immersions may be found to have historical or physical evidence of intentional injury. Abuse also should be considered when children are presented to care with a specious history of submersion injury but physical findings suggestive of other types of inflicted injury. The opposite situation is encountered when a child is brought to care *in extremis* without a history of drowning, but with clinical or pathologic evidence of immersion. Although neonaticide has been relatively neglected in the child abuse literature, drowning is often the mode of death in these events. Judgments also must be made whether child supervision leading to unintentional submersion is beneath community standards, meeting definitions of child neglect.

EPIDEMIOLOGY OF CHILDHOOD DROWNING

Drowning rates vary widely based on climate, culture, and environmental hazards. Pearn (35) observed freshwater immersion and drowning death rates of 10.43 and 5.17/ 100,000, respectively, in children younger than 16 years in a total population study of Brisbane, Australia, from 1971 to 1975. The immersion rate for toddlers reached 50.01/ 100,000, and 45% of these died. Sixty percent of the drownings were in pools, whereas 23% occurred in other bodies of water, and 17% in bathtubs. Hawaii had a lower immersion rate of 3.1/100,000 children from 1973 to 1977, but the ready access to salt-water recreation led to 41% of the incidents occurring in salt water (39). In King County, Washington, the annual incidence and mortality rates are 5.5 and 2.6/100,000 children (44). Rates are highest at 12.8 in preschoolers, with 43% of immersions in children younger than 5 years. The region has many bodies of cold natural water (50% of immersions) and a moderate presence of public and private, unguarded pools (33% of immersions). Twelve percent of these drownings occurred in the family bathtub. However, in contrast to the incidence throughout childhood, 24% of the immersions younger than 5 years occurred in the bath. In spite of abundant salt water, few (2%) instances of salt-water immersion were noted, probably because the salt water is cold enough to discourage swimming. In the British Isles, immersion (1.5/100,000) and immersion death rates (0.7/100,000) are lower, but a greater number of children were younger than 5 years (68%) (19). The garden pool (19%) poses a hazard nearly equal to that of natural bodies of water (20%), but still less than pools intended for swimming (27%). Bathtub immersions accounted for 14% of all immersions and 68% of these in children younger than 5 years. In California, Arizona, and Florida, drowning is the leading cause of unintentional injury death younger than 5 years (56). Florida has one of the highest drowning rates in the world (93/100,000 children younger than 12 years) (48). Although the private swimming pool is the single leading site of immersion in Florida, the canals, ponds, and lakes built to drain the low and marshy land combined to cause 41% of immersions. Swimming pool drowning in preschoolers follows an inverse socioeconomic status incidence pattern more than most childhood injuries. Because access to private pools is greater in higher income families, their rate of drowning also is increased (35,56).

Intentional Submersions

Pearn and Nixon (32,36–38) were the first to report intentional drowning as a pattern of child abuse (1977). Three bathtub submersion cases were described. Abuse was recognized in one from maternal confession and one due to a previous abuse report from neighbors. In one case, the child sustained a subsequent compound skull fracture while in the father's care. They noted that the usual unintentional bathtub immersion involves a child between ages 9 and 15 months, accompanied only by another young child in the bath. Lower socioeconomic status families with several children were most often involved in these submersions. They expressed

the opinion that bathtub submersions in older children were more often inflicted. Subsequent authors also noted a high frequency of epilepsy as a cause of submersions in older children (8,44,50). Kemp et al. (20) suggested that bathtub drownings outside the ages of 8 to 24 months are more concerning for abuse (20). Neither Pearn nor Kemp emphasized that immersion injuries at younger ages than 8 to 9 months are more likely to be inflicted, but few reports of accidental or inflicted bathtub submersions for younger infants can be found. However, it seems reasonable that parents are unlikely to leave an infant unattended in the tub before the infant is able to sit competently. The caretaker's overestimate of the older infant's ability to sit safely and of preschool peers to supervise the child is what leads to unintentional submersion. Jensen (17) found all but one of the 33 injuries (due to submersions of all causes) in children younger than 1 year to be in those older than 6 months. Further, all but one of the bathtub submersion deaths occurred while a younger-than-2-years child victim was bathing with a 10-month to 7-year-old peer, without direct adult supervision. One child was 47 months old, but had a known seizure disorder and was bathing unsupervised with his twin sib. Fifty-nine percent of the nonfatal bathtub submersion victims were both younger than 2 years and bathing with another child, but not directly supervised by an adult. Lavelle's (24) youngest bathtub injury due to abuse or severe neglect was 4 months old. Twenty-eight percent of her reported events occurred while the victim was bathing with a peer who was younger than 4 years. Seventy-five percent of the victims were younger than 2 years. One drowning victim among 12 child homicides reported by Hodge was 3 months old (15). He did not specify whether that child drowned in the bathtub, but another child died of a beating that preceded his being placed in the tub. Quan's (44) three cases of abuse or neglect submersions were children younger than 5 years in the bathtub. Although Gillenwater (12) reported that five of 16 inflicted immersions were younger than 1 year, the specific ages were not noted. Review of the original data indicates that one bathtub immersion victim was a newborn, two were 4 months old, and one each was 2.5, 3, and 3.25 years old. Only three of the nine bathtub drownings were from the usual 8- to 24-month-old range of unintentional bathtub victims. The victim was often the youngest child of a large sibship. Nixon and Pearn (32) reported that the socioeconomic status of the families of children with inflicted immersions did not differ from that of unintentional submersion victims (12).

> A 3-year-old who was being watched by his 15-year-old sibling soiled his clothes. The sib ran a bath, undressed him, and put him in the tub. On returning from a phone call, the sibling found the child submerged in 3 inches of water. Medics could not revive him. Feces were found in the tub, on the toilet, and on the floor. The tub water was very cold. Legal investigation revealed that the child had been suffocated before immersion.

Kemp (19) described two infants younger than 2 months that slipped from their parent's arms during a bath and were briefly immersed without injury. This outcome for unintentional submersion is reassuring when compared with the cumulative 52% mortality for inflicted cases (Table 17.1).

Inflicted bathtub immersions can be difficult to recognize because of the absence of associated injuries (2,32). Diagnosis usually depends on discrepancies in the history, caretaker confessions, or concerns expressed by others. Bowel or toilet-training accidents may trigger the event (36). Only one of Kemp's 10 cases had associated injuries of abuse at the time of the immersion (20). A second child subsequently sustained inflicted trauma. Lavelle (24) thought six bathtub immersion victims had been abused. However, she did not state how often individual children had associated injuries. In two cases each, there were bruising and fractures, and in one, retinal bleeding. However, in the combined group of children diagnosed with either abuse or severe neglect, physical findings of abuse and/or severe neglect were found in 38%, and one fourth of them had prior protective services involvement. One of her case descriptions also included abusive physical findings. Gillenwater (12) found physical evidence consistent with or suggestive of abuse in 14 of 16 inflicted immersion victims. Although he did not specifically state it in the original article, review of his data showed that eight of the nine children with bathtub immersions had physical evidence of abuse, as did both summaries of bathtub cases in the report. Ten of the 16 inflicted immersions of all types had histories inconsistent with the event; four, a previous history of abuse; three, an admission by a perpetrator or an eyewitness report; and one, a positive radiologic finding of abuse.

TABLE 17.1. *Bathtub submersion case series and child abuse*

Author	Study years	Bathtub immersions (n)	Due to abuse (n)	Fatalities (n)
Pearn, 1979	1973–1977	7	1	0
Quan	1974–1983	16	3	—
Devos	1934–1983 (9 due to carbon monoxide poison)	12	1	1
Kemp	1988–1989	44	10	6
Lavelle	1982–1992	21	6	—
Schmidt	1980–1993	12	2	2
Gillenwater	1983–1991 (56% of 16 inflicted submersions were in the tub)	34	9	3
Total		146	32 (22%)	12 (52%)[a]

[a]Denominator includes only studies reporting number of fatalities associated with abuse.

Her mother's stories varied as to whether a 14-month-old had been alone or with a 2-year-old sibling in a tub or whether both had last been seen outside the tub. She found the infant submerged in the tub and sought aid from a neighbor. At the hospital, resuscitation was unsuccessful. Bilateral retinal bleeding, left frontal ecchymoses with accompanying subgaleal bleeding, and two areas of occipital ecchymoses were present. Forearm, upper thigh, and buttock bruises were noted. Both palms had healing linear burn scars attributed to touching an oven. A healing clavicle fracture, with no accompanying history to account for it, was found on skeletal radiography (12).

The three inflicted bathtub immersion deaths described by Greist (14) had additional physical evidence of abuse, including bruising and scars. Perrot (40) found eight of 170 autopsies of apparent sudden infant death syndrome (SIDS) victims to have died of unnatural death. One occurred when a 4-month-old child's mother "blacked out" after placing her supine on a towel in a bathtub containing 2 to 3 inches of water. When she revived, she found the infant prone and apneic with its nose submerged. At autopsy, a parietal hematoma and free intraperitoneal air were attributed to attempts to remove the child from the tub and revive her. The authors declared this death as due to accidental immersion.

Brewster (6) found that 7% of the homicides of children aged between 1 day and 1 year in the United States Air Force occurred by drowning. One of 12 child homicides seen at a Philadelphia emergency department during the early 1980s was due to drowning (15). One additional child was brought with a history of drowning, but died of inflicted head injury, unaccompanied by evidence of drowning. In a death review study of 384 children from birth to 5 years old in Missouri from 1983 to 1986, the authors concluded that 121 had definitely been abused, 25 had probably been abused, and 109 had possibly been maltreated (9). Fewer than half of the definitely abused children had been previously recognized. Five of the probable and 16 of the possible maltreatment deaths [total 21 (16%) of 134] were due to drowning. The rate of

drowning in the definitely abused group of children was not specified.

Bodies of water other than the bathtub have been involved in inflicted immersions. Adelson (2) observed one homicidal drowning to have been in a brook. One of Greist's (14) homicidal drownings occurred in a natural hot spring. Another liveborn newborn was delivered and drowned in a toilet. The final non-bathtub victim was held prone with her mouth open and asphyxiated by water poured into her mouth. Five of the inflicted submersions reported by Gillenwater (12) occurred in natural bodies of water, one in a swimming pool and one in a toilet. The following case was judged "probably inflicted" because of the developmental stage of the child.

Her mother surmised that an 8-month-old child had climbed out of her infant walker and tipped headfirst into the toilet. The infant was found wedged and apneic; the toilet seat was down. She survived 3 days. Autopsy was negative for trauma, except for a knee contusion and tongue-tip abrasion.

Resnick (46) reported that in 17 (13%) of 131 of his literature review of filicide, the mode of death was drowning. However, only a small proportion (fewer than 12%) of the filicide victims followed the classic pattern of child abuse. Much more common were "altruistic" killings (49%), with 38% of them accompanied by suicide of the perpetrator. In the murder–suicides, the perpetrator, overidentifying the child with him- or herself, wished to save the child from a similar adulthood fate. The other altruistic killings fit a pattern of euthanasia. Twenty-four percent of the killings resulted from acute perpetrator psychosis. Eleven were intended to dispose of an unwanted child, and two were intended to punish or seek revenge on a spouse. This contrasts with the higher frequency of "unwanted child" and lower incidence of altruistic and "psychotic" killings in neonaticide; *vida infra.*

Toddlers have been recognized to fall head first into and sustain drowning events in 3- to 5-gallon pails (17,18,27,55,56). The top-heavy toddlers are waist high to the rim of a bucket. Curiosity leads them to look and fall in head first. The buckets are stable when filled with water, so that the wedged child is unable to escape. The children reported in individual case series range from 9 to 16 months old. A larger series using reports to the Consumer Product Safety Commission (CPSC) range from 7 to 15 months old (27). None of these authors noted inflicted instances of pail drownings. To fall into the pail, the child must either be at least a "cruiser" or be placed in it. Although the 7-month-olds from the Mann study may have been early cruisers, the data abstract format of the CPSC reports would have been unlikely to have details about child development. Certainly the child's individual developmental ability should be reviewed to decide whether the unintentional injury scenario is plausible. Toddlers can sustain similar unintentional immersions in toilets.

Neonaticide

Neonaticide has extensive historic roots. Lacking other means of birth control, societies either sanctioned or ignored parental killing of newborns. The victim might be simply unintended and unwanted, malformed, of reduced viability, or simply the wrong sex (26). Pinkham (41), from late 19th century, reported that 29 (28%) of 104 homicidal deaths in Massachusetts resulted from infanticide. He cited one "notorious case" of a neonate thrown from the dock in Lynn; this had been reported in the press. He also described in detail the medicolegal evaluation of an infant found dead in a privy. Resnick (47) reviewed the case literature of neonaticide in an attempt to understand its psychiatric underpinnings. Drowning, suffocation, strangulation, head trauma, exposure, and stabbing were the common methods of death in 37 cases of neonaticides. Drowning most often occurred in the toilet. The baby was killed by its mother in 34 instances, by its father in two, and by both parents in one. Motivations were divided between murder of an unwanted infant (29), psychotic acts (four), altruistic (one), and accidental (one) motivations. Altruistic murders were intended to relieve suffering, and accidental

murders in this study and his 1969 study (46) of older children contained many motivations including classic "battered child syndrome." The unwanted infant cases often involved young, unmarried primiparous women who either denied pregnancy or naively anticipated a stillbirth. There was a lack of preparation for both the birth and the murder. Many of the mothers were afraid to reveal the pregnancy to their mother and/or family. Included among these were instances of incest. A second group of mothers were older, egotistic, and promiscuous women who disposed of an encumbering infant with premeditation. Some of these were married women whose newborn were not conceived with their husbands. Common among both motivations was a lack of empathy with the neonate and failure to view it as a person. Finkelhor (11) also commented on the predominance of young mothers with unintended pregnancies and no prenatal care in the killing of unwanted newborns. Drowning was a prototypic mode. Greist's (14) case number four was a premature infant delivered in the toilet to a 17-year-old, unwed mother. Walther's (57) forensic postmortem study of 89 stillborns and liveborns found a violent cause of death during the postmortem examination of 20. Two additional children also had postmortem evidence of prenatal death. Histology and scene investigation led to the determination of violent causes of death in 11 of the remaining 67 cases not diagnosed at autopsy. Five of the children died after birth in the toilet, a pail, or another water container. After investigation, the cause of death remained unclear because of the advanced state of decomposition of 49 infants who had been left in water or otherwise concealed for prolonged periods. A violent cause of death was found for 33 of the 40 for whom a pathologic determination could be made.

In neonaticide as in drowning in general, local customs and the local environment contribute to patterns of injury. In the Hokkaido district of Japan, 24 (57%) of 42 cases of neonaticide were by drowning (52). This most often occurred in the cistern under the toilet. In all, 29 bodies were discovered in the toilet, and two in the bath. Some had been killed by other means than drowning before disposal.

PATHOLOGY OF DROWNING

One of the difficulties of assessing drowning as a cause of death is the lack of consistent and specific pathologic findings. As Knight (22) so aptly indicated: "Many corpses are recovered from water, but not all have drowned." Death of natural disease may precede or occur after entering the water. Natural disease also may decrease endurance, leading to a drowning death. Other injuries in the water can cause death, and other effects of immersion, such as vagal-induced bradycardia in the intoxicated victim due to cold-water exposure, may cause death. Review of 58 childhood drowning deaths by Smith (53) found no inflicted events, but six who died of natural causes. In four cases, epileptic events lead to the immersion. One child died of a ruptured intracranial aneurysm and one of a coronary anomaly. Devos (7) reported carbon monoxide poisoning to be a frequent cause of unintentional bathtub immersion deaths in Belgium. Although children in the U.S. are less likely to be as exposed to this environmental hazard, this mode of death could remain unrecognized without careful scene investigation and a high level of suspicion.

The final common pathway in drowning is asphyxial injury, although cold stress and electrolyte abnormalities often participate (22). Fresh-water drowning often includes washout of pulmonary surfactant, with alveolar overdistention. Betz (5) observed that alveolar macrophages also are washed out in the pulmonary edema fluid, but that the number of residual macrophages is not different between drowning victims and other fatalities. Frothy, often bloody, pulmonary fluid is commonly observed. It is not until the macrophages per area of alveolar lining are quantitated morphometrically that differences can be noted between drowning and other causes of death. This reflects the macrophage washout plus "emphysema aqueosum": the alveolar overdistention of the drowning vic-

tim. Such morphometric analysis is not suitable for routine case evaluation. Attempts to diagnose drowning by differences in electrolytes and chemistries on the right and left side of the circulation also have yielded inconsistent and unreliable results (22). Certainly aspirated or swallowed water is absorbed into the circulation, and in fresh-water drowning, hyponatremia may occur. This finding has been observed in infant swimming/drown-proofing programs (23).

> A breast-fed infant was admitted to the hospital at age 3 and 6 weeks with altered consciousness, seizures, and hyponatremia (114 mEq/L and 133 mEq/L). During the first hospitalization, a computed tomography scan of the brain, renal and endocrine studies, as well as breast milk electrolytes were normal. Further history revealed that the family had been supplementing the child with tap water by bottle, and the hyponatremia was attributed to that. Concerns about her father's rough play with and yelling at the baby led to protective services referral for parenting skills. Both parents had childhood histories of abuse and rejection. On the second hospitalization, respiratory distress led to finding a right upper lobe infiltrate as well as multifocal pulmonary atelectasis on the chest film. She was again hospitalized after an apneic event a week later. Pneumogram demonstrated moderate gastroesophageal reflux, and she was discharged on therapy for reflux.
>
> Three weeks later, she presented in irreversible shock with abdominal bruising, rib fractures, and a lacerated liver. In retrospect, she had been in her father's presence at the onset of all four events. Her father subsequently admitted immersing her in water when she was fussy. The hyponatremia likely resulted from aspiration of water, as did the pulmonary infiltrates of the second hospitalization.

Lung weights in drowning are inconsistently increased, and fluid may exude from the cut surface of the lung (22). "Dry lung" drowning may result from laryngospasm or in cases of reflex bradycardia. Intrapulmonary hemorrhage may be noted (22).

Attempts have been made to document drowning by the presence of foreign materials in the lung and body. Diatoms are present in most fresh- and salt-water bodies. They commonly enter the lungs with aspiration of water, and then pass into the circulation. Unfortunately the potential for specimen contamination is great, and their presence in the lungs may be a postmortem artifact of water entry (22). They are less likely to enter the circulation and other body tissues after death. Because there are a great number of diatom species with differing structure, they may have a role in matching victims with a specific body of water of immersion through identifying species homology (43). Similarly other foreign materials [silt, weeds, sand, bath salts, which may contain fluorescein (29), toilet paper (14), and cesspool contents (52)] have been described as links between a victim and a specific body of water. Middle-ear hemorrhage has been proposed as an indication of drowning (25), but it appears too nonspecific (22). In neonaticide, the first pathologic consideration is not whether the infant died by drowning, but whether the child was born alive.

Pathologic and scene evaluation also should consider whether caretakers have given a false history of unintentional drowning to obscure findings of other inflicted injury.

> Medics were called to the home of a 26-month-old foster child who had been found apneic in the bathtub after being left alone an indeterminate time. They, however, observed her to be lying on the floor beside the tub. She was dry and was wearing a dry diaper. Fresh hair-dryer grid-imprint burns were observed on her face, and granulating scald burns were seen at the angles of her mouth. Multiple bruises were observed about her face and body. Hair was avulsed from her scalp, and petechiae noted at the empty follicles. Right-sided retinal hemorrhage was present. She was resuscitated, but died a day later. At autopsy, an occipital scalp contusion, an acute subdural hemorrhage, and massive brain swelling were observed. The left humerus had a well-healed shaft fracture and deformity suggestive of a healed proximal metaphyseal injury. No evidence of drowning was seen at autopsy. Her foster mother subsequently plead guilty to charges of physical assault.

NEGLECT IN DROWNING

Most neglect fatalities result from common childhood unintentional injuries (34). Drowning represents a classic injury scenario in which caretakers must balance the child's needs for education about safety and independence of activity with needs for safety supervision. The younger child lacks the cognitive ability to learn how to avoid hazards, whereas the older child can incorporate safety learning. The older child needs to begin independent exploration of the world. If there is misunderstanding by the caretaker of the child's ability on this scale of protection versus independence or an imbalance between the caretaker's actions and the child's needs, problems result. At the younger end of the scale, the caretaker fails to protect the child from hazards it is unable to understand or avoid. At the older end of the scale, the child's learning and independence are stunted, and a symbiotic relationship of the parent with the overprotected child may develop. One of the commonest causes of fatal, unintended injury is drowning. Lapses in supervision expose the children to hazards beyond their mastery. Within these supervision lapses are those that are common or fit the community standard for most caretakers. Alternatively, individual events may represent pervasive patterns of lack of supervision or significantly fail to meet community standards of supervision. The former might result in unintentional or "accidental" child injury or death, whereas death or injury in the latter case would be termed injury due to "child neglect." Child neglect accounts for a number of child deaths similar to the number from child abuse (3,28). Among child deaths from neglect, drowning is frequent. At least nine (26%) of 34 cases of fatal neglect reported by Margolin (28) were the result of drowning. Six resulted from bathtub and two from bucket drownings. Lavelle (24) reported that 67% of 21 bathtub immersions constituted either simple or severe neglect. Feldman (10) observed that clinicians had sufficient concern to refer 25% of 12 bathtub immersions to protective services. Three of four reported neglect fatalities from Oregon during 1985 and 1986 resulted from drowning (34).

The peak ages for unintentional bathtub immersions are 8 to 24 months (20,37). Santer (49), surveying medically indigent families in Chicago, found that 89% of children between ages 35 and 59 months and 6% of those younger than 3 years sometimes bathe without supervision. This suggests that the supervisory milieu in which unintentional drowning occurs affects many infants. Bathtub drowning incidents, whether ruled neglect or not, follow a similar pattern of occurring in families with more children in the family (10,38). The younger child is left to bathe with preschool-age peers. All of Lavelle's (24) bathtub submersions had been left unattended by an adult, and 28% had a peer younger than 4 years in the bathtub with them. Margolin (28) found fatal neglect to involve older children more than did fatal abuse (ages 2.8 vs. 1.8 years), with fatalities from either form of maltreatment infrequent after age 3 years. Fatal neglect occurred in larger families (mean, 4.9 vs. 3.5 family members) with more children (mean, 3.3 vs. 1.8 children). A single parent (44% vs. 31%) frequently headed families of both fatal neglect and fatal abuse victims. Lavelle (24) also found 43% of bathtub drowning victims to be from a single-parent home. These incidents are commonest in lower socioeconomic status families (10,37) with significant psychosocial problems (24,37). Besharov (4) observed that neglect is 4 times as likely to involve low-income families on public assistance and single-parent families (45% of reports). The household routine may be upset, whereas in inflicted bathtub immersions, a frustrating event, such as a toileting accident or a child crying, may trigger the abusive event (32).

Health professionals who were provided scenarios of childhood submersions were only slightly more likely than not to consider neglectful a "welfare mother who left a one and four year old alone in the bathtub" and a "father who left a 16 month old alone in the tub in order to answer the phone" (10). Further, they were slightly less likely to report the incident to protective services. Clinicians were even less likely to consider a "three year old child who wandered off at a picnic and drowned in a lake" to have been neglected.

However, parental impairment seemed most likely to result in a neglect diagnosis. A "two year old who drowned in the family pool while under the care of his intoxicated father" elicited clinicians' strongest opinion of neglect. These judgments that most drownings are not neglect contrast with the opinion of Reece and Grodin (45). They thought lack of infant bath supervision to constitute "passive abuse." They thought that cases of drowning at younger than 1 year should be considered and managed as "nonaccidental" injury. Margolin (28) also equated any fatal childhood injury in the absence of direct caretaker supervision with neglect. All of the neglect deaths he reported, except four involving failure to follow medical advice and two from failure to seek medical care expeditiously, resulted from injury fatalities. Although others have also observed neglect deaths from malnutrition, exposure to the elements, and failure to provide needed medical care, this raises the problem of screening for risk of unintentional injury fatality due to neglect. He suggested that 61% of the families would have been identified by three items on Polansky's Childhood Level of Living Scale (42). However, the items suggested, such as "mother sometimes leaves child in the care of an insufficiently older sibling" seem to lack precision and be likely to encompass the majority of families.

Besharov (4) stated that protective services involvement is not warranted in injury due to neglect, unless the pattern of neglect was pervasive. Alter (1) also described neglect as a sustained pattern of inadequate parenting, which must be judged in light of community standards. She suggested that the danger to the child be quantified by documenting the degree of injury, age of the child, and frequency with which the child was exposed to hazard, in making decisions to involve protective services. Further qualitative judgments about parental behavior—its willfulness, the other attributes, and effectiveness of the parent child interaction, level of parental social deviance, and willingness to change—should be included in decision making. Feldman (10) suggested that clinicians consider the utility of reporting in borderline cases of neglect. Reports and requests for home evaluation to public health nursing, rather than initially to protective services, might in some cases allow better information gathering and preventive intervention. In any case, the focus should be less on establishing blame for past neglect than on identifying behavior that creates future risk to the child or its family. Evaluators should seek solutions to these risks.

CONCLUSION

As in any other type of childhood injury, the clinician should consider whether the injury scenario is behaviorally and developmentally plausible. The child should be examined for other indications of maltreatment. The strengths, weaknesses, and coping style of the family should be considered. If those procedures are followed, child abuse or neglect may be recognized as the cause of a childhood immersion event. This knowledge is required for the clinician to intervene appropriately to protect the victim and its siblings.

REFERENCES

1. Alter CF. Decision-making factors in cases of child neglect. *Child Welfare* 1985;64:99–111.
2. Adelson L. Slaughter of innocents: study of forty-six homicides in which the victims were children. *N Engl J Med* 1961;264:1345–1349.
3. Anderson R, Ambrosino R, Valentine D, et al. Child deaths attributed to abuse and neglect: an empirical study. *Child Youth Services Rev* 1983;5:75–89.
4. Besharov DJ. *Recognizing child abuse: a guide for the concerned.* New York: The Free Press/Macmillan, 1990: 99–107, 108–113.
5. Betz P, Nerlich A, Penning R, et al. Alveolar macrophages and the diagnosis of drowning. *Forensic Sci Int* 1993;62:217–224.
6. Brewester DR, Nelson JP, Hymel KP, et al. Victim, perpetrator, family, and incident characteristics of 32 infant maltreatment deaths in the United States Air Force. *Child Abuse Negl* 1998;22:91–101.
7. Devos C, Timperman J, Piette M. Deaths in the bath. *Med Sci Law* 1985;25:189–200.
8. Diekema DS, Quan L, Holt VL. Epilepsy as a risk factor for submersion injury. *Pediatrics* 1993;91:612–616.
9. Ewigman B, Kivilahan C, Land G. The Missouri Child Fatality Study: underreporting of maltreatment fatalities among children younger than five years of age, 1983 through 1986. *Pediatrics* 1993;91:330–337.
10. Feldman KW, Monestersky C, Feldman GK. When is

childhood drowning neglect? *Child Abuse Negl* 1993; 17:329–336.
11. Finkelhor D. The homicides of children and youth: a developmental perspective. In: Kantor KG, Jasinski xx, eds. *Out of darkness: contemporary perspectives on family violence.* Thousand Oaks, CA: Sage Publications, 1997:17–34.
12. Gillenwater JM, Quan L, Feldman KW. Inflicted submersion in childhood. *Arch Pediatr Adolesc Med* 1996; 150:298–303.
13. Gregg GS, Elmer E. Infant injuries: accident or abuse? *Pediatrics* 1969;44:434–439.
14. Griest KJ, Zumwalt RE. Child abuse by drowning. *Pediatrics* 1989;83:41–46.
15. Hodge D, Ludwig S. Child homicide: emergency department recognition. *Pediatr Emerg Care* 1985;1:3–6.
16. Holter JC, Friedman SB. Child abuse: early case finding in the emergency department. *Pediatrics* 1968;42: 128–138.
17. Jensen LR, Williams SD, Thurman DJ, et al. Submersion injuries in children younger than 5 years in urban Utah. *West J Med* 1992;157:641–644.
18. Jumblic MI, Chamblis M. Accidental toddler drowning in 5-gallon buckets. *JAMA* 1990;263:1952–1953.
19. Kemp A, Sibert JR. Drowning and near drowning in children in the United Kingdom: lessons for prevention. *Br Med J* 1992;304:1143–1146.
20. Kemp AM, Mott AM, Sibert JR. Accidents and child abuse in bathtub submersions. *Arch Dis Child* 1994;70: 435–438.
21. Kempe CH, Silverman FN, Steele BF, et al. The battered-child syndrome. *JAMA* 1962;181:17–24.
22. Knight B. Immersion deaths. In: Knight B, ed. *Forensic pathology.* New York: Oxford University Press, 1991: 360–373.
23. Kropp RM, Schwartz JF. Water intoxication from swimming. *J Pediatr* 1982;101:947–948.
24. Lavelle JM, Shaw KN, Seidl T, et al. Ten-year review of pediatric bathtub near-drownings: evaluation for child abuse and neglect. *Am J Emerg Med* 1995;25:344–348.
25. Liu C, Babin RW. A histological comparison of the temporal bone in strangulation and drowning. *J Otolaryngol* 1984;13:44–46.
26. McGowan J. Little girls dying: an ancient and thriving practice. *Commonwealth* 1991;118:481–482.
27. Mann NC, Weller SC, Rauchschwalbe R. Bucket-related drownings in the United States, 1984-1990. *Pediatrics* 1992;89:1068–1071.
28. Margolin L. Fatal child neglect. *Child Welfare* 1990;69: 309–319.
29. Mukaida M, Kimura H, Takada Y. Detection of bathsalts in the lungs of a baby drowned in a bathtub. *Forensic Sci Int* 1998;93:5–11.
30. Muscat JE. Characteristics of child homicide in Ohio, 1974-84. *Am J Public Health* 1988;78:822–824.
31. National Safety Council. *Accident facts, Itasca, Illinois.* 1998 edition 10-11.
32. Nixon J, Pearn J. Non-accidental immersion in the bath: another aspect of child abuse. *Br Med J* 1977;1:271.
33. O'Neill JA Jr, Meacham WF, Griffin PP, et al. Patterns of injury in the battered child syndrome. *J Trauma* 1973;13:332–339.
34. Oregon Department of Human Services. *Fatal child abuse and neglect in Oregon, 1985 and 1986.* Oregon Children's Services Division, 1988.

35. Pearn J, Nixon J. Freshwater drowning and near-drowning accidents involving children. *Med J Aust* 1976;2: 942–946.

36. Pearn J, Nixon J. Attempted drowning as a form of nonaccidental injury. *Aust Pediatr J* 1977;13:110–113.

37. Pearn J, Nixon J. Bathtub immersion accidents involving children. *Med J Aust* 1977;1:211–213.

38. Pearn J, Nixon J. Bathtub drownings: report of seven cases. *Med J Aust* 1977;1:211–213.

39. Pearn JH, Wong RYK, Brown J III, et al. Drowning and near drowning involving children: a five-year total population study from the city and county of Honolulu. *Am J Public Health* 1979;69:450–454.

40. Perrot LJ, Nawojczyk S. Nonnatural death masquerading as SIDS (sudden infant death syndrome). *Am J Forensic Med Pathol* 1988;9:105–111.

41. Pinkham JG. Some remarks upon infanticide, with report of a case of infanticide by drowning. *Boston Med Surg J* 1883;109:411–413.

42. Polansky N, Chalmers MA, Buttenweiser E, et al. Assessing adequacy of child caring: an urban scale. *Child Welfare* 1978;57:439–449.

43. Pollanen M. Diatoms and homicide. *Forensic Sci Int* 1998;91:29–34.

44. Quan L, Gore EJ, Wentz K, et al. Ten-year study of pediatric drownings and near-drownings in King County, Washington: lessons in injury prevention. *Pediatrics* 1989;83:1035–1040.

45. Reece RM, Grodin EJ. Recognition of nonaccidental injury. *Pediatr Clin North Am* 1985;32:41–57.

46. Resnick PJ. Child murder by parents: a psychiatric review of filicide. *Am J Psychiatry* 1969;126:73–82.

47. Resnick PJ. Murder of the newborn: a psychiatric review of neonaticide. *Am J Psychiatry* 1970;126: 58–64.

48. Rowe MI, Arango A, Allington G. Profile of pediatric drowning victims in a water-oriented society. *J Trauma* 1977;17:587–591.

49. Santer LJ, Stocking CNB. Safety practices and living conditions of low-income urban families. *Pediatrics* 1991;88:1112–1118.

50. Saxena A, Ang LC. Epilepsy and bathtub drowning: important neuropathological observations. *Am J Forensic Med Pathol* 1993;14:125–129.

51. Scott PH, Eigen H. Immersion accidents involving pails of water in the home. *J Pediatr* 1980;96:282–284.

52. Shionono H, Maya A, Tabata N, et al. Medicolegal aspects of infanticide in Hokkaido District, Japan. *Am J Forensic Med Pathol* 1986;7:104–106.

53. Smith NM, Byard RW, Bourne AJ. Death during immersion in water in childhood. *Am J Forensic Med Pathol* 1991;12:219–211.

54. Smith SM, Hanson R. 134 battered children: a medical & psychological study. *Br Med J* 1974;3:666–670.

55. Sturner WQ, Spruill FG, Smith RA, et al. Accidental asphyxial deaths involving infants and young children. *J Forensic Sci* 1976;21:483–487.

56. Walker S, Middelkamp N. Pail immersion accidents. *Clin Pediatr* 1981;20:341–343.

57. Walther G, Faust G. Kausalitatsprobleme beim Nachweis der Totung des Neugeborenen. *Z Rechtsmed* 1970; 67:109–118.

56. Wintermute GJ. Childhood drowning and near-drowning in the United States. *Am J Dis Child* 1990;144:663–669.

18

Unusual Manifestations of Child Abuse

*Rebecca R.S. Socolar and †Desmond K. Runyan

*Departments of *Pediatrics and *,†Social Medicine,
University of North Carolina School of Medicine at Chapel Hill;
*University of North Carolina Hospitals; and †Department of Pediatrics,
North Carolina Children's Hospital, Chapel Hill, North Carolina*

The task of describing unusual manifestations of child abuse is complex. First, there is the problem of how to define a manifestation of abuse. This could mean the perpetrated behaviors, or the consequences of those behaviors, such as physical and psychological signs in the child. Second, there is the problem of how to define "unusual." Unusual might mean infrequent manifestations of abuse or bizarre variations of common manifestations. Our judgment about what is rare is usually determined by clinical experience rather than by epidemiologic data.

Rare or unusual forms of child maltreatment have a history of becoming more widely recognized and losing the appellation "rare." Child maltreatment itself was once thought to be quite rare. David Gill (23) reported on the 6,000 officially reported cases of child abuse in the United States in 1967. Sexual abuse also was considered rare; in 1955, the total number of incest cases in the U.S. was estimated to be 500, and in 1969, the estimated number was 5,000 (25). Annual maltreatment incidence estimates now border on 49/1,000 children per year by parent self-report, and the total number of cases identified by professionals is 5.7/1,000 children per year (81). In the U.S., there are more than 1 million substantiated cases per year.

In the 1940s, 1950s, and 1960s, fractures were recognized as a manifestation of child abuse (11,76), and the battered child syn-

drome was described (42). At that time, these were new and unusual findings, and were reported as such in the literature. In literature from the 1960s and 1970s, early case reports of some unusual types of maltreatment were later recognized to represent more common manifestations. For example, in 1975, Kempe (41) listed a number of manifestations of child abuse as uncommon manifestations of the battered child syndrome, including human bites, handprint bruising, intramural hematoma of the bowel, and whiplash–shaken infant syndrome. Today these would be not considered to be uncommon manifestations of physical abuse. A review of the literature in the subsequent decades reveals that sometimes reports of findings that were originally viewed as unusual or bizarre have come to be incorporated into standard knowledge about maltreatment and are covered in some detail in other chapters. In addition, some forms of abuse that are fairly uncommon have been the subject of numerous reports in the literature. For example, Munchausen syndrome by proxy (MSBP) was once considered an unusual manifestation of abuse; it has now become the topic of a separate chapter in this volume, although epidemiologic estimates of the frequency still characterize this problem as one of relatively low frequency.

The purpose of a catalog of unusual manifestations is not to titillate the reader but to help extend the differential diagnostic possibilities for the clinician and to help ensure that maltreatment is included among the diagnostic possibilities when an unusual clinical presentation is noted. In this chapter we address perpetrated behaviors of abuse and summarize a variety of reported forms of maltreatment organized by organ system to assist the clinician in the recognition of unusual physical manifestations of maltreatment.

BEHAVIORS AND CULTURE

Determining what is rare or unusual is filtered through the lens of culture. What is "rare" in one culture may be more common and carry quite a different connotation in others. A specific behavior or form of abuse may appear to be uncommon not because the experience is uncommon within a culture or ethnic group of people but because that group is a relatively small part of the larger society. Alternatively, a behavior may be normative in the larger society but be very uncommon and unacceptable within a minority cultural group. For example, in the 1995 Gallup poll survey, "Disciplining Children in America," 4% of U.S. parents reported "slapping" a child on the face, head, or ears, whereas 47% reported "spanking" a child in the last year (22). Similar data from India found that 57% of parents had slapped their child on the face or head, whereas 57% had used "spanking" (38). When a group of investigators planning an international study of maltreatment convened focus groups of parents and professionals in three countries, focus groups in three different countries independently suggested that an instrument designed to assess the frequency of child abuse should include items such as "twisting his or her ear"; "hit him/her on the head with knuckles"; "threaten to invoke ghosts, evil spirits, or harmful people"; "put chili pepper, hot pepper, or spicy food in mouth"; and "force the child to stand or kneel in a painful area such as hot sand or with an added burden." These types of items had not risen to the top as possible means of discipline for the Parent–Child Conflict Tactics Scale developed in the U.S. (78).

Pilot data for the international study, from one rural area in one developing country, found that 3% of parents had used inflicting a burn as punishment, something that none of the 1,000 U.S. parents surveyed by the Gallup Organization in 1995 acknowledged. The item on putting hot pepper in the mouth or on the tongue that was suggested by the focus groups was not included in the U.S. survey. Unpublished conflict tactics scale data from a second developing country suggested some of the same manifestations of maltreatment were seen there. Interestingly, several cases of the use of pepper as punishment have been reported as unusual manifestations of maltreatment in the U.S. In both developing countries, there were reports of a relatively high frequency of forcing the children to stand in one place with an added burden or in hot sand. In one of the countries, nearly 2% of the children had been tied up off the ground by a parent (Table 18.1).

These data from other countries help to put the U.S. experience in context. It is likely that forms of maltreatment that are more common in other countries will be seen in the U.S., although perhaps at lower rates. It is difficult to know the extent to which the rates reported here represent true differences in behavior in different countries, as opposed to different willingness to report behaviors. It seems likely that societal norms affect actual behavior as well as willingness to report about behaviors.

In addition to the type of abuse and the involved organ system, other aspects of abuse might make it unusual. For example, in some cases, the implement used for the abuse is what is unusual, such as an air weapon, needles, or a candle; in other cases, a characteristic of the perpetrator or victim is the unusual feature, such as male perpetrators of MSBP, perpetrators with mental illness, or twin victims of the shaken baby syndrome. To avoid duplication, we have categorized these various other aspects of perpetrators, victims, and behavior by type of abuse and organ system that was affected and report these.

TABLE 18.1. *Unusual forms of maltreatment used by parents in population surveys (self-report)*

	Behavior rate U.S.[a] (last year)	Rate for rural area country 1[b] (last 6 mo)	Rate for urban area country 2[c] (last 6 mo)
Slapped face	46/1,000	578/1,000	210/1,000
Burned or scalded	0/1,000	12/1,000	5.9/1,000
Threatened with knife or gun	0/1,000	12/1,000	0/1,000
Choked	0/1,000	16/1,000	7.4/1,000
Beat-up	2/1,000	Not asked	27/1,000
Kicked	3/1,000	104/1,000	56/1,000
Hot pepper in mouth	Not asked	26/1,000	7.7/1,000

[a]Gallup Poll data.
[b]Unpublished data from the WorldSAFE consortium in a Lesser Developed Country from a poor rural village, from Runyan D, Hunter W, unpublished manuscript.
[c]Unpublished data from the WorldSAFE consortium in a Lesser Developed Country from an urban slum, from Runyan D, Hunter W, unpublished manuscript.

PHYSICAL ABUSE

Skin

Microwave Burns

The cases of two children, 5 weeks old and 14 months old, with full-thickness burns as a result of being placed in microwave ovens have been reported (3). The 5-week-old infant had burns over 11% of her body surface, was hospitalized for 33 days, and survived after four surgeries including amputations, escharotomies, and skin grafts (Fig. 18.1). Biopsies showed characteristic microwave burn patterns (see Chapter 2), with sparing of the subcutaneous fat level between burned dermis/epidermis and muscle. The 14-month-old toddler had second- and third-degree burns of the midback, which required skin grafting, but these lesions would not have been recognized as the result of microwave burns had the baby-sitter not confessed. The child recovered fully with no evidence of any long-term physical or psychological sequelae at approximately age 10 years.

Grease Burns

A review of 215 hospitalized cases of burns caused by hot grease/oil (57) revealed only one case of child abuse, although 4% to 8% of all pediatric burns are reported to be caused by hot grease or oil (62). This suggests that abuse by burning a child with grease is un-

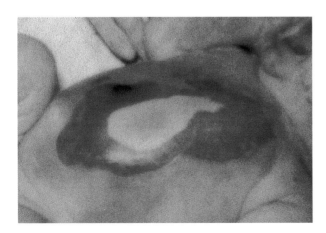

FIG. 18.1. Ventral burns. There are full-thickness burns to left abdomen and thorax and partial-thickness burns to left anterior thigh. Extensive circumferential burns of right foot and left hand are not seen. This infant presumably was placed on her back in microwave oven.

usual. Hot water is reported to be the thermal medium that burns 82% of child abuse burn victims (67), whereas flame and hot solids are the medium of burn in 8% to 10% of child abuse burns.

Subcutaneous Emphysema

A 2-month-old girl presented with extensive swelling of her head and neck as well as subcutaneous emphysema over her scalp, neck, and chest, with crepitus (5). Further studies revealed a hypopharyngeal perforation that caused pneumomediastinum and subcutaneous emphysema. In addition, she had multiple rib fractures. There now have been several reported cases of subcutaneous emphysema associated with perforations of the hypopharynx or esophagus of abused children (see later under Gastrointestinal/Thoracic).

Tattooing and Scarring

Cases of children who were given tattoos or scars have been reported, including a 7-year-old boy whose arm was forcibly tattooed with his name, two children with other signs of abuse who had been tattooed on their hands, and a 9-year-old girl who had a cross cut in her forehead when her mother heard voices that told her to cut crosses in her forehead and her daughter's forehead (39).

Gastrointestinal/Thoracic

Hypopharynx and Esophagus

Twenty-two cases of traumatic perforation of the hypopharynx have been reported since 1984 (68) (see Chapter 8). Although this seems to be a relatively rare manifestation of abuse, it has now been reported multiple times. Examples include (53) infants for whom laryngoscopy revealed hemorrhagic lesions of the posterior pharyngeal wall, and radiography revealed interstitial emphysema. Toddlers have been reported as well and, as with infants (80), frequently have other substantial injuries in addition to the pharyngeal/esophageal perforation (56,69). Often

these inflicted perforations result in associated infections (1,24).

One case of esophageal foreign bodies associated with a child fatality has been described (59). In this case, coins were repeatedly inserted into the esophagus of a 5-month-old infant. The child was seen initially at 4 months with numerous coins in the esophagus, and a history given that a piggy bank had spilled into the crib and the child ingested the coins. The child was hospitalized, and seven coins were retrieved by esophagoscopy. One month later, the child was brought dead on arrival to the same emergency department with multiple fractures of extremities and three coins in the esophagus. The mechanism of death was not clear.

Small Bowel

When intestinal intramural hematomas secondary to child abuse were first described (17), they were thought to be unusual. By now, intramural duodenal hematomas have been described numerous times, and jejunal hematomas are recognized as less common than duodenal, but still not rare. Strictures of the duodenum and jejunum have been described as an unusual complication of hematomas and perforations secondary to child abuse in a 15-month-old (75).

Pancreas

After pseudocysts of the pancreas secondary to child abuse were first described (9), it was not long before it was recognized that pseudocysts of the pancreas were due to child abuse more commonly than the literature had previously indicated (63,71). More than 25 years after pseudocysts of the pancreas were first described in cases of abuse, they are still considered relatively rare.

Chylothorax and Chylous Ascites

An 11-month-old with respiratory distress had chest radiography that showed complete opacification of the right lung field. Thoracentesis revealed odorless, sterile, creamy fluid. There were multiple fractures of ribs, spine, and long bone, as well as a probable inflicted burn (27).

Chylous ascites is an extremely rare complication of abdominal trauma in children. Some of the first cases of posttraumatic chylous ascites in children were first reported in the 1960s, and recognized as a manifestation of child abuse in the 1970s (10). Since that time, there have been several reports of chylous ascites secondary to child abuse (32,60). The diagnosis is made by the milky appearance of fluid obtained from paracentesis, a sterile culture, the presence of fat globules on Sudan stain, and an alkaline pH. It is estimated that child abuse accounts for approximately 10% of all cases of chylous ascites in children (7). The leakage caused by trauma has consistently been found at the root of the mesentery of the small bowel rather than at the thoracic duct or cisterna chyli.

Cardiac Lacerations

Six cases of fatal abusive cardiac lacerations in children from age 9 weeks to 2.5 years were reported (14). All were the result of severe blunt-force trauma, and all had evidence of other significant trauma. In five cases, the right atrium was lacerated; the left ventricle was lacerated in the remaining case. The authors pointed out that this type of injury is the result of motor vehicle accidents or very violent assault, and not minor trauma.

Head/Neurologic

Shaken Baby/Shaken Impact Syndrome

This is a common form of maltreatment, but some unusual variations of the syndrome have been reported. A case of a 6-week-old infant with a traumatic aneurysm as a complication of shaking with impact has been described (48). Initially the infant presented with a large left subdural hemorrhage, interhemispheric hemorrhage, and cerebral edema. The infant improved for 20 days and then developed seizures again. A repeated

computed tomography (CT) scan showed parafalcine subarachnoid blood and fresh intraventricular hemorrhage. Ultimately, a saccular traumatic aneurysm was removed. A reviewer of this article made the point that the phenomenon of traumatic aneurysm is different from rebleeding in an old subdural (36). In the case of traumatic aneurysm, the location of the bleeding is different, and the subdural hemorrhage had resolved before the second clinical deterioration occurred.

Ear

The tin-ear syndrome is defined by the clinical triad of isolated ear bruising, hemorrhagic retinopathy, and a small ipsilateral subdural hematoma with severe cerebral swelling. This injury is thought to be caused by blunt injury to the ear that results in significant rotational acceleration of the head, and represents an unusual manifestation of child abuse (see Chapter 3). Four cases of this injury have been reported, all in children aged 2 to 3 years, and all with a fatal outcome (29).

Intracranial Foreign Body

A 2-month-old baby presented with a 4-mm circular laceration on his forehead with a history that the baby pulled a coffee table over onto his head (12). Radiographs showed an intracranial airgun pellet. The father then changed his story and reported that his air pistol had gone off accidentally. The mother, who was interviewed separately, said that the father held the pistol several inches from the baby's head and said "shut up or I'll shoot you," and then fired the weapon. The skeletal survey was negative, and the infant recovered well after surgical removal of the pellet.

Spinal Cord Injury

Spinal cord injury without spinal fracture and without head injury is a rare presentation of child abuse, and may escape detection unless other signs of abuse are detected (see Chapter 7). Isolated spinal cord injury is usually due to hyperflexion/hyperextension injuries. Cervical magnetic resonance imaging (MRI) examination can provide specific information about the trauma, but is not routinely recommended to evaluate the shaken baby/shaken impact syndrome (45). The case of a 15-month-old girl with unexplained quadriplegia has been reported (64). At presentation there were fresh and old suggestive bruises, an old facial burn, and an old clavicular fracture, in addition to flaccid quadriplegia with an MRI that showed fusiform swelling of the midcervical spinal cord with hematomyelia. The child survived, but quadriplegia persisted with an MRI after 2 months that showed atrophy of the spinal cord where it had previously been swollen (Fig. 18.2). It should be noted that spinal cord injury without radiographic abnormality is limited to infants, because at this age, the spinal column can be deformed to the point of spinal cord injury without fracture of vertebrae or rupture of ligaments. In addition, thorough postmortem examination demonstrates upper cervical cord lesions in a substantial fraction of infants who die of their head injuries, but these injuries are seldom recognized before death.

Nose

Two reports involving four children ranging in age from 6 months to 8 years indicated that mothers became obsessed with nasal hygiene to the point of significant injury to the nasal tip, columella, and distal septum (21) (Fig. 18.3). There is a report of successful surgical correction in two of the children, although one child showed signs of failure of nasal growth (61). In each case, other causes such as congenital aplasias, congenital syphilis, and leishmaniasis were ruled out.

Teeth

Dental injuries that occur as the result of blunt trauma to the face are frequent manifestations of abuse (see Chapter 6). There has been a case report of three children in a family of six (ages 13 and younger) who were each found to have multiple missing permanent incisors (13). Eventually it was discovered that their parents were extracting teeth as punishment. Although the loss of a single tooth could have been the result of accidental trauma, the loss of multiple teeth at the ages of the children seen in this family did not have a plausible medical explanation.

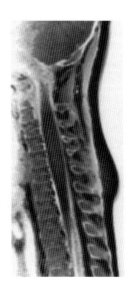
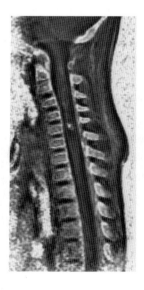

A,B

FIG. 18.2. A: A sagittal T1-weighted image of the cervical spine demonstrated fusiform swelling of the midcervical spinal cord (black arrowheads). **B:** A sagittal T2-weighted image of the cervical spine exhibited several globular (*white arrowhead*) and linear low-signal lesions within the substance of the spinal cord that were interpreted as hematomyelia.

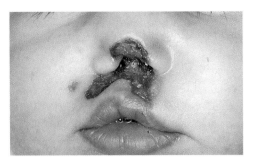

FIG. 18.3. Nasal destruction in a 6-month-old infant.

Skeletal

Pelvis

Fractures of the pelvis are seldom reported in abused children (see Chapter 7). If there is no history of a motor vehicle crash or other severe trauma, then intentional trauma should be considered the etiology for these injuries, because the force required to produce such an injury is tremendous. The case of a 4-year-old girl who was brought to the hospital in full cardiopulmonary arrest was described (66). Multiple injuries including skin bruising, abrasions, and scars were noted all over the body, as well as laceration of the external genitalia, hymen, and vagina. Radiographs showed multiple humeral fractures and a questionable area over the left acetabulum/pubic ramus. At autopsy this area was confirmed as a fracture of the superior pubic ramus and anterior acetabular margin. Pelvic fractures are rare in abused children, but pelvic fractures are associated with signs of sexual abuse as well as physical abuse. Radiography of the pelvis may be helpful in selected cases of sexual abuse that involved signs of significant blunt-force trauma to the soft tissues overlying the pelvis (44).

Spine

Spinal injury is an uncommon manifestation of child abuse, and when seen, it occurs in young children. The average age in reports of these injuries is 22 months, with half of them younger than 1 year (16). Cervical spine injuries occur in 1% to 2% of abusive head injury, and should be considered in any infant who has a severe shaking injury. However, despite the tremendous acceleration and deceleration forces on the head in the prevalent nonaccidental shaking injuries, cervical spine injuries are unusual (77). A report of thoracolumbar spondylolisthesis, bilateral pedicle fractures, and spinal cord trauma in a 12-month-old demonstrated that spinal fracture and spinal cord injury may occur simultaneously in abuse cases, although this is rare (77). Another report described twin infant girls with hyperflexion–extension injuries of the lower cervical spine that resulted in cervical spine fracture–dislocation and cord compression (73). Reports of hangman's fracture (C-2 fracture) are rare. A recent one described a 6-month-old infant with a hangman's fracture and multiple other fractures including 27 rib fractures, clavicular and acromion fractures, and metaphyseal chip fractures of femurs and tibias (46). A hangman's fracture results from forced hyperextension of the neck, and has occurred in conjunction with the shaken baby syndrome.

Hands and Feet

Fractures of the hands and feet are unusual compared with other fractures in abused children, but when found, particularly in infants, are highly suggestive of abuse. A recent review of abused children younger than 2 years found that these fractures were often subtle radiographic findings that require high-detail imaging systems. Buckle fractures of the phalanges likely resulted from forced hyperextension (58).

Systemic: Inhalants, Ingestions, Withholding Nourishment

Cocaine

A number of reports of cocaine intoxication emerged in the 1980s (6,18,72). Although it is unclear which of these cases was due to breast-feeding, intentional administration, accidental ingestion, or passive inhalation of crack vapors, any of these represents abuse or supervisory neglect (see Chapter 13). Cocaine intoxication may not be an unusual form of abuse/neglect. Of all children younger than 5 years seen in one urban emergency room, 2.5% had cocaine metabolites in their urine (43). Thus in this setting, this form of abuse/neglect could not be considered unusual. Clinical presentations of cocaine intoxication that were reported included tachycardia, hypertension, and a range of neurologic symptoms from drowsiness, tremulousness, and unsteady gait to seizures.

Pepper

Fatal pepper aspiration has been reported several times in the literature (2,15). Both abusive and accidental incidents have been reported. In cases of abuse, the pepper was given as punishment to children ranging in age from 4 months to 10 years. About half of the children had evidence of previous abuse, and about half of families initially gave incorrect histories. Mechanical obstruction and mucosal edema were the two mechanisms of death. The prevalence of this form of abuse is unknown, particularly if it is nonfatal. About two in 10,000 calls to poison centers are related to black pepper ingestions (15).

Withholding Water and Water Intoxication

Hypernatremic dehydration from water deprivation has been reported as a form of abuse in children ranging from 2 to 8 years old, often in children who are enuretic, either as a form of managing the enuresis or to punish the child for wetting (65). The degree of hypernatremia in each case was extreme (with serum sodium concentrations ranging from 183 to 201 mEq/L), and required hospitalization. On the other end of the hydration spectrum is the account of water intoxication produced by forcing a garden hose into a 4-year-old boy's mouth and making him swallow large quantities of water. He developed hyponatremia (serum saline concentration

was 117 mEq/L) accompanied by coma and convulsions, but he survived (55).

Other Unusual Poisoning

Poisoning may be one of the more common mechanisms for perpetration of MSBP (see also Chapter 14). However, the incidence of MSBP by any mechanism is unknown and is thought to be uncommon. Various substances have been used to poison or infect children who are victims of MSBP, including prescription and nonprescription drugs (20,82). In addition, a case of choral hydrate poisoning causing coma in a 3-year-old girl on four separate occasions, in the context of MSBP, has been described (49). Ipecac poisoning of three children younger than 2 years, resulting in symptoms including chronic vomiting and diarrhea as well as other gastrointestinal, neurologic, and cardiovascular symptoms has been described. In each case the perpetrator was the biologic mother (52), and each was thought to represent MSBP. Another early case of MSBP involved the intentional poisoning of two siblings by prescription drugs (35).

Other substances besides pepper and water withholding or intoxication have been used as punishment. A case of fatal child abuse has been reported in which a 6-year-old was forced by the live-in baby-sitter to consume large doses of sodium bicarbonate to make the child vomit as punishment. Included in the ingestion were vinegar, dishwashing liquid, and red pepper. Multiple electrolyte abnormalities ensued, and the child was removed from the ventilator after 6 days of flat line electroencephalogram (EEG) (34).

Other Trauma

Needles

Insertion of needles into various body parts as a form of abuse has been described. An 11-year-old boy from India presented to the hospital with an acute abdomen presumed to be secondary to appendicitis. Radiographs of the abdomen revealed seven needles in the abdomen and one in the right lower chest. He reported that this stepmother disliked him and had inserted a sewing needle in his abdomen once a week, and threatened to kill him if he complained (79). A report of three children with abusive needle injuries included a 4-week-old infant who died of pneumonia and was found to have three sewing needles embedded in the occipital lobe. The sibling of this infant had four needles in the soft tissues of the head, neck, and forearm. A third baby had four needles removed from the abdomen (19).

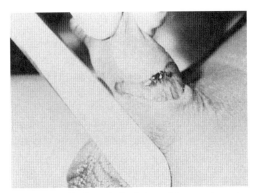

FIG. 18.4. Patient 1. Incision at base of penis.

Pencils

A 4-year-old boy had a deep penetrating wound of the right hand inflicted with a pencil. Although initially the parents said the wound was accidental, questioning of the child revealed that it was inflicted by the mother because the boy had failed to complete his homework properly (50).

Other Systemic Manifestations of Trauma due to Child Abuse

Myositis with elevation of creatinine phosphokinase (CPK) levels is a known manifestation of muscle trauma. It is unclear how common this manifestation of abuse may be. A case was reported of a 2-year-old boy with myositis secondary to the battered child syndrome; it was not recognized as abuse until there had been multiple emergency department visits, fractured bones, and intracranial bleeding (8). Hemoglobinuria has been reported in two children (20 and 32 months old) after severe beatings. One went on to develop transient oliguria, and the other, transient renal failure (71).

Genitourinary

Penis

Inflicted incisions of the penis have been reported in a 6-month-old and a 3-year-old boy. In each case the inconsistent or conflicting histories provided did not adequately explain the injury. In one case, the incision was clean but involved all skin layers, and in the other, there was a gaping wound at the base of the shaft (51) (Fig. 18.4).

Penile strangulations have been reported in cases of parents who have become frustrated with nocturnal enuresis. Patients have presented with penile edema, ulceration, or urethral fistula. Three cases of penile strangulation have been reported from Turkey, ages 4 to 7 years; one was due to ligation with thread, and two, to ligation with hair (28). When the penis is ligated, the urethra may be completely or partially transected. The degree of damage is variable and is correlated with the duration of strangulations.

Unusual Perpetrators

Munchausen Syndrome by Proxy

The incidence rate for MSBP (see also Chapter 14) and the prevalence of various methods used for inducing MSBP are unknown. Although confirmed cases of MSBP remain rare, it seems likely that many cases of MSBP go unreported, and so it is uncertain how unusual the diagnosis or its various manifestations might be. We do know that the perpetrator of MSBP is almost always the mother (74). Meadow (54), in the largest series reported of fathers as perpetrators, described 15 men, 12 of whom were acting out the need to assume a sick role by proxy or were engaged in attention-seeking behavior.

Mental Illness Related

Folie á deux is an uncommon disorder in which the dominant person imposes his or her delusions on a younger/more submissive person. Several cases have been reported of fatal or near-fatal child abuse at the hands of parents with folie á deux. In each case, there had not been a previous diagnosis of psychopathology in either parent. When the abuse occurred, it was based on shared religious delusions, with subsequent diagnoses of psychotic disorder in at least one parent (47). Several of the cases reported involved "beating the faith" into a child or ridding a child of Satan by beating or killing the child.

NEGLECT

Neglect has been associated primarily with poverty and parental problems with emotional health and substance abuse (see Chapter 13). Neglect secondary to religious beliefs and practices is an uncommon but pernicious form of child maltreatment.

In a case of fatal child neglect of an adolescent with ulcerative colitis, a 15.5-year-old girl had intermittent abdominal cramps and watery diarrheal stools 6 months before her death (37). Her devout Christian Scientist parents allowed her to be evaluated by a gastroenterologist 4 months before her death because of the urging of other family members. The parents refused the recommended therapy and instead instituted a liquid health-food diet and sought the care of a chiropractic/health food clinic. Eventually she presented to the hospital obtunded and with severe anemia, electrolyte abnormalities, malnutrition, and fatal gram-negative sepsis.

A review of the cases of 172 children who died between 1975 and 1995 in the U.S. whose parents withheld medical care because of religious beliefs revealed that most of the fatalities were from conditions for which survival rates with medical care would have exceeded 90% (4) (Table 18.2). The denominations represented most commonly for the fatalities reviewed were Faith Assembly; First Church of Christ, Scientist (Christian Scientist); Church of the First Born; Faith Tabernacle; and End Time Ministries. The incidence of nonfatal medical neglect due to religious beliefs and practices is unknown, but it is likely to be higher than 172 cases over 20 years.

SEXUAL ABUSE

Foreign Bodies and Objects

The prevalence of the use of objects to perpetrate sexual abuse is undetermined. A case was reported of a 20-month-old girl who was sexually assaulted by a male baby-sitter with a candle. The parents took the child for an evaluation after she moaned and cried all night. Surgeons removed a 12×2-cm wax candle from her peritoneal cavity. Other injuries included a tear in the perineum and posterior fourchette, ruptured levator ani muscle, and perforation of the posterior vaginal fornix (26).

Sometimes it is hard to determine whether injuries of the genitalia are accidental or inflicted. Sharp penetrating injuries to the hymen have been seen secondary to abuse and accidents. Four cases of girls who had genital injuries caused by sharp objects including three accidental injuries from a nail, sharp projections from the edge of a swimming pool, and a toy vacuum cleaner, and one abusive injury from a sharp wooden object have been reported (33).

Vaginal foreign bodies are rare in prepubertal girls, with an incidence of about 0.017% in a general clinic, and 1.4% to 4% in the presence of a vaginal discharge. A review of cases of girls presenting to a general pediatric clinic with vaginal foreign bodies including paper, hair, cotton, and a plastic cap indicated that sexual abuse was suspected or confirmed in 11 of 12 cases (30). It is unclear whether vaginal foreign bodies are related to sexual abuse in any given case, but it is an uncommon manifestation of sexual abuse.

Rectovaginal Trauma

Severe trauma, including perforation of the vagina, is unusual in sexually victimized chil-

TABLE 18.2. *Child fatalities associated with religion-motivated medical neglect*

Diagnoses	n	Ages (years unless specified)	Expected outcome
General or miscellaneous			
Cachexia, gastric aspiration	1	9	Excellent
Dehydration	6	4 mo, 5 mo, 1, 5, 8, 12	Excellent
Diabetes, type 1	12	3, 7, 10, 10, 11, 12, 12, 13, 13, 15, 15, 16	Excellent
Epilepsy, withheld medications	1	17	Excellent
Burns, 50% total burn surface area	1	1	Good
Hydrocephaly, myelomeningocele	1	2 mo	Excellent
Foreign-body aspiration	1	2	Good
Renal failure	3	15, 15, 15	Excellent
Trauma, motor vehicle accident	1	2	No benefit
Infections			
Diphtheria	3	3, 4, 9	Excellent
Laryngotracheobronchitis	1	18 mo	Excellent
Measles (with complications)	7	1, 5, 9, 9, 13, 14, 16	Excellent
Meningitis, *H. influenzae*	9	4 mo, 1 (7), 4	Excellent
Meningitis, *S. pneumoniae*	4	2 mo, 5 mo, 1, 7	Excellent
Meningitis, bacterial, nonspecified	1	1	Excellent
Meningitis, posttraumatic	1	15	Excellent
Pericarditis, *S. pneumoniae*	1	1	Excellent
Pertussis	1	1 mo	Excellent
Pneumonia (varying etiologies)	22	1 mo to 2 yr	Excellent
Pneumonia/myocarditis	1	1	Good
Rocky Mountain spotted fever	1	4	Excellent
Toxic shock syndrome, staphylococcus	1	17	Excellent
Abdominal surgical disorders			
Intussusception	3	8 mo, 9 mo, 14	Excellent
Appendicitis, ruptured	7	5 to 14	Excellent
Small bowel obstruction	1	6	Excellent
Strangulated hernia	1	6	Excellent
Volvulus	2	9 days, 26 mo	Excellent
Congenital heart lesions:			
Common atrioventricular canal	1	7 mo	Good
Double-outlet right ventricle	1	12	No benefit
Ventricular septal defect, pneumonia	2	9 mo, 10 mo	Excellent
Tumors			
Ewing's sarcoma	1	13	Good
Leukemia, acute lymphocytic	3	4, 5, 7	Good
Leukemia, nonspecified	1	2	Fair
Lymphoma, Burkitt's	1	13	Good
Lymphoma, non-Hodgkin's	1	3	Good
Neuroblastoma	1	1	Fair
Osteogenic sarcoma	3	6, 12, 14	Fair
Posterior fossa, nonspecified	1	2	Fair
Rhabdomyosarcoma	2	4 and 5	Fair
Wilms' tumor	1	2	Good
Total	113		

dren. The case of a 4-year-old with a rectovaginal fistula has been reported. The child had been abused by penile penetration of her mouth, vagina, and anus, and digital penetration of her vagina and anus 2 months earlier. A large defect of the posterior rim of the hymen and thickened perineal tissue was present on physical examination. In the knee–chest position, yellow mucoid material was visualized throughout the vagina and anus, and a fistula required a diverting colostomy and a vaginal flap to repair the defect (40). Perforation of the vagina was certainly present at the time of the abuse.

Genital Care Practices

Rarely children are subjected to bizarre, invasive, and/or abusive genital-care practices including painful washing, frequent and ritualistic inspections, application of creams/medicines, and enlistment of medical intervention for supposed genital or urinary problems. A record review of 790 children seen in a clinic specializing in abuse evaluation found 17 cases with abnormalities due to unusual genital-care practices; all were girls (31). The behaviors involved in genital-care practices fell into three categories: (a) a ritualistic excessive parental focus on the child's genitals; (b) parents giving a long history of genital problems in their children that may have been the result of parental fabrication or inducements of disorders; and (c) overt sexual abuse in which the father used cream on the daughter's genitalia as an excuse for the genital touching. Explanations given by parents for their behavior included that they had been washed this way or thought these hygiene practices were necessary to stop odor, or that at some point, an event such as a diaper rash or other medical problem occurred that legitimized their behavior in their own minds.

CONCLUSION

The litany of inhumanity to children in this chapter is sobering and painful. Fortunately, most of the cases reported here are uncommon. Despite high work loads, most clinicians and child-protection social workers will see few of these manifestations of abuse or neglect in their careers. Case reports are published because of the variation from normal and the information they can shed on the diagnostic process or prognosis. Caution should be taken against generalizing case reports as characteristic of the underlying phenomena. Although a compilation of case reports may serve some purpose, it cannot be used as epidemiologic data. As child abuse has become better recognized, the state of our knowledge may have matured to the point that what is currently considered unusual, may actually be so. However, in the decades to come, it may be that we again recognize that some of what we currently consider to be unusual, is not so.

REFERENCES

1. Ablin DS, Reinhart MA. Esophageal perforation with mediastinal abscess in child abuse. *Pediatr Radiol* 1990;20:524–525.
2. Adelson L. Homicide by pepper. *J Forensic Sci* 1964;9:391–395.
3. Alexander RC, Surrell JA, Cohle SD. Microwave oven burns to children: an unusual manifestation of child abuse. *Pediatrics* 1987;79:255–260.
4. Asser SM, Swan R. Child fatalities from religion-motivated medical neglect. *Pediatrics* 1998;101:625–629.
5. Bansal BC, Abramo TJ. Subcutaneous emphysema as an uncommon presentation of child abuse. *Am J Emerg Med* 1997;15:573–575.
6. Bateman DA, Heagarty MC. Passive freebase cocaine ("crack") inhalation by infants and toddlers. *Am J Dis Child* 1989;143:25–27.
7. Benhaim P, Strear C, Knudson M, et al. Posttraumatic chylous ascites in a child: recognition and management of an unusual condition. *J Trauma Injury Infect Crit Care* 1995;39:1175–1177.
8. Ben-Youssef L, Schmidt TL. Battered child syndrome simulating myositis. *Pediatr Orthop* 1983;3:392–395.
9. Bongiovi JJ, Logosso RD. Pancreatic pseudocyst occurring in the battered child syndrome. *J Paediatr Surg* 1969;4:220–226.
10. Boysen BE. Chylous ascites: manifestation of the battered child syndrome. *Am J Dis Child* 1975;129:1338–1339.
11. Caffey J. Multiple fractures in the long bones of infants suffering from chronic subdural hematoma. *Am J Roentgenol* 1946;56:163–173.
12. Campbell-Hewson GL, D'Amore A, Busuttil A. Non-accidental injury inflicted on a child with an air weapon. *Med Sci Law* 1998;38:173–176.
13. Carrotte PV. An unusual case of child abuse. *Br Dent J* 1990;168:444–445.
14. Cohle SD, Hawley DA, Berg EE, et al. Homicidal cardiac laceration in children. *J Forensic Sci* 1995;40:212–218.
15. Cohle SD, Trestrail JD, Graham MA, et al. Fatal pepper aspiration. *Am J Dis Child* 1988;142:633–636.
16. Diamond P, Hansen C, Christofersen M. Child abuse presenting as a thoracolumbar spinal fracture dislocation: a case report. *Pediatr Emerg Care* 1994;10:83–86.
17. Eisenstein EM, Delta BG, Clifford JH. Jejunal hematoma: an unusual manifestation of the battered-child syndrome. *Clin Pediatr* 1965;4:436–440.
18. Ernst AA. Unexpected cocaine intoxication presenting as seizures in children. *Ann Emerg Med* 1989;18:774–777.
19. Fearne C, Kelly J, Habel J, et al. Needle injuries as a cause of non-accidental injury [Letter]. *Arch Dis Child* 1997;77:187.
20. Feldman KW, Christopher DM, Opheim KB. Munchausen syndrome/bulimia by proxy: ipecac as a toxin in child abuse. *Child Abuse Negl* 1989;13:257–261.
21. Fischer H, Allasio D. Nasal destruction due to child abuse. *Clin Pediatr* 1996;35:165–166.

22. Gallup O. *Disciplining children in America.* Princeton, NJ: Gallup Organization, 1995.

23. Gill D. *Violence against children: physical abuse in the United States.* Cambridge: Harvard University Press, 1970.

24. Golova N. An infant with fever and drooling: infection or trauma? *Pediatr Emerg Care* 1998;13:331–333.

25. Greenberg N. The epidemiology of childhood sexual abuse. *Pediatr Annu* 1979;8:16–28.

26. Gromb S, Lazarini HJ. An unusual case of sexual assault on an infant: an intraperitoneal candle in a 20-month-old girl. *Forensic Sci Int* 1998;94:15–18.

27. Guleserian K, Gilchrist B, Luks F, et al. Child abuse as a cause of traumatic chylothorax. *J Pediatr Surg* 1996; 31:1696–1697.

28. Gultekin EY, Ozdamar AS, Gokalp A, et al. Penile strangulation injuries. *Pediatr Surg Int* 1996;11: 279–280.

29. Hanigan WC, Peterson RA, Njus G. Tin ear syndrome: rotational acceleration in pediatric head injuries. *Pediatrics* 1987;80:618–622.

30. Herman-Giddens MD. Vaginal foreign bodies and child sexual abuse. *Arch Pediatr Adolesc Med* 1994;148: 195–200.

31. Herman-Giddens ME, Berson NL. Harmful genital care practices in children. *JAMA* 1989;261:577–579.

32. Hilfer CL, Holgersen LO. Massive chylous ascites and transected pancreas secondary to child abuse: successful non-surgical management. *Pediatr Radiol* 1995;25: 117–119.

33. Hostetler B, Muram D, Jones CE. Sharp penetrating injuries to the hymen. *Adolesc Pediatr Gynecol* 1994;7:94–96.

34. Huntington RW, Weisberg HF. Unusual form of child abuse [Letter]. *Forensic Sci* 1977;22:5–6.

35. Hvizdala EV, Gellady AM. Intentional poisoning of two siblings by prescription drugs. *Clin Pediatr* 1978;17: 480–482.

36. Hymel KP. Review's note. *Child Abuse Q Med Update* 1999;6:6.

37. Jackson DL, Korbin J, Younger S, et al. Fatal outcome in untreated adolescent ulcerative colitis: an unusual case of child neglect. *Crit Care Med* 1983;11:832–833.

38. Jain D. India safe. Presented at the International Conference on Child Abuse Research, New Hampshire, 1997.

39. Johnson CF. Symbolic scarring and tattooing: unusual manifestations of child abuse. *Clin Pediatr* 1994;33: 46–49.

40. Kellog ND, Para JM. A rectovaginal fistula in a sexually assaulted child. *Clin Pediatr* 1996;35:369–371.

41. Kempe CH. Uncommon manifestations of the battered child syndrome. *Am J Dis Child* 1975;129:1265.

42. Kempe CH, Silverman FN, Stelle BF, et al. The battered child syndrome. *JAMA* 1962;181:105–112.

43. Kharasch S, Vinci R, Glotzer D, et al. Unsuspected cocaine exposure in young children. *Am J Dis Child* 1991; 145:204–206.

44. Kleinman P. Editor's note. *Q Child Abuse Med Update* 1999;6:7.

45. Kleinman PK. Spinal trauma. In: Kleinman PK, ed. *Diagnostic imaging of child abuse.* 2nd ed. St. Louis: Williams & Wilkins, 1998:161.

46. Kleinman PK, Shelton YA. Hangman's fracture in an abused infant: imaging features. *Pediatr Radiol* 1997; 27:776–777.

47. Kraya NAF, Patrick C. Folie á deux in a forensic setting. *Aust N Z Psychiatry* 1997;31:883–888.

48. Lam CH, Montes J, Farmer JP, et al. Traumatic aneurysm from shaken baby syndrome: case report. *Neurosurgery* 1996;39:1252–1255.

49. Lansky LL. An unusual case of childhood chloral hydrate poisoning. *Am J Dis Child* 1974;127:275–276.

50. Lee ACW, So KT, Wong HL, et al. Penetrating pencil injury: an unusual case of child abuse. *Child Abuse Negl* 1998;22:749–752.

51. Lukschu M, Bays J. Inflicted incision of the penis. *Child Abuse Negl* 1996;20:979–981.

52. McClung HJ, Murray R, Braden NJ, et al. Intentional ipecac poisoning in children. *Am J Dis Child* 1988;142: 637–639.

53. McDowell HP, Fielding DW. Traumatic perforation of the hypopharynx: an unusual form of abuse. *Arch Dis Child* 1984;59:888–889.

54. Meadow R. Munchausen syndrome by proxy abuse perpetrated by men. *Arch Dis Child* 1998;78:210–216.

55. Mortimer JG. Acute water intoxication as another manifestation of child abuse. *Arch Dis Child* 1980;55: 401–403.

56. Morzaria S, Walton JM, MacMillan A. Inflicted esophageal perforation. *J Pediatr Surg* 1998;33:871–873.

57. Murphy JT, Purdue GF, Hunt JL. Pediatric grease burn injury. *Arch Surg* 1995;130:478–482.

58. Nimkin K, Spevak MR, Kleinman PK. Fractures of the hands and feet in child abuse: imaging and pathologic features. *Radiology* 1997;203:233–236.

59. Nolte KB. Esophageal foreign bodies as child abuse: potential fatal mechanisms. *Am J Forensic Med Pathol* 1993;14:323–326.

60. Olazagasti J, Fetzgerald J, White S, et al. Chylous ascites: a sign of unsuspected child abuse. *Pediatrics* 1994;94:737–739.

61. Orton CI. Loss of columella and septum from an unusual form of child abuse. *Plast Reconstr Surg* 1975;56: 345–346.

62. Parish RA, Novack AH, Heimbach DM, et al. Pediatric patients in a regional burn center. *Pediatr Emerg Care* 1986;2:165–167.

63. Pena DJ, Medovy H. Child abuse and traumatic pseudocyst of the pancreas. *J Pediatr* 1973;83:1026–1028.

64. Piatt J, Steinberg M. Isolated spinal cord injury as presentation of child abuse. *Pediatrics* 1995;96: 780–782.

65. Pickel S, Anderson C, Holliday MA. Thirsting and hypernatremic dehydration: a form of child abuse. *Pediatrics* 1970;45:54–59.

66. Prendergast NC, deRoux SJ, Adsay NV. Non-accidental pediatric pelvic fracture: a case report. *Pediatr Radiol* 1998;28:344–346.

67. Purdue GF, Hunt JL, Prescott PR. Child abuse by burning: an index of suspicion. *J Trauma* 1988;28:221–224.

68. Reece RM. Editor's note. *Child Abuse Q Med Update* 1999;6:5.

69. Reece RM. Unusual manifestations of child abuse. *Pediatr Clin North Am* 1990;37:905–921.

70. Reece RM, Arnold JE, Splain J. Pharyngeal perforation as a manifestation of child abuse: report of three cases. *Child Maltreat* 1996;1:364–367.

71. Rimer RL, Roy S. Child abuse and hemoglobinuria. *JAMA* 1977;238:2034–2035.

72. Rivkin M, Gilmore HE. Generalized seizures in an in-

fant due to environmentally acquired cocaine. *Pediatrics* 1989;84:1100–1102.

73. Rooks VJ, Sisiler C, Burton B. Cervical spine injury in child abuse: report of two cases. *Pediatr Radiol* 1998; 28:193–195.

74. Rosenberg DA. Web of deceit: a literature review of Munchausen syndrome by proxy. *Child Abuse Negl* 1987;11:547–563.

75. Shah P, Applegate KE, Buonomo C. Stricture of the duodenum and jejunum in an abused child. *Pediatr Radiol* 1997;27:281–283.

76. Silverman FN. The roentgen manifestations of unrecognized skeletal trauma in infants. *Am J Roentgenol* 1953; 69:413–427.

77. Smith W. Editor's note. *Q Child Abuse Med Update* 1998;5:5.

78. Straus M, Hamby S, Finkelhor D, et al. Identification of child abuse with the Parent Child Conflict Tactics Scale (PCCTS): development and preliminary psychometric data from a national sample of American parents. *Child Abuse Negl* 1998;22:249–270.

79. Swadia ND, Thakore AB, Patel BR, et al. Unusual form of child abuse presenting as an acute abdomen. *Br Surg* 1981;68:668.

80. Tavill MA, Trimmer W, Austin MB. Pediatric esophageal perforation secondary to abusive blunt thoracic trauma. *Int J Pediatr Otorhinolaryngol* 1996;35: 263–269.

81. Theodore A, Runyan D. A medical research agenda for child maltreatment: negotiating the next steps. *Pediatrics* 1999;104:168–177.

82. Valentine JL, Schexnayder S, Jones JG, et al. Clinical and toxicological findings in two young siblings and autopsy findings in one sibling with multiple hospital admission resulting in death. *Am J Forensic Med Pathol* 1997;18:276–281.

19

Pathology of Fatal Abuse

Robert H. Kirschner and *Harry Wilson

*Departments of Pathology and Pediatrics, University of Chicago; and University of Chicago
Hospitals, Chicago, Illinois; *Department of Pathology, Providence Memorial Hospital, El Paso, Texas*

Forensic pathologists and clinicians working in the field of child abuse and neglect have now reached consensus on many issues regarding mechanisms and timing of injuries, cause of death, and manner of death of victims of abuse. In this chapter we try to reflect this consensus and the weight of the evidence that supports it, as well as our personal experience in the field. The discussion emphasizes those aspects of child death investigation that we believe are most important, and those that cause the greatest diagnostic dilemmas for the pathologist. However, this chapter is not meant to be an encyclopedic review of fatal child abuse injuries or a reference only for pathologists. Rather it is directed to all individuals working in the field of abuse and neglect who have a voice in improving our system of child death investigation. In addition, much of the discussion in this chapter will apply both to the living, seriously injured infant or child and to the child who has died of alleged abuse. The chapter follows the format of the first edition of this text, but has been revised to reflect not only the increased literature and experience in the field, but also the contemporary medicolegal climate.

Historically, child abuse deaths generally went unrecognized, and an accurate assessment of numbers from the past is not possible. Presently, approximately 2,000 abuse and neglect fatalities occur annually, 90% in children younger than 5 years, and 41% among infants (123). From 1979 to 1988, the fatality rate remained relatively stable, and reports of a recent increase may reflect variations in survey technique (123). Inflicted injury is the leading cause of infant deaths due to trauma, and now ranks fourth among causes of death in children younger than 4 years. One half of these homicides occur by the fourth month of life (4,136). Strong evidence exists of persistent underreporting because of inadequate death investigation, including failure to perform autopsies in children who die suddenly, lack of information sharing between agencies, and reporting systems that often fail to recognize abuse or neglect as contributing to a child's death (53,81).

A number of socioeconomic and demographic risk factors for infant homicide and other fatal infant injuries have been described, including childbearing at an early age (136), low birth weight, prematurity, high parity, low maternal education, male sex of the infant, and isolation (26,161). However, injuries and deaths due to abuse occur within all communities and social groups in the United States. Unfortunately, abuse is less likely to be recognized, reported, thoroughly investigated, or prosecuted when the perpetrator is from a middle or upper socioeconomic class or has recognized "status" in the community.

Deaths that occur suddenly and/or unexpectedly in both previously healthy children and ill children require careful investigation. These include all deaths that occur out of the hospital as well as inpatient deaths in which the cause is not clearly natural. Such deaths must be reported to the local medical examiner or coroner, and appropriate jurisdiction established. A death certificate should not be signed without direct and accurate medical knowledge of the cause and manner of death for that infant or child. Except for hospitalized children with a recognized serious illness, an autopsy is usually necessary to make that determination (42,109). An example from the personal experience of one of the authors (R.H.K.) emphasizes this point.

A 2-year-old boy with a confirmed history of cardiac complications of Kawasaki disease, including multiple coronary artery aneurysms and thromboses, was found dead at home. The family had been warned that the child was unlikely to survive beyond his third birthday, and the child's pediatrician and pediatric cardiologist were willing to sign the death certificate. A medical examiner's autopsy was performed, motivated primarily by interest in the remarkable cardiac abnormalities (Fig. 19.1). The cause of death, however, was not Kawasaki coronary artery disease, but intracranial injuries from inflicted head trauma. Subsequent police investigation revealed that on the night the child died, a resident in a neighboring apartment had heard the child crying, a thud from the child being thrown against a wall, and then silence.

THE DEATH INVESTIGATION

Like many other clinical syndromes that at first were puzzling but now are easily recognized, the fatally battered child usually presents no diagnostic problem to the forensic pathologist. Concomitant with an increasing awareness of the more subtle manifestations of abuse and neglect in living children (122,193), we now recognize a spectrum of fatal injuries, the causation of which often cannot be determined by autopsy or laboratory studies alone. These subtle forms of abuse are most common in infants, who are especially vulnerable because of their relative isolation, small size, lack of verbal skills, and frequent dependence on a sole caretaker. Progress in recognizing the more subtle forms of abuse owes much to the increasing collab-

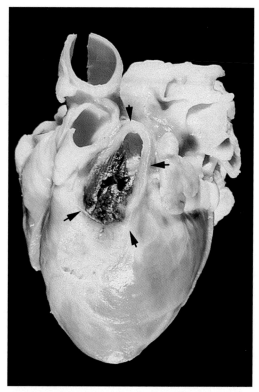

FIG. 19.1. Kawasaki heart disease in a 2-year-old who died at home. An obliquely cut coronary artery (delimited by *arrows*) is nearly the size of the great vessels, and is partially occluded by thrombus. Because physicians had predicted the child would die of his disease by age 3 years, a death certificate was almost issued without performing an autopsy. The actual cause of death was inflicted head trauma.

oration of forensic pathologists with forensic pediatricians and other pediatric specialists with a focus on abuse and neglect. Many such deaths that were previously misdiagnosed as natural or accidental deaths are now properly ascribed to abuse or neglect, other children in the family are protected, and the abusive caretakers successfully prosecuted.

The establishment of child fatality review teams to evaluate the often complex nature of fatal abuse and neglect also has contributed to the successful investigation of child deaths. Such teams have been formed both as the result of state and local legislation, and at a grass-root level by professionals concerned about improving the status of child death investigation in their communities (50). More than 95% of the nation's population now live in jurisdictions served by such teams, most of which have been established since 1988 (88). These advances have challenged pathologists to improve the skills and methods used to diagnose the cause and manner of death correctly in infants and children who have died suddenly and unexpectedly. Toward this end, protocols for child death autopsy and investigation have been developed (158,175) and are widely available from various professional societies and state governmental agencies.

Perhaps the most significant advancement in child death investigation in recent years has been the emphasis placed on the nonlaboratory aspects of the investigation. It is no longer sufficient to wait until the pathologist emerges from the autopsy room before deciding what further investigation to undertake. Rather, a better understanding of child abuse and neglect on both a case-specific and global basis requires a multidisciplinary, multiagency approach. Because the medical examiner or coroner has the ultimate responsibility for determining the cause and manner of death and signing the death certificate, he or she should coordinate the death investigation and take the responsibility that all necessary information is obtained. The major components of this investigation are described later.

Requirement for Qualified Personnel

Sudden, unexpected deaths in infants and children represent a diagnostic challenge for the pathologist. Although most such deaths prove to be from natural causes, the possibility of fatal abuse necessitates that the autopsy be performed by a pathologist experienced in forensic pathology, preferably board certified in the specialty. A pathologist who does not deal routinely with deaths related to trauma lacks the necessary experience to recognize certain injuries or to interpret mechanisms of injury. Conversely, some forensic pathologists lack expertise in pediatric pathology and are unfamiliar with growth and nutrition standards, metabolic diseases, and genetic disorders. More important, they may lack familiarity with the clinical presentation of acquired diseases and injuries in infants and young children. This may lead to significant misinterpretation of autopsy findings with respect to the timing of injuries and determination of cause and manner of death.

When the cause of death in a child is obscure, the expertise of various pediatric specialists may be essential to arrive at a correct diagnosis. Pathologists performing pediatric forensic autopsies should have a close working relationship with a radiologist trained to interpret infant skeletal films, a neuropathologist, and a pediatrician experienced in the evaluation of child abuse and neglect. In addition, the pathologist should consult other pediatric specialists and pathology subspecialty colleagues as necessary. In view of the limited number of such specialists throughout the U.S., physicians, attorneys, and law-enforcement personnel should not hesitate to contact their regional medical schools, medical examiner's office, or appropriate professional organizations for assistance in identifying medical specialists with the requisite knowledge and experience.

Review of Records

Before the autopsy begins, all available records should be reviewed, and other necessary records should be requested or subpoenaed. This includes all investigative reports pertaining to the death, paramedic reports, police reports, hospital emergency department records, child-protection agency records, previous hospital and/or physician's records (including birth records), results of laboratory examinations, and radiographs. Birth records can provide information regarding gestational age or other medical problems that might increase the risk for sudden death. The birth certificate provides important information regarding the names of both parents, the mother's maiden name, and prior addresses. This latter information may be particularly important when searching for previous interactions of the family with social service, police, or other agencies, and can be used to detect discrepancies in historical information obtained from the caretaker.

The observations and reports of paramedics, often the first responders on the scene, can provide critical information about the injured child, the surrounding environment, and verbal exchanges among family members, witnesses, and others. The type of treatment administered by paramedics during transport may be important in reaching a decision about the cause of the injuries. In particular, inquiry should be made as to whether prehospital resuscitation was attempted, and if so by whom. The recorded body temperature of the infant when transported also is important. Hypothermia may reflect cerebral dysfunction secondary to head injury (179) or cold-water immersion (73), although these are not often considered in the initial differential diagnosis of hypothermia. Because the paramedics run sheet is unlikely to contain all of this information, a personal conversation soon after the event is often best.

When children die in hospital after an emergency admission, the medical record may be incomplete, particularly with respect to specific injuries noted on the child. Attention is properly directed at treatment, and the description of bruises, abrasions, and other skin lesions may be sketchy. Clinicians should be encouraged to document injuries with high-quality photographs as soon as possible after admission (Fig. 19.2). If death occurs after some days, injuries may have healed or been obscured by subsequent treatment. Contemporaneous photographs also may prevent later courtroom disputes regarding the nature of the injuries. It is important to discuss with the attending physician, as soon as possible after the death of the child, his or her recollection of the injuries, clinical status, medical history, and family situation. The pathologist should determine whether in-hospital resuscitation was attempted, and if so on how many occasions.

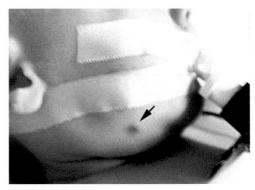

FIG. 19.2. Small bruise of right cheek (*arrow*) in 6-month-old shaking victim was the only external evidence of injury. The photograph was taken shortly after admission to hospital to document that the injury was not iatrogenic. The child died the following day, and at autopsy had typical findings of shaken baby syndrome.

Family History

Before the postmortem examination, the pathologist should inquire into the child's personal and family history, including developmental, medical, and social history, and the illness or death of other siblings. Unexplained deaths of previous siblings or deaths of "sudden infant death syndrome" (SIDS) should alert the pathologist to the possibility of serial suffocation by a parent, or, less likely, a rare metabolic disorder.

Many medical examiners and coroners maintain an infant death file cross-indexed for the mother's maiden name, family name(s) of all her children, and fathers' names. Such an index is useful when searching for previous, undisclosed infant deaths within the same family. Unfortunately, when families move from one jurisdiction to another, there is no effective way of tracking these prior deaths. Attempts to form regional or national child death registries have not succeeded, and would probably involve a significant infringement of privacy rights and face serious court challenge. Ideally, it would be most useful to know of previous infant or child deaths in the same family, involving the same caretaker, or in the same location.

Agency Investigation and Collaboration

Developing good working relationships among personnel from the principal agencies involved is critical to the investigation process. This may require considerable effort. The medical examiner or coroner, police, child protective agency, and prosecutor must keep one another informed, share data, and otherwise cooperate in various stages of the investigation, as appropriate for each agency. Often, only by this means will the full story surrounding the death of an infant or child be known. This collaboration will not succeed, however, in the face of excessive claims of record confidentiality, excessive investigative secrecy, agency indifference to a child's death, or "turf" issues. Fortunately, with increasing cooperation during the past decade in most jurisdictions, many of the initial fears regarding sharing of information have diminished as those involved have come to recognize the benefits of a collaborative approach to child death investigation.

Scene and Circumstance Investigation

Scene investigation is important in establishing the cause and manner of infant deaths. In 1986, Bass et al. (15) conducted independent death-scene investigations in 26 consecutive cases in New York City in which a presumptive diagnosis of SIDS had been made. They discovered strong circumstantial evidence of accidental death in six cases, and various other possible causes of death, including abuse in 18 cases. Although the validity of the results was questioned at the time of their publication (70,178), the impact of the study has been great, virtually mandating scene investigations in all infant death cases since the time of its publication. Subsequent experience has confirmed the value of this process.

The scene investigation is best performed as soon as possible after the death. In most circumstances when the infant has been removed from the residence, a life-size doll can be used to identify the location and position in which the child was found. Photographs should be taken, not only of the location where the fatal event occurred, but also of the surrounding environment. If this investigation is undertaken before the autopsy, a return visit is sometimes necessary, based on the postmortem findings. A moribund child may be brought to the hospital, die hours or days later, or go on to survive. This in-hospital survival does not diminish the necessity of a scene investigation.

The scene investigator should be someone trained to recognize the unique circumstances of infant deaths, and whose report will reflect information about sleep position, type of bedding, covers, and room temperature. Results of several studies now suggest that rebreathing of expired air in a restricted, but not occlusive, microenvironment may lead to suffocation in young infants (72,98,160,182). These findings and others strongly indicate that the differentiation of SIDS from accidental or intentional suffocation usually cannot be made from autopsy findings alone; this determination also depends on other aspects of the investigation.

When an infant has been using a home apnea monitor, the investigator must try to determine if the infant was attached to the monitor, whether the monitor was functioning properly, and if the alarm sounded. If a discrepancy is noted between the caretaker's story and the apparent functional state of the monitor, the monitor should be retained as evidence and, if necessary, evaluated by an independent, qualified laboratory. It should be noted that noncompliance with proper monitoring occurs in most families using such devices (126). Paradoxically, in families in which an infant's repeated apnea spells are later attributed to Munchausen syndrome by proxy, home monitor compliance is high (155).

The home environment, including its cleanliness, safety hazards, pets, quantity and quality of food, medications, and so on, may provide important information, particularly when evidence exists that neglect may have contributed to the death. Investigators must be sensitive to socioeconomic factors that may place certain children at greater risk for accidental death in the home. Toddler drownings in industrial buckets (95,120), for example, are more common in the inner city than in the suburbs, where swimming pool drownings represent a significant hazard. The scene investigation is essential in determining whether situational neglect (i.e., leaving an infant or child alone in a situation that is dangerous for the developmental age of the child) played a role in the death of the child. The scene investigation also is necessary to assess possible caretaker impairment because of age, physical disability, intoxication, mental disorder, or retardation.

When a child has been badly battered, the cause of death is usually obvious, but an attempt should be made to recover implements that might have been used to inflict the fatal injuries or previous injuries noted on the child. It is particularly important to photograph all objects, furniture, or locations that the caretaker claims the child may have struck, fallen against, or fallen from; a tape measure or yardstick should be included in the photographs. When the child has died as a result of bathtub scald burns, the dimensions of the tub, the height of the faucet, the hot-water temperature, and the length of time required to reach that temperature after turning on the faucet should be measured.

The investigator should make a record of persons present in the hours preceding death and at the time of death, including all adults and other children. These persons, including the children, should be interviewed individually as soon as possible. Careful, nonthreatening interrogation is of utmost importance. The circumstances of alleged falls, bathtub injuries, and other types of burns should be reconstructed by the involved caretaker. Accidental injuries can often be distinguished from inflicted injuries by such a reenactment and confirmation by a pediatrician that the child's actions were either appropriate or inappropriate for his or her developmental stage and the circumstances of injury.

In fatal abuse cases, lack of consistency between history and injuries is usually obvious, but at times, the reported circumstances may be equivocal. The story also may change in an attempt to fit the injuries to the circumstances as the suspected caretaker is confronted with the extent of injuries discovered at autopsy. De-

nial by all caretakers of any knowledge of how an infant's injury occurred is highly indicative of abuse by one or more of the caretakers. Often the caretaker provides a story with truthful elements, but facts are inverted, shaded, or omitted in an attempt to conceal the true circumstances of injury or death. In Table 19.1 we list common suggestive stories provided by caretakers to explain lethal injuries. Many of these recur with such regularity as to be almost predictable. The history of an infant falling from a sofa to the floor is so common that we labeled these deadly items of furniture "killer couches" (Fig. 19.3). It is discouraging to see how often these stories are still accepted at face value by physicians, other health care professionals, and child-protective workers.

Injury Time Window

The time window of responsibility for the child's injuries must be determined by coordinating (a) the medical time window determined from the medical records and gross and microscopic autopsy findings, (b) the circumstantial time window based on who was with the victim at particular times, and (c) the func-

TABLE 19.1. *Common suspicious stories (a dirty dozen + one)*

1. Child fell from a low height (<4 ft) such as couch, crib, bed, or chair
2. Child fell and struck head on floor or furniture, or hard object fell on child
3. Unexpectedly found dead (age and/or circumstances not appropriate for SIDS)
4. Child choked while eating and was therefore shaken or struck on chest or back
5. Child suddenly turned blue or stopped breathing, and was then shaken
6. Sudden seizure activity
7. Aggressive or inexperienced CPR to a child who suddenly stopped breathing
8. Alleged traumatic event day or more before death
9. Caretaker tripped or slipped while carrying child
10. Injury inflicted by sibling
11. Child left alone in dangerous situation (e.g., bathtub) for just a few moments
12. Child fell down stairs
13. Self-inflicted injuries

SIDS, sudden infant death syndrome; CPR, cardiopulmonary resuscitation.

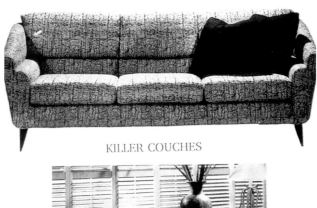

KILLER COUCHES

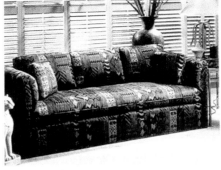

FIG. 19.3. Falls from sofas, beds, and other household furniture do not cause life-threatening injuries. If this occurred, the Consumer Product Safety Commission undoubtedly would have banned such "killer couches" long ago.

tional time limit. The functional limit is that time when the victim was last known to be well (i.e., eating, playing, and normally active for its age). Because coma can mimic sleeping, the last time the child was awake and alert is an important marker. In most child abuse–related deaths, witnesses, physical evidence, and obvious motive are lacking. The case therefore rests on the synthesis of the medical evidence, the circumstances, and the functional time limit to determine the responsible party. In some cases, it may be useful to develop this timeline of reported observations regarding the child's behavior and activities for a period of 1 to 2 days before the death of the child. In subsequent sections, we discuss the criteria for establishing the medical time windows for injuries under various circumstances.

THE AUTOPSY

Autopsies involve a process of observation, documentation, and interpretation. The child death autopsy more than any other requires the maximal skills of the pathologist, and wherever possible, a forensic pathologist with pediatric autopsy experience should perform the postmortem examination (110, 158,175). Most general pathologists are less familiar with the special requirements of both the forensic and the pediatric autopsy than they are with the usual hospital autopsy, and are often uncomfortable in interpreting the findings of a child death autopsy. Table 19.2 identifies the essential questions a pathologist may be expected to answer regarding the sudden death of an infant or child. These questions often cannot be answered from the autopsy alone, but require knowledge of the environment in which the child lived, the medical and family history of the child, and the circumstances of the fatal event.

It is particularly important that documentation of the autopsy findings be thorough and accessible to review by other pathologists,

TABLE 19.2. *Pediatric autopsies: questions to be answered by pathologist*

1. Was death due to injury, neglect, or complications of injury or neglect?
2. If related to injury, what was the mechanism of injury?
3. Was the injury consistent with the alleged history or circumstances of injury? If not, why not?
4. When did the injury occur in relation to the time of death?
5. Did a delay in seeking medical care contribute to death? If so, was this an "unreasonable" delay?
6. Did death result from a single episode or multiple episodes of injury?
7. Were drugs or poisons involved in the death?
8. If neglect was involved, what form did it take?
9. If there is evidence of failure to thrive, was this due to metabolic disorder, other disease, or neglect?
10. To what extent did environmental, nutritional, and social factors contribute to death?

clinicians, law-enforcement personnel, and attorneys. The complete forensic autopsy of a child abuse victim may include incisions and procedures not common in a routine hospital autopsy. The pathologist should be sensitive to the feelings of the child's family, but must not forego necessary components of the autopsy because of pressure from family members or funeral directors. To do so might compromise the death investigation. However, there is no reason why any autopsy procedure should prevent an open-casket viewing, should the family so choose.

Identification

When an infant or child is the victim of a homicide, positive identification is required before anyone can be charged with the death. Usually, identification can be confirmed by a relative or other person who knew the child. In some jurisdictions, verification of identification through footprints is required before homicide charges are lodged. If the body is decomposed, mummified, or skeletonized, radiologic, dental, or anthropologic identification is necessary. If these efforts fail because of lack of appropriate antemortem records for comparison, DNA technology can be applied

to establish the relationship of the deceased child to a putative parent.

Time-of-Death Determination

Time of death may be especially important when there has been more than one caretaker, or a caretaker's story appears discrepant. Questions regarding time of death also are frequently asked by parents who placed their infant in bed for the night, only to discover the child dead in the morning, an apparent victim of SIDS. However, the pathologist must be cautious when making any estimate regarding time of death. Terminal body temperature and environmental conditions have significantly greater influence in infants than in adults on the development of postmortem changes such as rigor mortis and lividity. When, as is often the case, the pathologist does not examine the body until many hours after death, it may be helpful to view photographs taken at the time of discovery of the body or pronouncement of death, if such are available, for evidence of the pattern of lividity. In light-skinned infants, dependent lividity may become evident in less than 1 hour and prominent within 3 hours. Rigor mortis also becomes evident more rapidly than in adults, and disappears more rapidly.

Estimating the time of death from body temperature also is subject to sufficient error that it may lead investigators astray, and one should be conservative in using such measurements. The presence or absence of food in the stomach should be correlated with the feeding history and the reported time of the last meal. As with adults, gastric-emptying time in infants depends on the type of meal and the quantity ingested; it is usually less than 2 hours, but may extend beyond that time. The time of death is most accurately determined by interviewing witnesses who can reliably state when the child was last seen alive, and at what time he or she was found dead. However, so many variables are involved in the determination that it is prudent to be circumspect in one's opinion.

When there has been an attempt to conceal the death of a child, a not uncommon event in newborns, discovery of the body may be delayed for days to years, and the body will be decomposed or skeletonized. In such instances, a forensic entomologist may provide valuable information regarding the time of death based on examination of the life stages of flies and other insects found on and around the body (68). Where possible, the entomologist should visit the death scene before removal of the body to recover evidence personally. Because such specialists are few and far between, every forensic facility should establish a protocol to preserve representative life stages of insect specimens for later analysis.

Skeletonized remains are best examined by a forensic anthropologist, who can determine stature and age range by using standardized anthropologic, dental, and radiologic tables. Most anthropologists concur that accurate sex determination in prepubertal skeletons is not possible (16). Snow et al. (168) however, analyzed the exhumed skeletal remains of 136 children (ages 0 to 12 years; mean age, 6 years) murdered by the infamous Atlacatl Battalion of the El Salvadoran Army in the 1981 massacre at El Mozote, El Salvador. They were approximately 80% correct in skeletal sex assignment based on comparison with the children's clothing, which is usually gender specific from infancy onward in that country. This corresponds to previous data that cited a range of 73% to 81% accuracy of sex assignment between 2 and 8 years of age (108).

Photography

Color photography is an integral part of the child abuse autopsy. If the body has not been removed from the scene, it should first be photographed in its environment before transport to the medical examiner's office. Photographs are used to document all injuries, congenital anomalies, and dysmorphic features. When possible, the body should be photographed before being undressed, before washing the unclothed body if there is blood, dirt, or other foreign matter on the body, and then after cleaning the body. In addition, individual lesions or groups of lesions must be photographed at close range by using a macro lens and appropriate label and scale.

The pathologist must remember that these photographs may be used in court. The photographs must accurately portray the body and the injuries as they would appear to a layperson seeing the child in a nonmedical context. Photographs that show a background of extraneous blood, dirty instruments, or internal organs may be barred from a jury as inflammatory. Color transparency film is preferable to print film because it has better color balance, permits greater enlargement by projection, and is thus easier to interpret when viewed at a later date. Electronic flash provides the best lighting source. Polaroid photographs are not a substitute for a 35-mm photography system in the autopsy suite, the pediatric emergency department, or the clinic because of their lack of resolution and color balance (149).

Reflective ultraviolet (UV) photography in the near-UV range (320 to 400 nm) is used in some jurisdictions to enhance recent injury patterns on the skin and to detect older injuries that are no longer visible on the skin surface. The technique has been used particularly by forensic odontologists to enhance bite marks, but it also has been used to document older bruises in child abuse cases. Epidermal response to UV light has been documented as late as 3 months after injury, but great individual variability has been noted in the intensity and duration of this response (107). In our opinion, the results using UV or near-UV light to demonstrate cutaneous injuries do not warrant its broad application, and there is a significant risk that an artefact of the lighting may be misinterpreted as injury.

In the past few years, digital photography has become more widely used, and the resolution of high-quality digital cameras is approaching that of film. Its limits become most apparent when enlarged images are projected onto a screen. Among the advantages of digital photography are the ability to determine the quality of the photograph immediately, its ease of storage and recall within an office computer system, the ability to transmit images to any location, and the ease of comparison of multiple images. The ease with which such images can be manipulated has caused some concern within the medicolegal community, but ultimately the integrity of any photograph is dependent on the integrity of the person producing the image.

Radiologic Documentation

The increasingly knowledgeable approach to child abuse is particularly reflected in advances in the radiologic recognition of intentional injury (100,102). Newer imaging techniques and improved diagnostic skills have helped to define subtle injuries to the brain and skeletal system that previously escaped detection (3,100). These advances have important application to the autopsy. For example, small metaphyseal fractures, spinous process fractures, and digital fractures are unlikely to be seen on the usual postmortem "babygram," but they can be identified by using a complete skeletal survey with appropriate cone-down views. The radiographs serve as a guide to the pathologist, who should excise the involved bones or bone segments. These specimens are radiographed separately, photographed, and submitted for histologic evaluation after gross examination. This combination of techniques provides the best basis for aging of the injuries. When long bones are removed, appropriate-length dowels can be inserted to retain the normal configuration of the limb. Radiologic examination does not relieve the pathologist of his or her responsibility to look for fractures. Acute rib fractures and linear skull fractures may not be visible radiographically, but they are obvious on careful gross examination.

Postmortem radiographs also will alert the pathologist to the presence of small foreign bodies or other radiodense materials that otherwise might escape detection within the gastrointestinal tract, pulmonary tree, soft tissues, or other organs. The standards of the American College of Radiology for skeletal surveys in children should be used in postmortem imaging (6,101). As an adjunct to the prescribed skeletal survey, there has been

some interest in the use of postmortem computerized tomography (CT) or magnetic resonance imaging (MRI) scans (78). There is little evidence that such modalities are of more than limited benefit.

Hospital radiographs, and CT and MRI scans when available, should be reviewed before autopsy. These images are of particular value in cases of head injury, in which progressive cerebral edema, neurosurgical intervention, and respirator brain changes may obscure the original injuries. When there has been prolonged hospitalization between the time of injury and death, the findings at autopsy may be totally nonspecific. In such cases, the hospital radiologic studies may be the only graphic representation of the child's injuries. The neuroradiologic and skeletal manifestations of child abuse are discussed in Chapters 4 and 7, respectively.

Recovery of Evidence

With rare exception, fatal abuse occurs in the child's usual environment, and the victim is normally in intimate contact with the person who may be the suspected abuser. Trace evidence may be of limited value. Furthermore, the body and the death scene are usually "contaminated" by therapeutic intervention and by numerous outsiders at the scene. When the death scene is found undisturbed by first responders, without evidence of attempted resuscitation by the caretaker, this, in and of itself, causes suspicions. It implies previous awareness that the child is dead. The expected and natural response of a caretaker who finds a child unresponsive is to call for help and to make some attempt at resuscitation. Paramedics, who are usually the first responders on the scene, will institute cardiopulmonary resuscitation (CPR) unless they have clear evidence, such as rigor mortis, that the child has been dead for a prolonged period. CPR is often continued in the hospital emergency department, invasive procedures are often performed, and the body may be partially washed, particularly if stool, vomitus, or other body fluids are present. In the circumstances surrounding resuscitation, valuable evidence may be ignored or lost.

The child's diaper or underpants, clothing, covers, and associated paraphernalia are likely to be displaced, left at the home, or discarded in the hospital emergency department. All items worn by the child or removed from the home should be brought to the autopsy suite for examination by the pathologist, preferably in the presence of an evidence technician from the appropriate police jurisdiction, for evidence of vomitus, urine, feces, and blood stains. The cleanliness of the clothing should be described, and medications, formula, milk, or other items that might have been ingested should be recovered. The pathologist should search for hairs, fibers, or other trace evidence that might be on the body and the clothing, and retain such evidence as appropriate. When indicated, appropriate toxicologic tests should be conducted on formula, milk, or other food items. When evidence exists that a contaminated commercial product may have been involved in the death through spoilage or tampering, the appropriate local and/or federal government agencies and the manufacturer should be notified immediately.

Nutrition and Hygiene Assessment

The general appearance of the child should be documented, with attention to determinants of age and appropriate growth and development, such as weight, body length, head circumference, and stature. These values are then compared with standard growth charts as well as with the child's previous growth measurements, including birth weight and length. If a child was premature, a correction must be made for gestational age. This can be done by determining foot length from the birth-record footprint and reference to appropriate prenatal growth charts. Standard infant growth charts offer the most objective standard for assessing failure to thrive, and should be consulted in every pediatric forensic autopsy. For example, an infant whose weight for height is below the 5th percentile or whose weight is below the

5th percentile when the weight for height is below the 10th percentile has nutritional wasting. Height below the 5th percentile strongly suggests stunted growth if weight for height is below the 25th percentile (175). The infant and childhood years are a period of rapid growth. A plateau in a child's growth or loss of weight before death must be viewed with concern, and an appropriate explanation must be sought at autopsy.

The general state of hygiene can be assessed by skin cleanliness, including the presence of stool, food, and secretions on skin surfaces. Poor hygiene may be manifested by severe chronic diaper rash, lichenification and pigment changes of the perineal skin, chronic seborrhea of the scalp, and dirt in the skin creases. Accusations of neglect may be leveled at parents whose infants died with a coincident moderate to severe acute diaper rash, but without other evidence of abuse or neglect. Such accusations are unfair and only add to the parents' guilt feelings. Diaper rash can progress rapidly, particularly in the presence of diarrhea, or when caused by a yeast infection. Assessment of dental development and oral hygiene also is necessary. Bottle caries in older infants may indicate situational neglect.

Dehydration with electrolyte derangements can be a cause of unexpected death in an infant, but the ability to evaluate the state of hydration at autopsy is limited. A recent antemortem body weight, if available, can provide information about acute weight loss attributable to dehydration. Sunken eyes, depressed fontanelle, and dry mucosal and serosal membranes may be indicators of moderate to severe dehydration. Skin turgor is generally not a good indicator in the dead child. Refrigerated bodies develop significant postmortem drying artefact, which may mimic dehydration when a small infant is left in a refrigerator overnight. Elevated vitreous humor sodium and urea nitrogen levels, however, are reliable criteria of dehydration, and are discussed in greater detail later. Dehydration usually reflects an acute condition, but severe dehydration is a common finding in the fatal outcome of chronic failure to thrive.

Organic failure to thrive may be associated with metabolic disorders, congenital anomalies, infections, especially tuberculosis and acquired immune deficiency syndrome (AIDS), or other chronic diseases. Nonorganic failure to thrive can result from chronic abuse, nutritional deprivation, and emotional neglect. It is common to have components of both organic and nonorganic failure to thrive in the same child (83,192). Cause and manner of death in such children are among the most difficult problems for the pathologist to solve. Review of all previous medical records, scene investigation, and interview with the primary caretaker are necessary. Frequently the medical records reflect uncertainty on the part of the child's physician as to the cause of the failure to thrive, even after hospitalization. One factor may be a lack of postnatal health care, or lack of continuity of care, characterized by visits to various emergency departments or health clinics for acute care only.

A 2-month-old term male infant, appropriate for gestational age at birth, was brought dead on arrival to a hospital emergency department. The only history was that the child, whose mother was a prostitute and intravenous drug abuser, did not feed well. A forensic autopsy revealed patchy acute bronchopneumonia (*Hemophilus influenzae* and *Streptococcus pneumoniae* on postmortem lung culture), bilateral otitis media, and severe failure to thrive. The infant's height and weight had decreased 2 SD on the growth chart since birth. Nutritional and medical neglect were suspected. Further studies by a pediatric pathologist revealed pulmonary *Pneumocystis* infection and depletion of lymphoid tissues. A diagnosis of AIDS was suspected. Blood from the infant was not available, but the diagnosis was confirmed by subsequent human immunodeficiency virus (HIV) testing of the mother. The death of this infant with failure to thrive was attributed to congenital HIV infection, aggravated by the failure of a mother to seek appropriate medical attention for an obviously sick child. Although this child had a terminal disease, death was hastened by maternal neglect.

To establish nutritional neglect as the sole cause of failure to thrive, it is necessary to rule out preexisting organic disease. Significant congenital and acquired disorders (e.g., degenerative neurologic disorders, hydrocephalus, congenital heart disease, renal anomalies, and metabolic storage diseases) are readily recognized by careful autopsy technique. In practice, autopsy rarely reveals a previously undiagnosed organic cause for failure to thrive. Therefore starvation related to neglect is likely to be the diagnosis when the autopsy findings are otherwise negative and the child had no documented medical history of disease. Autopsy clues to support this conclusion are identified in Table 19.3. Not surprisingly, this diagnosis is rarely made beyond infancy, because the older child is able to forage for food and drink unless shackled or kept in a locked room or closet. The issue of failure to thrive is further addressed in Chapter 12.

Documentation of Injuries

The multitude of injuries that can be inflicted on children are well described elsewhere in this book and in the literature, and it is not our intention to catalogue all of them here. In contrast to accidental injuries, inflicted injuries are inconsistent with the al-

TABLE 19.3. *Autopsy clues for failure to thrive due to neglect*

1. Poor hygiene
2. Loose skin folds; dry thin skin
3. Chronic rash with scabbing and scarring; other cutaneous lesions
4. Sparse hair; occipital or "hat band" alopecia
5. Severe growth retardation in the absence of previously diagnosed organic disease
6. Emaciation; evidence of kwashiorkor or marasmus
7. Fixed positional soft-tissue and bony deformations and cutaneous pressure ulcerations
8. Dehydration with dry mucous and serous membranes; markedly increased vitreous sodium and urea nitrogen
9. Empty gastrointestinal tract
10. Lack of subcutaneous and deep fat; decreased skeletal muscle mass; atrophy of thymus and nonreactive lymph nodes

leged circumstances, lack independent witnesses, and are usually not appropriate to the child's age. Such injuries may be scant or numerous, of different ages, produced by a variety of blunt trauma and other forms of injury, and involve any part of the body. Certain types of injuries are more commonly seen in particular age groups, and the abuse is often triggered by behavior patterns characteristic of the age group. In the infant younger than 1 year, persistent crying or crankiness may lead to shaking or near-suffocation in an attempt to quiet the child. Undoubtedly, some caretakers learn through experience or hearsay that one or the other of these methods is an effective, if dangerous, way to control an infant's crying. Thus near-suffocation or shaking may be used repeatedly until the infant is seriously injured or killed. In the 1- to 2-year-old, toilet training may become the focus of abuse, leading to beatings or scald burns as a form of punishment. In the older child, "misbehaving" may lead to a variety of punishments. As the infant matures, suffocation, occult head injury, and rib fractures become less common; severe beatings, burns, and abdominal injuries become more common.

Many autopsy protocols fail to describe injuries in a manner readily interpretable by subsequent readers. Because the autopsy report is likely to be used in legal proceedings, it is preferable to describe injuries in common language, avoid medical jargon, and record them in an organized tabulated form (e.g., separately describing external injuries and internal injuries) by separating the description of injuries into various anatomic regions of the body, and by separately describing recent injuries, healing injuries, and healed injuries. This type of grouping not only facilitates later review by physicians, but also assists attorneys, judges, and juries in understanding the injuries. These comments apply as well to recording injuries in medical charts. A comparison of emergency department records between 1980 and 1995 reported that documentation of physical abuse showed little improvement despite increased awareness of abuse during this 15-year period and the introduction of a structured reporting form (115).

A further problem is the mistaken diagnosis of abuse by physicians. Dermatologic conditions, blood dyscrasias, osteogenesis imperfecta, accidental injuries, and the sequelae of folk treatments applied to the skin have all been mistaken for abuse (99,157,180,181). Medical personnel who are unfamiliar with usual postmortem changes such as purging of fluids from the nose and mouth, dependent lividity, and congealing of subcutaneous fat due to a decrease in body temperature may examine a dead child brought to a hospital emergency department. Mongolian spots and postmortem roach bites may be misinterpreted as evidence of injury. If these erroneous opinions are given to police officers, criminal charges may be pending against a caretaker before the pathologist has even begun an autopsy.

A 1-year-old child, clothed in infant pajamas, was brought dead on arrival to a hospital emergency department. The pediatrician-on-call noticed circumferential injuries of both wrists, which he interpreted to be rope burns (Fig. 19.4) The police were notified, and charges of abuse were filed against the parents. At autopsy, the injuries were identified as postmortem roach bites. Excursion of the roaches above the wrists was prevented by the elastic in the sleeves of the pajamas. The infant died of natural causes, but a juvenile

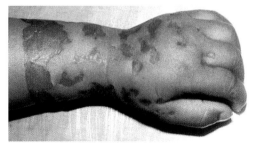

FIG. 19.4. Postmortem roach bites of wrist and hand mistaken for rope burns. The elastic cuff of the infant's pajama top prevented the roaches from proceeding farther up the arm. The lesions were bilateral.

court hearing proceeded because of the original charges.

This case is not unique, but is becoming increasingly uncommon with better training of medical and nursing personnel. When an infant or child has died, it is best to await the results of an autopsy before commenting on the cause of death. The pathologist must recognize the artefacts of resuscitation, reserve judgment regarding injuries, and proceed in a systematic way to evaluate and record his or her findings. Whereas the mistaken diagnosis of abuse is always possible, it is far more frequent today to find irresponsible medical experts who falsely invoke esoteric diseases as the cause of injury or death of children who have clearly been abused.

Cutaneous Injuries

Child abuse injuries may be scant or numerous, of different ages, produced by a variety of blunt trauma and other forms of injury, and involve any part of the body (12,52,55, 173). Contusions caused by blows are the most common form of abuse in all age groups and are often clustered on the chest, abdomen, or back. Although accidental injuries are 15 times more common than abuse-related injuries in infants (151), the benign nature of such injuries occurring in and around the home has been demonstrated repeatedly (29, 32,80,91,147). The cutaneous manifestations of accidental falls are usually confined to the forehead, bony prominences of the face and extremities, and the palms; abrasions and superficial lacerations are common in these circumstances. The axiom "Those who don't cruise, don't bruise" briefly summarizes the status of the younger infant (173). Within this context, even an apparently innocuous injury in a younger infant who has died unexpectedly must be viewed with suspicion, and significant injury must be considered abuse related until proven otherwise.

When describing injuries, each the type of trauma (contusion, abrasion, laceration, burn, etc.) should be identified, and its dimensions, shape, and color recorded. Although it is ap-

propriate to note the color of bruises, dating their age based on color is at best an imprecise exercise and should be avoided (112,162, 172). Fresh bruises are most readily identified, not only by color, but also by associated tissue swelling that recedes after the first day. Deep bruises may take days to appear, whereas superficial bruises may occur almost immediately and disappear within a few days. Anatomic location and skin complexion also influence the appearance of bruises. Therefore bruises inflicted on a child at the same time and by the same mechanism may be of different color and resolve at different rates.

When blunt trauma injuries are identified or suspected at autopsy, the standard of care requires the pathologist to make lengthwise incisions through the skin and subcutaneous tissues of the involved regions to determine the depth to which hemorrhage extends. This effort provides an indication of the severity of the blunt force used and also may reveal significant soft tissue injury not apparent from examination of the skin surfaces. This is particularly true in children who die acutely, before deep bruises have had the opportunity to diffuse closer to the skin surface. The standard of care also requires that head hair be shaved to examine bruises of the scalp. Faint bruises and abrasions may become more distinct after the autopsy, resulting from postmortem "aging" of the injury and drainage of blood from vessels. Reexamining the body 24 hours later may accentuate injuries that were difficult to distinguish at first examination. Samples of representative lesions should be taken for histologic evaluation. The presence of varying aged lesions establishes a pattern of continued abuse as opposed to a single episode of injury.

If patterned injuries are noted, scene investigation should include a search for the implement or implements that are consistent with the patterns on the body. It is unusual to find an injury with a unique pattern, so one should be cautious in specifically identifying an alleged weapon as responsible for an injury. A suspected weapon, however, may show evidence of trace amounts of blood or tissue to link it to the assault. Loop marks caused by a belt, cord, or similar implement are probably the most common patterned injuries of abuse.

Examination of the oral cavity, including the teeth, tongue and buccal mucosa, nares, and ear canals is an often neglected part of the autopsy. Special forensic techniques are necessary to document and sample injuries of these regions adequately. Figure 19.5 shows ulcerated bite marks of the tongue in a chronically abused child. These injuries were judged microscopically to be at least 1 week old, consistent with the age of several bruises noted on the face, and part of an extensive pattern of abuse.

Burns are a common form of abuse, and scald burns have significant mortality. In one prospective study, there were four deaths among 30 deliberately scalded children (mean age, 22.5 months) with burns of the buttocks. The infants who died had burns involving an average of 32.3% of their total body surface area (148); sepsis from stool contamination of the burns was thought to be the significant factor leading to death. Inflicted scald burns tend to be symmetrical, often involving the hands or feet in a glove or stocking pattern, and to have sharp margins. The injuries are inconsistent with the alleged circumstances and usually inappropriate for the infant's age. If the infant survives in hospital beyond 24 hours, the appearance of the burns at death may be quite different from their original appearance (Fig. 19.6A and B) During scene investigation, the caretaker should be asked to

recreate the incident by using a mannikin of similar size to the child, using water at a temperature similar to that of the alleged circumstances.

Certain infectious and inflammatory skin conditions may mimic burns. Among the more common errors, impetigo may be mistaken for cigarette burns (and vice versa), and phytophotodermatitis and other dermatotoxic and hypersensitivity reactions may be mistaken for scald burns (82). Although such problems are more commonly encountered by clinicians, the authors are aware of a case of staphylococcal scalded-skin syndrome and a case of necrotizing myositis mistaken for abuse at autopsy.

Bite-Mark Injuries

Perhaps no other type of forensic evidence causes as much controversy as that of bite-mark evidence. Because the skin is an elastic substrate that is easily distorted by movement of the assailant or the victim, bite marks usually form imperfect and incomplete impressions. The forensic odontologist must evaluate the evidence and attempt to determine the probability of a bite mark corresponding to or excluding the dentition of one or more suspects. It is important, therefore, that the dental consultant be experienced in bite-mark interpretation, and preferably certified by the American Board of Forensic Odontology. However,

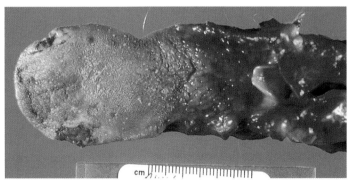

FIG. 19.5. Bilateral, ulcerated bite marks of the tongue bite, histologically at least 1 week of age, in a chronically abused child. Such injuries may be missed if a complete forensic autopsy is not performed.

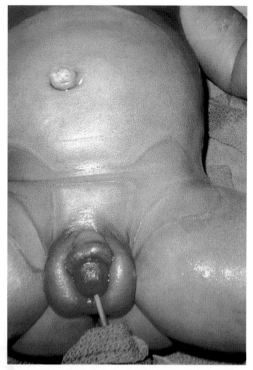

A

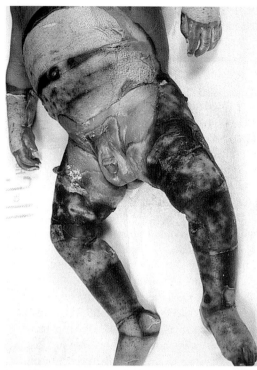

B

FIG. 19.6. Infant with scald burns inflicted in a bathtub. He survived for 10 days in hospital. **A:** Photograph taken at time of admission shows the sharp margins of the burn with sparing of the groin region. **B:** At autopsy, the appearance of the burn is much different, but the sharply demarcated burn patterns remain obvious.

even in the best of hands, the reliability of bite-mark evidence remains open to question.

Bite marks occurring in the setting of child abuse may be found anywhere on the body, particularly in infants. Depending on the amount of force and location, they may not appear typical to the untrained eye, particularly on such regions as the fingers or toes. If bite marks are suspected, a forensic odontologist should be consulted before proceeding further, because the autopsy procedure is likely to distort these injuries. Failure to observe this rule may cause irretrievable loss of evidence. The skin is not washed before bite-mark examination to preclude loss of serologic evidence from the saliva of the perpetrator. Because bite marks are often found on victims who have sustained multiple cutaneous injuries, a careful examination of the body is necessary to distinguish possible bite marks from other abrasions and contusions. Bite marks should not be excised, except by the odontologist as part of his or her examination. Photographs and impressions should be made by using accepted forensic techniques.

The police and prosecutor should be advised that bite-mark evidence is available, so that a search warrant or court order may be prepared to allow dental impressions to be made of the suspected abuser(s). Recognition and processing of such evidence may provide a link to the perpetrator of the abuse. It is important to remember that retarded or disturbed children may bite themselves, and that children may be bitten by an older sibling or other child.

Intrathoracic Injuries

Intrathoracic injuries are usually obvious at autopsy, but subtle injuries may be missed if a thorough examination is not performed. This is more likely to occur if the pathologist is not familiar with routine forensic procedures for examination of the oral cavity and upper respiratory tract. In such cases, evidence related to ingestion, suffocation, or aspiration of foreign material may be lost. Rib fractures, common in child abuse, may either be missed or overcalled by the inexperienced pathologist who mistakes the costochondral junctions for healing fractures. The similarity between the normal structure and pathologic lesion is shown in Fig. 19.7. In a 1984 clinical study, rib fractures were documented on chest radiograph in 15% of abused children. The authors concluded, "in the absence of roentgenographic evidence for other bone disease, unexplained rib fractures [are] specific for abuse" (56). Our experience has been similar with respect to both clinical and autopsy evaluation, in which resuscitation efforts may be falsely invoked as a cause of rib fractures. Intrathoracic injuries other than rib fractures are uncommon, even in infants, although pulmonary contusions may result from abusive compression of the chest, usually in association with multiple rib fractures.

Cardiac injury is rare. Abusive cardiac trauma usually presents as a laceration of the heart, most commonly at the junction of the vena cava with the right atrium, but also may involve the left ventricle (40).

An 11-month-old, previously healthy baby girl became unresponsive while in the care of her baby-sitter, who called 911 after allegedly initiating CPR. The child was reportedly found unresponsive on the floor, having been seen alert and happy only moments earlier. Autopsy revealed scattered abrasions of the face and several small contusions of varying ages of the chest and abdomen inconsistent with accidental injuries. The right atrium was lacerated at its junction with the inferior vena cava, and 80 to 100 mL of blood was present within the pericardial sac. Two other children in the care of this baby-sitter had had injuries of abuse, including the sister of the deceased who had sustained a serious skull fracture and fracture of the wrist when she allegedly tripped while running. Three forensic pathologists and a pediatrician with extensive child abuse experience all testified as to the nonaccidental nature of the child's injuries. The defense retained a forensic pathologist who claimed that the child had died of a "viral" illness, although no evidence of such was noted clinically or at autopsy. He attributed the atrial laceration to CPR. The jury failed to bring a conviction.

This child was afebrile and had no symptoms of viral illness. Whereas a pathologist unaccustomed to the normal exuberant appearance of lymphoid tissue in the lungs, gastrointestinal tract, and lymph nodes of infants might mistake this normal histologic pattern for evidence of a viral reaction, the presence of a viral infection would not explain sudden death in the absence of other findings. Although a cardiac arrhythmia might cause sudden death at any age, such an event is extremely rare in infancy in the absence of congenital heart disease. Similarly, despite thousands of episodes of CPR of infants by untrained persons, we are unaware of any documented cases of cardiac laceration during this procedure. A single case report of cardiac laceration allegedly after CPR provides a sketchy clinical history that is open to question (145). The force necessary to produce such an injury is clearly beyond the bounds of therapeutic chest compression. It is most likely

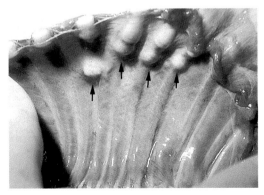

FIG. 19.7. Four healing rib fractures (*arrows*) on the excised ribs of an abused infant show areas of callus lateral to the costochondral junctions. The costochondral junctions are prominent in infants, as seen in this photograph, and may be mistaken for healing fractures by inexperienced pathologists.

caused by stomping on the child or by severe, prolonged compression with the hands.

Rarely, blunt trauma to the precordium may cause contusion of the myocardium. In a case from our files, a 5-month-old infant was resuscitated by paramedics after a blow to the sternum inflicted by the infant's baby-sitter, apparently with a telephone handset. A ventricular septal hematoma was subsequently demonstrated on CT scan. The sitter claimed that the infant had rocked his infant seat to the edge of a countertop, tipped it over, and fallen to the floor with the seat landing on top of him. The chest injury was inconsistent with such a scenario, and biomechanical investigation of the incident proved that a 5-month-old infant would not have had the size, strength, or coordination to have rocked or tipped the infant seat.

Fatal cardiac arrest also may result from so-called "commotio cordis" or cardiac concussion. In this form of trauma, a sharp, sudden blow to the sternum causes ventricular fibrillation. Maron et al. (121) reported 25 cases in children and young adults (ages 3 to 19) who died after being struck in the chest by a baseball, hockey puck, or similar object during sports activity. It is the timing of the blow that is significant. Using an experimental pig model and 30-mph impact by a wood sphere of baseball size and weight, Link et al. (116) showed that to produce its fatal effect, the blow must be coincidentally timed with a 15- to 30-msec window on the upslope of the T wave. A similar blow delivered at other times in the cardiac cycle produced at most a transient heart block. We have seen several cases of children who have similarly collapsed and died after receiving an inflicted blow to the sternum of only moderate force but with fatal consequences. Although such cases are classified as homicides, there is usually no evidence of chest wall contusion, and there is no evidence of physical trauma to the heart.

Abdominal Injuries

Blunt trauma to the abdomen, usually seen in the older infant or young child, is second only to head trauma as a leading cause of fatal abuse. Three major types of injuries are common: (a) laceration of a solid organ, most commonly the liver, and less commonly the spleen, pancreas, or kidney; (b) intramural hematoma or laceration of a segment of the gastrointestinal tract, particularly the small intestine; and (c) laceration of the bowel mesentery. The mechanism of injury is usually a sharp blow or kick to the abdomen, producing displacement or compression of the affected organ and leading to a shearing or crushing injury. Increased intraabdominal pressure may also lead to a blow-out injury of a distended stomach or loop of bowel. Less commonly, a child may receive abdominal injury by being thrown against a wall, floor, or other hard surface. The mechanism of death in these cases is intraabdominal hemorrhage or peritonitis, depending on the type of injury. These injuries do not occur as a result of accidents within the home, such as tripping while running, falling down stairs, or falling out of bed (32,80,91,118,186).

Unlike fatal head trauma, in which significant symptoms develop immediately, the child with abdominal trauma may appear relatively symptom free for several hours after injury. An immediate response to the pain of the inflicted injury will have occurred, but often will not be reported. The onset of serious abdominal symptoms may be insidious, particularly in the preverbal child, and is characteristic of injuries such as duodenal perforation or other retroperitoneal injury. The child with an injury such as a small liver or mesenteric laceration also may initially appear relatively asymptomatic, with persistent slow accumulation of blood in the abdominal cavity until collapse suddenly occurs due to hypovolemic shock. The blood volume of a young child is approximately 75 mL/kg body weight; the extent of blood loss into the abdominal cavity may be calculated on this basis, and may be as great as one third of the total blood volume. In the child with peritonitis, several days may elapse between injury and death, which can occur if the caretaker ignores the child's obvious need for medical care.

When a child dies of inflicted abdominal trauma associated with a lacerated liver, there may be a claim that the injury was sustained during resuscitation. Even vigorous, inexpert resuscitation in a young child will rarely, if ever, produce hepatic injury. If it does occur, the laceration will be superficial, located in the midline on the superior surface of the liver, and associated with only minimal hemorrhage, as opposed to the significant hemorrhage characteristic of lethal inflicted injury (Fig. 19.8) Similarly, attorneys defending a man who had fatally injured a 17-month-old child in his care argued that multiple abdominal bruises, a large mesenteric laceration, and partial avulsion of the small bowel were caused by overvigorous resuscitation efforts applied to the lower abdomen. Figure 19.9 demonstrates this child's massive injury. Although it was obvious that such a claim was clearly absurd, it was still necessary to explain to a jury that the contusions of the bowel wall, tissue reaction, inflammation, significant intraabdominal hemorrhage, and fecal spillage were all inconsistent with resuscitation injury.

The presence of peritonitis and associated adhesions may complicate the task, but it is essential that the pathologist perform complete dissection of the gastrointestinal tract when there is evidence of trauma to the bowel.

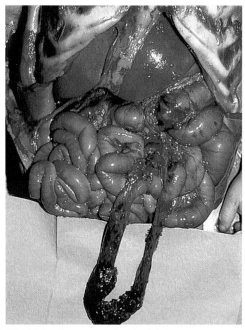

FIG. 19.9. Severe abdominal injury with lacerations of the mesentery, avulsion of a segment of the jejunum, and multiple contusions of the bowel due to repeated punches to the abdomen.

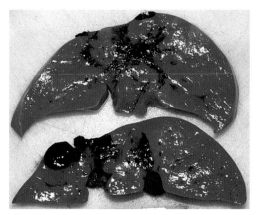

FIG. 19.8. Lacerations of the liver with acute intrahepatic and subcapsular hematomas due to blunt abdominal trauma. Partial clotting of the blood indicates that the child survived for several hours. Externally, there were multiple contusions in the right upper quadrant of the abdomen.

Sampling of injuries is best done after the bowel has been fixed in formalin, when the full extent of the trauma is often better appreciated. If previous surgical intervention included partial bowel resection, the surgical specimen and associated histologic slides should be retrieved and examined. Interpretation of the age of injuries requires sampling for microscopy not only of the lesion itself but also of inflamed peritoneal surfaces and other tissues secondarily involved by hemorrhage or infection. To the extent possible, internal injuries should be correlated with cutaneous lesions, which also should be sampled for microscopic evaluation.

Autopsies of battered children may reveal previously undiagnosed healed liver or mesenteric lacerations from prior episodes of abuse. In one such case, exploratory laparotomy of a young child with peritoneal signs revealed inflammation and granulation tissue at the base of the mesentery, which was misinterpreted at the time of surgery as retroperitoneal fibromatosis. The child later died after further abuse, and review of hospital records showed evidence of contusions of the abdomen that had previously been dismissed as "usual childhood bruising."

Because of the time lag between injury, onset of symptoms, and death, the outcome of an investigation may depend in large part on the ability of the pathologist to date an injury or injuries. He or she must resist pressure to expand or contract the injury time window derived through gross and microscopic examination to conform to theories of the police, prosecutors, or defense attorneys. Conversely, pathologic dating of evolving intraabdominal injuries is often imprecise. A pathologist who is unwilling to admit uncertainty or error, or whose conclusions are judged by medical colleagues to be persistently idiosyncratic, quickly loses the confidence of the attorneys and police with whom he or she must work.

Musculoskeletal Injuries

Significant injuries to muscle tissues are unusual even in fatal abuse associated with severe beatings. However, some children may die after such a beating, without evidence of internal injuries. The problem of fatal abuse without "fatal" injuries is considered later in the chapter.

Skeletal fractures are a prominent component of child abuse injuries. Skull fractures are most common, followed by long-bone fractures, but in extreme circumstances, even the lumbar spine may be affected (58). Isolated cervical spinal cord damage without spinal column fracture also has been reported as the result of abuse (140). Toddlers and older children may fall and fracture limbs or sustain uncomplicated skull fractures in a fall from a moderate height. These age-appropriate accidental fractures conform to the clinical history, and are benign. However, any skeletal fracture in a deceased infant or child, absent a confirmed history of motor vehicle accident or fall from an upper-story window, should be considered abuse until proven otherwise. Fractured bone(s) should be excised

by the pathologist for further gross and microscopic examination after appropriate radiologic documentation. The differential diagnosis of abusive fractures versus osteogenesis imperfecta (OI) rarely occurs at autopsy. However, this question may arise in living infants with one or more fractures, (1,22,59) and lead to extensive (and expensive) diagnostic testing. A full discussion of the topic is beyond the scope of this chapter. However, one does not expect OI to be associated with multiple bruises, subdural hematomas (SDHs), cerebral injury, or damage to internal organs. Such findings indicate abuse, even in a child with proven OI.

The concept of "temporary" brittle-bone disease (128,137), coincidentally characterized by fractures typical of abuse (e.g., rib and metaphyseal fractures), but lacking features common to OI, remains totally unsubstantiated (22,35). Unfortunately, it is being raised as a defense in child abuse cases. Thorough investigation, appropriate laboratory and radiologic studies, and documentation of all injuries are necessary to deflect this medically irresponsible hypothesis, which has become one of several courtroom diagnoses unknown in a normal medical setting. The fact that the term "temporary" refers to the recognition that when the injured infant is removed from the custody of the abusive caretaker, the "brittle-bone disease" goes into complete remission, provides a clue as to its true etiology.

Sexual Abuse Injuries

When sexual abuse is suspected at autopsy, oral, rectal, and vaginal swabs are taken for DNA analysis and antigenic typing of seminal fluid. The protocol to be used should be determined in consultation with local crime laboratory personnel so that appropriate supplies and materials for the studies will be available when needed. Careful examination of the oral cavity, external genitalia, perineum, and anal region is necessary to establish evidence of acute or chronic injury from sexual abuse. Toluidine blue can be used to aid in the detection of perianal and anal trauma (18). A photographic record of the findings is essential for documentation because some inflammatory, infectious, and congenital lesions may be confused with abuse (17,77,117). If there is any question about the findings, appropriate pediatric specialists should be consulted.

The anal sphincter may relax after death, giving a false impression of recent anal penetration, and congealing of subcutaneous fat may produce a gaping of the vulvar tissues that suggests vaginal penetration. These changes are demonstrated in Fig. 19.10A. This 6-month-old infant was pronounced dead in a hospital emergency department. A report was made to the medical examiner's office recounting probable sexual abuse after a nurse had cleaned the genital and perineal regions of adherent stool. The changes were produced by the efforts to clean the baby before releasing it to the medical examiner. In comparison, Fig. 19.10B shows healed lacerations and incipient rectal prolapse in an infant who was subjected to repeated rectal penetration.

Although external examination may have revealed no evidence of sexual abuse, a further search should be made during internal examination for foreign bodies or trauma within the vagina or rectum, or for evidence of perforation into the peritoneal cavity. Absence of sexual abuse is recorded as an essential negative finding. If evidence of trauma is found, special dissection is necessary. In the male, the rectum, anus, and perianal tissues are excised *en bloc*; in the female, the dissection also includes the perineum, uterus, vagina, and vulva. The bladder and urethra are usually incorporated within this block. After removal, the anus (and vagina) are opened, and the injuries are photographed. The tissues are then fixed in formalin and subsequently sectioned for microscopic examination. When these dissections are done properly, the remaining pelvic tissues can be sewn shut so as to leave little evidence of the exenteration.

Cardiopulmonary Resuscitation and Other Therapy

Prolonged hospitalization may obscure evidence of injury, and even brief hospitalization and therapy may alter the appearance of injuries. All findings related to therapy should be identified and described separately, including excoriations related to prolonged intubation, tape marks on the face, pressure purpura in the occipital region, and ecchymoses associated with cutaneous needle-puncture sites. Resuscitation efforts may produce contusions of the chest, (Fig. 19.11) but internal iatrogenic injuries are rare. In one study of 211 children younger than 12 years who had CPR,

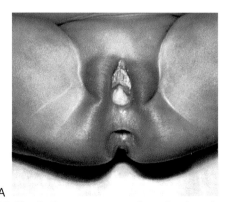
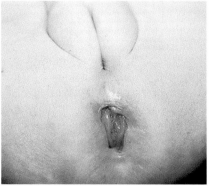

A   B

FIG. 19.10. A: Postmortem gaping of vulvar tissues and relaxation of anal sphincter reported as child abuse. The findings resulted from the cleansing of the area by an emergency department nurse. **B:** By comparison, chronic anorectal trauma with incipient rectal prolapse in a sexually abused infant who had repeated rectal penetration.

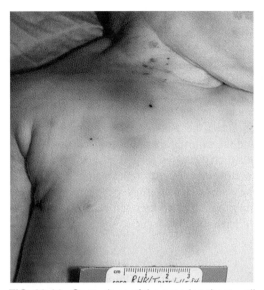

FIG. 19.11. Contusions of the anterior chest wall associated with resuscitation attempts. Needle-puncture marks are evident on the right side of the neck and in the right infraclavicular region. Histologically, there was no vital reaction associated with the contusions.

only seven (3%) had injuries regarded as medically significant, such as pneumothorax, pulmonary hemorrhage, or retroperitoneal hemorrhage. The iatrogenic etiology of the injuries in these cases was obvious (27). In two other studies, among a total of 170 infants who received CPR, none had CPR-related rib fractures (56,171). Those who suggest vigorous or inexpert CPR as the cause of a child's injuries must offer a reasonable explanation for the three components of this factitious syndrome: (a) sudden cardiorespiratory arrest in a previously healthy infant, (b) injuries that are not observed in infants receiving CPR for medically documentable causes of cardiac arrest, and (c) injuries that occur only in the presence of a lone caretaker.

Numerous clinical and pathological studies also have confirmed that retinal hemorrhages do not result from CPR (64,96,134), and medical controversy on this issue has been resolved. According to Levin (114), there is only one well-documented case of proven retinal hemorrhage in an infant after resusci-

tation where none was noted before resuscitation: a single, small hemorrhage in an infant who sustained 75 minutes of in-hospital CPR. The hemorrhage in this extremely rare occurrence should not be confused with the multiple, severe retinal hemorrhages of inflicted head trauma.

A brain-dead child maintained on a respirator will develop a "respirator brain." The features include cerebral edema, progressive softening of the brain, clot formation within the dural sinuses, and occasional focal subarachnoid hemorrhage. Low-grade infection may develop within the middle or inner ears, which in an infant may normally show evidence of mild chronic inflammation. These changes must not be mistaken for a primary disease process. Similarly, pneumonia can develop within hours when a comatose child requires use of a respirator, and the pathologist must take care not to identify this secondary phenomenon as the cause of death.

A 15-month-old, previously healthy male infant was brought into a hospital emergency department in a coma and seizing after an alleged fall from a couch at home. He had been in the care of his mother's boyfriend at the time of the incident. Treating physicians noted a small bruise on the right ear, cerebral edema (right more than left), and retinal hemorrhages; tympanic membranes were judged normal by three examiners. The clinical diagnosis was blunt head trauma related to abuse. The child died after 3 days of care on a respirator. Autopsy revealed cerebral edema, a small SDH, clot within the transverse sinus interpreted as thrombosis, and mild inflammation of the middle ears. The pathologist listed the cause of death as transverse sinus thrombosis secondary to middle ear infection, and the manner of death as natural. The police were forced to release the assailant, who had been in custody since the day of the assault. Fortunately, later review of the case by other pathologists, including the authors, led to his indictment and conviction.

Surgical intervention may interfere with the recognition of blunt-trauma injury of the scalp in regions contiguous with a craniotomy. Abdominal surgery does not usually interfere with identification of cutaneous injuries to the abdominal wall, but resection and repair of tissues and organs may alter intraabdominal anatomy. Preautopsy review of operative reports or discussion with the operating surgeon is essential, and examination and histologic sampling of surgical specimens are often helpful in reconstructing the original injuries.

There is rarely any reason for a pathologist to deny permission for postmortem organ retrieval for transplantation when an abused child has been declared brain dead and the family consents to the procedure. Almost all such children have died of head injury, and their visceral organs are likely to be normal. The pathologist can attend the organ harvest or request that the transplant surgeon report any abnormal internal findings. Harvesting of bone, corneas, and/or skin should be deferred until after autopsy. We are not aware of a situation anywhere in the country in which prosecution was impaired because of organ harvesting from a child abuse victim.

Microscopic Examination

Microscopic examination of tissues includes routine sections of internal organs and sections of representative injuries. The pathologist must be familiar with the normal histo-logic appearance of neonatal and infant organs. Often examiners misinterpret the significance of various lymphoid/inflammatory cells within various organs. Probably the most common error is the overinterpretation of interstitial cellularity and peribronchiolar lymphoid aggregation within the lungs as evidence of pneumonia. Another common error is the misinterpretation of normally occurring small lymphoid aggregates in the infant heart as evidence of myocarditis.

Microvesicular fat within the liver also is a common finding, and was reported in the livers of 21 infants and children who died suddenly of trauma or natural causes (25). Although the study was done with reference to the reliability of fatty change in the liver as a marker for Reye syndrome, the findings have significance for the interpretation of various metabolic, nutritional, and toxic conditions. In our experience, children dying of these disorders, including most cases of Reye syndrome, invariably show far more fat within hepatocytes than is seen in trauma victims or children dying of other natural causes (Fig. 19.12).

The healing process evolves more rapidly in young children than in adults, and this fact must be considered when dating the age of injuries. Although more accurate than gross examination, dating of injuries by microscopic examination is imprecise, and the pathologist

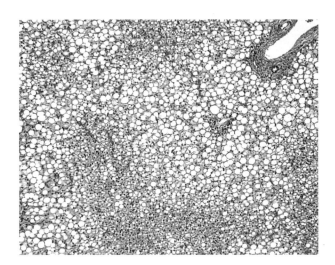

FIG. 19.12. Macrovesicular and microvesicular fatty liver in an infant with a medium-chain fatty acid oxidation disorder. Whereas not all cases show changes as prominent as this, the amount of fat far exceeds that seen in normal infant livers.

should give an appropriate time range during which the injuries might have occurred. This time window expands as the interval between injury and death increases. Although special histologic stains for collagen and hemosiderin may assist in this evaluation (45), age, nutrition, immune system status, and inherent individual differences are important variables that affect healing. Furthermore, an overreliance on microscopic examination may lead a pathologist to give undue weight to a lesion that is so minute that it could not have any possible clinical significance.

Inflammatory response and wound healing in the severely malnourished child may be inhibited (174), and children who are comatose may show an impaired response to systemic and cutaneous injury (106). The cause of the coma does not appear to be a factor in determining this altered time sequence, but the pathologist must be aware that it can occur. In all cases, pathologists must avoid claiming greater precision in microscopic aging of lesions than is possible based on the inherent biologic variability of the species.

LABORATORY STUDIES

Postmortem Chemistry

Vitreous electrolytes provide the most objective information regarding dehydration, and these levels should be determined routinely in sudden infant deaths. In cases of suspected shaken baby syndrome or other head trauma in which the eyes must be examined for retinal hemorrhages, an equal volume of formalin can be instilled into the vitreous chamber after removal of vitreous fluid. One to 2 mL of fluid can be obtained from almost any infant, and should be analyzed by using pediatric micromethodology. A laboratory that performs vitreous analyses should first establish a "normal range" for electrolytes in this fluid before reporting results. The pathologist is responsible for interpreting the variables that may affect the values obtained.

Vitreous sodium, urea nitrogen, and creatinine values closely parallel antemortem serum values, and remain stable after death in the absence of decomposition. Vitreous potassium levels, like serum potassium levels, increase rapidly after death and do not reflect the antemortem serum concentration. Vitreous chloride levels remain stable, but have a normal range approximately 20 mEq/L greater than normal antemortem serum values. An elevated vitreous glucose concentration correlates with antemortem hyperglycemia, but a low glucose value is of little diagnostic significance because glucose is depleted rapidly after death. If factitious hypoglycemia resulting from administration of exogenous insulin is suspected, then serum total insulin and C-peptide concentrations should be determined by using the usual radioimmunoassay methods. These proteins, as well as albumin, globulins, and hemoglobin, remain stable for at least 24 hours after death under normal circumstances, permitting reliable postmortem analysis.

Normal vitreous electrolytes are an important negative finding. A vitreous sodium level greater than 155 mEq/L and a urea nitrogen value greater than 30 mg/dL indicate a contracted intravascular water content. An elevated vitreous creatinine value indicates renal damage. A serum sodium concentration in excess of 160 mEq/L can have severe clinical consequences (41). Dehydration in the absence of an appropriate clinical history must be regarded as suggestive; a vitreous sodium concentration of more than 175 mEq/L in the absence of a credible history of severe vomiting and/or diarrhea must be regarded as diagnostic of abuse or neglect until proven otherwise.

Hypernatremia as a form of abuse is probably far more common than is reported (36,141). Meadow (124) reviewed 12 cases of intentional salt poisoning, most of which were in the first 6 months of life. The mother was the perpetrator in 10 of 12 cases. Three typical cases in our experience involved toddlers from 2 to 3 years of age admitted to hospital with serum sodium concentrations in the range of 190 to 205 mEq/L. One child died in the emergency department, after water restriction for several days while in the care of a baby-sitter; two others died as inpatients and

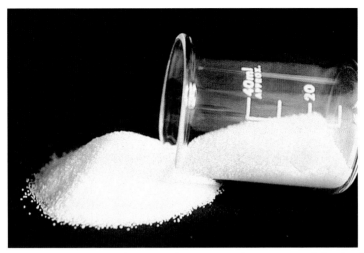

FIG. 19.13. Beaker containing 30 g of salt, to demonstrate the excess salt load a 2-year-old child was forced to ingest as punishment for misbehaving. Death was caused by hypernatremia.

also had evidence of physical abuse. All had been forced to eat salt or drink salt water as a form of punishment. In one such case, the parents claimed the child had been playing with a salt shaker and accidentally ingested the salt. The excess salt load, calculated to be 30 grams, is illustrated in Fig. 19.13, a photograph prepared to demonstrate graphically that the claim of accidental ingestion was untrue. In none of these children did the pediatric house staff or attending physicians suspect the true cause of the hypernatremia, but in all cases, considered hypothalamic tumor high on the differential diagnosis list.

Dilutional hyponatremia due to water intoxication has been reported in infants fed diluted formula for a long period (97), and fatalities have occurred in children forced to drink large quantities of water as a form of punishment (9).

Toxicology

The yield from toxicologic screening in infant deaths remains relatively low despite a marked increase in the birth of drug-intoxicated infants in recent years (57,183). Cocaine or its major metabolite, benzoylecgonine, is the drug most frequently recovered,

and Mirchandani et al. (130) in 1991 reported 16 such cases in Philadelphia. This figure met with some skepticism at the time, but subsequent experience in other jurisdictions has been similar. The presence of any concentration of either cocaine or its metabolite benzoylecgonine should be considered sufficient to cause or contribute to the death of any live-born infant in whom an unrelated, obvious cause of death is not present. One must be cautious, however, of identifying cocaine intoxication as a cause of death on fetal death certificates, given the numerous maternal and fetal factors that can produce a stillbirth in the absence of this drug.

Additional substances that are frequently part of routine screening include alcohol, opiates, acetaminophen, phencyclidine, and aspirin, but the yield for these drugs will be below that for cocaine. Toxicologic results must be interpreted within the context of the other autopsy findings. Clearly, the presence of any illicit drug, alcohol, prescription drug not prescribed for the child, or inappropriate over-the-counter medication is cause for concern. Poisoning may result from intentional efforts to harm the child (66,152), toxins in herbal remedies (13), or carelessness on the part of the caretaker with respect to use or storage of substances harmful to children. Apparent toxic postmortem serum concentrations of prescribed drugs such as digoxin, however, may reflect only artefact due to postmortem redistribution of the drug, and not indicate antemortem toxicity (105).

Inaccurate laboratory procedures may lead to serious error and unnecessary grief for parents. An 8-year-old boy drowned in a recreation center swimming pool in a northern Illinois county, and the boy's parents alleged negligence in the guarding of the pool. An autopsy was performed, and the county toxicology laboratory reported the presence of cocaine in the blood. The examining pathologist, not experienced in forensic pathology, subsequently misinterpreted aspirated small food particles within bronchioles as intravascular foreign matter consistent with intravenous drug abuse. Cocaine intoxication was listed as the underlying cause of death. Review of the gas chromatograms by an experienced forensic toxicologist showed them to be virtually uninterpretable, but demonstrating no evidence of cocaine or any other drug.

Both the toxicologist and the pathologist in this case failed to consider how unlikely it would be to find an 8-year-old intravenous drug abuser. The pathologist, biased by incorrect laboratory results, produced an incorrect microscopic evaluation of the lungs. A lawsuit brought by the parents of the dead child against the county was settled out of court.

Clearly, precautions are needed to assure proper handling and processing of toxicology specimens. This of itself is not sufficient. The interpretation of results, including therapeutic and toxic tissue concentrations and physiologic and toxic effects of a substance on the body, is the responsibility of both the pathologist and the toxicologist if the findings, positive or negative, are to withstand challenge.

Metabolic and Genetic Disorders

The sudden, unexpected death of an infant or child and a subsequent "negative" autopsy often raises the question of a subtle or "undiscovered" metabolic disorder. This idea may be proposed in an attempt to offer an alternative diagnosis to suffocation when multiple "SIDS" deaths have occurred among siblings. Indeed, inborn errors of fatty acid oxidation occasionally cause death after minimal symptoms so as to mimic SIDS (133,150), or after a clinical course like that of Reye syndrome (153). Hale and Bennett (74) reported that among more than 100 confirmed cases of medium-chain acyl-coenzyme A (CoA) dehydrogenase (MCAD) deficiency, nearly 20% had originally been misdiagnosed as SIDS or "near-miss" SIDS, and that cases of children with other forms of fatty acid oxidation disorders initially misdiagnosed as SIDS also had been reported. The frequency of the homozygous state for the gene mutation G-985 responsible for 80% to 90% of the cases of MCAD deficiency is about 1 in 18,500 births (21,74). This fact indicates that MCAD deficiency might be implicated in approximately 5% of sudden, otherwise unexplained deaths. Miller et al. (127) extracted DNA from paraffin-embedded autopsy tissues of 67 SIDS victims. They detected no G-985 homozygotes and three G-985 heterozygotes, findings not statistically different from those of their 70 newborn controls (one heterozygote). They concluded that mutation G-985 MCAD deficiency is probably not a significant factor in the etiology of SIDS. Later studies indicate that approximately 5% of all sudden infant deaths are probably caused by a fatty acid oxidation disorder (23,24).

Other genetic diseases, congenital disorders, or inborn errors of metabolism, such as amino acidemias, also may mimic SIDS, or rarely be mistaken for child abuse (180). Shoemaker et al. (164) reported the case of a mother who was charged with the ethylene glycol poisoning of her infant. Reexamination of the postmortem serum showed that the gas chromatographic peak originally identified as ethylene glycol was actually propionic acid, and that the child had died of methylmalonic acidemia, an inborn error of branched-chain amino acid metabolism. Glutaric aciduria type 1, a disorder with variable degenerative neurologic signs, may occasionally present with subdural hemorrhages or fluid collection in the context of progressive cerebral atrophy (191). It is hypothesized that an enlargement of the subdural space secondary to atrophy may place extra strain on bridging veins, causing occasional rupture. This is an entirely different mechanism for intracranial injury than shaken baby syndrome, in which there is acceleration force injury to an otherwise normal brain. There is no evidence that infants with this disorder who do not have cerebral atrophy are more susceptible to subdural hemorrhage, nor are these infants more susceptible to retinal hemorrhages, fractures, or other trauma characteristic of abuse.

The absence of severe fatty change in the liver is good evidence against a disorder of fatty acid oxidation, and the absence of organic acids on gas chromatography rules out a lethal amino acidemia. Less than 1 mL of blood is necessary to test for these disorders, and freezing samples of blood, urine, liver, and heart at $-7°C$ permits testing at a later date. Dried blood samples also may be used to test for many genetic disorders.

Microbiology

Microbiologic studies in the absence of gross evidence of infection are unlikely to be positive except in the young infant, in whom sepsis or pneumonia may remain occult at autopsy. Routine bacteriologic culture of the cerebrospinal fluid (CSF; by cisternal puncture or spinal tap) and blood as a first step in the autopsy will detect those otherwise occult infections. Blood cultures taken more than 24 hours after death are almost certain to be contaminated by intestinal flora, and are, therefore, not worthwhile. However, a spleen culture obtained under sterile conditions can often clarify the issue of postmortem contaminants. Postmortem testing for most sexually transmitted diseases also is unreliable if not done in the immediate postmortem period. Such testing, however, should not be performed by emergency department personnel who first see the dead child without the specific permission of the medical examiner.

Probing of the vaginal or rectal regions may produce artefactual injury or distort existing injuries.

Testing for gonococcal infections requires special transport media and immediate plating in a laboratory that is qualified to handle such specimens. The incidence of misidentification of *Neisseria* strains is high in laboratories that use commercial systems for gonococcal identification (89).

Viral cultures are expensive and have a generally poor yield at autopsy. It is usually more beneficial to test serum for viral antibody titers. Testing for HIV should be done when the maternal history is positive or the autopsy findings or circumstances otherwise suggest the likelihood of HIV infection.

SPECIAL PROBLEMS IN CHILD AUTOPSIES

From time to time, every pathologist is faced with a death in which abuse is strongly suspected or is obvious, but the actual cause of death is unknown or obscure after autopsy. In other cases, the immediate cause of death may be obvious, but its relation to the abuse may be uncertain; and in still other cases, the diagnosis of fatal abuse may be obvious, but the timing of the injury may be in dispute. Deaths also occur in children in whom the medical diagnosis of abuse is incorrect or cannot be proven. The pathologist must be able to assist in the resolution of these cases.

Correct determination of the cause (or causes) of death has important legal ramifications, because the medical examiner/coroner also must determine the manner of death (i.e., whether death is of natural causes, an accident, suicide, or homicide). Ultimately, if no decision is reached, the manner of death is classified as undetermined. The pathologist involved in child autopsies must have a clear understanding of the concept of medicolegal causation. It is often best to ask the question, "Within a reasonable degree of medical and scientific certainty, is it probable (that is, more likely than not), that this child would have died on this day and at this time if he or she had not suffered the observed (inflicted) injuries?" If the answer to this question is "No," then the manner of death is homicide. In this section, we attempt to provide information that will reduce the number of cases in which the answer is "I don't know."

Perinatal Deaths

Perinatal death investigation poses particular medical and legal issues for the forensic pathologist, which only can be summarized in this chapter. For those seeking more information, an excellent and comprehensive review of the forensic aspects of the subject is provided by Knight (104).

There is often considerable medical and pathological uncertainty with respect to the circumstances and status of perinatal deaths. Many cases represent births in concealed nonmedical settings after concealment of the pregnancy. In such instances, delivery of an infant into an unsafe environment, such as a toilet, may cause death by drowning. When a neonatal death is concealed by secret disposal of the body, the pathologist is faced with the question of whether this was a live birth, and if so, was death related to natural causes, intentional injury, or the result of abandonment. In other cases, the pregnant mother may have been assaulted or had accidental trauma that is alleged to have contributed to fetal or neonatal demise.

Newborns can remain relatively hearty at moderate temperatures, without food or water, as illustrated by the survival of 44 newborns buried for 7 to 10 days in the debris of a collapsed hospital in the 1985 Mexico City earthquake (43). In another example of neonatal durability, a newborn baby girl survived for 3 hours after being placed in a home freezer after her birth. Her body temperature was 50°F at the time of admission to a hospital emergency department. The mother, who claimed that she thought the baby had died at birth, was subsequently charged with attempted murder (38).

The pathologist must start with the presumption of stillbirth, and provide evidence of a live birth; an unsuccessfully resuscitated stillborn remains a stillborn. He or she must subsequently determine the cause and manner of death of any liveborn infant. If the infant is stillborn, the cause of death is entered on a fetal death certificate, which does not call for a manner-of-death determination. In cases of trauma to the pregnant mother, the specific maternal factors that contributed to fetal demise should be listed on the death certificate. Common complications of direct abdominal trauma are premature rupture of the membranes, premature labor, and placental abruption; uterine rupture is less common but can occur. Direct trauma to the fetus is infrequent, but may be seen in motor vehicle collisions or in severe assaults in which there is extensive blunt trauma to the abdomen.

The complete perinatal autopsy should include placental examination whenever possible. Body weight, crown–heel length, crown–rump length, and foot length assist in determining gestational age and fetal maturity. The external examination includes recording facial configuration, skin creases, and other topographic features. Evidence of trauma is evaluated as in any other autopsy. Birth trauma such as cephalohematomas or fractures of the clavicle must be differentiated from postbirth trauma, such as rib fractures and skull fractures. Clavicular fractures occur in approximately 3% of hospital deliveries (94). Other fractures are rare, although we have observed fatal depressed skull fracture and cervical spine dislocation due to incorrect application of forceps by inexperienced physicians. We are not aware of data regarding the frequency of accidental fractures associated with unassisted out-of-hospital deliveries, but we have not seen any such fractures associated with death of an infant.

Fractures, contusions, lacerations, or cutting and stabbing wounds can be seen in neonatal homicides. Attempts to remove a nuchal cord may result in scratch marks of the neck resembling strangulation. The cord should also be examined for evidence of abrasion or laceration, however, to avoid overlooking an effort to pass off signs of strangulation as attempts by the mother to remove a nuchal cord. Similarly, stab wounds of the infant may be alleged to have occurred during attempts to cut the umbilical cord.

The internal examination includes notation of organ weights and maturity. Signs of live birth are evaluated. In a nondecomposed infant, the presence of an air bubble in the stomach on radiologic examination indicates either live birth or postpartum resuscitation attempts. If the lungs and sections of lungs float in water in the absence of attempted resuscitation or decomposition, the infant was probably live born. It also is true that nonaerated, atelectatic lungs do not always indicate stillbirth. Milk or colostrum in the stomach is proof of live birth. Microscopically, meconium or squamous alveolar debris does not indicate live birth, but lungs with alveolar hyaline membranes are characteristic of a living infant.

Signs of maceration are diagnostic of intrauterine death, and preclude live birth. These include a red floppy body with loose joints, a collapsed head with poorly cohesive brain, skin slippage and blistering, generalized organ autolysis, and serosanguinous body cavity effusions.

Infants may be live born but die shortly after birth because they are lethally malformed, of previable gestational age, or septic. An infant may be full term and live born, but cannot be resuscitated because of perinatal asphyxiation from a variety of causes including placental anomalies, nuchal cord, and meconium aspiration. A diagnosis of neonaticide requires that the live-born infant would still be alive but for abandonment or neglect, purposeful asphyxiation, inflicted trauma, or intoxication or poisoning. In all cases, blood and other tissues should be preserved for possible toxicologic tests, testing for genetic disorders, and DNA analysis when the infant is unknown or a question of maternity and/or paternity arises.

Fatal Abuse Without "Fatal" Injury

Occasionally, the pathologist is faced with a dead infant or child who has obvious signs of physical abuse or neglect but no identifiable "fatal" injuries. This can occur in one of several ways: (a) failure to seek medical attention for complications of an otherwise nonlethal inflicted injury; (b) superimposed illness in a child whose immune responses are impaired by the stress of chronic abuse or severe neglect; (c) abuse of a child already impaired by acute or chronic illness; (d) sudden death resulting from acute or chronic abuse; or (e) failure to seek medical attention for an obvious life-threatening illness or surgical condition.

A common example in the first category is the child who dies of sepsis or pneumonia as a result of failure of a caretaker to seek medical attention for an inflicted scald burn, which subsequently becomes infected. In such cases, the linear relation between the burn injury, the subsequent infection, and the terminal sepsis is obvious. This example implies a probable element of medical neglect, but such a finding is not necessary to make a determination of fatal abuse.

A more difficult type of case is that in which the child shows multiple injuries of abuse inflicted up to several days before death, the cause of death is often pneumonia or other infection, but no direct linkage is identified. Many of these children have been chronically abused, and healing and/or healed injuries are often present. To the experienced forensic pathologist, the relation of injury to fatal disease is familiar, although not anatomically demonstrable. Repeated episodes of abuse produce sufficient physical and psychological stress to impair the child's immune system, lowering resistance to infection. This relation has been well documented under a variety of circumstances (106,184,189). These deaths are properly labeled homicides, based on the probability that the child would not have contracted an infection and/or died had he or she not been abused. It is not coincidence or "bad luck" that this child died, but a foreseeable result of abuse.

Similarly, an acutely or chronically ill child who is subsequently abused is more likely to die as a result of the additional stress. No studies to quantitate this increased risk have been performed, however, and each situation must be evaluated on its own merits. One must ask, given the child's underlying state of health, whether it is more likely than not that this child would have died at this particular time absent any abuse (i.e., is this a coincidental association of a natural disease process in a child who "just happens" to be abused?). Before answering that question, the pathologist must consider the usual risk of death for a child of this particular age and state of health from the particular infection or other disease process. The role of the inflicted injuries in causing death is then considered within that context. If the injuries aggravated the underlying disease or further impaired the child's health to any extent, the manner of death should be classified as homicide.

Perhaps even more difficult is the child abuse case that involves significant soft-tissue injuries, usually inflicted almost immediately before death, where autopsy reveals no anatomic cause of death. We have seen this phenomenon in infants and children up to 10 years of age. Some children may show extensive subcutaneous hemorrhage from a severe beating or beatings, with injuries primarily to the back, buttocks, and legs, and no evidence of significant head injury. Other children may have less numerous injuries; one young infant who had been anally assaulted showed no other evidence of trauma, although asphyxiation could not be completely ruled out. Autopsy in these children has revealed no internal injuries, although mild to moderate cerebral edema may be noted.

A 3-year-old girl was beaten by her mother on the arms, lower back, buttocks, and thighs, by hand and with a plastic wagon handle. No history of abuse was recorded, but the child's mother was 1 month postpartum and had shown signs of postpartum depression. Approximately 30 minutes after the beating, the child collapsed and died. Autopsy revealed several small bruises consistent with pinch marks on both arms, as well as confluent bruising of the buttocks and thighs (Fig. 19.14A). Incision into the injured regions showed extensive subcutaneous hemorrhage and focal intra-

muscular hemorrhage (Fig. 19.14B). No internal injuries or evidence of aspiration of gastric contents was noted. Microscopic examination of internal organs was unremarkable.

The common feature in all such cases is severe physical and psychologic stress related to pain. The pain is produced by injuries that are repetitive, anticipated, and extended over many minutes to hours, unlike accidental injury, which is almost always sudden, of short duration, nonrepetitive, and lacking in the emotional impact that accompanies abuse. In the absence of an anatomic cause, the pathologist must establish a probable pathophysiologic mechanism to explain the death. Several proposed mechanisms may lead to death in these cases. Strong experimental and clinical evidence supports the concept of stress cardiomyopathy as the mechanism of death. The release of high levels of catecholamines induced by stress damages the myocardium, and may be reflected microscopically by areas of focal myocardial cell necrosis (Fig. 19.15) (31). The absence of such foci does not negate the diagnosis. Release of myoglobin, tissue lipases, or other enzymes into the blood might similarly provoke sudden cardiovascular collapse. Extensive hemorrhage into areas of soft-tissue injury has been reported to produce significant anemia or exsanguination, and may play a role in some deaths (193), but we did not consider it to be a factor in our cases. In none of the cases we have reviewed or in which we have performed the autopsy did we find evidence of fat emboli within the lungs or brains, but that also is a potential mechanism of death.

When an otherwise nonabused child dies of a treatable but neglected illness or surgical condition, investigation must focus on the motivation, awareness, and state of mind of the caretaker. Meningitis and other bacterial infections in young infants may lead to death before the parent is fully aware of the seriousness of the illness. In other cases, parental impairment, ignorance, or indifference may contribute to a delay in treatment. At the far end of the spectrum are those parents who deliberately reject essential medical care, including immunizations, for religious reasons, and

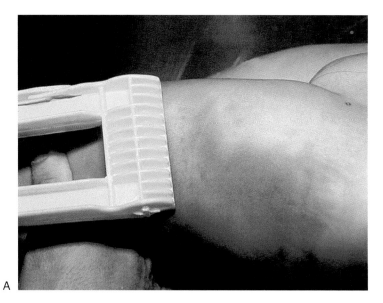

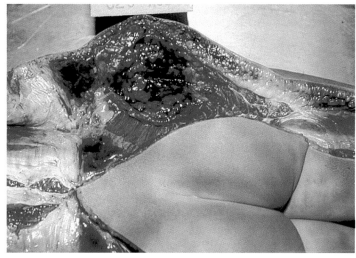

FIG. 19.14. Confluent bruising of the buttocks and thighs of a 3-year-old girl who died of shock after a severe beating. **A:** A plastic wagon handle used to beat the child is compared with the patterned bruising of the left thigh. Note that the wagon handle was partially broken by the force of the beating. **B:** Incision into the buttock shows hemorrhage extending through the subcutaneous tissues into the gluteus muscle.

whose children die as a result. Asser and Swan (10) documented 172 such fatalities between 1975 and 1995, and the numbers are probably much higher. Unfortunately, existing laws in many states are currently inadequate to protect children from this form of abuse.

The extreme example of fatal abuse without fatal injury is the child who is asphyxiated without leaving any telltale signs. This situation is discussed in the next section.

Negative Autopsy

The search for the cause or causes of SIDS and its relation to accidental or intentional suffocation, subtle metabolic disorders, respi-

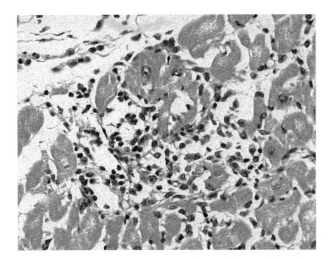

FIG. 19.15. Stress cardiomyopathy. Microscopic section of the heart of a 4-year-old, chronically abused child who died after a beating. There is focal myocardial cell necrosis characterized primarily by a mixed lymphocytic–plasmacytic infiltrate.

ratory disorders, and so on, led to a revised definition of SIDS in 1991. This new definition includes a required death-scene investigation and complete review of the child's clinical history, in addition to a "negative" autopsy, before establishing the diagnosis (187). This effort to redefine SIDS has had important implications for the entire process of child death investigation.

A negative autopsy of a previously healthy, appropriately aged infant who is found dead in bed, presumably dying during sleep, is consistent with a diagnosis of SIDS. Appropriate scene and circumstance investigation and negative medical, family, and social history confirm this diagnosis. The criteria that define a negative autopsy are listed in Table 19.4. Within the 2- to 4-month peak age range for SIDS, approximately 75% to 80% of all sudden infant deaths fall into this category. Given that this is a diagnosis of exclusion, the concern is always present that a subtle fatal injury, such as suffocation, or unrecognized metabolic disorder has been missed. This situation is unlikely, however, if careful attention is given to all the aspects of the autopsy investigation.

As a fatal event, suffocation of the young infant, whether accidental or homicidal, usually produces no distinct pathologic changes observable at autopsy. At times, punctate petechial hemorrhages are observed on the head and neck and in the sclerae and conjunctivae.

This variable finding is suggestive but not diagnostic of asphyxiation. The infant who has been febrile or septic may show similar petechial hemorrhages at postmortem examination. Some pathologists (103,177) have placed emphasis on the presence of significant numbers of intrathoracic petechiae on the thymus and pleural surfaces as characteristic of SIDS, and few or absent petechiae as suggestive of suffocation. In our experience, more than 50% of documented SIDS cases show only minimal to moderate numbers of intrathoracic petechiae. It is true that large numbers of petechiae are not seen in cases of suffocation, but the predictive value of this observation is minimal. Acute pulmonary emphysema and patchy atelectasis at autopsy, in the absence of CPR,

TABLE 19.4. *Criteria for "negative" autopsy*

1. Complete autopsy without significant gross or microscopic findings
   a. Absence of significant fatty change in heart, liver, and skeletal muscle
   b. Absence of significant inflammation in heart, lungs, and brain
   c. Usual skeletal muscle and lymphoid tissue architecture
2. Normal vitreous electrolytes
3. Negative toxicologic and microbiologic studies
4. Negative metabolic and genetic testing, as required
4. Negative scene and circumstance investigation
5. Negative medical and family history, including history of previous infant and child deaths

also is suggestive of asphyxiation, and the simultaneous appearance of this finding and conjunctival and/or scleral petechial hemorrhages strongly indicates death by asphyxiation (19).

Another autopsy finding that may suggest a diagnosis other than SIDS, especially in the absence of resuscitation efforts, is cerebral edema. Although not frequently emphasized in the differential diagnosis of SIDS, cerebral edema is not usually a feature of this disorder. Its presence suggests direct trauma or a prolonged event of dying, as might be seen in asphyxiation or some metabolic, toxic, or encephalopathic disorder. Careful attention to the assessment of the existence of cerebral edema is warranted at autopsy.

Any previous family involvement with a child-protective services department is cause for concern. A maternal psychiatric history, marital difficulties, frequent visits to pediatric emergency departments, nonorganic failure to thrive, and reports of previous apneic episodes witnessed by only one parent are all warning signs of possible abuse. A caveat is necessary, however. In most large metropolitan regions, the prevalence of SIDS within census tracts is nearly inversely proportional to average income and other indicators of quality of life. Most SIDS infants were born prematurely and are small for age (almost all below the 25th percentile and many below the 3rd); approximately 30% have had prenatal/perinatal cocaine intoxication (135). Although the incidence of SIDS among black inner-city infants is almost 2 to 3 times that of black or white suburban children, no evidence exists that subtle infant homicide contributes to this difference.

SIDS occurs in young, sleeping infants. The "back to sleep" campaign of recent years has led to a decrease in the frequency of prone sleeping from 70% to approximately 20%, and has been associated with a significant decrease in the SIDS rate (5). Infants who die suddenly in a parent's arms, while in a high chair, or while being given a bath have not died of SIDS, and should not be labeled as such. We view all such deaths as being suggestive if autopsy and investigation yield no substantive findings. The cause of death should be certified as "undeter-

mined," and the manner of death labeled "undetermined." Occasionally, an infant who has died suddenly will have a history of alleged episodes of apnea, often with associated cyanosis, hypotonia, choking, or seizures. In the absence of a specific medical or autopsy diagnosis, these apparent life-threatening events (ALTEs) are very likely to have been manifestations of factitious apnea, and the dead infant was probably asphyxiated (125,170).

The extent of the problem was most dramatically demonstrated by Southall et al. (170). They used covert video surveillance (CVS) for in-hospital monitoring of 39 infants with suggestive ALTEs, in 33 of whom abuse was documented. These patients had 41 siblings, 12 of whom had previously died suddenly and unexpectedly. Eleven of the deaths had been classified as SIDS, but after CVS, four parents confessed to suffocating eight of the siblings.

Even in the absence of other suggestive findings, if a previous unexplained infant death, including SIDS, has occurred in the same family, and no further evidence is forthcoming, the manner of death is classified as undetermined. It is now common practice among medical examiners that if a third infant death occurs in the same family without an obvious natural disease process, the cause of death is classified as "asphyxiation," and the manner of death as "homicide." SIDS occurs in approximately 1:500 to 1:1,000 live births, and minimal evidence exists that the risk increases with subsequent births within a SIDS family. Even should the risk of subsequent SIDS deaths in a family increase by 10-fold, the likelihood of three deaths in one family would be no greater than 1:1,250,000. One recent review of the literature that proposed an increased risk of subsequent SIDS in a family with one such death failed to consider the probability of homicide in many cases (85). There is also no documented evidence of SIDS as the etiology of simultaneous deaths of twins. When such an event occurs an environmental, infectious, or human factor must be sought (14,119,144).

The discussion in this section has focused on the infant because the infant is more susceptible to fatal abuse, and particularly to sub-

TABLE 19.5. *Diagnoses consistent with a "negative" gross and microscopic examination at autopsy*

1. Sudden infant death syndrome (appropriate age group)
2. Cardiac arrhythmia
3. Viremia or culture-negative bacteremia; gram-negative shock
4. Seizure disorder
5. Endogenous or exogenous hyperthermia and hypothermia
6. Asphyxiation of various types including birth asphyxia, suffocation, drowning
7. Electrocution
8. Undetected drug or poison

tle abuse that leaves no identifiable anatomic marker. A negative gross and microscopic examination can occur under a variety of circumstances, as outlined in Table 19.5. At any age, negative findings at autopsy most likely reflect a natural cause of death, and in most instances, the circumstances will indicate a cardiac arrhythmia. However, sudden death also may occur in children with seizure disorders, even in the absence of a clinical seizure, particularly if blood levels of seizure medication are subtherapeutic or absent. When homicide is suspected in the death of an older child, complete toxicologic studies are essential. Suffocation without associated injury becomes more difficult with advancing age, although the clues may be subtle. Figure 19.16

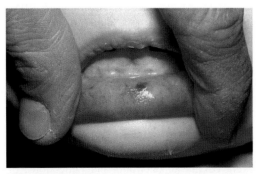

FIG. 19.16. Small contusion of the buccal mucosa of the lower lip in a 1-year-old who had been suffocated. This was the only sign of injury other than a few petechial hemorrhages of the conjunctivae.

demonstrates a small contusion on the buccal mucosa of the lower lip of a 1-year-old allegedly found unresponsive. This injury and a few scattered petechiae in the conjunctivae were the only signs of suffocation.

The relation of ALTEs, SIDS, and child abuse is addressed at greater length elsewhere in the literature (125,146,170) and in the next chapter.

Traumatic Head Injury

Differentiating accidental from inflicted head injury is not usually a difficult process in older children and adults. The amount of force required to produce significant injury is such that contusions, abrasions, and/or lacerations of the scalp will mark the impact site(s). The number and location of these external injuries, and their relation to the underlying injuries of the skull and brain permit the forensic pathologist to distinguish between injuries caused by falls and those inflicted by blows. Typically, falls produce deceleration injury characterized by cerebral contusions on the surface of the brain opposite the point of impact (i.e., contre-coup injury). Inflicted trauma is usually associated with cerebral contusions directly below the impact site (i.e., coup injuries). Skull fractures and/or intracranial hemorrhage are a frequent component of both accidental and inflicted trauma in older children. Severe accidental trauma occurs in documentable circumstances (e.g., fall from window, motor vehicle accident) and is often verifiable by independent witnesses.

Several features distinguish the infant younger than 1 year with respect to severe and lethal head injury. Unlike the older child, there may be significant head trauma without evidence of impact to the scalp. For example, scalp lacerations are uncommon in infants even in the presence of skull fractures, and subgaleal hemorrhages are a more constant marker for impact than are visible contusions of the scalp (Fig. 19.17A and B). Furthermore, the thin pliable skull of the young infant transmits force more diffusely than does the more rigid skull of the older child. Thus

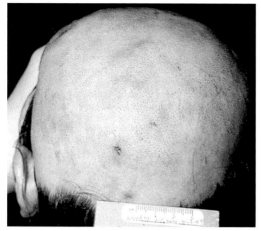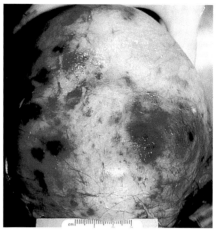

A B

FIG. 19.17. A: Scattered, faint scalp contusions of an abused child repeatedly struck on the head with a spoon. These injuries would not be apparent if the scalp hair had not been shaved. **B:** The extent of bruising is better appreciated in the subgaleal region, after reflection of the scalp. Despite the multiple blows, there was no internal head injury.

cerebral contusions are less common, and one rarely sees a typical pattern of coup or contre-coup injuries. The subdural space in the young infant is narrower and less tolerant of space-occupying lesions. Finally, the un-myelinated infant brain with its higher water content more rapidly produces life-threatening cerebral edema than the brain in the older child. Between the ages of 1 and 2 years, as the skull and brain mature, the response to head injury shows a transition from the infantile to the more adult form.

The experience of physicians who diagnose and/or treat pediatric trauma strongly indicates that injuries of inflicted head trauma are disproportionate to the alleged circumstances of injury, and that with rare exception, severe or fatal cerebral injury is inconsistent with accidental trauma in the home. In this section, we discuss the clinical and pathologic evidence that supports this conclusion (32,44,67, 86,111,147).

Falls

Despite the seeming fragility of infants and young children, they are highly resistant to fatal head trauma from accidental falls. This has been documented in numerous studies dating back many years (20,37,71,80,132,151,186). Galileo, in his *Discourses and Mathematical Demonstrations Concerning Two New Sciences,* published in 1638, asked rhetorically in a discussion of size and strength of materials, "Do not children fall with impunity from heights which would cost their elders a broken leg or perhaps a fractured skull?" (169). More recently, Chadwick et al. (32) examined the outcome of head injuries due to a fall in 317 children brought to a children's trauma center in San Diego. Seven deaths occurred in 100 children who allegedly fell 4 feet or less, no deaths in 65 children who fell 5 feet to 9 feet, and only 1 death among 117 children who fell 10 feet to 45 feet. The height of the fall was unknown in the other 34 children, all of whom survived. The histories in those children who died after short falls were false, and these children all died as a result of abuse. In another study, the medical records of 151 children who fell from buildings were reviewed, including 108 who fell two stories. There was significant morbidity in the latter group, but there were no fatalities (113).

When children fall while restrained or otherwise encumbered in car seats (139), shopping carts (167), or baby walkers (166), protective righting reflexes are restricted, and more serious injuries may occur, although fatalities are still rare. Data from the U.S. Consumer Product Safety Commission for the years 1990 through 1992 showed that among 63,200 children younger than 5 years who fell from shopping carts, fewer than 3% required hospitalization for their injuries (167). Falls down stairs in baby walkers represent a more significant risk of harm to infants. The emergency department at one large academic children's hospital treated 271 infants with such injuries during a 3-year period. Ten children were admitted with skull fracture, but there were no fatalities (166).

Simple linear skull fractures without significant neurologic sequelae occasionally occur from falls around the home. Such falls can occur from upper bunk beds, from ladders, from trees, or from porch railings. These fractures are nondiastatic, usually parietal, and represent no danger to the child. There will be minimal to moderate associated subgaleal hemorrhage. Most important, these benign fractures are associated with age-appropriate activity. Accidental falls in the home that produce potentially serious injury are so rare as to be reportable. For example, a 7-month-old infant had a depressed right parietal skull fracture when she fell 24 inches from a bed to the floor, landing on a small toy car whose roof contours corresponded to the size and contours of the skull depression. The child was neurologically normal on admission to hospital and recovered uneventfully (185).

In a prospective study of head trauma in 608 infants presenting to a pediatric emergency department, only 5% had radiographically documented intracranial injury, and only half of those infants showed clinical evidence of cerebral injury. There was a 2% risk of intracranial injury in falls reported to be less than 3 feet, but no unfavorable outcomes. Patients with no reported history of trauma, all of whom were suspected victims of abuse, were significantly more likely to have intracranial injury than were infants with any other mechanism of injury (69). Furthermore, In a study of 173 cases of abusive head trauma at an academic children's hospital, the

clinical diagnosis was initially missed in 54 (31.2%) of the victims, particularly if the victim was white and from an intact family (90). Despite an obvious discordance between reported history (or lack of history) and fatal outcome, this same failure to diagnose abuse is seen among some pathologists as well as among clinicians.

Given the benign nature of accidental falls, it is instructive to look at the very limited literature that suggests otherwise, and is often cited by those who postulate an accidental cause for inflicted head trauma. In 1984, Aoki and Masuzawa (7) reported 26 cases of SDH and retinal hemorrhages presenting with seizures, in which the mother alleged that the child (23 boys/three girls; average age, 8.1 months) had fallen to the floor from a sitting or standing position. The histories were accepted at face value, and the authors concluded that minor trauma could produce significant, and even fatal, injuries. Two years later, the same authors reported six cases with similar findings, but with external bruising, and concluded that these were due to abuse, and in an oblique recognition that their earlier cases were also abusive head trauma, conceded that retinal hemorrhage and SDH in the absence of external injuries were interpreted differently in the U.S. and Japan (8).

In 1989, Hall et al. (75) reported on the mortality of childhood falls after reviewing records at the Cook County, Illinois, Medical Examiner's Office for the years 1983 through 1986 (75). They reported that 50% of the deaths were from "minor" falls in the home, while playing, or from falls down stairs. Unfortunately, the lead authors, who were not affiliated with the Medical Examiner's Office, relied on "a brief summary. . .available in most of the charts." to draw their conclusions. This "summary" represented the caretaker's initial story, and did not reflect hospital records or subsequent police investigation. The opinions in the article were at wide variance with the factual findings and forensic opinions in the reported cases.

Howard et al. (84) conducted a 20-year retrospective review of all head-injured children up to age 18 months admitted to a hospital in London with SDH. Although only 28 cases were reviewed ("[17] were Caucasian, 10 were non-Caucasian and one was of mixed race") the authors claimed to discern a "race-dependent pattern of SDH pathophysiology," and a racial predilection among nonwhites for subdural hemorrhage after trivial falls. In addition to this highly suspect finding, these authors did not differentiate between motor vehicle accident victims, known assault victims, and victims of alleged falls with respect to severity of injury outcome. Retinal hemorrhages were highly associated with inflicted head trauma, but the authors' data must be regarded as otherwise uninterpretable.

Recognizing the exception posed by encumbered falls, if free falls of the type encountered within the home were potentially lethal, it is unlikely the human race would have survived. Based on our clinical experience with documented accidental trauma, it is appropriate to compare the forces necessary to produce fatal cerebral injury with those that would be sustained in a motor vehicle accident or fall from an upper-story window. When a parent or other caretaker indicates that severe head trauma has resulted from a fall in the home, or occurred without his or her knowledge, the story must be presumed to be false. Although not all abusive head trauma leads to permanent neurologic injury or death, when an infant or young child presents in such a state, the probability of abuse is extremely high.

Shaking/Impact Lesions

Serious or lethal head injury may result from shaking, impact, or a combination of shaking and impact (30,48,109). External injuries may be minimal or absent (11), and the history given by the caretaker must be carefully recorded because the story is likely to change if inconsistencies are discovered. In the most difficult clinical circumstances, a previously healthy, afebrile infant may present to the hospital with the rapid onset of unexplained coma, cerebral edema, no external evidence of injury, and no evidence of subdural or retinal hemorrhages. The differential diagnosis must include infection, metabolic disease, drug intoxication, or, rarely, carbon monoxide poisoning. When studies for these disorders prove negative, the diagnosis should focus on near-asphyxiation, blunt head trauma, or shaking without its other usual manifestations of subdural hemorrhage and retinal hemorrhages.

The autopsy in such a case may reveal only cerebral edema, with no evidence of subgaleal hemorrhage, skull fracture, or cerebral contusions. Absence of any scalp, cranial, or localized cerebral injury supports a diagnosis of asphyxiation. Small contusional tears or lacerations within the subcortical white matter of the brain indicate deceleration injury, such as might be caused by violent shaking, or by striking the head against a firm padded surface. Striking an infant's head against a surface or striking the head with a hand or other object will usually produce subgaleal hemorrhage, even in the absence of external bruising. Each contusion or subgaleal hemorrhage represents a separate impact site. Careful documentation of these hemorrhages is important, as they may represent the only anatomic markers of inflicted trauma. Infants with skull fractures and significant brain injury who survive more than a few minutes will usually show swelling overlying the fracture site due to hemorrhage and edema within soft tissues. At times, however, soft-tissue swelling may be absent, particularly in the occipital region.

Shaken baby syndrome (SBS) is the result of a violent shaking force, with or without impact, that causes a whiplash action of the relatively unstable infant's head on its neck. It usually produces a triad of injuries that includes cerebral edema, subdural hemorrhage, and retinal hemorrhages. No other medical condition fully mimics all of its features (48). Fatal shaking events are usually characterized clinically by almost immediate loss of consciousness, often preceded by seizures or apnea. Irritability, lethargy, inability to feed, and vomiting are common components of less severe shaking episodes. It is the type of shaking that an independent lay observer would recognize as likely to cause serious harm: rapid acceleration–deceleration of the head in an angular/rotational manner on an unstable neck. Shaking a baby who has allegedly stopped breathing to start it breathing again, or shaking a baby that has aspirated food or some foreign object does not cause the SBS. There is absolutely no medical evidence that infant immunizations cause SDH or other signs of SBS. However, an infant who is irritable or cries at length after an immunization injection is susceptible to being shaken and otherwise abused by a caretaker.

The shaking may produce slight to moderate hemorrhage in the cervical paraspinous muscles, but this is not a constant feature. Epidural or subdural hemorrhage in the cervical canal also is a variable feature; spinal cord injury is unusual. Shaken babies may show other evidence of injury, such as rib fractures or bruises of the chest, arms, or legs where the infant has been grabbed, and associated fractures of a clavicle, humerus, femur, or tibia. It has been our experience that in the unusual case in which such symptoms progress over a period of a few hours to unresponsiveness and coma rather than to recovery, there is likely to be evidence of multiple shaking episodes on CT scan, MRI, or autopsy.

A variation of SBS is the "tin-ear" syndrome, in which the infant is struck on the side of the head, producing contusion of the ear and rotational acceleration of the head that produces ipsilateral cerebral edema and subdural hemorrhage, and hemorrhagic retinopathy (76).

Duhaime et al. (49) have claimed that shaking alone is unlikely to produce the injuries observed in SBS, and that an impact component is probably necessary. Their conclusions were based on the findings in 13 autopsies, a biomechanical model using specially constructed dolls, and comparison of their data with that obtained from studies involving subhuman primates. Although there can be no doubt that shaking with impact generates far more force than shaking alone (49,86), there is considerable evidence based on confessions

(87), witnessed events, and the absence of blunt trauma to the head in many SBS autopsies that shaking alone is sufficient to cause death (2,22,63). Those who support the necessity of impact, on all occasions, dismiss confessions as being unreliable, and point to the possibility of impact on a soft surface not producing injury to the scalp. This academic dispute should not be construed, however, to indicate that there is any disagreement that the diagnostic triad of SBS represents serious inflicted injury.

SBS is more common in younger infants. It may, however, be seen at any age if there is great enough disparity between the size of the victim and the size of the perpetrator. A documented shaking fatality involving an adult victim is particularly illustrative (138,142). For several years, Israeli security agents used violent shaking as one of many techniques to interrogate Palestinian detainees. During one such episode that involved a rather small man (44 kg) being shaken by two large agents, the victim suddenly began to froth at the mouth and lapsed into unconsciousness. On arrival at hospital, CT scan showed cerebral edema and subdural hemorrhage, and the patient died within hours. At autopsy, in addition to the intracranial findings, there were extensive retinal hemorrhages, diffuse axonal injury on microscopic examination of the brain, and bruises of the upper chest. There was no evidence of impact either by history or at autopsy. One of us (R.H.K.) subsequently had the opportunity to interview more than one dozen Palestinians who were subjected to the same form of interrogation. They reported symptoms ranging from dizziness, to severe and persistent headache, nausea, vomiting, confusion, and disorientation. In September 1999, on petition from attorneys representing Palestinian detainees, the Israeli High Court of Justice prohibited the security services from further use of shaking as an interrogation technique.

Ultimately in any particular case, it is irrelevant from a medicolegal standpoint whether shaking or impact produces the fatal force; each is a form of abusive head trauma. In this regard, many physicians prefer to use the term shaking–impact syndrome as being more inclusive, but use of the term SBS should not imply lack of a possible impact component, only a lack of a recognizable impact site on the head.

Epidural, Subdural, and Subarachnoid Hemorrhage

Epidural hematomas are uncommon in infants. They usually result from the brief linear contact forces that are commonly associated with accidental falls, with or without skull fracture, and are rarely seen in inflicted head trauma (139,165). An epidural hematoma can expand with time and cause increased intracranial pressure that is associated with delayed symptom onset.

SDH of SBS is not usually a significant space-occupying lesion in young infants, as shown in Fig. 19.18, but the torn bridging veins are manifestations of the extreme forces involved. Autopsy will occasionally reveal evidence of organizing or organized SDH (Fig.

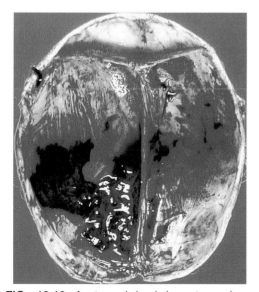

FIG. 19.18. Acute subdural hematoma in a shaken baby. This was not a significant space-occupying lesion, but the infant also had marked cerebral edema, as well as retinal hemorrhages.

19.19) and/or old contusions of the brain. These should be evaluated histologically. The timetables for estimating resolution of these injuries in children are not well established, but are much shorter than in older children or adults. Infants may die weeks or months after cerebral injury without recovery. Cerebral atrophy will be noted at autopsy, and the timing of the trauma and its cause will not be possible from postmortem examination alone. In such cases it is important to review medical records, radiographs, CT scans, and other documents relevant to the time of injury before reaching a conclusion as to cause and manner of death.

There is a lack of clinical evidence, based on our experience and that of others (30,48,69,109), to support the hypothesis put forth at times in the courtroom that a child has died of a "rebleed" of an organizing or chronic SDH. Many infants are shaken on more than one occasion and may have SDHs of varying ages even in the absence of external evidence of abuse (30,90,131). The claim that trivial trauma has reactivated the bleeding of a prior subdural (which would be of low-pressure capillary or venous origin) and led to rapid progression of clinical symptoms and death, lacks pathologic credibility. In several cases that we have reviewed, the "rebleed" diagnosis was based on a misinterpretation of the pathology specimen, and there was no gross or microscopic evidence of prior SDH. In other cases, where prior SDH was present, the immediate findings were not those of rebleeding within an expanding chronic SDH, but findings of a new site of hemorrhage induced by significant trauma. The acute hemorrhage, like the prior subdural, was usually not a significant space-occupying lesion, and was invariably associated with extreme cerebral injury and bilateral retinal hemorrhages.

When there is no gross evidence of a prior SDH, pathologists who support the rebleed theory claim that they can detect microscopic evidence of an organizing subdural. In all of the cases we have examined, the microscopic rebleed diagnosis is due to lack of understanding on the part of the pathologist of the

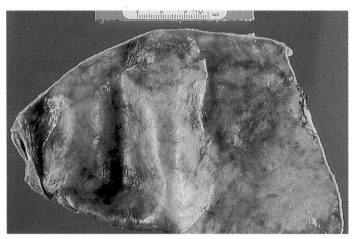

FIG. 19.19. Old subdural membrane in an infant who died of shaken baby syndrome. This is probably the marker of a prior episode of shaking. The brown color is due to hemosiderin staining. Such a lesion will not give rise to rebleeding, nor predispose an infant to a new, acute subdural hematoma from trivial trauma.

normal microscopic anatomy of infant meninges, and the disruptive effect of subdural hemorrhage on normal meningeal tissues (Fig. 19.20A and B). Furthermore, there is evidence that subdural neomembranes may be found in 31% of infants dying of SIDS (154). The etiology of these neomembranes is uncertain, but they appear to develop in the perinatal period, and may be related to the usual forces involved in the head molding that occurs at birth. They do not imply inflicted trauma, have no known sequelae, and totally resolve, suggesting that they represent part of the normal growth and development of the dural membranes.

Perinatal head trauma may be put forward as an explanation for the discovery of inflicted injuries in a young infant. However, in a California study of more than 580,000 singleton births, the rate of clinically evident neonatal intracranial hemorrhage in full-term infants was quite low, ranging from 1 of 664 delivered by forceps to 1 of 2,750 delivered by cesarean section before labor. The rate for spontaneous vaginal delivery was 1 per 1,900 live births (176). Injuries too minimal to be detected at birth or resolved before hospital discharge would not present as catastrophic head trauma days or weeks after hospital discharge.

Focal subarachnoid hemorrhage (SAH) involving the cerebral hemispheres and cerebellum is a common finding in both inflicted and accidental traumatic brain injury. At autopsy, it is usually easily distinguishable from primary traumatic SAH arising from a lacerated basilar artery, from spontaneous SAH arising from a ruptured saccular aneurysm, or from a ruptured vascular malformation (Fig. 19.21). Whereas saccular aneurysms account for approximately 80% of cases of nontraumatic SAH in the adult population (51), they are rare in infants and have a propensity to bleed after trauma (143). Ruptured aneurysms and disorders associated with multiple intracranial vascular malformations can usually be diagnosed on careful gross examination of the brain at autopsy. Microscopic examination is often needed to confirm isolated vascular malformations, which may be confused with child abuse in rare circumstances (190).

Occasionally when there is extensive SAH, blood may leak into the subdural space through ruptured leptomeninges. This should not be mistaken for primary SDH; it will usually be at the base of the brain or over a lateral surface of a cerebral hemisphere, and the site of rupture through the meninges is often evident. A common mistake among pathologists is to misin-

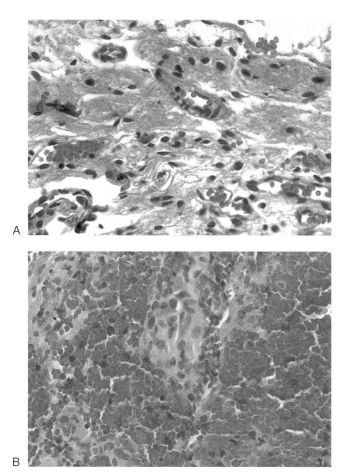

A

B

FIG. 19.20. A: Normal infant lepto-meninges: meningocytes, fibroblasts, and numerous capillaries are prominent. B: Acute subdural hemorrhage. Fragments of meninges intermixed with fresh blood that were misinterpreted by a pathologist as an organizing subdural with rebleed.

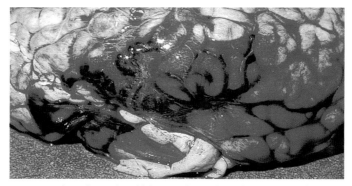

FIG. 19.21. Acute, traumatic subarachnoid hemorrhage in a baby with inflicted head trauma. The hemorrhage involves the right frontal, temporal, and parietal lobes. A portion of the arachnoid has been peeled away from the temporal lobe, exposing the underlying cortex.

terpret marked congestion of the meninges as SAH, when examining a brain at autopsy. After formalin fixation, the congested appearance is minimized, and the diagnosis of SAH evaporates. If, however, the brain is examined only in the fresh state, and not preserved, the erroneous diagnosis may persist.

Care also should be taken in cases of early meningitis, in which meningeal vascular congestion and stasis with extravasated blood may be mistaken for SAH. Microscopic examination will clarify the gross findings.

Retinal Hemorrhages

Severe retinal hemorrhages (RHs) are virtually pathognomonic of violent shaking/impact, and are frequently associated with retinal detachment and formation of retinal folds (11,28, 46–48,93,114,129,156). They are characteristic of inflicted acceleration/deceleration injury, at least in part due to the susceptibility of the retinal vessels to these particular lines of force (47). For example, among 140 children who had accidental head trauma that included skull fractures and/or intracranial hemorrhage, including 52 children younger than 2 years old, only two children who were rear-seat passengers in a motor vehicle collision showed evidence of RH (93). Multiple studies have shown that RHs occur in fewer than 3% of accidental pediatric head injuries, and are usually associated with extreme force (93,114). In those cases, the hemorrhages are usually few and confined to the posterior pole of the eye. The rarity of RH in accidental household trauma is demonstrated by the report of Christian et al. (39), who documented only three such cases, all with unilateral, posterior-pole RHs, among 1,617 children with head injury admitted to their hospital during a 4-year period.

As discussed earlier, resuscitation does not cause RHs. Vaginal delivery may produce RHs in the neonate, but these rarely persist beyond the first week of life. Increased intracranial pressure with papilledema may be associated with small posterior-pole hemorrhages confined to the region of the optic disk. Convulsions do not cause RHs (159), and Terson syn-

drome (retinal and vitreous hemorrhage in association with subarachnoid hemorrhage) appears to be very unusual in children (114). The reader is referred to Chapter 5 for a more complete review of this subject.

Cerebral Injury

It is trauma to the brain, and not the mass effect of the SDH, that causes death in infants. Not only is inflicted brain injury likely to be more serious than accidental injury, but such infants are far more likely to have evidence of prior injury. In a prospective study of 40 children aged 0 to 6 years admitted to hospital for traumatic brain injury, nine of 20 with inflicted injury had CT/MRI evidence of prior head injury versus 0 of 20 with accidental injury; 14 of 20 had RHs versus none in the accidental group; and Glasgow outcome scales were significantly worse for the inflicted injury group (54). Furthermore, among infants admitted to a pediatric intensive care unit with apparently similar injuries, the morbidity of those with inflicted trauma was much greater (79).

Death of inflicted head trauma is usually caused by diffuse axonal injury (DAI) with associated contusional tears or lacerations of the cortex, and global hypoxia/ischemia, which may be secondary to apnea induced by the head trauma (60,92). Cerebral edema is the common manifestation of these injuries. Unlike those in the brains of older children and adults, contusion injuries in infants do not usually correspond to the point of impact on the cortical surface, but extend along lines of force through the brain. These may be represented as small, hemorrhagic tears at the junction of the gray matter and white matter, and more infrequently as areas of hemorrhage deeper within the white matter. Because the young infant brain is almost gelatinous, artefactual tears, lacking evidence of hemorrhage, may occur when the brain is removed at autopsy and must not be confused with antemortem lesions. Microscopically, DAI is usually evident if the victim survives for a time. In infants, standard neurologic stains may not reveal the axonal spheroids or "retraction balls" diagnostic of DAI unless survival has extended for 12 to 24 hours, but newer immunohistochemical stains for β-amyloid precursor protein (B-APP) and 68-kDa neurofilament protein may be positive within 1 to 2.5 hours of injury, and are more sensitive than routine hematoxylin–eosin staining (65,163). The specificity of these latter staining techniques is not sufficient, however, to differentiate axonal damage of acceleration–deceleration injury from that of hypoxic/ischemic injury.

Despite our medical knowledge of this subject, inflicted head trauma deaths may be difficult to prosecute for several reasons. First, there is often no external evidence of injury, leading to speculation about mysterious natural causes or trivial accidental injury. Second, treating doctors in many smaller hospitals may lack experience diagnosing and treating abusive head trauma, or have an established professional relationship with the abusive adult, and be reluctant to testify with respect to the nature of the injury. Third, there may be irresponsible medical testimony with respect to causation and timing (33,34). Finally, juries are often reluctant to believe that a parent or other caretaker would inflict serious harm on a child.

Timing of Head Injuries

As discussed earlier, severe head trauma in infants produces immediate symptoms. We are not aware of a single case, in our experience or in the literature, of a seriously or fatally abused infant with head trauma in whom a lucid interval was documented by an independent witness (30,48,61,62,109,188). Because coma can mimic sleeping in the undisturbed child, the last time the child was awake and alert is an important marker. It should be noted, however, that if a comatose child is lifted from its bed, it should be immediately obvious that the usual reflexes, positioning, and breathing patterns are absent.

Clinically, an older child may appear to recover briefly after head impact and become comatose some hours later due to evolving SDH or cerebral edema. This so-called lucid period, during which the signs of increasing intracranial pressure may not be obvious to the casual observer, occurs because the subdural space is large enough to accommodate moderate brain swelling or bleeding before intracranial pressure increases sufficiently to compromise cerebral function. Unless there is an inordinate delay in seeking medical care, such injuries are rarely fatal. It is the misapplication of clinical knowledge regarding older children and adults with SDH that has led to the myth of the lucid interval in serious and fatal inflicted head trauma in infants.

Willman et al. (188) monitored the clinical progression of fatal head injury in 95 children with documented accidental injuries (188). Of these, 66 had a Glascow coma scale of 3 or 4 at the scene of injury, and 81 had decreased to that level by the time of their arrival at the hospital emergency department. Only one child, with an epidural hemorrhage, had a lucent interval. The average age of the study group was 8.5 years, and only four were younger than 2 years. This reflects the probability of older children being more likely to be involved in outdoor activities that are associated with fatal accidental head trauma. When an independent witness is present, similar findings have been reported for abused infants (62).

The father of a young infant retrieved his sleeping son from the apartment of a baby-sitter. It was agreed that the child appeared normal at that time. After returning home, the father changed the child's diaper, held it, and rocked the baby for several minutes when it cried. During this time, he noticed nothing unusual. More than 1 hour after returning home, he called 911, claiming that the child had stopped breathing. The infant died several hours later in hospital, and autopsy revealed two large subgaleal hemorrhages, SDH, cerebral edema, and RHs. The prosecution experts and one defense expert agreed that a layperson without special medical knowledge or skills would be able to distinguish between coma and sleep when actively handling an infant. One defense expert claimed that the baby's injuries had occurred earlier in the evening at the baby-sitter's, and that the father had failed to recognize that his "sleeping" son was actually in a coma. The parent was convicted of first-degree murder.

In another case in which the injuries were more severe, treating physicians were reluctant to determine the time of injury. A moribund 3-month-old infant was admitted to hospital with a comminuted, depressed skull fracture, RHs, and fracture of the left femur due to abuse. During the 18 hours before his admission, he had been in the care of several different relatives, but had been reported as alert and acting normally until he suddenly became unresponsive while solely in the care of his father. None of the treating physicians was willing to narrow the injury time frame to less than 18 hours, and the case remained unresolved for several months. The father confessed when faced with a forensic opinion that the onset of symptoms was necessarily concomitant with the time of injury.

We have seen numerous cases in which a so-called lucid period is invoked to explain how an infant with massive head trauma can remain asymptomatic for hours after an injury that would quickly incapacitate an adult. At times, this explanation is used to avoid facing the reality that the perpetrator is someone who does not fit the appropriate abuser profile, often because of their socioeconomic status. Physicians in some hospitals refuse to recognize abuse by suburban parents. In other cases, there is a failure to prosecute abusers because of their social status, or prosecution has failed because juries refused to believe the perpetrator guilty of horrendous acts, despite the best efforts of the prosecutor. It should never be forgotten that any parent or other caretaker of an infant or young child can potentially become the lethal abuser of that child during a momentary violent loss of control.

A 17-month-old boy was dropped off by his mother at a baby-sitter's house at 7:20 a.m. in apparent good health. The mother, separated from her husband, had been accused of abusing her children. The baby-sitter was married and had a stable home environment. At 7:45,

the child was seen by other parents to be sitting in the kitchen eating cereal. At 8:25, the baby-sitter called the mother to report that the child had fallen. The child was admitted to hospital with an extensive left parietal skull fracture and occipital fractures, cerebral contusions, and RHs. The baby-sitter claimed no knowledge of the parietal fracture, but stated that the occipital fracture might have occurred when the child fell backward and struck a coffee table. She was indicted for murder. Medical evidence and eye-witness testimony ruled out the mother as the offender, but local newspapers attacked the district attorney for indicting the baby-sitter rather than the mother, claiming that the latter fit the profile of an abuser. All treating physicians and two forensic pathologists identified the injuries as occurring while the child was in the care of the sitter. A retired neurologist with no expertise in child abuse testified for the defense. He claimed that the infant might have had the first injury at home, had a prolonged lucid period that ended when he fell against the coffee table and had the second skull fracture. Unfortunately, this testimony led to a hung jury, and there was no conviction.

DETERMINATION OF MANNER OF DEATH

The determination of the manner of death—natural, accident, homicide, suicide, undetermined—is the responsibility of the medical examiner or coroner. Table 19.6 is a summary of how to correlate the autopsy findings and the results of investigation to arrive at this determination. We recognize that such a table is an oversimplification of the process of death investigation and can be used only as a guideline in arriving at an appropriate conclusion. Fortunately, most cases can ultimately be resolved, but a few may remain unresolved, leading to an "undetermined" classification, particularly when the death involves allegations of neglect, the infant shows evidence of failure to thrive, or the home environment is marginal. Those professionals involved in child death investigation, includ-

TABLE 19.6. *Sudden death in infants and children: determination of manner of death*

Autopsy	Investigation	Manner
I. Natural disease process No injury	a. Negative b. Inconclusive (e.g., FTT, impaired parent, possible neglect) c. Positive (intentional neglect, MSBP)	a. Natural b. Undetermined or natural c. Homicide

II. Negative autopsy
  No disease
  No injury
	a. Negative
	b. Inconclusive (Prior abuse or neglect; prior SIDS or unexplained death)
	c. Positive (2 or more prior SIDS or unexplained deaths), physical evidence, confession
		a. Natural
		b. Undetermined
		
		c. Homicide

III. Fatal injury	a. Negative (circumstances documented, consistent with accident) b. Inconclusive investigation c. Positive (inconsistent with injuries)	a. Accident b. Undetermined c. Homicide
IV. "Nonfatal" injury Aggravating disease process	a. Confirmed accidental injury, medical complication b. Injury due to abuse, medical complication c. Inconclusive investigation d. Injury due to abuse, no anatomic cause of death	a. Accident b. Homicide c. Undetermined d. Homicide or undetermined

FTT, failure to thrive; MSBP, Munchausen syndrome by proxy; SIDS, sudden infant death syndrome.

ing the pathologist and those who may assist him or her in arriving at a manner of death, must remain cognizant of the significant social and economic difficulties faced by many families, and strive to maintain a sense of balance, impartiality, and compassion. Every child has the right, however, to be shielded from harm and to receive the physical and emotional care necessary to permit normal growth and development.

REFERENCES

1. Ablin DS, Sane SM. Non-accidental injury: confusion with temporary brittle bone disease and mild osteogenesis imperfecta. *Pediatr Radiol* 1997;27:111–113.
2. Alexander R, Sato Y, Smith W, et al. Incidence of impact trauma with cranial injuries ascribed to shaking. *Am J Dis Child* 1990;144:724–726.
3. Alexander RC, Schor DP, Smith WL. Magnetic resonance imaging of intracranial injuries from child abuse. *J Pediatr* 1986;108:975–979.
4. American Academy of Pediatrics Committee on Child Abuse and Neglect and Committee on Community Health Services. Investigation and review of unexpected infant and child deaths. *Pediatrics* 1999;104:1158–1160.
5. American Academy of Pediatrics Task Force on Infant Sleep Position and Sudden Infant Death Syndrome. Changing concepts of sudden infant death syndrome: implications for infant sleeping environment and sleep position. *Pediatrics* 2000;105:650–656.
6. American College of Radiology: ACR Standards. *Standards for skeletal surveys in children.* Res 22. Reston, VA: American College of Radiology, 1997:23.
7. Aoki N, Masuzawa H. Infantile acute subdural hematoma: clinical analysis of 26 cases. *J Neurosurg* 1984;61:273–280.
8. Aoki N, Masuzawa H. Subdural hematomas in abused children: report of six cases from Japan. *Neurosurgery* 1986;18:475–477.
9. Arieff AI, Kronlund BA. Fatal child abuse by forced water intoxication. *Pediatrics* 1999;103:92–95.
10. Asser SM, Swan R. Child fatalities from religion-motivated medical neglect. *Pediatrics* 1998;101:625–629.
11. Atwal GS, Rutty GN, Carter N, et al. Bruising in non-accidental head injured children; study of the prevalence, distribution and pathology in 24 cases. *Forensic Sci Int* 1998;96:215–230.
12. Ayoub C, Pfeifer D. Burns as a manifestation of child abuse and neglect. *Am J Dis Child* 1979;133:910–914.
13. Bakerink JA, Gospe SM Jr, Dimand RJ, et al. Multiple organ failure after ingestion of pennyroyal oil from herbal tea in two infants. *Pediatrics* 1996;98:944–947.
14. Bass M. The fallacy of the simultaneous sudden infant death syndrome in twins. *Am J Forensic Pathol Med* 1989;10:200–205.
15. Bass M, Kravath RE, Glass L. Death-scene investigation in sudden infant death. *N Engl J Med* 1986;315:100–105.
16. Bass WA. *Human osteology: a laboratory and field manual.* 3rd ed. Columbus, MO: Missouri Archeological Society, 1987.

17. Bays J, Jenny C. Genital and anal conditions confused with child sexual abuse trauma. *Am J Dis Child* 1990; 144:1319–1322.

18. Bays J, Lewman LV. Toluidine blue in the detection at autopsy of perianal and anal lacerations in victims of sexual abuse. *Arch Pathol Lab Med* 1992;116:285–286.

19. Betz P, Hausmann R, Eisenmenger W. A contribution to a possible differentiation between SIDS and asphyxiation. *Forensic Sci Int* 1998;91:147–152.

20. Billmire ME, Myers PA. Serious head injury in infants: accident or abuse? *Pediatrics* 1985;75:340–342.

21. Blakemore AIF, Singleton H, Pollitt RJ, et al. Frequency of the G985 MCAD mutation in the general population. *Lancet* 1991;337:298–299.

22. Block RW. Child abuse: controversies and imposters. *Curr Probl Pediatr* 1999;29:249–276.

23. Boles RG, Buck EA, Blitzer MG, et al. Retrospective biochemical screening of fatty acid oxidation disorders in postmortem livers of 418 cases of sudden death in the first year of life. *J Pediatr* 1994;132:924–933.

24. Boles RG, Martin SK, Blitzer MG, et al. Biochemical diagnosis of fatty acid oxidation disorders by metabolite analysis of postmortem liver. *Hum Pathol* 1994; 25:735–741.

25. Bonnell HJ, Beckwith JB. Fatty liver in sudden childhood death: implications for Reye's syndrome? *Am J Dis Child* 1986;140:30–33.

26. Brenner RA, Overpeck MD, Trumble AC, et al. Deaths attributable to injuries in infants, United States, 1983-1991. *Pediatrics* 1999;103:968–974.

27. Bush CM, Jones JS, Cohle SD, et al. Pediatric injuries from cardiopulmonary resuscitation. *Ann Emerg Med* 1996;28:40–44.

28. Buys YM, Levin AV, Enzenauer RW, et al. Retinal findings after head trauma in infants and young children. *Ophthalmology* 1992;99:1718–1723.

29. Carpenter RF. The prevalence and distribution of bruising in babies. *Arch Dis Child* 1999;80:363–366.

30. Case ME, Graham MA, Handy TC, et al. National Association of Medical Examiners' ad hoc Committee on Shaken Baby Syndrome: Position paper on fatal abusive head injuries in infants and young children. *Am J Forensic Med Pathol* (in press).

31. Cebelin MS, Hirsch CS. Human stress cardiomyopathy: myocardial lesions in victims of homicidal assaults without internal injuries. *Hum Pathol* 1980;11:123–132.

32. Chadwick DL, Chin S, Salerno C, et al. Deaths from falls in children: how far is fatal? *J Trauma* 1991; 10:1353–1355.

33. Chadwick DL, Kirschner RH, Reece RM, et al. Shaken baby syndrome: a forensic pediatric response. *Pediatrics* 1998;101:321–323.

34. Chadwick DL, Krous HF. Irresponsible testimony by medical experts in cases involving the physical abuse and neglect of children. *Child Maltreat* 1997;2: 313–321.

35. Chapman S, Hall CM. Non-accidental injury or brittle bones. *Pediatr Radiol* 1997;27:106–110.

36. Chesney RW, Brusilow S. Extreme hypernatremia as a presenting sign of child abuse and psychosocial dwarfism. *Johns Hopkins Med J* 1981;148:11–13.

37. Chiaveillo C, Christoph R, Bond R. Stairway-related injuries in children. *Pediatrics* 1994;94:679–681.

38. Chicago Tribune, April 3, 1993; Section 2, p. 1.

39. Christian CW, Taylor AA, Hertle RW, et al. Retinal hemorrhages caused by accidental household trauma. *J Pediatr* 1999;135:125–127.

40. Cohle SD, Hawley DA, Berg KK, et al. Homicidal cardiac lacerations in children. *J Forensic Sci* 1995;40: 212–218.

41. Conley SB. Hypernatremia. *Pediatr Clin North Am* 1990;37:365–372.

42. Cote A, Russo P, Michaud J. Sudden unexpected deaths in infancy: what are the causes? *J Pediatr* 1999; 35:437–443.

43. DeMaio DJ, DeMaio VJM. Neonaticide, infanticide, and child homicide. In: *Forensic pathology.* New York: Elsevier Science, 1989.

44. DiScala C, Sege R, Li G, et al. Child abuse and unintentional injuries. *Arch Pediatr Adolesc Med* 2000;154: 16–22.

45. Dorandeu A, Perie G, Jouan H, et al. Histological demonstration of haemosiderin deposits in lungs and liver from victims of chronic physical child abuse. *Int J Legal Med* 1999;112:280–286.

46. Drack AV, Petronio J, Capone A. Unilateral retinal hemorrhages in documented cases of child abuse. *Am J Ophthalmol* 1999;128:340–344.

47. Duhaime AC, Alario AJ, Lewander WJ, et al. Head injury in very young children: mechanisms, injury types, and ophthalmologic findings in 100 hospitalized patients younger than 2 years of age. *Pediatrics* 1992;90: 179–185.

48. Duhaime AC, Christian CW, Rorke LB, et al. Nonaccidental head injury in infants: the "shaken baby syndrome." *N Engl J Med* 1998;338:1822–1829.

49. Duhaime AC, Gennarelli TA, Thibault LE, et al. The shaken baby syndrome: a clinical and biomechanical study. *J Neurosurg* 1987;66:409–415.

50. Durfee MJ, Gellert GA, Tilton-Durfee D. Origins and clinical relevance of child death review teams. *JAMA* 1992;267:3172–3175.

51. Edlow JA, Caplan LR. Avoiding pitfalls in the diagnosis of subarachnoid hemorrhage. *N Engl J Med* 2000; 342:29–36.

52. Ellerstein NS. The cutaneous manifestations of child abuse and neglect. *Am J Dis Child* 1979;133:906–909.

53. Ewigman B, Kivlahan C, Land G. The Missouri Child Fatality Study: underreporting of maltreatment fatalities among children younger than five years of age, 1983 through 1986. *Pediatrics* 1993;91:330–337.

54. Ewing-Cobbs L, Kramer L, Prasad M, et al. Neuroimaging, physical, and developmental findings after inflicted and noninflicted traumatic brain injury in young children. *Pediatrics* 1998;102:300–307.

55. Feldman KW. Patterned abusive bruises of the buttocks and pinnae. *Pediatrics* 1992;90:633–635.

56. Feldman KW, Brewer DK. Child abuse, cardiopulmonary resuscitation, and rib fractures. *Pediatrics* 1984;73:339–342.

57. Fulroth R, Phillips B, Durand DJ. Perinatal outcome of infants exposed to cocaine and/or heroine in utero. *Am J Dis Child* 1989;143:905–910.

58. Gabos PG, Tuten HR, Leet A. Fracture-dislocation of the lumbar spine in an abused child. *Pediatrics* 1998; 102:473–477.

59. Gahagan S, Rimsza ME. Child abuse or osteogenesis imperfecta: how can we tell? *Pediatrics* 1991;88:987–992.

60. Gennarelli TA. Mechanisms of brain injury. *J Emerg Med* 1993;11:5–11.

61. Gilles EE, Nelson MD Jr. Cerebral complications of nonaccidental head injury in children. *Pediatr Neurol* 1998;19:119–128.

62. Gilliland MGF. Interval duration between injury and severe symptoms in non-accidental head trauma in infants and young children. *J Forensic Sci* 1998;43:723–725.

63. Gilliland MGF, Folberg R. Shaken babies: some have no impact injuries. *J Forensic Sci* 1996;41:114–116.

64. Gilliland MGF, Luckenbach MW. Are retinal hemorrhages found after resuscitation attempts? A study of the eyes of 169 children. *Am J Forensic Med Pathol* 1993;14:187–192.

65. Gleckman AM, Bell MD, Evans RJ, et al. Diffuse axonal injury in infants with nonaccidental craniocerebral trauma: enhanced detection by beta-amyloid precursor protein immunohistochemical staining. *Arch Pathol Lab Med* 1999;123:146–151.

66. Goebel J, Grense DA, Artman M. Cardiomyopathy from ipecac administration in Munchausen syndrome by proxy. *Pediatrics* 1993;92:601–603.

67. Goldstein B, Kelly MM, Bruton D, et al. Inflicted versus accidental head injury in critically injured children. *Crit Care Med* 1993;21:1328–1332.

68. Greenberg B. Flies as forensic indicators. *J Med Entomol* 1991;28:565–577.

69. Greenes DS, Schutzman SA. Clinical indicators of intracranial injury in head-injured infants. *Pediatrics* 1999;104:861–867.

70. Gross EM, Leffers B. Investigation of SIDS [Letter]. *N Engl J Med* 1986;315:1675.

71. Gruskin KD, Schutzman SA. Head trauma in children younger than 2 years. *Arch Pediatr Adolesc Med* 1999;153:15–20.

72. Guntheroth WG, Spiers PS. Sleeping prone and the risk of sudden infant death syndrome. *JAMA* 1992;267:2359–2362.

73. Gustavson E, Levitt C. Physical abuse with severe hypothermia. *Arch Pediatr Adolesc Med* 1996;150:111–112.

74. Hale DE, Bennett MJ. Fatty acid oxidation disorders: a new class of metabolic diseases. *J Pediatr* 1992;121:1–11.

75. Hall JR, Reyes HM, Horvat M, et al. The mortality of childhood falls. *J Trauma* 1989;29:1273–1275.

76. Hanigan WC, Peterson RA, Njus G. Tin ear syndrome: rotational acceleration in pediatric head injuries. *Pediatrics* 1987;80:618–622.

77. Hanks JW, Venters WJ. Nickel allergy from a bed-wetting alarm confused with herpes genitalis and child abuse. *Pediatrics* 1992;90:458–460.

78. Hart BL, Dudley MH, Zumwalt RE. Postmortem cranial MRI and autopsy in suspected child abuse. *Am J Forensic Med Pathol* 1996;17:217–224.

79. Haviland J, Russell RIR. Outcome after severe non-accidental head injury. *Arch Dis Child* 1997;77:504–507.

80. Helfer RE, Slovis TL, Black M. Injuries resulting when small children fall out of bed. *Pediatrics* 1977;60:533–534.

81. Herman-Giddens ME, Brown G, Verbiest S, et al. Underascertainment of child abuse mortality in the United States. *JAMA* 1999;282:463–467.

82. Hill PF, Pickford M, Parkhouse N. Phytophotodermatitis mimicking child abuse. *J R Soc Med* 1997;90:560–561.

83. Homer C, Ludwig S. Categorization of etiology of failure to thrive. *Am J Dis Child* 1981;135:848–851.

84. Howard MA, Bell MA, Uttley D. The pathophysiology of infant subdural hematomas. *Br J Neurosurg* 1993;7:355–365.

85. Hunt CE. Sudden infant death syndrome and subsequent siblings. *Pediatrics* 1995;95:430–432.

86. Hymel KP, Bandak FA, Partington MD, et al. Abusive head trauma? A biomechanical approach. *Child Maltreat* 1998;3:116–128.

87. *Independent Record,* Helena, Montana: September 5, 1999.

88. Inter-Agency Council on Child Abuse and Neglect/National Center on Child Fatality Review website: www.ican-ncfr.org

89. Janda WM. Sexually transmitted diseases in children: the role of the clinical microbiology laboratory. *Clin Microbiol Newsl* 1991;13:9.

90. Jenny C, Hymel KP, Ritzen A, et al. Analysis of missed cases of abusive head trauma. *JAMA* 1999;281:621–626.

91. Joffe M, Ludwig S. Stairway injuries in children. *Pediatrics* 1988;82:457–461.

92. Johnson DL, Boal D, Baule R. Role of apnea in nonaccidental head injury. *Pediatr Neurosurg* 1995;23:305–310.

93. Johnson DL, Braun D, Friendly D. Accidental head trauma and retinal hemorrhage. *Neurosurgery* 1993;33:231–234.

94. Joseph PR, Rosenfield W. Clavicular fractures in neonates. *Am J Dis Child* 1990;144:165–167.

95. Jumbelic MI, Chambliss M. Accidental toddler drowning in 5-gallon buckets. *JAMA* 1990;263:1952–1953.

96. Kanter TK. Retinal hemorrhage after cardiopulmonary resuscitation or child abuse. *J Pediatr* 1986;108:430–432.

97. Keating JP, Schears GJ, Dodge PR. Oral water intoxication in infants: an American epidemic. *Am J Dis Child* 1991;145:985–990.

98. Kemp JS, Thach BT. Sudden death in infants sleeping on polystyrene-filled cushions. *N Engl J Med* 1991;324.1858–1864.

99. Kirschner RH, Stein RJ. The mistaken diagnosis of child abuse: a form of medical abuse? *Am J Dis Child* 1985;139:873–875.

100. Kleinman PK. Diagnostic imaging in child abuse. *AJR Am J Roentgenol* 1990;155:703–712.

101. Kleinman PK. Postmortem imaging. In: *Diagnostic imaging of child abuse.* 2nd ed. St. Louis: Mosby, 1998:242–246.

102. Kleinman PK, Blackbourne BD, Marks SC, et al. Radiologic contributions to the investigation and prosecution of cases of fatal infant abuse. *N Engl J Med* 1989;320:507–511.

103. Knight B. Sudden death in infancy. In: *Forensic pathology.* 2nd ed. New York: Oxford University Press, 1996:447–455.

104. Knight B. Infanticide and stillbirth. In: *Forensic pathology.* 2nd ed. New York: Oxford University Press, 1996:435–446.

105. Koren G, Beatie D, Soldin S, et al. Interpretation of elevated postmortem serum concentrations of digoxin in infants and children. *Arch Pathol Lab Med* 1989;113:758–761.

106. Krause PJ, Woronick CL, Burke G, et al. Depressed neutrophil chemotaxis in children suffering blunt trauma. *Pediatrics* 1994;93:807–809.

107. Krauss TC. Close-up medical photography: forensic considerations and techniques. In: Wecht C, ed. *Legal medicine 1989.* Salem, NH: Butterworth Legal Publishers, 1990:93–111.

108. Krogman WM, Iscan MY. Skeletal age: early years. In: *The human skeleton in forensic medicine.* Springfield, IL: Charles C Thomas, 1986:50–102.

109. Krous HF, Byard RW. Shaken infant syndrome: selected controversies. *Pediatr Dev Pathol* 1999;2:497–498.

110. Kumar P, Taxy J, Angst DB, et al. Autopsies in children: are they still useful? *Arch Pediatr Adolesc Med* 1998;152:558–563.

111. Lallier M, Bouchard S, St-Vil D, et al. Falls from heights among children: a retrospective review. *J Pediatr Surg* 1999;34:1060–1063.

112. Langolis NE, Gresham GA. The ageing of bruises: a review and study of the time. *Forensic Sci Int* 1991; 50:227–238.

113. Lehman D, Schonfield N. Falls from heights: a problem not just in the Northeast. *Pediatrics* 1993;92: 121–124.

114. Levin AV. The ocular findings in child abuse focal points. *Clin Modules Ophthalmol* 1998;16:1–13.

115. Limbos MP, Berkowitz CD. Documentation of child physical abuse: how far have we come? *Pediatrics* 1998;102:53–58.

116. Link MS, Wang PJ, Pandian NG, et al. An experimental model of sudden death due to low-energy chest-wall impact (commotio cordis). *N Engl J Med* 1998;338:1805–1811.

117. Loening-Baucke V. Lichen sclerosus et atrophicus in children. *Am J Dis Child* 1991;145:1058–1061.

118. Lyons TJ, Oates RK. Falling out of bed: a relatively benign occurrence. *Pediatrics* 1993;92:125–127.

119. Malloy MH, Freeman DH. Sudden infant death syndrome among twins. *Arch Pediatr Adolesc Med* 1999; 153:736–740.

120. Mann NC, Weller SC, Rauchschwalbe R. Bucket-related drownings in the United States, 1984 through 1990. *Pediatrics* 1992;89:1068–1071.

121. Maron BJ, Poliac LC, Kaplan JA, et al. Blunt impact to the chest leading to sudden death from cardiac arrest during sports activities. *N Engl J Med* 1995;333: 337–342.

122. Marshall WN, Puls T, Davidson C. New child abuse spectrum in an era of increased awareness. *Am J Dis Child* 1988;142:664–667.

123. McClain PW, Sacks JJ, Froelke RG, et al. Estimates of fatal child abuse and neglect, United States, 1979 through 1988. *Pediatrics* 1993;91:338–343.

124. Meadow R. Non-accidental salt poisoning. *Arch Dis Child* 1993;68:448–452.

125. Meadow R. Unnatural sudden infant death. *Arch Dis Child* 1999;80:7–14.

126. Meny RG, Blackmon L, Fleischmann D, et al. Sudden infant death and home monitors. *Am J Dis Child* 1988; 142:1037–1040.

127. Miller ME, Brooks J, Forbes N, et al. Frequency of medium-chain acyl-CoA dehydrogenase deficiency G-985 mutation in sudden infant death syndrome. *Pediatr Res* 1992;31:305–307.

128. Miller ME, Hangartner TN. Temporary brittle bone disease: association with decreased fetal movement and osteopenia. *Calcif Tissue Int* 1999;64:137–143.

129. Mills M. Fundoscopic lesions associated with mortality in shaken baby syndrome. *J AAPOS* 1998;2:67–71.

130. Mirchandani HG, Mirchandani IH, Hellman F, et al. Passive inhalation of free-base cocaine ("crack") smoke by infants. *Arch Pathol Lab Med* 1991;115:494–498.

131. Morris MW, Smith S, Cressman J, et al. Evaluation of infants with subdural hematoma who lack external evidence of abuse. *Pediatrics* 2000;105:549–553.

132. Musemeche CA, Barthel M, Cosentino C, et al. Pediatric falls from heights. *J Trauma* 1991;31:1347–1349.

133. Nuoffer JM, deLonley P, Costa C, et al. Familial neonatal SIDS revealing carnitine-acylcarnitine translocase deficiency. *Eur J Pediatr* 2000;159:82–85.

134. Odom A, Christ E, Kerr N, et al. Prevalence of retinal hemorrhages in pediatric patients after in-hospital cardiopulmonary resuscitation: a prospective study. *Pediatrics* 1997;99:E3.

135. Ostrea EM, Brady M, Gause S, et al. Drug screening of newborns by meconium analysis: a large scale, prospective, epidemiologic study. *Pediatrics* 1992;89:107–113.

136. Overpeck MD, Brenner RA, Trumble AN, et al. Risk factors for infant homicide in the United States. *N Engl J Med* 1998;339:1211–1216.

137. Paterson CR, Burns J, McAllion SJ. Osteogenesis imperfecta: the distinction from child abuse and the recognition of a variant form. *Am J Med Genet* 1993; 45:187–192.

138. Physicians for Human Rights. *Israel and the occupied territories: shaking as a form of torture.* Boston: Physicians for Human Rights, 1995.

139. Piatt J, Hulka F. An infant in a car seat on a washing machine: epidural hematoma. *Pediatrics* 1994;94: 556–557.

140. Piatt JH, Steinberg M. Isolated spinal cord injury as a presentation of child abuse. *Pediatrics* 1995;96: 780–782.

141. Pickel S, Anderson C, Holliday MA. Thirsting and hypernatremic dehydration: a form of child abuse. *Pediatrics* 1970;45:54–59.

142. Pounder DJ. Shaken adult syndrome. *Am J Forensic Med Pathol* 1997;18:321–324.

143. Prahlow JA, Rushing EJ, Barnard JJ. Death due to a ruptured berry aneurysm in a 3.5 year old child. *Am J Forensic Med Pathol* 1998;19:391–394.

144. Ramos V, Hernandez AF, Villanueva E. Simultaneous death of twins: an environmental hazard or SIDS? *Am J Forensic Med Pathol* 1997;18:75–78.

145. Reardon MJ, Gross DM, Vallone AM, et al. Atrial rupture in a child from cardiac massage by his parent. *Ann Thorac Surg* 1987;43:557–558.

146. Reece RM. Fatal child abuse and sudden infant death syndrome: a critical diagnostic decision. *Pediatrics* 1993;91:423–429.

147. Reece RM, Sege R. Childhood head injuries. *Arch Pediatr Adolesc Med* 2000;154:11–16.

148. Renz BM, Sherman R. Abusive scald burns in infants and children: a prospective study. *Am Surg* 1993;59: 339–342.

149. Ricci LR. Photographing the physically abused child: principles and practice. *Am J Dis Child* 1991;145: 275–281.

150. Rinaldo P, Stanley CA, Hsu BYL, et al. Sudden neonatal death in carnitine transporter deficiency. *J Pediatr* 1997;131:304–305.

151. Rivara FP, Kamitsuka MD, Quan L. Injuries to children younger than 1 year of age. *Pediatrics* 1988;81: 93–97.

152. Rivenes SM, Bakerman PR, Miller MB. Intentional caffeine poisoning in an infant. *Pediatrics* 1997;99: 736–738.

153. Roe CR, Millington DS, Maltby DA, et al. Recognition of medium-chain acyl-CoA dehydrogenase deficiency in asymptomatic siblings of children dying of sudden infant death or Reye-like syndromes. *J Pediatr* 1986;108:13–18.

154. Rogers CB, Itabashi HH, Tomiyasu U, et al. Subdural neomembranes and sudden infant death syndrome. *J Forensic Sci* 1998;43:375–376.

155. Rosen CL, Frost JD, Glaze DG. Child abuse and recurrent infant apnea. *J Pediatr* 1986;109:1065–1067.

156. Royal College of Ophthalmology. The Ophthalmology Child Abuse Working Party: child abuse and the eye. *Eye* 1999;13:3–10.

157. Rutty GN, Smith CM, Malia RG. Late-form hemorrhagic disease of the newborn: a fatal case with illustration of investigations that may assist in avoiding the mistaken diagnosis of child abuse. *Am J Forensic Med Pathol* 1999;20:48–51.

158. Sadler DW. The value of a thorough protocol in the investigation of sudden infant deaths. *J Clin Pathol* 1998;51:689–694.

159. Sandramouli S, Robinson R, Tsaloumas M, et al. Retinal haemorrhages and convulsions. *Arch Dis Child* 1997;76:449–451.

160. Scheers NJ, Dayton CM, Kemp JS. Sudden infant death with external airways covered. *Arch Pediatr Adolesc Med* 1998;152:540–547.

161. Scholer SJ, Mitchel EF, Ray WA. Predictors of injury mortality in early childhood. *Pediatrics* 1997;100: 342–347.

162. Schwartz AJ, Ricci L. How accurately can bruises be aged in abused children? Literature review and synthesis. *Pediatrics* 1996;97:254–256.

163. Shannon P, Smith CR, Deck J, et al. Axonal injury and neuropathology of shaken baby syndrome. *Acta Neuropathol* 1998;95:625–631.

164. Shoemaker JD, Lynch RE, Hoffmann JW, et al. Misidentification of propionic acid as ethylene glycol in a patient with methylmalonic acidemia. *J Pediatr* 1992;20:417–421.

165. Shugerman RP, Paez A, Grossman DC, et al. Epidural hemorrhage: is it abuse? *Pediatrics* 1996;97:664–668.

166. Smith GA, Bowman MJ, Luria JW, et al. Baby-walker related injuries continue despite warning labels and public education. *Pediatrics* 1997;100:e1.

167. Smith GA, Dietrich AM, Garcia CT, et al. Epidemiology of shopping cart-related injuries to children: an analysis of national data for 1990 to 1992. *Arch Pediatr Adolesc Med* 1995;149:1207–1210.

168. Snow CC, Kirschner RH, Fitzpatrick JJ, et al. Report of forensic investigation: El Mozote, El Salvador. In: Betancur B, Planchart RF, Berganthal T, eds. *Report of the truth commission on El Salvador.* New York: United Nations, 1993: Appendix I.

169. Sobel D. *Galileo's daughter: a historical memoir of science, faith and love.* New York: Walker and Company, 1999:308.

170. Southall DP, Plunkett MC, Banks MW, et al. Covert video recording of life-threatening child abuse: lessons for child protection. *Pediatrics* 1997;100:735–760.

171. Spevak MR, Kleinman PK, Belanger PL, et al. Cardiopulmonary resuscitation and rib fractures in infants: a postmortem radiologic-pathologic study. *JAMA* 1994;272:617–618.

172. Stephenson T, Bialas Y. Estimation of the age of bruising. *Arch Dis Child* 1996;74:53–55.

173. Sugar NF, Taylor JA, Feldman KW. Bruises in infants and toddlers: those who don't cruise don't bruise. *Arch Pediatr Adolesc Med* 1999;153:399–403.

174. Tanegashima A, Yamamato H, Yada I, et al. Estimation of stress in child neglect from thymic involution. *Forensic Sci Int* 1999;12:55–63.

175. Task Force for the Study of Non-Accidental Injuries and Child Deaths. *Protocol for child death autopsies.* Cook Cuounty, IL: Illinois Department of Children and Family Services and Office of the Medical Examiner, Cook County, Illinois, 1987.

176. Towner D, Castro MA, Eby-Wilkens E, et al. Effect of mode of delivery in nulliparous women on neonatal intracranial injury. *N Engl J Med* 1999;341:1709–1714.

177. Valdes-Dapena M. A pathologist's perspective on sudden infant death syndrome-1991. *Pathol Annu* 1992; 27(pt 1):133–164.

178. Valdes-Dapena MA, Mandell F, Merritt TA. Investigation of SIDS [Letter]. *N Engl J Med* 1986; 315:1675.

179. Wahl N, Woodall B. Hypothermia in shaken infant syndrome. *Pediatr Emerg Care* 1995;11:233–234.

180. Wardinsky TD. Genetic and congenital defect conditions that mimic child abuse. *J Fam Pract* 1995;41: 377–383.

181. Wardinsky TD, Vizcarrondo FE, Cruz BK. The mistaken diagnosis of child abuse: a three-year USAF Medical Center analysis and literature review. *Milit Med* 1995;160:15–20.

182. Waters KA, Gonzalez A, Jean C, et al. Face-straight-down and face-near-straight-down positions in healthy, prone-sleeping infants. *J Pediatr* 1996;128: 616–625.

183. Weathers WT, Crane MM, Sauvain KJ, et al. Cocaine use in women from a defined population: prevalence at delivery and effects on growth in infants. *Pediatrics* 1993;91:350–354.

184. Weiner H. New concepts about the organism and its perturbation by stressful experience. In: *Perturbing the organism: the biology of stressful experience.* Chicago: University of Chicago Press, 1992:246–284.

185. Wheeler DS, Shope TR. Depressed skull fracture in a 7 month old who fell from bed. *Pediatrics* 1997; 100:1033–1034.

186. Williams RA. Injuries in infants and small children resulting from corroborated free falls. *J Trauma* 1991; 31:1350–1352.

187. Willinger M, James LS, Catz C. Defining the sudden infant death syndrome (SIDS): deliberations of an expert panel convened by the National Institute of Child Health and Human Development. *Pediatr Pathol* 1991; 11:677–684.

188. Willman KY, Bank DE, Senac M, et al. Restricting the time of injury in fatal inflicted head injuries. *Child Abuse Negl* 1997;21:929–940.

189. Wilson NW, Ochs HD, Peterson B, et al. Abnormal an-

tibody responses in pediatric trauma patients. *J Pediatr* 1989;115:24–27.

190. Weissgold DJ, Budenz Dl, Hood I, et al. Ruptured vascular malformation masquerading as battered/shaken baby syndrome: a nearly tragic mistake. *Surv Ophthalmol* 1995;39:509–512.

191. Woelfle J, Kreft B, Emons D, et al. Subdural hemor-

rhage as an initial sign of glutaric aciduria type 1: a diagnostic pitfall. *Pediatr Radiol* 1996;26:779–781.

192. Wright CM, Talbot E. Screening for failure to thrive: what are we looking for. *Child Care Health Dev* 1996; 22:223–234.

193. Zumwalt RE, Hirsch CS. Subtle fatal child abuse. *Hum Pathol* 1980;11:167–174.

20

Fatal Child Abuse and Sudden Infant Death Syndrome

Robert M. Reece and *Henry F. Krous

*Department of Pediatrics, Tufts University School of Medicine; Child Protection Program,
Department of Pediatrics, The Floating Hospital for Children at New England Medical Center; and
Institute for Professional Education, Massachusetts Society for the Prevention of Cruelty to Children,
Boston, Massachusetts; *Department of Pathology, Children's Hospital-San Diego, San Diego,
California; and *Departments of Pathology and Pediatrics, University of California
at San Diego, LaJolla, California*

Distinguishing sudden infant death syndrome (SIDS) from death due to inflicted injury is a challenge to professionals required to make that decision. The pediatrician or family physician must know which course to follow in relating to the family. If child abuse is suspected, the physician must fulfill mandated legal obligations to report the case to the appropriate authorities. If the reason for death is SIDS, a sympathetic and supportive role is required. Complicating this decision is the polarization between two camps: those who believe that a sympathetic approach to parents losing their baby is the highest priority, and those whose training and experience have convinced them that fatal child abuse is distressingly common. In the final analysis, a nonaccusatory approach to the caretakers is best, because all parties are treated fairly. Coroners, medical examiners, and pathologists have the added responsibility of rendering a medicolegal opinion as to the cause and manner of death. All agree that the state of our knowledge in this area is incomplete and ambiguity exists in some cases. The purpose of this chapter is to present the scientific evidence about SIDS and fatal child abuse so that the correct determination can be made and to help to reduce the areas of ambiguity.

The subject of crib death was described in the Bible (I Kings 3:19,22) and was known to happen even before biblical history. For centuries, it was accepted as a natural phenomenon, defying explanation. Since the 1950s, spurred by parents suffering the loss of infants to this poorly explained condition, the scientific community entered a period of fruitful research about why these infants were dying suddenly and unexpectedly. At the same time, the medical community, which had previously repressed the abhorrent concept of caretakers harming their children, was being informed by new literature describing this phenomenon. In 1946, Caffey (39) published his seminal article on multiple fractures and subdural hematomas, and in 1953 Silverman (178) postulated that these injuries were the result of unrecognized trauma. In 1961, Adelson (3) added to the factual information about fatal child abuse. In 1962, Kempe et al. (96) coined the phrase the "battered child syndrome" and further raised the consciousness of the medical community about the unpleasant truth that infants and children were being physically abused and killed. The stage was being set for a controversy about death in infancy, its causes, and the possibility of a caretaker's culpability for those deaths.

High-profile cases of serial child homicides focused attention on fatal child abuse as a reason for some sudden, unexpected deaths in infants. Criminal charges were brought against Waneta Hoyt in upstate New York, charging her with having suffocated five children, all having been initially declared as being due to SIDS. Two of these children were among five cases included in the report of Steinschneider in 1972 (195). He had studied these children in his laboratory at Syracuse and reported his findings in an article that claimed that SIDS was the result of prolonged apnea, using these two deaths from SIDS as examples of this disorder. This article, heralded as a breakthrough despite the small numbers and questionable data interpretation, elevated prolonged apnea to the top of the list of hypotheses for SIDS. This in turn spurred the development of research about apnea and subsequently the proliferation of the concept of testing for apnea and home-monitoring programs. In their book, *The Death of Innocents,* Firstman and Talan (62) skillfully analyzed this case, the implications it had for the SIDS research community, and the impact it had on pediatric practitioners and hundreds of thousands of their families. The media accounts of the Hoyt case raised the public awareness about the possibility of infant murders being mistaken for crib death or other medical illness. For those parents who had lost babies to SIDS and for many health care providers, the suggestion that even some SIDS deaths were actually child murders was painful and unacceptable. They feared that by raising the old specter of infanticide, the 25-year effort of parents and professionals to provide compassion for families losing their babies to SIDS would evaporate. It is apparent that an objective and integrated approach to the ascertainment of death in sudden unexpected infant deaths must occur.

WHAT IS SUDDEN INFANT DEATH SYNDROME?

Definition

SIDS is defined as "the sudden death of an infant under 1 year of age which remains unexplained after the performance of a complete postmortem investigation, including an autopsy, an examination of the scene of death and review of the case history" (216). Because the proportion of SIDS cases having an atypical clinical presentation, potentially unsafe sleeping environment, and/or more "severe" pathologic findings at postmortem examination is increasing (*vide infra*), the need to refine and stratify the definition is becoming more important (28,76,198).

Incidence and Epidemiology

SIDS occurs most frequently in infants who are between ages 2 and 4 months (21). Fewer than 5% of cases occur during the first month of life, and the number of SIDS deaths decreases progressively after the third to fourth months of life. Approximately 90% of SIDS deaths occur by age 6 months (21). In most studies, SIDS occurs more often in male infants (60% to 70%). It occurs more frequently in the winter months in both the northern and southern hemispheres, suggesting that temperature alone is not a causative factor. Little and Peterson (119) suggested the possibility that colder outdoor temperatures may encourage overdressing an infant, producing a microclimate of overheating. Because hyperthermia and overheating have been implicated by some authors as etiologic factors (153), this concept is interesting, but these authors concluded that the "meaning of climate and ambient temperature pattern for risk of SIDS death remains to be elucidated."

The overall incidence of SIDS has declined dramatically in developed countries of the world, yet it remains the most common cause of postneonatal infant death (197). The National Center for Health Statistics reported that there were 5,476 SIDS cases in the United States in 1988, representing an overall rate of 1.4 deaths per 1,000 live births. This means that in 1988, SIDS was the second leading cause of death in infancy, including the neonatal period, accounting for 14.5% of all deaths among white infants and representing a rate of 1.24 per 1,000 live births. In contrast, for African-American infants, SIDS was the leading cause of death, accounting for 12.8% of all deaths and representing a rate of 2.26 per 1,000 live births. By 1995, the number of cases declined to approximately 3,000 deaths (9), now yielding a rate of approximately 0.5 deaths per 1,000 live births.

Sleeping Position

SIDS incidence rates in the U.S., western Europe, Australia, and New Zealand have declined after the implementation of public awareness initiatives, such as the "Back to Sleep" campaign in the U.S.(50,63,94,132). These initiatives recommend the use of the supine, rather than prone or side infant sleep position; that mothers avoid excessive swaddling or wrapping of their babies; and not to smoke cigarettes during their pregnancies or expose their babies to smoke after their births. These campaigns have not reached all segments of the population. Willinger et al. (217) have reported that significant predictors of prone placement included maternal African-American race, mother's age between 20 and 29 years, residence in the mid-Atlantic or southern states, mothers with a previous child, and infants younger than 8 weeks. In this study, it was encouraging that the prevalence of infants placed in the prone sleep position declined by 66% between 1992 and 1996, and at the same time, SIDS rates declined approximately 38%.

Ethnicity

Ethnicity affects SIDS rates. African-American (29), Alaskan natives (2), and most, but not all, Native American infants have higher SIDS rates than do white and Asian infants (67,68). However, in some studies, the excess mortality among black infants disappears when adjusted for maternal education and income (111). A recent report indicated a dramatic decrease in the SIDS rates (8.9 to 3.00/1,000 live births) among American Indians and Alaska natives (157). Kraus and Bultreys (110) concluded from their studies on the effect of various factors on the rate of SIDS

within certain populations that SIDS rates and socioeconomic status (SES) are inversely related, but SES may act as a confounder, effect modifier, or intermediate variable.

Cigarette Smoking

Smoking seems to have emerged as the major risk factor of SIDS since supine sleep position has replaced the prone position (30,121, 163). Maternal smoking before and/or during gestation and after delivery all increase the risk of SIDS (6,34,42,77,106,119,129,130, 133,140,152,177,202,204). Paternal smoking also increases the risk of SIDS (163), but this association may be a reflection of a higher rate of passive smoke exposure by a coexisting smoking mother. At postmortem examination, pericardial levels of cotinine, a nicotine metabolite, are higher in SIDS cases than in controls (129).

Substance Abuse during Pregnancy

Infants of illegal substance-abusing mothers (ISAM) also are reported to be at higher risk of SIDS compared with control subjects (17,18,40,44,45,48,148,201). In a study from Los Angeles County, the SIDS rate was 8.87 cases per 1,000 ISAM compared with 1.22 cases per 1,000 infants for the non-ISAM general population, a very significant statistical difference (212). The significantly greater incidence of SIDS in male infants, higher winter months' occurrence, and African-American infants and non-Hispanic white infants in the non-ISAM population was not observed in the ISAM group. Conversely, symptomatic apnea was reported significantly more frequently before SIDS for the ISAM than for the non-ISAM population (22% vs. 5.4%; $p = 0.022$). In another study from New York City, the SIDS rate in drug-exposed infants was 5.83 per 1,000 infants compared with 1.39 per 1,000 who were not drug-exposed (91). When known associated high-risk variables were controlled, the risk ratio for SIDS was calculated, and methadone, heroin, methadone and heroin, cocaine, and cocaine and methadone or heroin were 3.6, 2.3, 3.2, 1.6 and 1.1, respectively, compared with the ratio for the non–drug-exposed group. In infants whose mothers do not use illegal drugs during pregnancy, SIDS rates differ according to ethnicity, being higher in African-Americans than in whites. As in the Los Angeles study, however, ethnic SIDS rates in this New York study were similar in infants if the mothers used drugs during pregnancy.

In a study in Detroit, 44% of 2,964 infants screened by meconium sampling had positive results for cocaine, opiates, or cannabinoids. Studies of mortality rates during the first 2 years of life showed no difference between the drug-positive and drug-negative groups, and the incidence of SIDS was no different between the two groups.

Immunizations

Diphtheria–tetanus–pertussis (DTP) vaccine does not increase the risk of SIDS (31,84,134).

Co-sleeping

Co-sleeping as a potential risk factor for SIDS has generated controversy. More than 100 articles in the medical literature have been devoted to this issue. McKenna et al. (136–138) hypothesized that the comparatively sensory-rich co-sleeping environment might be protective against SIDS in some contexts. After studying mother–infant pairs, these investigators concluded that bed-sharing promoted infant arousals (137), reduced stage 3 to 4 sleep, and the mother's responsiveness to infant arousals during bed-sharing may contribute to the protective effects of bed-sharing. From an epidemiologic viewpoint, however, investigators in the New Zealand Cot Death Study found that bed-sharing significantly increased the risk of SIDS, particularly among infants of mothers who smoked (171). More recent, prospective studies from this same group led to the conclusion that the risk of SIDS was increased if the mother also smoked (135,170). Suffice it

to say that the issue is unresolved and remains intensely controversial.

Twins and SIDS

In most studies, SIDS is seen to be 2.5 times more common in multiple births with twins and triplets than in singleton births. This is probably due to the lower mean birth weight of twins as compared with singletons. Sudden unexpected death in both twins has been the subject of numerous articles (19,109,179,187,205). In a summary of the world's literature concerning this phenomenon (1956 to 1988), Beal (19) reported that six (1%) of 625 surviving twins had subsequently died of SIDS. In a large study in 1999, Malloy and Freeman (122) studied twin pairs over a 5-year period in the U.S. to determine whether there was an increased risk of SIDS in this population. There were 767 matched twin pregnancies in which one or both twins died of SIDS. Compared with twin pregnancies (170) in which no SIDS deaths occurred, the victims of SIDS both had lower mean birth weights and gestational ages and were likely to be associated with African-American race and lower than a 12th grade maternal education status. In the 767 SIDS twin deaths, there were only seven sets in which both twins died, and in only one of these sets were the deaths on the same day. The authors concluded that, independent of birth weight, twins do not appear to be at greater risk for SIDS compared with singleton births (122).

The value of the postmortem examination and death-scene investigation cannot be overstated in all SIDS deaths, but particularly in deaths in twins. This is particularly true in cases of simultaneous deaths of twins. Data concerning the rate of simultaneous deaths in twins due to SIDS are difficult to interpret, but Beal's estimate, based on published series, is 12 of 637 twin infant pairs, or 2% of all twin sets in which SIDS occurs (19). Ramos et al. (155) reported on 45-day-old twins dying within hours of one another. After postmortem examination (including an autopsy and thorough death-scene investigation), they concluded that the combination of sublethal blood levels of carbon monoxide combined with overwrapping of bedclothes and mechanical obstruction of the upper airways caused the deaths. Simultaneous twin death is a statistical near impossibility, and accidental or nonaccidental causes are far more likely.

Recurrence of SIDS within a Family

Parents of infants who die of SIDS usually wish to have subsequent children. Therefore the possibility of recurrence of SIDS within the family is an important counseling issue for future pregnancies. Given that the cause(s) of SIDS remains unknown, the possibility of genetically transmitted inborn errors of metabolism or other genetically transmitted conditions is raised. It also provokes questions of a forensic nature. In a 14-year study of subsequent siblings of SIDS victims in Norway (85), and in a Washington state study over 16 years (150), the SIDS sibling risk was seen to be almost 4 times that of the SIDS risk among births at large. A comparison of SIDS occurrences in siblings of SIDS victims and in non-SIDS siblings in maternal age– and birth rank–matched control families, however, revealed no statistically significant difference in SIDS rates or in total infant mortality rates in families with a history of SIDS as compared with families in which there was no SIDS. Thus the notion was challenged that having a SIDS baby increases the likelihood of having another SIDS baby. With the exclusion from the SIDS statistics of some of the deaths now thought to be due to inborn errors of metabolism (see subsequent discussion), the chances for recurrent SIDS in families seem even less likely. It should be noted that these studies were reported before implementation of initiatives promoting back sleep position and avoidance of smoke exposure. There is a growing impression among pediatric and forensic pathologists that an increasingly higher proportion of SIDS cases are now of the atypical or nonclassic type. In this setting of socioeconomic deprivation, less-safe sleep environments, persistence of use of the prone sleep position, and continued exposure to tobacco smoke, the recurrence risk may be increased. Newer studies are urgently needed to address this issue.

Clinical Presentation

Two overlapping presentations of SIDS have been termed either "classic" or "typical" as opposed to "nonclassic" or "atypical." With the rapid decline in SIDS rates, it was not so long ago that most cases were of the classic type, but now an increasing proportion are complicated by a complex social milieu and poverty accompanied by chaotic living conditions and less than pristine postmortem findings. Consequently, the diagnosis of SIDS has become more difficult and argumentative.

Classic or typical SIDS cases are characterized by the sudden and unexpected death of an apparently healthy baby during sleep. Usually these infants had been fed before being put to bed. At varying intervals, the parents or other caretakers had checked the baby, who appeared to be normal, but was later discovered lifeless. No outcry had been heard, and the baby was in the position in which he or she had been placed at bedtime. Emergency personnel were contacted, and they often initiated cardiorespiratory resuscitation in the home and continued these measures until reaching the hospital, where the baby was pronounced dead. The remainder of the infant's medical history is usually unremarkable, although it is not uncommon that the infant had experienced a mild upper respiratory infection or had been seen recently for routine pediatric care. Some evidence of terminal motor activity, such as clenched fists, may be seen, and some serosanguinous discharge coming from the nose and mouth may be noted. The face and dependent portions of the body may have reddish blue mottling, a condition caused by postmortem lividity. The scene investigation does not betray an unsafe sleep environment, and the postmortem examination is unrevealing of a cause of death.

In nonclassic or atypical SIDS, the infant often lives in lower socioeconomic conditions and not infrequently has a medical history of recent upper respiratory infection, or gastrointestinal illness accompanied by low-grade fever, poor eating, and diarrhea. The sleep site may not have been completely safe because of an unstable bed, soft sleep surfaces, or the presence of pillows and/or over-stuffed toys. The infant may have been in a chaotic co-sleeping situation with adults. The postmortem examination may show some abnormalities, such as pulmonary inflammation, that some, but not all, pathologists would consider sufficiently severe to be the cause of death. These cases are often the subject of considerable controversy at child death review committees.

Theories of Etiology

Sudden unexpected death at any age is a catastrophic event, typically having its cause centered in the central nervous, cardiovascular, or respiratory system. It is thus not surprising that the hypotheses of causation of SIDS have focused on these three organ systems. However, nearly 30 years after the definition of SIDS was first formulated and during which time literally thousands of research studies have been published, no single theory has been proven to explain SIDS. If anything, the published research makes it ever more likely that SIDS is an event encompassing several, although probably a relatively few disorders with a final common pathway. Controversy still exists whether SIDS represents a developmentally abnormal infant responding inadequately to some environmental stress that would not be lethal to a normal infant, or the inability of a normal infant to respond to an insurmountable environmental stress. The evidence now suggests that either possibility might exist in any one infant.

Neurologic Hypothesis

There are two principle hypotheses centering on neurophysiology and neuropathology in SIDS. The first focuses on an abnormality in the brain's regulation of respiration during sleep and/or stimulation of normal protective arousal during life-threatening events that occur in all infants. The second is known as the developmental hypothesis, in which case SIDS victims are neuroanatomically and neurophysiologically immature. Both conditions may operate simultaneously.

Abundant literature emphasizes abnormalities of respiration as the important event in SIDS (20,72,73,90,160,161). Respiration as well as autonomic activity, sleep, and arousal are regulated in the brainstem, which, therefore, has been a site of intensive investigation in SIDS (59,100). In SIDS, gliosis, hypomyelination, increased dendritic spine density, increased synaptic density, and neurotransmitter abnormalities have been observed in, but not restricted to, brainstem nuclei related to cardioventilatory control (97,100). Filiano and Kinney (59,60) have linked these neuropathologic findings with the epidemiology of SIDS in a triple-risk model wherein SIDS results from the intersection of (a) a vulnerable infant who possesses some underlying abnormality, (b) a critical period in development, and (c) exogenous stressor(s). Implicit in this model is that the infant, by virtue of its young age, confronts an exogenous stressor specific to its peculiar vulnerability and dies suddenly and unexpectedly. Implicit also is that all three factors must intersect for death to occur. This model also is attractive given the likelihood that the cause of SIDS varies from infant to infant.

The arcuate nucleus has received particular attention in the attempt to unravel the role of the brainstem in SIDS. Evidence suggests that the infant's vulnerability lies in this structure (98,99,145,186). It lies along the human ventral medullary surface and may connect with the caudal raphae, which is involved in respiratory and cardiovascular control (218). Perhaps this line of research began with the report of a 5-month-old infant with congenital central hypoventilation syndrome who died suddenly and was found at postmortem examination to lack arcuate nuclei (64). Subsequently, Filiano and Kinney (61) described two cases of SIDS whose brainstems revealed severe hypoplasia of the arcuate nucleus but no other degenerative or necrotizing abnormalities. This observation was followed by a series of studies documenting a significant decrease in muscarinic cholinergic (101) and kainate (145) and sertonergic (Kinney et al.) receptors, but not opioid receptors (98) in the arcuate nucleus of SIDS victims. Muscarinic cholinergic binding was decreased when compared with that of infants dying acutely of known causes but not when compared with those controls with chronic hypoxemic conditions. These ventral medullary surface muscarinic cholinergic and kainate receptors are thought to be directly involved in CO_2 responsiveness, and therefore their deficiency is possibly catastrophic when an infant is confronted with hypercapnia or asphyxia.

Investigators proposed that the maturational regulation of the arcuate nucleus is abnormal in SIDS brains, such that there is a developmental deficiency of neurons and/or neuropil with an associated deficiency of neurotransmitter-receptor binding. The finding of severe hypoplasia in some SIDS cases indicates a failure in the proliferation and/or migration of neuroblasts destined to become arcuate neurons. Cell counts are needed to determine if there is a subtle deficiency of neuron number in a larger group of SIDS cases. It has been suggested that there may be a lag in neurotransmitter maturation, regardless of a deficiency of neuron number; for example, an underlying common signal of neurotransmitter maturation may be at fault. This may explain the apparently asymptomatic behavior of most SIDS victims, and explains why eliminating an external stressor (e.g., prone sleeping position) may reduce the incidence of SIDS. The model also explains why the overwhelming majority of infants who sleep prone do not die of SIDS, as they are "normal" and do not have an underlying vulnerability.

The concept that an external stressor precipitates sudden death is derived from epidemiologic studies indicating that minor respiratory or gastrointestinal illness occurs around the time of death in some SIDS victims, as well as symptoms suggestive of more severe illness in the 2 days before death (103,115). Exogenous stressors associated with SIDS, such as fever and infection, tend to cause an increased rate of CO_2 production, alter the demand for cardiac output and/or thermoregulation, and/or decrease arousal. The prone sleeping position is associated with the spontaneous face-down sleeping position in infants (9). The face-down position is associated with rebreathing exhaled gases and increased end-tidal CO_2 in normal infants, particularly those sleeping on soft bedding where pockets of exhaled gas form and trap CO_2 (84). The prone position also may lead to partial or complete upper airway obstruction, by repositioning the mandible and occluding the pharynx, by compressing the nose directly, or by reflex laryngeal closure as part of the "diving" response. At least 26% of SIDS victims are found in the face-down position, and 71% are found in the prone position (50).

It is reasonable to propose that the underlying vulnerability in at least a subset of SIDS victims is an abnormality in the arcuate nucleus cell populations of the ventral medulla. The critical developmental period concerns maturation of homeostatic control. Although changes in cardioventilatory function and state organization continue throughout life, a relatively stable configuration is achieved by the end of the sixth month of life, the end of the period during which infants are at most risk for SIDS. It is possible that the external stressor is hypoxia or hypercapnia that results from upper airway obstruction and/or asphyxial rebreathing in the face-down (prone) sleeping position. A normal infant's nervous system detects progressive hypercapnia and hypoxia, and responds by arousal and a series of protective reflexes and behaviors to ensure airway patency. Because of the underlying abnormality in the ventral medulla, the vulnerable SIDS infant fails to arouse, cry, increase ventilation, and move his or her head in response to the hypercapnia and hypoxia: death results. If the arcuate nucleus abnormality is eventually shown to be a defect of timing of arcuate development, then the triple-risk model serves as a conceptual framework that merges the cardioventilatory/arousal hypothesis with the developmental hypothesis in SIDS.

Airway Obstruction, Apnea, and Respiratory Control Hypotheses

Upper Airway Obstruction

The theory of upper airway obstruction has been postulated by several investigators over the years (190,202). In 1971, Cross and Lewis (43) suggested a common "march of events" taking place, commencing with a "mild nasal infection in a baby who is an obligate nose breather." Because of the failure to respond to increasing carbon dioxide levels, they argued, the baby finally dies. The defect in this theory is that obligate nasal breathing diminishes around age 4 to 6 weeks, which is before the high SIDS incidence period of 2 to 4 months. Other authors (20,21,113,115) suggested high negative intrathoracic pressure as the cause of the prominent intrathoracic petechiae, and claimed that this concept requires some obstructive phenomenon to produce that negative pressure. Pharyngeal obstruction, because of backward falling of the tongue, pharyngeal collapse during sleep, or neck flexion leading to obstruction have all been suggested as instrumental in producing upper airway obstruction.

Kahn et al. (88) described the polysomnograms they performed on 11 future SIDS babies. These records showed longer central apneic episodes and more episodes of obstructive and mixed sleep apneas among the SIDS infants, thus adding some credence to reports of increased obstructive breathing in SIDS victims. Southall et al. (185) suggested,

> The majority of abnormal apneic episodes occurring during infancy have the respiratory patterns and evidence of ventilatory perfusion mismatch characteristic of the condition, called prolonged expiratory apnea. Epidemiologic and postmortem pathologic investigations into SIDS would be compatible with this as the final mechanism of death in a significant proportion of cases. Sleep-related upper airway

obstruction is an occasional cause of cyanotic episodes but more frequently presents with a constellation of recognizable clinical features that have not been reported from inquiries done after SIDS deaths. It is unlikely, therefore, that this cause of abnormal apnea is a major mechanism for SIDS. Because prolonged expiratory apnea may follow an infection with pertussis, respiratory syncytial virus (7,33), or other respiratory viruses, contact with these infections should be avoided. Finally, adverse prenatal factors, perhaps acting through disturbances in fetal oxygen exchange, viral infection, or through premature birth, are undoubtedly associated with an increased risk of SIDS.

McNamara and Sullivan (125) found obstructive sleep apnea in 19 (95%) of 20 infants of families who had histories of SIDS, apparent life-threatening events (ALTEs), or obstructive sleep apnea (OSA). When they studied a comparison group of 105 infants with no history of OSA, they found OSA in 31 (30%). They concluded that infants of families with multiple histories of SIDS, ALTE, or OSA are more likely to have OSA than are infants or families with only one case of SIDS or ALTE.

Gastroesophageal Reflux

Gastroesophageal reflux with reflex apnea from laryngospasm is posed as another mechanism and has led to preventive medical measures to reduce the number and amount of refluxes, and in extreme cases, to surgical fundal plication. The efficacy of this surgical procedure in preventing any cases of SIDS is unproven, and its use now for this purpose has few proponents.

The Apnea Hypothesis

In 1972, Steinschneider (195) described five infants who had been referred to him for cyanotic spells or apnea. Two of those patients (siblings) died, and in both, the diagnosis was initially SIDS. All had been documented as having had episodes of prolonged apnea, made worse by upper respiratory tract infections (195). However, the two infants who died and were called SIDS had no prolonged apnea observed in the hospital, and later the mother, Waneta Hoyt, confessed to having smothered them (62). However, this flawed research paper began a period of vigorous research about apnea as the etiology for SIDS. Guntheroth (74) postulated that a lack of an arousal response to apnea might be instrumental in SIDS. Shannon and Kelly (173) implicated sleep apnea as the mechanism for some "near miss SIDS" based on home monitoring results. Belief in the apnea hypothesis began to erode when Southall et al. (180) presented data on continuous electrocardiogram (ECG) and pneumogram monitoring of more than 9,000 infants, of whom 29 subsequently died of SIDS. Among those SIDS cases, no infant had shown abnormalities in the pneumograms, whereas those with abnormal pneumograms did not die. In 1991, Schechtman et al. (161) reported that the 24-hour pneumograms taken between 40 and 65 days of life in SIDS victims showed significantly fewer respiratory pauses than did age-matched control infants in both quiet sleep and rapid-eye-movement (REM) sleep; however, during the first month of life, the SIDS victims did not differ significantly from controls. This finding supported the view that some as yet undefined abnormality makes the future SIDS victim more vulnerable between ages 1 and 4 months. Current consensus is that SIDS victims seldom have a history of apnea, as manifested either clinically or by pneumography.

Cardiac Hypotheses

Prolonged QT interval, possibly resulting from a developmental abnormality in cardiac sympathetic innervation, has been advocated as a cause of SIDS. Schwartz et al. (166) found prolongation of the corrected QT (QT_c) interval in the three SIDS cases in their prospective study of 4,205 infants and proposed that some SIDS deaths could result from ventricular fibrillation induced by a sudden increase in sympathetic activity affecting a heart with reduced electrical stability. They suggested that maturational disparities in the right and left sympathetic neural pathways could produce an imbalance, thus triggering ventricular tachyarrhythmias in electrically unstable hearts and causing death (165). The markers of this abnormality (QT prolongation, heart-rate abnormalities), it was hoped, could allow early identification of some future SIDS victims. In a Milan, Italy, prospective study, Segantini et al. (172) examined the QT intervals prospectively in 8,000 infants, nine of whom died of SIDS, and four of whom died of other causes. Six of the nine SIDS infants had a prolonged QT_c; all four of the non-SIDS victims had normal QT_c. This study also showed that the QT_c normally increases from birth and then decreases over time, so that by age 6 months, it has returned to the same levels recorded at birth (172). This theory is consistent with a time-limited vulnerability. In a later study, Schwartz et al. (167) performed a prospective study of 34,442 newborn infants. At 1 year, a follow-up on 33,034 of these infants included 34 deaths, 24 of which were due to SIDS. ECGs performed on the third or fourth day of life revealed longer QT_c in the infants who died of SIDS than in the survivors and the infants who died of other causes. Moreover, 12 of the 24 SIDS victims but none of the other infants had a prolonged QT_c (defined as a QT_c >440 msec). This study has received intense criticism (82,83,124,181,203). Although the study is strengthened by the large number of cases and a single group analyzing the ECGs, it is weakened in part by the lack of blinded analyses, unknown aware (activity) or sleep states, and failure to list the other causes of death. Other questions about the study include (a) What caused the death of the control infants? (b) Were intrathoracic petechiae present in all cases of SIDS, only those with prolonged QT_c, or only those without prolonged QT_c? (c) Were the ECGs interpreted with computer or with visual measurements? (d) Were the ECGs blinded before review with respect to the cause of death? and (e) How does sudden death secondary to prolongation of the QT interval cause the formation of intrathoracic petechiae?

Southall et al. (180,182) were unable to show prolonged QT_c in two studies, and the dispute continues because of disagreements as regards methods. Morphologic studies of the conduction system have repeatedly shown it to be normal in SIDS infants (8,118,207). There have been ongoing discussions in the medical literature about the finding of prolonged QT interval in the Schwartz study. Most investigators commenting on this subject think more studies are needed on prolonged QT interval before it is accepted as a marker for SIDS. There is strong consensus that screening newborns for this abnormality would yield results too nonspecific to be useful. Further, treatment of infants with powerful medications for an unproven goal (prevention of SIDS), would be inadvisable (75,82, 83,124,181).

Environmental Factors

Overheating and hyperthermia have been suggested as factors in SIDS after descriptions of such infants being overdressed, overwrapped, and hot and sweaty when found (15,16,188–190). The mechanism suggested is that of "febrile apnea," the younger infant equivalent of a febrile seizure. Apnea has been associated with elevated ambient temperatures in premature babies (146), and this occurrence is cited as reason to believe the existence of the phenomenon in older infants. Hyperthermia as a factor contributing to SIDS deaths is gaining deserved attention, but more carefully crafted studies must be conducted to know the relative importance of this factor. One such study (153), using a case–control method, examined this issue in 41 SIDS victims by measuring thermal conditions at the death scene and at the scene of last sleep for control infants. A questionnaire also was administered to all the parents. The results showed that SIDS children had more excess thermal insulation for their given room temperature than did the matched controls ($p = 0.009$).

Byard et al. (38) reported on 30 cases of unexpected death by asphyxia caused by unsafe sleeping conditions. Deaths occurred from hanging from loose retainers, clothing, or curtain cords, positional asphyxia (wedging), and suffocation from plastic bed covers.

Other Theories

Other theories of etiology have had their advocates: elevated levels of fetal hemoglobin (85) have been reported, but have not been replicated (255). Infant botulism was reported in the late 1970s as the cause of death in a small subset of SIDS infants, and the spores of *Clostridium botulinum* were isolated from honey fed to nearly one third of infants found with the nonfatal results of that exposure (11,12). Nothing has appeared in the recent medical literature concerning infant botulism as a cause for SIDS, but feeding of honey has continued to be implicated in nonfatal infant botulism.

In 1989, Burchell et al. (35) reported finding increased hepatic glycogen levels in the livers of 10 infants who had died of SIDS. Eight of those infants had glucose-6-phosphatase deficiency (type 1a glycogen storage disease), and two infants had transport protein T2 deficiency (type 1c glycogen storage disease). Another metabolic abnormality, medium-chain acyl-CoA dehydrogenase deficiency (MCAD), allegedly accounts for death in 2% to 3% of infants in whom the diagnosis is SIDS (164). This disease is an autosomal recessive abnormality in fatty acid oxidation and usually presents with recurrent episodes of hypoglycemia and lethargy mimicking Reye syndrome, or with features clinically indistinguishable from SIDS. Mortality in MCAD is 60% in the first 2 years of life, but when recognized, the disease can be managed effectively. A single mutation in the MCAD gene accounts for more than 90% of the disease genes among whites, and a DNA test can be used to identify most MCAD-deficiency patients and carriers (164). Blood from the affected individual, or tissue or blood from both parents, can be used to identify carriers. At present, the defects in fatty acid β-oxidation known to be responsible for attacks of hypoketotic hypoglycemia, Reye-like syndrome, near-miss SIDS, and possibly SIDS are numerous (80).

PATHOLOGY

Although the autopsy has not elucidated the etiology of SIDS, and despite the presence of minor pathologic findings in many cases, it is still considered the *sine qua non* in determining the cause of sudden and unexpected death in infancy. In a recent study, Kumar et al. (117) reviewed the autopsy findings in 107 cases of postneonatal patients who had died during a 10-year period at a large suburban medical center. Sixty of these patients were younger than 1 year. In 34%, a new diagnosis was made at autopsy, whereas complete concordance was seen in 66%. This is a convincing argument about the value of conducting pediatric autopsies in general.

Sturner (196) described the need for careful examination of the "bed of death," thorough photography of the external aspects of the body and its coverings, including the orifices, as well as patterns of livor and external drainages and markings, before the body is washed or altered; extensive histologic study of the upper respiratory tract and lungs; the obtaining of consultation; and detailed review of the significance of findings before rendering a diagnosis.

Scene investigation is integral to the definition and accurate diagnosis of SIDS. It is the forensic pathologist's "medical history" and is analogous to the importance of the clinical history to the pathologist performing postmortem examinations in the hospital. Because the diagnosis of SIDS is one of exclusion, the postmortem examination does not reveal findings of sufficient severity to assign death to another cause. In this regard, it is vital that the scene where the infant was found lifeless be evaluated for environmental conditions, noxious gases, safety of the crib or bed and its sleep surface, and presence of harmful substances and medications. To facilitate the scene investigation, the Centers for Disease Control has produced and published *Guide-*

lines for the Scene Investigation of Sudden Unexpected Infant Death (86,87). These guidelines have been endorsed by the SIDS Global Strategy Task Force.

In the same vein, a standardized protocol has been developed for pathologists performing postmortem examinations on infants dying suddenly and unexpectedly (114). Endorsed by the Society for Pediatric Pathology, National Association of Medical Examiners, and the SIDS Global Strategy Task Force, this protocol prompts recording of positive and negative observations important to trying to reach a diagnosis in sudden unexpected infant death by use of a checklist and encourages narrative descriptions of abnormalities supplemented by microscopic, microbiologic, and toxicologic analyses as well as use of radiographic and photographic images when indicated.

Hanzlick (79) has listed the impediments interfering with high-quality death investigations. These include state variations in death-investigation requirements, lack of peer review, lack of standards, diversity, credentialing inconsistencies, coroner versus medical examiner systems, inadequate funding, manpower shortages, lack of government interest, legal influences on medical decisions, and operation of medical examiner/coroner offices outside of the usual health care delivery systems. He proposed a National Office of Death Investigation Affairs to facilitate improvements.

Actual autopsy findings in SIDS have been described extensively (4,20,206,208). The bodies of SIDS victims appear well nourished and well developed, but their weights are typically below the 50th percentile expected for age. It has been suggested that their growth rates are slow, but this notion has been challenged in a study comparing each of 78 autopsy-confirmed SIDS cases with two controls matched for postnatal age, season, neighborhood, and date of parental interview. No differences were observed between SIDS victims and controls with respect to the growth rates between their births and last live weights and between their last two live weights. Stratification of these infants by sex, gestational age, maternal smoking during pregnancy, breast versus bottle feeding, or age at death did not change the results.

A mucoid discharge, occasionally foamy and often tinged with blood, often is present around the nares and mouth. Fibers from bedclothes may be found in the hands, which are often clenched. Signs of resuscitation and postmortem changes must be distinguished from nonaccidental trauma. Reddish blue mottling of the skin indicative of postmortem lividity may alter dependent portions of the body. The blood in the heart is liquid and often oozes from venipuncture sites. The bladder and rectum are empty. Subtle anomalies reported by Vawter and Kozakewich (210) are neither diagnostic nor specific.

Intrathoracic petechiae, the most common abnormality seen with the naked eye, are identified in about 80% of SIDS cases (22,112). Despite opinion to the contrary (103), facial and conjunctival petechiae are not seen in SIDS, and their presence should provoke a search for another cause of death. Experimental evidence and observations in human postmortem examinations suggest petechiae limited to the thorax can result by breathing against an obstructed upper airway during the moments preceding death (22,58, 112,115). Alternatively, it also has been suggested that bronchiolar obstruction could cause the same finding. More recently, Poets et al. (151) identified intrathoracic petechiae in infants shown by monitoring to be gasping deeply before dying of SIDS.

The lungs are congested and variably edematous, but not consolidated. It is unlikely that pneumonia that cannot be seen with the naked eye is lethal. Given that infants may have considerable clinical and radiographic evidence of pneumonia and, even if ill, are nevertheless alive, it seems all the more improbable that microscopic pulmonary inflammatory infiltrates are lethal.

Microscopic examination of the lungs, heart, and leptomeninges may show mild, focal interstitial lymphocytic infiltrates in SIDS cases. These should not be interpreted as a lethal finding (37). These infiltrates in the heart are not accompanied by myocardial necrosis, thus precluding a diagnosis of myocarditis by using the Dallas criteria, and are seen with about equal frequency in other causes of sudden, unexpected infant death. Trivial microscopic inflammatory infiltrates also may be seen in the meninges but are not accompanied by brain swelling, encephalitis, or hemorrhage, and are not therefore a lethal finding.

A pathognomonic marker for SIDS has not been found. It is unlikely that such a marker will be found, given the likelihood that SIDS consists of more than one entity and has more than one cause. Nevertheless, it has been proposed that laryngeal basement membrane thickening is just such a marker (174–176). Krous et al. (116), in a recent study, have shown it is not a reliable postmortem marker in SIDS.

Accumulation of small lipid droplets collectively in the liver, renal tubular epithelium, and smooth, skeletal, and cardiac muscle does not occur in SIDS and warrants evaluation for metabolic disorders such as MCAD deficiency, of which the A985G mutation is the most common variant (32,142). Death during the first week of life is rare in SIDS, and if microscopic lipid accumulation is found in these tissues, then the G583A mutation variant of MCAD deficiency should be considered (32).

Hypoxic Tissue Markers

Naeye and Ladis (139–141) reported a series of subtle histopathologic findings in SIDS cases that became known as hypoxic tissue markers, which they interpreted to indicate that these babies experienced recurrent or prolonged hypoxia and hypoxemia before death. These markers consisted of increased pulmonary arteriolar muscle, periadrenal brown fat, and hepatic erythropoiesis in association with right ventricular hypertrophy and abnormalities in the adrenal medulla and carotid bodies. Brainstem gliosis completed the list of these alleged abnormalities. In a critical review of the publications of Naeye et al. and others attempting to confirm their work, Beckwith (24) found important flaws in the selection of the control cases, lack of standardization of microscopic tissue sections, deficiencies in the analytic methods, and indefensible conclusions drawn from the investigator's own data. With the exception of brainstem gliosis, none of these markers has been convincingly and repeatedly confirmed.

Death Certification

Death certification typically requires determination of both cause and manner, cause being the physiologic and/or anatomic abnormalities leading to death, and manner being natural, accidental, homicide, suicide, or undetermined. In the last few years, there has been a trend toward ascribing sudden, unexpected infant death unexplained by medical history review, scene investigation, and postmortem examination as undetermined with respect to both cause and manner. This is unfortunate because the diagnosis of SIDS is an admission of not knowing the cause of death, yet it is commonly accepted that the vast majority of these deaths are natural. At least there is insufficient information to designate these deaths as homicidal, yet "undetermined," as a manner of death, does not provide the benefit of lessening the guilt caretakers often feel about the infant's death. It leaves room for suspicion that they somehow escaped detection for a murder they might have committed.

Unfortunately, in some cases, soft suffocation and SIDS may be indistinguishable at postmortem examination. It has been said that differentiation depends on a confession. This seems like a harsh penalty, given that in the vast majority of cases, there is nothing to raise suspicion of homicide on the part of the caretakers. Even prior referral to child-protection service agencies does not discriminate homicide from SIDS in these cases (143).

DIFFERENTIATING BETWEEN SIDS AND CHILD ABUSE

"The causes of these deaths (SIDS) are probably multiple and virtually all of a natural origin. Unfortunately, some cases are homicide by soft smothering" (46,47). Despite the accusatory nature of this statement, the objective observer of sudden death in infancy must concede that inflicted injury sometimes causes death. After studying the problem of infant deaths in Sheffield, England, for more than 25 years, Emery (53) concluded, "filicide is the probable mechanism of death in approximately one in ten of the unexplained unexpected deaths." In the U.S., estimates as high as 5,000 deaths annually attributable to child abuse in children younger than 18 years come from reliable sources. As death-review teams become more common and we gain more information, this figure may be further clarified. The intense negative emotional response to DiMaio's statement derives from the persisting need to deny abhorrent behavior and the natural urge of health care professionals to protect innocent, grieving parents from heavy-handed false accusations of child abuse.

What is the landscape of this dispute? Is the provision of compassionate support to families losing an infant more important than the responsibility to discover when an infant has been the victim of fatal, inflicted injury? What does the literature tell us as clinicians to help us choose either a path of support for grieving parents or a path of prosecution for the conduct of a heinous crime? The literature often provides more questions than answers, but since the 1970s, we have learned a great deal about both SIDS and child abuse. The balance of this chapter is a description of the evolution of knowledge and opinion about sudden deaths in infancy in terms of their clinical, pathologic, and investigational dimensions. Further, we describe a systematic approach to the problem to assist the clinician, investigator, and pathologist in determining the exact cause and mechanism of a given death.

CHILD ABUSE FATALITIES

In 1961, Adelson (3) reported on 46 child homicides in Cuyahoga County, Ohio, from 1944 through 1960. Ten of those children were younger than 1 year. Of those, five drowned, and three died of starvation. The causes of death of the other two are not described. Adelson concluded, "Failure to perform autopsies on infants found dead (or said to have been found dead) because they are 'crib deaths' . . . will inevitably result in the missing of many cases of this type of homicide." In a follow-up article in 1991 (5), Adelson reported 194 child homicides in Cuyahoga County between 1976 and 1980; 16 occurred in infants between ages 1 month and 1 year, and seven occurred between ages 1 and 6 months. All were fatally and obviously battered, and no cases were likely to be confused with SIDS.

Emery and Taylor (56) described a 24-year period in Sheffield, England (1960 to 1984), during which postperinatal deaths (birth to 2 years) were investigated by gathering information about the death scene, obstetric and pediatric care, and autopsy findings, and by conducting an extensive home visit. Accidental suffocation was thought to be the cause of death in 10% of these cases, and the possibility of active intervention on the part of one or both parents was raised in another 10%, a rate consistently double that of overt child abuse in this age group. Specific data on infants between ages 1 month and 1 year were not reported.

Asch (13), a psychiatrist who, based on his experience but no actual data, hypothesized that "a large part" of the number of "mysterious and baffling" sudden infant deaths were "infanticides, perpetrated by the mother as a specific manifestation of a postpartum depression." Although Asch's assumption that large numbers of these deaths were the result of maternal postpartum depression was erroneous, data are convincing (107,108,109, 192–194) that at least in some cases, postpartum depression and other psychiatric disturbances, particularly in mothers who had histories of maltreatment themselves, have led to infanticide.

In 1977, Bass (14) reported on 15 infant deaths that occurred in a 30-month period in Wayne County, Michigan, from accidental asphyxia. Ten of these deaths were attributed to suffocation resulting from entrapment of the head and neck between crib slats or crib rail and mattress. Five cases involved strangulation when the pacifier cord, necklace, or nightgown became entangled on the crib post or on a toy attached to the crib rail. "Three other cases of crib asphyxia were considered to be SIDS by physicians, even though information indicating accidental asphyxia was available." Ellerstein (52) criticized Bass for ignoring the possibility of child abuse as a cause for strangulation, and advised that intentional injury should be part of the differential diagnosis in such cases.

In 1985, Christoffel et al. (41) examined 43 unexpected deaths in children brought to Children's Memorial Hospital in Chicago from 1980 to 1981. Nine of those deaths were the result of child abuse; in three cases, the correct diagnosis was established only by postmortem examination. The two factors having the highest predictive value for child abuse, according to the authors, were "dead on arrival" (DOA) and the subject's being younger than 1 year. An interesting observation, however, is that this study included six SIDS infants who arrived as DOA and were in the appropriate age group (1 to 7 months), and yet when all were subjected to postmortem examination, results in every instance were consistent with SIDS and were not to be confused with child abuse.

Alternatively, in the same journal issue, Kirschner and Stein (102) described 10 cases in which the diagnosis of child abuse was made on the basis of incomplete or erroneous medical observation. Five of those cases involved autopsy-proven SIDS. The clinical physical examinations had described conditions that were postmortem changes (e.g., lividity, sphincter dilation), misinterpreted skin markings (mongoloid pigmentation), or a physical finding often seen in SIDS deaths (serosanguinous discharge from the nose and mouth). Both articles underscored the need for appropriate evaluation both before and after death, including knowledgeable clinical physical examinations and thorough autopsies for all unwitnessed deaths.

A controversial article by Bass et al. (16) brought the dilemma of death ascertainment to a new level of debate. They described a series of 26 cases to which a diagnosis of SIDS had been assigned. The authors conducted death-scene and family investigations and concluded that overlying accounted for one death and was suspected in five others; hyperthermia caused three deaths; hyperthermia combined with asphyxiation claimed three infants; and poor judgment by the caretaker was a contributing factor in almost all the deaths.

Reaction to this publication came from several sources. The office of the Chief Medical Examiner of New York stated that the study was conducted without their knowledge; that 18 of the cases were subject to reevaluation at the time of the Bass study; and that four other cases were not attributed to SIDS after microscopic study. The absence of scientific method in the conduct of the study was clear. Speaking for the National SIDS Foundation, Valdes-Dapena et al. (209) agreed that death-scene investigations were important in the establishment of a diagnosis in cases of infant death, but that Bass et al. had overinterpreted the results of the study and that there was systematic bias to bolster the author's hypothesis that mechanical events have a role in causation. They also pointed out the absence of controls in the study. Other authors (123) noted that thousands of other infants living in the same conditions in the urban low-socioeconomic community served by the study hospital did not die, and that a control group was necessary to justify the conclusions drawn by the authors. No data were presented to support the authors' claim in one case of the diagnosis of shaken baby syndrome, which requires either radiographic or autopsy findings. Thach (199) observed that this series of SIDS patients was small, atypical because all of the patients presented to the hospital emergency department, and the patient population was drawn from an economically disadvantaged community. Thach went on to state that death-scene investigations, if conducted sensitively, might reveal potentially preventable causes of death. Death by overlying is practically unprovable by virtue of the fact that the two parties—caretaker and infant—are both asleep at the time of the supposed occurrence. Overlying is observed, he noted, in most mammalian species, and there is no reason to believe that the human being is the only exception to this biologic phenomenon. Accidental suffocation, he concluded, cannot be summarily excluded as the cause of some infant deaths.

In a report from Arkansas Children's Hospital covering the period between October 1983 and May 1987, eight of 170 cases referred to their hospital with a diagnosis of SIDS were selected for review because of concern that the diagnosis of SIDS was erroneous. All eight were rediagnosed after postmortem and death-scene investigation (147). The number of recategorized cases would have been greater, according to Perrot, had all 170 cases been subjected to such review (personal communication).

Emery et al. (55) reviewed the autopsy findings of 60 Madison, Wisconsin, infant deaths registered as SIDS victims between 1974 and 1985. The authors claimed that 10 of those infants had medical diagnoses sufficient to explain their deaths. This high rate (20%) has not been seen in any other such analyses and calls into question the criteria for making the decision that the medical diagnoses were indeed "sufficient." Two deaths were attributable to infanticide.

SUFFOCATION AND MUNCHAUSEN BY PROXY

Since 1977 and Meadow's introduction of the term Munchausen syndrome by proxy (MBP) (126), this form of parent-induced illness has been recognized as the etiology in numerous cases in which a bizarre and undiagnosable illness in a child has turned out to be parent induced (see Chapter 14). Because parent-induced apnea is the most frequent manifestation of MBP, it is now in the differential diagnosis when ALTEs are being evaluated.

In 1979, Berger (27) reported two cases of child abuse simulating near-miss SIDS. The first case involved a 5-month-old girl who had a history of apnea and cyanotic spells and was extensively evaluated in the hospital for 5 weeks. During an unattended bathing of the infant by the mother, the mother ran out of the bathroom calling for help, and the infant was found cyanotic and limp, with bleeding gums and fresh pinch marks on her nose. The second patient was a 6-week-old girl with apnea and cyanosis, also hospitalized for several weeks, who had "spells" only when her mother visited. On one of those visits, the mother was discovered holding her hand over the patient's nose and mouth. Rosen et al. (158) reported on two siblings with recurrent cardiorespiratory arrest who, when removed from the care of the mother, stopped having the episodes. In 1986, Rosen et al. (159) described six infants referred for evaluation of recurrent infant apnea requiring multiple resuscitation efforts. In two cases, the mothers were proven conclusively, by means of video surveillance, to be the perpetrators of the apneic episodes, and in a third, the mother had an overt psychiatric disorder. For these three infants, the apneic episodes stopped when they were placed with other caretakers. The three other infants died within 1 month of leaving the hospital. Southall et al. (184) reported two cases of apneic episodes induced by smothering and detected by covert video surveillance. Griffith and Slovik (70) reported two infants who were referred to a sleep-disorders center because of apnea and near-miss SIDS, both of whom turned out to be victims of MBP.

Meadow (127) reviewed and reported on 27 cases of young children suffocated by their mothers. Twenty-four of the children had histories of previous episodes of apnea, cyanosis, or seizure, and 11 had had 10 or more of these episodes either invented or caused by their mothers. Eighteen of the children were alive, and nine were dead. In the families of the 27 children were 18 children who had died suddenly and unexpectedly in early life. Thirteen of the siblings had histories of recurrent apnea, cyanosis, or seizures. Most of these deaths had been certified as SIDS. Meadow

drew the distinction between the features seen in this group of suffocated infants and in infants dying of SIDS (Table 20.1). In an article in 1999, Meadow (128) reported on 81 children from 50 families in which 42 deaths had been ascribed to SIDS and 29 another cause. Family and criminal courts had determined that all 81 of these children had been killed by their parents.

In 1991, Burchfield and Rawlings (36) described 10 hospitalized neonates from a variety of referring hospitals who had ALTEs or who died of unexplained causes in the hospital. Five of these patients died, and autopsies performed on four of the five yielded no adequate explanations for the deaths. Evaluation of the survivors also failed to reveal a cause for the ALTEs. Four of the survivors had severe neurologic impairment. These cases are puzzling because they occurred in the hospital, in the early morning hours, and presumably under good nursing supervision.

Southall et al. (183) reported their extraordinary experience with 39 children referred to them for the evaluation. While in the hospital, these children, ranging in age from 2 months to 44 months, were studied by means of covert video-surveillance. Thirty-six of these children had been referred for apparent life-threatening events (ALTE), one for suspected seizure disorder, one for failure to thrive, and one for suspected strangulation. The number of ALTEs reported by the parents ranged from two to more than 50 (median, seven). Forty-six children constituted a control group and were being investigated for ALTEs attributed to

TABLE 20.1. *Features seen in suffocated infants and in SIDS victims*

Features	Suffocation (%)	SIDS (%)
Previous apnea	90	<10
Previous unexplained disorder	44	<5
More than 6 months old	55	<15
Dead sibling	48	2

SIDS, sudden infant death syndrome.
From Meadow R. Suffocation, recurrent apnea, and sudden infant death. *J Pediatr* 1990;117:351–354, with permission.

proven medical conditions. Covert video-sur-veillance was accomplished by locating a video camera in four corners of the room and a microphone in the ceiling. The patients underwent continuous monitoring of transcutaneous oxygen saturation, and pulse oximetry, breathing movements, and ECG. The median time of surveillance was 29 hours. In 30 cases, covert video-surveillance revealed intentional suffocation of the child. It revealed abuse in 33 of the 39 cases. Frank bleeding from the nose or mouth was reported in 11 of 38 patients with ALTEs, but in none of the 46 control children. Of the 41 siblings of the patients undergoing surveillance, 12 had previously died suddenly and unexpectedly. Eleven of these had been classified as SIDS, but after video-surveillance, four parents admitted to suffocating eight of these children. One child had died of deliberate poisoning. In the 52 siblings of the 46 children in the control group, two had died: one of hypoplastic left heart at age 5 days, and the other of documented SIDS. Studies such as these underscore the need for comprehensive medical and scene investigation because the postmortem examination may yield only limited information.

SUBSTANCE ABUSE AND ITS RELATION TO CHILD FATALITIES

The relation between child abuse and substance abuse is well established. Wallace (211) found that among 70 crack-using women with children, 34.3% had the Bureau of Child Welfare involved in their children's lives as a result of the mother's crack use and the neglect or abuse that followed. Thirty percent of the children were placed with relatives, and 4.3% were in foster care. Relatives were caring for another 15%. Wallace concluded that the majority (53%) of crack-smoking mothers had become dysfunctional as parents and no longer cared for their children. She further stated, "Crack-related deterioration in mothers' ability to care for their children reveals a shocking decline in psychosocial functioning compared with a pre-crack level of functioning." Famularo et al. (57) showed a strong as-

sociation between substance abuse and child maltreatment. During the period of study, 67% of the abused or neglected children seen in a juvenile court system in Massachusetts lived with substance-abusing parents. The rates of fatal child abuse directly attributable to substance abuse are unknown, but logic instructs that a fatal outcome is a natural consequence in a proportion of these reported instances of maltreatment.

TWINS AND CHILD ABUSE

In 1982, Groothuis et al. (71), in a retrospective study of twins in Nashville, reported an increased incidence of child abuse in families with twins. Forty-eight families with twins were compared with control singleton births, matched for hospital of delivery, birth date, maternal age, race, and socioeconomic status. Three (2.4%) control and nine (18.7%) twin families had been reported for maltreatment. One child died, and eight children from six families were removed from their homes. When analyzing the variables in the families studied, the authors concluded that twin status had the greatest impact on the risk of subsequent child abuse, suggesting that the stress of rearing twins, added to the other elements of child-rearing in already marginally functioning families, was a significant determinant for subsequent abuse.

RADIOGRAPHIC STUDIES

The use of radiography as an ancillary study in postmortem examinations is routine in most jurisdictions. Kleinman (104) noted, "The babygram is an inadequate examination to assess for skeletal injuries, particularly when they are inflicted. The babygram should be strenuously condemned, as it not only may fail to identify critical forensic data, but the apparent absence of fractures may give unjustified reassurance that no trauma has occurred."
Belanger (26) described the elements of the skeletal survey. The skeletal survey consists of 19 images collimated to each anatomic body region with frontal views of the appen-

dicular skeleton and frontal and lateral views of the axial skeleton (Table 20.2).

In 1984, Kleinman et al. (105) subjected 12 cases of unexplained infant deaths to complete radiographic skeletal surveys by pediatric radiologists using high-resolution film–screen cassettes or direct-exposure techniques to yield maximal osseous detail. Autopsies were performed, supplemented with resection and high-detail radiography and histologic study of all noncranial sites of suspected osseous injury or sites of high risk of injury (distal femoral, proximal and distal tibia, and proximal humeral metaphyses). Eight of the infants were found to have been abused. Four of the abused infants had an initial history of apnea or other ALTEs. A history of having been shaken was noted in three cases. The cause of death in six of the eight cases was head trauma. In three of these infants, multiple rib fractures were found at autopsy, and in the other three, only postmortem evidence of head injury was found. In total, 34 bony injuries were found, including 13 metaphyseal injuries. Eleven of the 13 were evident on skeletal survey, 12 on specimen radiography, and all on histologic analysis. Fifteen posterior rib fractures were identified at autopsy, eight of which were not visible on skeletal survey because of their acuity. Three skull fractures and one thoracic spine fracture were found. Fractures of the clavicle, vertebrae, and long-bone diaphyses were indistinguishable from fractures re-

sulting from accidental injury. Kleinman et al. (105a) later studied 165 fractures in 31 fatally abused infants whose average age was 3 months. Fifty-one percent of these fractures were in the rib cage, and 44% in the long bones (of which 89% were classic metaphyseal lesions). Williamson and Perrot (215) reported results of the use of radiography in 108 infants who died. The radiographs consisted of frontal and lateral radiographs of the skull and trunk and frontal views of the extremities on each of the infants aged 7 days to 11 months. Seventy-three infants were diagnosed after postmortem examination as having SIDS. Three of the 35 in whom a specific cause for death was found were victims of child abuse. The 73 infants dying of SIDS had no findings of significance with regard to the skeleton or that would suggest or be confused with child abuse. In all of the child abuse cases, multiple fractures were seen. In this study, the absence of radiographic findings was consistent with the diagnosis of SIDS.

CHILD FATALITY REVIEW TEAMS

The first interagency child fatality review (CFR) team was formed in 1978 in Los Angeles County under the direction of Michael Durfee (ICAN, The Interagency Council on Child Abuse and Neglect). By 1999, CFR teams exist in 49 states. In California, nearly 100% of the population lives in communities served by CFR teams. The composition of these teams varies from place to place, but usually consists of, at the minimum, representatives from the medical examiner/coroner's office, the District Attorney's office, Child Protective Services, and a pediatrician familiar with pediatric diseases, child abuse, and childhood injury. This approach has been described in four manuals prepared by the Child Maltreatment Fatalities Project of the American Bar Association Center on Children and the Law and the American Academy of Pediatrics, supported by the Robert Wood Johnson Foundation (10,66,92,93).

Review of cases of child deaths has been shown to have a variety of applications. In a

---

TABLE 20.2. *The skeletal survey*

Anteroposterior skull
Lateral skull
Lateral cervical spine
Anteroposterior thorax
Lateral thorax
Anteroposterior pelvis
Lateral lumbar spine
Anteroposterior humeri
Anteroposterior forearms
Oblique hands
Anteroposterior femora
Anteroposterior tibias
Anteroposterior feet

Note: All positive sites should be viewed in at least two projections. From Kleinman PK. *Diagnostic imaging in child abuse.* St. Louis: Mosby, 1998, with permission.

report from Georgia (120), team members reviewed 255 cases of 1,889 childhood deaths. Agreement on the cause of death between the death certificate and the CFR was 87%. In 21 cases there was disagreement with the death certificate. Five of these cases were changed to child abuse based on the team's recommendations. Stronger child-passenger restraint laws and installation of a traffic signal at a dangerous intersection where a number of deaths had occurred were other results of the CFR activity.

In another report on the activities of a CFR, Herman-Giddens et al. (81) reviewed all child homicides in North Carolina from 1985 to 1994. Two hundred twenty were child abuse homicides, but the ICD code E967 (Homicide and Injury Purposely Inflicted by Other Persons/Child Battering and Other Maltreatment) was assigned to only 68 of the 220 cases. This underascertainment was almost 60%, so it can be said that the ascertainment of the cause and manner of death in children is being grossly neglected.

PERPETRATORS OF FATAL CHILD ABUSE: IS THERE A PROFILE?

In 37 of the 46 homicides reported by Adelson (3), the children were killed by their parents, close blood relatives, or by persons who stood *in loco parentis.* Eight were slain by non-related persons, and one assailant was never identified. Frankly psychotic assailants were identified in 17 cases, four were "borderline psychotic," and suicidal intent with the desire to "take the children" with them accounted for three cases. Nine children were killed by fathers during frustrated outbursts of emotion, four girls and one boy were killed during sexual assault, three infants died of starvation, and one child died of burns inflicted by a father throwing inflammable liquid onto the bed in which mother and child were sleeping. One child died of repeated beatings.

In a 1973 English study of 29 children killed by their fathers (169), Scott found the following characteristics. First, fatherhood was ambiguous, with nearly two thirds of the

fathers not married to their partners and more than one half not being the biologic father of the child. Second, the work and child-caring roles were reversed, with the father being the primary caretaker, for one fourth of these parents. Finally, the fathers had unrealistic expectations of the children, failing to see the behaviors of the victims as usual for infants and children, and viewing the infant as having adult motivations. Three fourths of the cases had unmistakable warnings of the subsequent outcome. In 27% of the cases, the fathers had records of violent crimes. Personality disorders, broadly characterized as "immature" or "aggressive," were seen in 75% of fathers. Most of the fathers had themselves experienced parental violence or hostility.

Korbin (108) examined the childhood histories of nine women imprisoned for fatal child abuse and found that all had a history of childhood abuse, and that "abuse in one's childhood is an enduring potentiating factor," but she cautioned of a preponderance of risk factors and a lack of compensating factors that compounded the effect of the women's childhood experiences. Five of these women had experienced spousal abuse and had a "dearth of support or compensatory factors." They also were seen as unable to seek and obtain effective assistance. Korbin (107) described the mothers' faulty perceptions of their children as being rejecting and having developmental abnormalities, either advanced or delayed. The author found that the mothers had provided warning signals to professionals and their personal networks before the abusive incidents.

These and other retrospective studies (42) have been criticized because of methodologic flaws. Later studies drawing a connection between child victimization and subsequent abusive parental behaviors also had poor study design. Evidence suggesting that childhood victimization does not lead to abusive parenting behavior was provided by Miller and Challas (131). In their longitudinal study over a 25-year period, they found that 45% of persons abused as children were rated as not being at risk of abusing their children. Egelund et al. (51) found that 70%

of 47 mothers who had themselves been abused as children were currently mistreating their children. Kaufman and Zigler (95) concluded from review of the extant literature that the link between being maltreated and becoming abusive was "far from inevitable." Widom (213,214) supported this contention, and Hunter and Kilstrom (84a) reported on 40 families in which this pattern was broken. They identified the mitigating factors in this change as relating to "a broad network of resources, a degree of self-differentiation, an attitude of realistic optimism, and the ability to marshall extra resources to meet crisis situations."

Schloesser et al. (162) studied 104 abuse-related fatalities occurring in Kansas from 1975 to 1980 and then from 1983 to 1989. Among their findings were these indicators: very young age of the parents at the first pregnancy; high rate of single parenthood; significantly lower educational achievement of victims' mothers; late, inadequate prenatal care; complications during pregnancy; and low birth weight among the victims.

Starling et al. (191) studied 151 head-injury victims and found that males were more often perpetrators of that form of abuse. Fathers accounted for 37%, mother's boyfriend 21%, female babysitters 17%, and mothers 13%. There was no determination of the identity of the perpetrator in some of the cases.

Studies of perpetrators such as these provide some useful information for the analysis of unexpected infant death. The construction of infallible profiles, however, invites misdiagnosis. The importance of these risk factors derives from their incorporation into the larger landscape of infant-death review.

The literature thus provides some parameters for making the distinction between SIDS and fatal child abuse. These may be grouped roughly into three categories: highly consistent with SIDS; less likely to be SIDS; and suggestive or diagnostic of abuse (Table 20.3).

To reach the best decision in these sometimes ambiguous cases, we recommend the following steps.

1. Accurate history taking by emergency responders and medical personnel at the time of death.
2. Examination of the dead infant at a hospital emergency department by qualified and competent individuals with child abuse expertise, even if the infant is known to be dead. Resuscitation paraphernalia must not be removed before examination by the medical examiner.
3. High-quality postmortem examinations within 24 hours of death, including indicated toxicologic and metabolic screening on infants dying unexpectedly and inexplicably.
4. Routine skeletal surveys in all infants dying inexplicably or from suggestive causes.
5. Prompt death-scene investigation by knowledgeable individuals, including careful and supportive interviews of the household members.
6. Detailed collection of previous medical records from all sources of medical care and personal interviews of key medical providers.
7. Detailed collection of medical history from caretakers by using a standardized medical history questionnaire.
8. Use of infant death-review teams organized locally to review the data collected.
9. Use of accepted diagnostic categories on death certificates as promptly as possible, including International Codes for Disease E codes, after review.
10. Recognition of all the diagnostic elements involved in the decision about infant deaths.
11. Maintenance of a supportive approach to parents during the death-review process.
12. Appropriation of adequate funds to support this critical process to ascertain the cause and manner of death and, secondarily, to encourage the protection of all infants and children.
13. Stimulation and support of more research into the etiology of both SIDS and child abuse.

TABLE 20.3. *Criteria for distinguishing SIDS from fatal child abuse and other medical conditions*

	Consistent with SIDS	Less Consistent with SIDS	Suggestive or Diagnostic of Child Abuse
History surrounding death	Apparently healthy infant fed, put to bed. Found lifeless. Silent death. EMS resuscitation unsuccessful.	Infant found apneic. EMS transports to hospital. Infant lives hours to days. Substance abuse. Family illness.	Atypical history for SIDS. Discrepant history. Unclear history. Prolonged interval between bedtime and death
Age at death	Most common age at death: 2–4 mo. Range, 1–12 mo. 90% of SIDS die before age 7 mo.	8–12 mo of age.	>12 mo.
Physical examination and laboratory studies	Pinkish frothy nasal discharge. Postmortem lividity in dependent areas of body. Possible marks on pressure points of body. No skin trauma. Well-cared-for baby.	Enlarged organs. Evidence of disease process in organs.	Skin injuries. Traumatic lesions on body or body cavities. Malnutrition. Physical signs of neglect. Fractures
History of pregnancy, labor, delivery and infancy	Normal. Prematurity or low birth weight. Multiple births (twins, triplets). History of cigarette smoking. Prone sleeping position. Overdressing leading to hyperthermia.	Recurrent illnesses, multiple hospitalizations. "Sickly" or "weak" baby. Specific diagnosis of organ system disease.	Unwanted pregnancy. Failed attempt at abortion. Little or no prenatal care. Out-of-hospital birth. Late arrival for delivery. No well-baby visits. No immunizations. Use of drugs/alcohol, tobacco during and after pregnancy. Baby described as hard to care for or to "discipline". Unusual feeding practices.
Death-scene investigation	Crib or bed in good repair. No dangerous bedclothes, toys, plastic sheets, pacifier strings, lambs wool, or pellet pillows. No cords or bands for possible entanglement. No apparent head/neck entrapment. Normal room temperature. No toxins, insecticides. Good evaluation. Heating system functioning normally.	Defective crib/bed. Use of inappropriate sheets, pillows, sleeping clothes. Presence of dangerous toys, plastic sheets, pacifier cords, pellet pillows, lambs wool. Pool ventilation, heat control. Presence of toxins, insecticides. Unsanitary conditions.	Chaotic, unsanitary, crowded living conditions. Evidence of drugs/alcohol. Signs of terminal struggle in crib, bedclothes. Bloodstains. Hostility, discord, accusations of caretakers. Admission of harm.
Previous infant deaths in family	First unexplained infant death in family.	One previous unexplained death in family	More than one previous unexplained death.
Autopsy findings	No adequate cause for death. Normal: skeletal survey; toxicology; blood chemistries; microscopic examination of tissues; metabolic screen. Presence of intrathoracic petechiae. Presence of dysmorphic, dysplastic, or anomalous lesions. Presence of gliosis of brainstem. Anal sphincter dilatation.	Changes in liver, adrenal, . myocardium. Few or no intrathoracic petechiae	Traumatic cause of death. Intracranial or visceral bleeding. External bruises, abrasions, or burns. No . intrathoracic petechiae. Malnutrition. Fractures. Subgaleal hematoma. Abnormal blood chemistries. Abnormal blood toxicology
Previous child-protective services or law-enforcement involvement	None	One	Two or more. One or more family members arrested for violent behavior. Restraining orders against a partner. History of domestic violence

SIDS, sudden infant death syndrome; EMS, emergency medical services; PM, postmortem; PE, physical examination; LBW, low birth weight; IC, intracranial; CPS, children's protective services; LE, law enforcement.

Adapted from Reece RM. Fata child abuse and sudden infant death syndrome: a critical diagnostic decision. *Pediatrics* 1993;91:423–429, with permission.

REFERENCES

1. AAP Task Force on Infant Positioning and SIDS, J. Kattwinkel, Chair. *Pediatrics* 1992;89:1120–1126.
2. Adams MM. The descriptive epidemiology of sudden infant deaths among natives and whites in Alaska. *Am J Epidemiol* 1985;122:637.
3. Adelson L. Slaughter of the innocents: a study of forty-six homicides in which the victims were children. *N Engl J Med* 1961;264:1345–1349.
4. Adelson L. Specific studies of infant victims of sudden death: sudden death in infants. In: Wedgewood RJ, Benditt EP, eds. *Proceedings of the Conference on Causes of Sudden Death in Infants. Seattle, WA.* Washington DC: Government Printing Office (PHS publ. no. 1412), 1963:1–40.
5. Adelson L. Pedicide revisited: the slaughter continues. *Am J Forensic Med Pathol* 1991;12:16–26.
6. Alm B, Milerad J, Winnergren G, et al. A case-control study of smoking and sudden infant death syndrome in the Scandinavian countries 1992-1995: the Nordic Epidemiological SIDS Study. *Arch Dis Child* 1998;78: 329–334.
7. Anas N, Boettrich C, Hall CB. The association of apnea and respiratory syncytial virus infection in infants. *J Pediatr* 1982;101:65–68.
8. Anderson RH, Bourton J, Burrow CT, et al. Sudden death in infancy: a study of cardiac specialized tissue. *Br Med J* 1974;2:135–139.
9. Anderson RN, Kochanek KD, Murphy SL. Report of final mortality statistics 1995. *Mon Vital Stat Rep* 1997;45(suppl):66–69.
10. Anderson TL, Wells SJ. *Data collection for child fatalities: existing efforts and proposal guidelines.* Chicago: American Bar Association,1992.
11. Arnon SS. Infant botulism: epidemiology in relation to sudden infant death syndrome. *Epidemiol Rev* 1981;3: 45–66.
12. Arnon SS, Damus K, Midura T, et al. Intestinal infection and toxin production by *Clostridium botulinum* as one cause of sudden infant death syndrome. *Lancet* 1978;1:1273–1277.
13. Asch SS. Crib deaths: their possible relationship to postpartum depression and infanticide. *Mt Sinai J Med* 1968;35:214–220.
14. Bass M. Asphyxial crib death. *N Engl J Med* 1977; 296:555–556.
15. Bass M. Sudden infant death syndrome. *N Engl J Med* 1982;307:891.
16. Bass M, Krovath RE, Glass L. Death scene investigation in sudden infant death. *N Engl J Med* 1986;315: 100–105.
17. Bauchner H, Zuckerman BS. Cocaine, sudden infant death syndrome and home monitoring. *J Pediatr* 1990; 117:904–906.
18. Bauchner H, Zuckerman B, McClain M, et al. Risk of sudden infant death syndrome among infants with in-utero exposure to cocaine. *J Pediatr* 1988;113:831–834.
19. Beal S. Sudden infant death syndrome in twins. *Pediatrics* 1989;84:1038–1044.
20. Beckwith JB. Observations on the pathologic anatomy of the sudden infant death syndrome. In: Bergman A, Beckwith JB, Roy CG, eds. *Proceedings of the Second International Conference on the Causes of Sudden Deaths in Infants.* Seattle: University of Washington Press, 1970:83–107.

21. Beckwith JB. The sudden infant death syndrome. *Curr Probl Pediatr* 1973;3:1–36.
22. Beckwith JB. Sudden infant death syndrome: a new theory. *Pediatrics* 1975;55:583–584.
23. Beckwith JB. *The sudden infant death syndrome.* Washington, DC: U.S. Department of HEW, publ. no. (HSA) 76-5137, Government Printing Office, 1976.
24. Beckwith JB. Chronic hypoxemia in the sudden infant death syndrome: a critical review of the data base. In: Tildon JT, Roeder LM, Steinschneider A, eds. *Sudden infant death syndrome.* New York: Academic Press, 1983:145–155.
25. Beckwith JB. Intrathoracic petechial hemorrhages: a clue to the mechanism of sudden infant death syndrome? *Ann N Y Acad Sci* 1988;533:37–47.
26. Belanger PL. Quality assurance and skeletal survey standards. In: Kleinman PK, ed. *Diagnostic imaging in child abuse.* St. Louis: Mosby, 1998:418–423.
27. Berger D. Child abuse simulating "near-miss" sudden infant death syndrome. *J Pediatr* 1979;95:554–556.
28. Berry PJ. Pathological findings in SIDS. *J Clin Pathol* 1992;45:11–16.
29. Black L, David RJ, Brouillette RT, et al. Effects of birth weight and ethnicity on incidence of sudden infant death syndrome. *J Pediatr* 1986;108:209–214.
30. Blair PS, Fleming PJ, Bensley D, et al. Smoking and the sudden infant death syndrome: results from 1993-1995 case-control study for confidential enquiry into stillbirths and deaths in infancy: Confidential Enquiry into Stillbirths and Deaths Regional Coordinators and Researchers. *Br Med J* 1996;313:195–198.
31. Bouvier-Cole MH, Flahaut A, Messiah A, et al. Sudden infant death and immunization: an extensive epidemiological approach to the problem in France, winter 1986. *Int J Epidemiol* 1989;18:121–126.
32. Brackett JC, Sims HF, Steiner RD, et al. A novel mutation in medium chain acyl-CoA dehydrogenase causes sudden neonatal death. *J Clin Invest* 1994;94: 1477–1483.
33. Bruhn FW, Mokrohisky ST, McIntosh K. Apnea associated with respiratory syncytial virus infection in young adults. *J Pediatr* 1977;90:382.
34. Bultreys MG, Greenland S, Kraus JF. Chronic fetal hypoxia and sudden infant death syndrome: interaction between maternal smoking and low hematocrit during pregnancy. *Pediatrics* 1990;86:535–548.
35. Burchell A, Bell JE, Busuttil A, et al. Hepatic microsomal glucose-6-phosphatase system and sudden infant death syndrome. *Lancet* 1989;2:291–294.
36. Burchfield DJ, Rawlings J. Sudden deaths and apparent life-threatening events in hospitalized neonates presumed to be healthy. *Am J Dis Child* 1991;145: 1319–1322.
37. Byard RW, Becker LE, Berry PJ, et al. The pathological approach to sudden infant death: consensus or confusion? Recommendations from the Second SIDS Global Strategy meeting, Stavangar, Norway, August 1994, and the Third Australian SIDS Global Strategy Meeting, Gold Coast Australia, May 1995. *Am J Forensic Med Pathol* 1996;17:103–105.
38. Byard R, Beal S, Bourne A. Potentially dangerous sleeping environments and accidental asphyxia in infancy and early childhood. *Arch Dis Child* 1994;71:497–500.
39. Caffey J. Multiple fractures in the long bones of infants suffering from chronic subdural hematoma. *AJR Am J Roentgenol* 1946;56:163–173.

40. Chasnoff IJ, Burns WJ, Scholl SH, et al. Sudden infant death syndrome in infants of substance-abusing mothers. *N Engl J Med* 1985;313:666–669.

41. Christoffel KK, Zieserl EJ, Chiaramonte J. Should child abuse and neglect be considered when a child dies unexpectedly? *Am J Dis Child* 1985;139: 876–880.

42. Cook RW. Smoking, intra-uterine growth retardation and sudden infant death syndrome. *Int J Epidemiol* 1998;27:238–241.

43. Cross KW, Lewis SR. Upper respiratory obstruction and cot death. *Arch Dis Child* 1971;46:211–213.

44. Davidson-Ward SL, Bautista D, Chan L, et al. Sudden infant death syndrome in infants of substance-abusing mothers. *J Pediatr* 1990;117:876–881.

45. Davidson-Ward SL, Schultz S, Krishna V, et al. Abnormal sleeping ventilating patterns in substance-abusing mothers. *Am J Dis Child* 1986;140:1015–1020.

46. DiMaio DJ, DiMaio VJM. Sudden infant death syndrome. In: DiMaio DJ, DiMaio VJM, eds. *Forensic pathology*. New York: Elsevier Science, 1989:289–297.

47. DiMaio VJM. SIDS or murder? *Pediatrics* 1988;81: 747–748.

48. Durand DJ, Espinoza AM, Nickerson BG. Association between prenatal cocaine exposure and sudden infant death syndrome. *J Pediatr* 1990;117:909.

49. Dwyer T, Ponsonby AL, Newman NM, et al. Prospective cohort study of prone sleeping position and sudden infant death syndrome. *Lancet* 1991;337:1244–1247.

50. Dwyer T, Ponsonby AL. The decline of SIDS: a success story for epidemiology. *Epidemiology* 1996;7: 323–325.

51. Egelund B, Jacobvitz D, Papatola K. Intergenerational continuity of abuse. In: Gelles R, Lancaster J, eds. *Child abuse and neglect:* biosocial dimensions. New York: Aldine Press, 1987:97–104.

52. Ellerstein NS. [Letter]. *N Engl J Med* 1977;296:1296.

53. Emery JL. Infanticide, filicide and cot death. *Arch Dis Child* 1985;60:505–507.

54. Emery JL. Child abuse, sudden infant death syndrome and unexpected infant death. *Am J Dis Child* 1993; 147:1097–1100.

55. Emery JL, Chandra S, Gilbert-Barness EF. Findings in child deaths registered as sudden infant death syndrome (SIDS) in Madison, Wisconsin. *Pediatr Pathol* 1988;8:171–178.

56. Emery JL, Taylor EM. Investigation of SIDS [Letter]. *N Engl J Med* 1986;315:1676.

57. Famularo R, Stone K, Barnum R, et al. Alcoholism and severe child maltreatment. *Am J Orthopsychiatry* 1986;82:888–895.

58. Farber JP, Catron AC, Krous HF. Pulmonary petechiae: ventilatory-circulatory interactions. *Pediatr Res* 1983; 17:230–233.

59. Filiano JJ, Kinney HC. Sudden infant death syndrome and brainstem research. *Pediatr Ann* 1995;24:379–383.

60. Filiano JJ, Kinney HC. A perspective on neuropathological findings in victims of sudden infant death syndrome. *Biol Neonate* 1990;15:194–197.

61. Filiano JJ, Kinney HC. Arcuate nucleus hypoplasia in the sudden infant death syndrome. *J Neuropathol Exp Neurol* 1992;51:394–403.

62. Firstman R, Talan J. *The death of innocents.* New York: Bantam Books, 1997.

63. Fleming PJ, Blair PS, Bacon C, et al. Environment of infants during sleep and risk of the sudden infant death syndrome: results of 1993-1995 case-control study for confidential enquiry into stillbirths and deaths in infancy: Confidential Enquiry into Stillbirths and Deaths Regional Coordinators and Researchers. *Br Med J* 1996;313:191–195.

64. Folgering H, Kuyper F, Kille JF. Primary alveolar hypoventilation (Ondine's curse syndrome) in an infant without external arcuate nucleus: case report. *Bull Eur Physiopathol Respir* 1979;15:659–665.

65. Geertinger P. *Sudden death in infancy:* American lecture *series.* Springfield, IL: Charles C Thomas, 1968.

66. Granik, LA, Durfee M, Wells SJ. *Child death review teams: a manual for design and implementation.* Chicago: American Bar Association, 1992.

67. Grether JK, Schulman J. Sudden infant death syndrome and birth weight. *J Pediatr* 1989;114:561–567.

68. Grether JK, Schulman J, Croen LA. Sudden infant death syndrome among Asians in California. *J Pediatr* 1990;116:525–528.

69. Griffin MR, Ray WA, Livengood JR, et al. Risk of sudden infant death syndrome after immunization with the diphtheria-tetanus-pertussis vaccine. *N Engl J Med* 1988;319:618–622.

70. Griffith JL, Slovik LS. Munchausen syndrome by proxy and sleep disorders medicine. *Sleep* 1989;12: 178–183.

71. Groothius JR, Altemeier WA, Robarge JP, et al. Increased child abuse in families with twins. *Pediatrics* 1982;70:769–773.

72. Guilleminault C, Ariagno RL, Forno LS, et al. Obstructive sleep apnea and near miss SIDS. I. Report of an infant with sudden death. *Pediatrics* 1979;63: 837–843.

73. Guilleminault C, Heldt G, Powell N, et al. Small upper airway in near-miss sudden infant death syndrome infants and their families. *Lancet* 1986;1:402–407.

74. Guntheroth WG. In: *Crib death. The sudden infant death syndrome.* Mount Kisko, NY: Futura Publishing, 1989:130–132.

75. Guntheroth WG, Spiers PS. Prolongation of the QT interval and the sudden infant death syndrome. *Pediatrics* 1999;103:813–814.

76. Guntheroth WG, Spiers PS, Naeye RL. Redefinition of the sudden infant death syndrome: the disadvantages. *Pediatr Pathol* 1994;14:127–132.

77. Haglund B, Cnattingius S. Cigarette smoking as a risk factor for sudden infant death syndrome: a population-based study. *Am J Public Health* 1990;80:29–32.

78. Hall CB, Kopelman AE, Douglas RG, et al. Neonatal respiratory syncytial virus infection. *N Engl J Med* 1979;300:393–396.

79. Hanzlick R. Impediments in death investigations. *Arch Pathol Lab Med* 1996;120:329–332.

80. Harpey J-P, Charpentier C, Paturneau-Jonas M. Sudden infant death syndrome and inherited disorders of fatty acid β-oxidation. *Biol Neonate* 1990;48:770–808.

81. Herman-Giddens ME, Brown G, Verbiest S, et al. Under-ascertainment of child abuse mortality in the United States. *JAMA* 1999;282:463–467.

82. Hodgman JE, Siassi B. Prolonged QT_c as a risk factor for SIDS. *Pediatrics* 1999;103:814–815.

83. Hoffman JIE, Lister G. The implications of a relationship between prolonged QT interval and the sudden infant death syndrome. *Pediatrics* 1999;103:815–817.

84. Hoffman HF, Damus K, Hillman L, et al. Risk factors for SIDS: results of the National Institute of Child

Health and Human Development SIDS Cooperative Study. *Ann N Y Acad Sci* 1988;53:13–30.

84a. Hunter RS, Killstrom N. Breaking the cycle in abusive families. *Am J Psychiatr* 1979;136:1320–1326.

85. Irgens LM, Skjaerven R, Peterson DR. Prospective assessment of recurrence risk in sudden infant death syndrome siblings. *J Pediatr* 1984;104:349–351.

86. Iyasu S, Hanzlick R, Rowley D, et al. Proceedings of "Workshop on Guidelines for Scene Investigation of Sudden Unexplained Infant Deaths," July 12-13, 1993. *J Forensic Sci* 1994;39:1126–1136.

87. Iyasu S, Rowley D, Hanzlick R. Guidelines for death scene investigation of sudden unexplained infant deaths: recommendations of the interagency panel on sudden infant death syndrome. *J SIDS Infant Mortality* 1996;1:183–202.

88. Kahn A. Polysomnographic studies of infants who subsequently died of sudden infant death syndrome. *Pediatrics* 1988;82:721–727.

89. Kahn A, Blum D, Muller MF, et al. Sudden infant death syndrome in a twin: a comparison of sibling histories. *Pediatrics* 1986;78:146–150.

90. Kahn A, Rebuffat E, Sottiaux M, et al. Recent advances in sudden infant death syndrome: possible autonomic dysfunction of the airways in infants at risk. *Lung* 1990;168(suppl):920–924.

91. Kandall SR, Gaines J, Habel L, et al. Relationship of maternal substance abuse to subsequent sudden infant death syndrome in offspring. *J Pediatr* 1993;123:120–126.

92. Kaplan SR. *Child fatality legislation in the United States.* Chicago: American Bar Association, 1992.

93. Kaplan SR, Granik LA, eds. *Child fatality investigative procedures manual.* Chicago: American Bar Association, 1992.

94. Kattwinkel J, Brooks JS, Keenan ME, et al. Changing concepts of sudden infant death syndrome: implications for infant sleeping environment and sleep position. *Pediatrics* 2000;105:650–656.

95. Kaufman J, Zigler E. The intergenerational transmission of child abuse. In: Cicchetti D, Carlson V, eds. *Child maltreatment theory and research on the causes and consequences of child abuse and neglect.* New York: Cambridge University Press, 1989:129–150.

96. Kempe CH, Silverman FN, Steele BF, et al. The battered child syndrome. *JAMA* 1962;181:105–112.

97. Kinney HC, Filiano JJ. Brainstem research in sudden infant death syndrome. *Pediatrician* 1988;15:240–250.

98. Kinney HC, Filiano JJ, Assmann SF, et al. Tritiated-naloxone binding to brainstem opioid receptors in the sudden infant death syndrome. *J Auton Nerv Syst* 1998;69:156–163.

99. Kinney HC, Filiano JJ, Sleeper LA, et al. Decreased muscarinic receptor binding in the arcuate nucleus in sudden infant death syndrome. *Science* 1995;269:1446–1450.

100. Kinney HC, Filiano JJ, Harper RM. The neuropathology of sudden infant death syndrome: a review. *J Neuropathol Exp Neurol* 1992;51:115–126.

101. Kinney HC, Panigrahy A, Rava LA, et al. Three-dimensional distribution of (^{3}H) quinuclidinyl benzilate binding to muscarinic cholinergic receptors in the developing human brainstem. *J Comp Neurol* 1995;362:350–367.

102. Kirschner RH, Stein RJ. The mistaken diagnosis of child abuse: a form of medical abuse? *Am J Dis Child* 1985;139:873.

103. Kleeman WJ, Wiechern V, Schuck M, et al. Intrathoracic and subconjunctival petechiae in sudden infant death syndrome (SIDS). *Forensic Sci Int* 1995;72:49–54.

104. Kleinman PK, ed. *Diagnostic imaging in child abuse.* St. Louis: Mosby, 1998.

105. Kleinman PK, Blackbourne BD, Marks SC Jr, et al. Radiologic contributions to the investigation and prosecution of cases of fatal infant abuse. *N Engl J Med* 1989;320:507–511.

105a. Kleinman PK, Marks SC Jr, Richmond JM, et al. Inflicted skeletal injury: a postmortem radiologic-histopathologic study in 31 infants. *AJR Am J Roentgenol* 1995;165:647–650.

106. Klonoff-Cohen HS, Edelstein SL, Lefkowitz ES, et al. The effect of passive smoking and tobacco exposure through breast milk on sudden infant death syndrome. *JAMA* 1995;273:795–798.

107. Korbin JE. Incarcerated mothers' perceptions and interpretations of their fatally maltreated children. *Child Abuse Negl* 1987;11:397–407.

108. Korbin JE. Childhood histories of women imprisoned for fatal child maltreatment. *Child Abuse Negl* 1986;10:331–338.

109. Kraus JF, Borhani NO. Post-neonatal sudden unexplained death in California: a cohort study. *Am J Epidemiol* 1972;95:497–510.

110. Kraus JF, Bultreys M. The epidemiology of sudden infant death syndrome. In: Kiely M, ed. *Reproductive and perinatal epidemiology.* Boca Raton: CRC Press, 1991:219–249.

111. Kraus JF, Greenland S, Bultreys M. Risk factors for sudden infant death syndrome in the US Collaborative Perinatal Project. *Int J Epidemiol* 1989;18:113–120.

112. Krous HF. The microscopic distribution of intrathoracic petechiae in sudden infant death syndrome. *Arch Pathol Lab Med* 1984;108:77–79.

113. Krous HF. Pathological considerations of sudden infant death syndrome. *Pediatrician* 1988;15:231–239.

114. Krous HF. Instruction and reference manual for the international standardized autopsy protocol for sudden unexpected infant death. *J SIDS Infant Mortality* 1996;1:203–246.

115. Krous HF, Jordan J. A necropsy study of distribution of petechiae in non-sudden infant death syndrome. *Arch Pathol Lab Med* 1989;108:75–76.

116. Krous HF, Valdes-Dapena M, McClatchey M, et al. Laryngeal basement membrane thickening is not a reliable postmortem marker for SIDS: results from the Chicago Infant Mortality Study. Fifth SIDS Research Conference, Rouen, France, 1998.

117. Kumar P, Taxy J, Angst EB, et al. Autopsies in children: are they still useful? *Arch Pediatr Adolesc Med* 1998;152:558–563.

118. Lie JT, Rosenberg HS, Erickson EE. Histopathology of the conduction system in the sudden infant death syndrome. *Circulation* 1976;53:3–8.

119. Little RE, Peterson DR. Sudden infant death syndrome epidemiology: a review and update. *Epidemiol Rev* 1990;12:241–246.

120. Luallen JJ, Rochat RW, Smith SM, et al. Child fatality review in Georgia: a young system demonstrates its potential for identifying preventable childhood deaths. *South Med J* 1998;91:414–419.

121. MacDorman MF, Cnattingius S, Hoffman HJ, et al. Sudden infant death syndrome and smoking in the United States and Sweden. *Am J Epidemiol* 1997;146:249–257.

122. Malloy MH, Freeman DH. Sudden infant death syndrome among twins. *Arch Pediatr Adolesc Med* 1999; 153:736–740.
123. Mandell F. *Pediatr Alert* July 17, 1986.
124. Martin RJ, Miller MJ, Redline S. Screening for SIDS: a neonatal perspective. *Pediatrics* 1999;103:812–813.
125. McNamara F, Sullivan CE. Obstructive sleep apnea in infants: relation to family history of sudden infant death syndrome, apparent life-threatening events, and obstructive sleep apnea. *J Pediatr* 2000;136:318–323.
126. Meadow R. Munchausen syndrome by proxy: the hinterland of child abuse. *Lancet* 1977;2:343–345.
127. Meadow R. Suffocation, recurrent apnea and sudden infant death. *J Pediatr* 1990;117:351–357.
128. Meadow R. Unnatural sudden infant death. *Arch Dis Child* 1999;80:7–14.
129. Milerad J, Rajs J, Gidlund E. Nicotine and cotinine levels in pericardial fluid in victims of SIDS. *Acta Paediatr* 1994;83:59–62.
130. Milerad J, Sundell H. Nicotine exposure and the risk of SIDS. *Acta Pediatr Suppl* 1993;82:70–72.
131. Miller D, Challas G. Abused children as adult parents: a twenty-five year longitudinal study. Paper presented at the National Conference for Family Violence Researchers, Durham, NC, 1981.
132. Mitchell EA, Brunt JM, Everard C. Reduction in mortality from sudden infant death syndrome in New Zealand 1986-1992. *Arch Dis Child* 1994;70:291–294.
133. Mitchell EA, Ford RP, Stewart AW, et al. Smoking and the sudden infant death syndrome. *Pediatrics* 1993; 91:893–896.
134. Mitchell EA, Stewart AW, Clements M. Immunisation and the sudden infant death syndrome: New Zealand Cot Death Study Group. *Arch Dis Child* 1995;73: 498–501.
135. Mitchell EA, Tuohy PG, Brunt JM, et al. Risk factors for sudden infant death syndrome following the prevention campaign in New Zealand: a prospective study. *Pediatrics* 1997;100:835–840.
136. Mosko S, McKenna J, Dickel M, et al. Parent-infant cosleeping: the appropriate context for the study of infant sleep and implications for sudden infant death syndrome (SIDS) research. *J Behav Med* 1993;16: 589–610.
137. Mosko S, Richard C, McKenna J. Infant arousals during mother-infant bed sharing: implications for infant sleep and sudden infant death syndrome research. *Pediatrics* 1997;100:841–849.
138. Mosko S, Richard C, McKenna J, et al. Maternal proximity and infant CO_2 environment during bedsharing and possible implications for SIDS research. *Am J Phys Anthropol* 1997;103:315–328.
139. Naeye RL. Pulmonary arterial abnormalities in the sudden infant death syndrome. *N Engl J Med* 1973; 289:1167–1170.
140. Naeye RL. Hypoxemia and the sudden infant death syndrome. *Science* 1974;186:837.
141. Naeye RL, Ladis B, Drage JS. Sudden infant death syndrome. *Am J Dis Child* 1976;130:1207–1210.
142. Nagao M. Frequency of 985A-to-G mutation in medium-chain acyl-CoA dehydrogenase gene among patients with sudden infant death syndrome, Reye syndrome, severe motor and intellectual disabilities and healthy newborns in Japan. *Acta Paediatr Jpn* 1996; 38:304–307.
143. O'Halloran RL, Ferratta F, Harris M, et al. Child abuse reports in families with sudden infant death syndrome. *Am J Forensic Med Pathol* 1998;19:57–62.
144. Ostea EM, Ostea AR, Simpson PM. Mortality within the first 2 years in infants exposed to cocaine, opiate or cannabinoid during gestation. *Pediatrics* 1997; 100:79–83.
145. Panigrahy A, Filiano JJ, Sleeper LA, et al. Decreased kainite binding in the arcuate nucleus of sudden infant death syndrome. *J Neuropathol Exp Neurol* 1997;56: 1253–1261.
146. Perlstein PH, Edwards NK, Sutherland JM. Apnea in premature infants and incubator-air temperature changes. *N Engl J Med* 1970;282:461–466.
147. Perrot LJ, Nawojczyk S. Non-natural death masquerading as SIDS (sudden infant death syndrome). *Am J Forensic Med Pathol* 1988;9:105–111.
148. Peterson DR. SIDS in infants of drug dependent mothers. [Letter]. *J Pediatr* 1980;96:784.
149. Peterson DR. Clinical implications of sudden infant death syndrome epidemiology. *Pediatrician* 1988;15: 198–203.
150. Peterson DR, Sabotta EE, Daling JR. Infant mortality among subsequent siblings of infants who died of sudden infant death syndrome. *J Pediatr* 1986;108: 911–914.
151. Poets CF, Meny RG, Chobanian MR, et al. Gasping and other cardiorespiratory patterns during sudden infant deaths. *Pediatr Res* 1999;45:350–354.
152. Ponsonby AL, Couper D, Dwyer T. Features of infant exposure to tobacco smoke in a cohort study in Tasmania. *J Epidemiol Commun Health* 1996;50:40–46.
153. Ponsonby AL, Dwyer T, Gibbons LE, et al. The infant thermal environment and sudden infant death syndrome: a case-control study. *Br Med J* 1992;304: 277–282.
154. Ponsonby AL, Dwyer T, Gibbons LE, et al. Factors potentiating the risk of sudden infant death syndrome associated with the prone position. *N Engl J Med* 1993;329:377–382.
155. Ramos V, Hernandez A, Villanueva E. Simultaneous death of twins: an environmental hazard or SIDS? *Am J Forensic Med Pathol* 1997;18:75–78.
156. Reece RM. Fatal child abuse and sudden infant death syndrome: a critical diagnostic decision. *Pediatrics* 1993;91:423–429.
157. Robertson LD, Deroo LA, Gaudina JA, et al. Decrease in infant mortality and sudden infant death syndrome among Northwest American Indians and Alaskan Natives, Pacific Northwest 1985-1996. *MMWR* 1999;48: 181–184.
158. Rosen CL, Frost JD, Bricker T, et al. Two siblings with recurrent respiratory arrest: Munchausen syndrome by proxy or child abuse? *Pediatrics* 1983;71:715–720.
159. Rosen CL, Frost JD, Glaze DG. Child abuse and recurrent infant apnea. *J Pediatr* 1986;109:1065–1067.
160. Schechtman VL, Harper RM, Wilson AJ, et al. Sleep apnea in infants who succumb to the sudden infant death syndrome. *Sleep* 1988;11:413–424.
161. Schechtman VL, Harper RM, Wilson AJ, et al. Sleep apnea in infants who succumb to the sudden infant death syndrome. *Pediatrics* 1991;87:841–846.
162. Schloesser P, Pierpont J, Poertner J. Active surveillance of child abuse fatalities. *Child Abuse Negl* 1992;16:3.
163. Schoendorf KC, Kiely JL. Relationship of sudden infant death syndrome to maternal smoking during and after pregnancy. *Pediatrics* 1992;90:905–908.

164. Schulman JD. Letter from the Genetics and IVJ Institute. 3020 Javier Rd, Fairfax, VA: 22031 (1-800-654-GENE).
165. Schwartz PJ. The quest for the mechanisms of the sudden infant death syndrome: doubts and progress. *Circulation* 1987;75:677–683.
166. Schwartz PJ, Montemerlo M, Facchini P, et al. The QT interval throughout the first six months of life: a prospective study. *Circulation* 1982;66:496–501.
167. Schwartz PJ, Stramba-Badiale M, Segantini A, et al. Prolongation of the QT interval and the sudden infant death syndrome. *N Engl J Med* 1998;338:1709–1714.
168. Scott PD. Fatal battered baby cases. *Med Sci Law* 1973;13:197–206.
169. Scott PD. Parents who kill their children. *Med Sci Law* 1973;13:120–126.
170. Scragg R, Mitchell EA. Side sleeping position and bed sharing in the sudden infant death syndrome. *Ann Med* 1998;30:345–349.
171. Scragg R, Mitchell EA, Taylor BJ, et al. Bed sharing, smoking, and alcohol in the sudden infant death syndrome: New Zealand Cot Death Study Group. *Br Med J* 1993;307:1312–1318.
172. Segantini A, Varisco T, Monza E, et al. QT interval and the sudden infant death syndrome: a prospective study. *J Am Coll Cardiol* 1986;7:118A.
173. Shannon DC, Kelly DH. SIDS and near SIDS. *N Engl J Med* 1982;306:959–1028.
174. Shatz A, Hiss J, Arensburg B. Basement membrane thickening of the vocal cords in sudden infant death syndrome. *Laryngoscope* 1991;101:484–486.
175. Shatz A, Hiss J, Arensburg B. Myocarditis misdiagnosed as sudden infant death syndrome (SIDS). *Med Sci Law* 1997;37:16–18.
176. Shatz A, Hiss J, Hammel I, et al. Age-related basement membrane thickening of the vocal cords in sudden infant death syndrome (SIDS). *Laryngoscope* 1994;104:865–868.
177. Shiono PH, Klebanoff MA, Rhoads GG. Smoking and drinking during pregnancy: their effects on preterm birth. *JAMA* 1986;255:82.
178. Silverman FN. The roentgen manifestations of unrecognized skeletal trauma in infants. *AJR Am J Roentgenol* 1953;69:413–427.
179. Smialek JE. Simultaneous sudden infant death syndrome in twins. *Pediatrics* 1986;77:816–821.
180. Southall DP. Identification of infants destined to die unexpectedly during infancy: evaluation of predictive importance of prolonged apnoea and disorders of cardiac rhythm or conduction. *Br Med J* 1983;286:1092–1096.
181. Southall DP. Examine data in Schwartz article with extreme care. *Pediatrics* 1999;103:819–820.
182. Southall DP, Arrowsmith WA, Alexander JR. QT interval measurements before sudden infant death syndrome. *Arch Dis Child* 1986;61:327–333.
183. Southall DP, Plunkett MCB, Banks MW, et al. Covert video recordings of life-threatening child abuse: lessons for child protection. *Pediatrics* 1997;100:735–760.
184. Southall DP, Stebbins VA, Rees SV, et al. Apnoeic episodes induced by smothering: two cases identified by covert video surveillance. *Br Med J* 1987;294:1637–1641.
185. Southall DP, Stevens V, Franks CI, et al. Sinus tachycardia in term infants preceding sudden infant death. *Eur J Pediatr* 1988;147:74.
186. Sparks DL, Hunsaker JC. Increased ALZ-50-reactive neurons in the brains of SIDS infants: an indicator of greater neuronal death? *J Child Neurol* 1991;6:123–127.
187. Spiers PS. Estimated rates of concordance for the sudden infant death syndrome in twins. *Am J Epidemiol* 1974;100:1–7.
188. Stanton AN. Overheating and cot death. *Lancet* 1984;2:1199–1201.
189. Stanton AN, Oakley JR. Pattern of illnesses before cot death. *Arch Dis Child* 1983;58:878–888.
190. Stark AR, Thach BT. Mechanisms of airway obstruction leading to apnea in newborn infants. *J Pediatr* 1976;89:982–985.
191. Starling S, Holden JR, Jenny C. Abusive head trauma: the relationship of perpetrators to their victims. *Pediatrics* 1995;95:259–262.
192. Steele BF. Parental abuse of infants and small children. In: Anthony EJ, Benedek T, eds. *Parenthood: its psychology and psychopathology.* Boston: Little, Brown, 1970:xx–xx.
193. Steele BF. Psychodynamic factors in child abuse. In: Helfer ME, Kempe RS, Krugman RD, eds. *The battered child.* 5th ed. Chicago: University of Chicago Press, 1997:73–103.
194. Steele BF, Pollock C. A psychiatric study of parents who abuse infants and small children. In: Helfner RE, Kempe CH, eds. *The battered child.* 1st ed. Chicago: University of Chicago Press, 1968.
195. Steinschneider A. Prolonged apnea and the sudden infant death syndrome: clinical and laboratory investigations. *Pediatrics* 1972;50:646–654.
196. Sturner WQ. Common errors in forensic pediatric pathology. *Am J Forensic Med Pathol* 1998;19:317–320.
197. Sudden infant death syndrome: United States, 1983-1994. *MMWR* 1996;45:859–863.
198. Taylor EM, Emery JL. Categories of preventable unexpected infant deaths. *Arch Dis Child* 1990;65:535–539.
199. Thach BT. Sudden infant death syndrome: old causes rediscovered? *N Engl J Med* 1986;315:126–128.
200. Thach BT, Davies AM, Koenig JS. Pathophysiology of sudden upper airway obstruction in sleeping infants and its relevance for SIDS. *Ann N Y Acad Sci* 1988;533:314–328.
201. Thomas DB. Narcotic addiction and the sudden infant death syndrome [Letter]. *Med J Aust* 1988;149:562.
202. Tonkin SL, Beach D. The vulnerability of the infant upper airway. In: Harper RM, Hoffman HJ, eds. *Sudden infant death syndrome risk factors and basic mechanisms.* New York: PMA Publishing Corp 1988:417–422.
203. Tonkin SL, Clarkson PM. A view from New Zealand: comments on the prolonged QT theory of SIDS causation. *Pediatrics* 1999;103:818–819.
204. Toubas PL, Duke JC. Effects of maternal smoking and caffeine habits on infantile apnea: a retrospective study. *Pediatrics* 1986;78:159–163.
205. Valdes-Dapena MA. *Sudden unexplained infant death, 1970-1975: an evolution in understanding.* U.S. Department of HEW, publ. (HSA) 80-5255. Washington DC: Government Printing Office, 1980.
206. Valdes-Dapena M. The pathologist and sudden infant death syndrome. *Am J Pathol* 1982;106:118–131.
207. Valdes-Dapena MA, Green M, Basavanand N, et al. The myocardial conduction system in sudden death in infancy. *N Engl J Med* 1973;289:1179–1180.
208. Valdes-Dapena M, Huff D. *Perinatal autopsy manual.* Washington, DC: Armed Forces Institute of Pathology, 1983.

209. Valdes-Dapena M, Mandell F, Merritt TA. [Letter]. *N Engl J Med* 1986;315:1675–1676.
210. Vawter GF, Kozakewich HPW. Aspects of morphologic variation amongst SIDS victims. In: Tildon JT, Roeder LM, Steinschneider A, eds. *Sudden infant death syndrome.* New York: Academic Press, 1983: 163–170.
211. Wallace BC. *Crack cocaine: a practical treatment approach for the chemically dependent.* New York: Brunner/Magel, 1991.
212. Ward SL, Bautista D, Chan L, et al. Sudden infant death syndrome in infants of substance-abusing mothers. *J Pediatr* 1990;117:876–881.
213. Widom CS. Does violence beget violence? A critical examination of the literature. *Psychol Bull* 1989;106: 3–28.
214. Widom CS. The cycle of violence. *Science* 1989;244: 160–166.
215. Williamson SL, Perrot LL. The significance of post-mortem radiographs in infants. *J Forensic Sci* 1990; 35:365–367.
216. Willinger M, James LS, Catz C. Defining the sudden infant death syndrome (SIDS): deliberations of an expert panel convened by the National Institutes of Child Health and Human Development. *Pediatr Pathol* 1991; 11:677–684.
217. Willinger M, Hoffman HJ, Wu KT, et al. Factors associated with the transition to nonprone sleep positions of infants in the United States: the National Infant Sleep Position Study. *JAMA* 1998;280:329–335.
218. Zec N, Filiano JJ, Kinney HC. Anatomic relationships of the human arcuate nucleus of the medulla: a Dil-labeling study (published erratum appears in *J Neuropathol Exp Neurol* 1997;56:509–522).
219. Zumwalt RE, Hirsch CS. Subtle fatal child abuse. *Hum Pathol* 1980;11:167–174.

21

Medicolegal Aspects of Child Abuse

John E.B. Myers

McGeorge School of Law, University of the Pacific, Sacramento, California

The medical profession plays a key role in protecting abused and neglected children. This chapter is a discussion of the impact of law on medical practice related to child abuse and neglect.

FORENSIC IMPLICATIONS OF CHILDREN'S DISCLOSURE: STATEMENTS DURING PHYSICAL EXAMINATIONS AND INTERVIEWS

Many children disclose abuse to medical professionals. The diagnostic importance of children's disclosure statements is described elsewhere in this text. Children's statements during examinations and interviews have forensic as well as medical significance. This section provides a description of the critical forensic importance of documenting children's disclosure statements, and addresses the use of suggestive and leading questions with children.

Children's Statements Describing Abuse Are Hearsay

Professionals are aware of the forensic importance of medical and laboratory evidence of abuse. Professionals may, however, be less cognizant of the important legal implications of children's words during examinations and interviews. If children's statements are properly documented, they may be admissible in subsequent legal proceedings (i.e., the child's words become legal evidence of abuse or ne-

glect). In some cases, the child's statements to professionals are the most compelling evidence of maltreatment. Suppose, for example, that while 4-year-old Beth is being examined by a physician, the child points to her genital area and says, "Daddy put his pee-pee in me down there. Then he took it out and shook it up and down until white stuff came out." Beth's words are compelling evidence of abuse. In subsequent criminal proceedings against Beth's father, the prosecutor calls the examining physician as a witness and asks the physician to repeat Beth's words and to describe her pointing gesture for the jury. Before the doctor can speak, however, the father's defense attorney objects that Beth's words and gesture are hearsay. The rule in all states is that hearsay is inadmissible in criminal and civil litigation unless the particular hearsay statement meets the requirements of an exception to the rule against hearsay.

To determine whether Beth's description of abuse is hearsay, analyze Beth's words in terms of the following definition. A child's words are hearsay if three requirements are fulfilled: (a) the child's words were intended by the child to describe something that happened; and (b) the child's words were spoken before the court proceeding at which the words are repeated by someone who heard the child speak; and (c) the child's words are offered in court to prove that what the child said actually happened (20–22).

Analysis of Beth's words describing abuse reveal that they are hearsay. First, Beth in-

545

tended to describe something that happened. Second, Beth spoke before the proceeding where the prosecutor asks the physician to repeat Beth's words. Finally, the prosecutor offers Beth's words to prove that what the child said actually happened.

Beth's words are not the only hearsay, however. Her gesture pointing to her genital area also is hearsay. The gesture was nonverbal communication intended by Beth to describe the abuse.

The judge will sustain the defense attorney's hearsay objection unless the prosecutor persuades the judge that Beth's words and gesture meet the requirements of an exception to the rule against hearsay. In this, as in many other child abuse cases, the prosecutor's ability to convince the judge that the child's hearsay statement meets the requirements of an exception depends as much on the conduct of the physician as on the legal acumen of the prosecutor. If the doctor knew what to watch for and document when Beth disclosed the abuse, the prosecutor has a better chance of persuading the judge to allow the doctor to repeat Beth's powerful hearsay statement.

Although the rule against hearsay has many exceptions, only a few play a day-to-day role in child abuse and neglect litigation. Five hearsay exceptions are briefly discussed.

The Excited Utterance Exception

An excited utterance is a hearsay statement that relates to a startling event. The statement must be made while the child is under the acute emotional stress caused by the startling event. Excited utterances can be used in court even though they are hearsay. Judges consider all relevant circumstances to determine whether a hearsay statement is an excited utterance. Professionals can document the following important factors:

1. *Nature of the event.* Some events are more startling than others, and judges consider the likely impact a particular event would have on a child of similar age and experience.

2. *Amount of time elapsed between the startling event and the child's statement relating to the event.* The more time that passes between a startling event and a child's statement describing it, the less likely a judge is to conclude that the statement is an excited utterance. Although passage of time is important, time alone is not dispositive. Judges have approved delays ranging from a few minutes to several hours. Elapsed time is considered along with other factors indicating presence or absence of excitement.

3. *Indications the child was emotionally upset when the child spoke.* Judges consider whether the child was crying, frightened, or otherwise upset when the statement was made. If the child was injured or in pain, a judge is more likely to find an excited utterance.

4. *Child's speech pattern.* In some cases, the way the child speaks (e.g., pressured or hurried speech) indicates emotional excitement.

5. *Extent to which the child's statement was spontaneous.* Spontaneity is a critical factor in the excited utterance exception. The more spontaneous the statement, the more likely it meets the requirements of this exception.

6. *Number and type of questions used to elicit the child's statement.* Asking questions does not necessarily destroy the spontaneity required for the excited utterance exception. As questions become leading, however, spontaneity may dissipate, undermining applicability of this exception.

7. *First safe opportunity.* In many cases, abused children remain under the control of the abuser for minutes or hours after the abusive incident. When the child is finally released to a trusted adult, the child has the first safe opportunity to disclose what happened. A child's statement at the first safe opportunity may qualify as an excited utterance even though considerable time has elapsed since the abuse occurred.

Fresh Complaint of Sexual Assault

A child's initial disclosure of sexual abuse may be admissible in court under an ancient legal doctrine called fresh complaint of rape or sexual assault. In most states, a child's fresh complaint is not, technically speaking, hearsay.

Statements to Professionals Providing Diagnostic or Treatment Services

Most states have an exception to the hearsay rule for certain statements to professionals providing diagnostic or treatment services. The professional may be a physician, nurse, or technician. This exception is commonly called the diagnosis or treatment exception. The exception includes the child's statement describing medical history. Also included are statements describing present symptoms, pain, and other sensations. Finally, the exception includes the child's description of the cause of illness or injury.

In many cases, the child is the one who provides the information that is admissible under the diagnosis or treatment exception. On occasion, however, an adult describes the child's history and symptoms to a professional. As long as the adult's motive is to obtain treatment for the child, the adult's statements are admissible under this exception.

The primary rationale for the diagnosis or treatment exception is that hearsay statements to professionals providing diagnostic or treatment services are reliable. Reliability exists because the patient has a strong incentive to be truthful with the professional. This rationale is applicable for many older children and adolescents. Some young children, however, may not understand the need for accuracy and candor with health care providers. When a child does not understand that personal well-being may be affected by the accuracy of what is said, the primary rationale for the diagnosis or treatment exception evaporates, and the judge may rule that the child's hearsay statement does not satisfy the exception.

The diagnosis or treatment exception has its clearest application with children receiving traditional medical care in a hospital, clinic, or physician's office. Most children have at least some understanding of doctors and nurses, and of the importance of telling the clinician "what really happened." Judges are less certain about the applicability of the diagnosis or treatment exception with psychotherapy. In psychotherapy, the child may not understand the importance of accuracy, thus undermining the rationale of the exception. If, however, the child understands the need for accuracy with the mental health professional, most judges conclude that the exception applies.

To increase the probability that a child's statements satisfy the diagnosis or treatment exception to the rule against hearsay, the professional can take the following steps:

1. Discuss with the child the clinical importance of providing accurate information, and of being completely forthcoming. For example, the physician might say, "Hello, I'm Dr. Jones, I'm a doctor and I'm going to give you a check-up to make sure everything is okay. While you are here today, I'll ask you some questions so I can help you. It's important for you to listen carefully to my questions. When you answer my questions, be sure to tell me everything you know. Okay? Tell me only things that really happened. Don't pretend or make things up. Will you do that for me? Your answers to questions help me to do my job as a doctor, so it is important for you to tell me only things that really happened."

2. The diagnosis or treatment exception requires that information supplied to the professional be pertinent to diagnosis or treatment. Thus it is important to document how information disclosed by the child is pertinent to diagnosis or treatment.

3. If the child identifies the perpetrator, the professional should document why knowing the identity of the perpetrator is pertinent to diagnosis or treatment. For example, knowing the identity of the perpetrator may be important to determine whether it is safe to send the child home. The physi-

cian needs the perpetrator's identity if sexually transmitted disease is a possibility.

4. Document the foregoing factors in the child's chart.

The Residual and Child Hearsay Exceptions

Many states have a hearsay exception known as a residual or catch-all exception, which allows use in court of reliable hearsay statements that do not meet the requirements of one of the traditional exceptions, such as the excited utterance exception. A majority of states also have a special hearsay exception for statements by children in child abuse cases. These "child hearsay exceptions" and residual exceptions allow use in court of children's reliable hearsay statements that do not fit into another exception.

When a child's hearsay statement is offered under a residual or child hearsay exception, the most important question is whether the statement is reliable. Professionals who interview, examine, and treat children play an indispensable role in documenting the information judges consider when determining whether children's statements are sufficiently reliable to be admitted under a residual or child hearsay exception. Professionals can document the following information:

1. *Spontaneity.* The more spontaneous the child's statement, the more likely a judge will find it reliable.
2. *Statements elicited by questioning.* The reliability of a child's statement may be influenced by the type of questions asked. When questions are suggestive or leading, the possibility increases that the questioner influenced the child's statement. It should be noted, however, that suggestive questions are sometimes necessary to elicit information from children, particularly when the information is embarrassing (10,12,16,22,24,27,30).
3. *Consistent statements.* Reliability may be increased if the child's description of abuse is consistent over time. Consis-

tency regarding core details is most important. Inconsistency regarding peripheral details is marginally relevant.
4. *Child's affect and emotion when hearsay statement is made.* When a child's emotions are consistent with the child's statement, the reliability of the statement may be enhanced.
5. *Play or gestures that corroborate the child's hearsay statement.* The play or gestures of a young child may strengthen confidence in the child's statement. For example, the child's use of anatomic dolls may support the reliability of the child's statement (22).
6. *Developmentally unusual sexual knowledge.* A young child's developmentally unusual knowledge of sexual acts or anatomy supports the reliability of the child's statement (7,8,21,22).
7. *Idiosyncratic detail.* Presence in a child's statement of idiosyncratic details of sexual acts points to reliability. Jones and McQuiston (13) wrote, "[i]diosyncracy in the sexual abuse account is exemplified by children who describe smells and tastes associated with rectal, vaginal, or oral sex."
8. *Child's belief that disclosure might lead to punishment of the child.* Children hesitate to make statements they believe may get them in trouble. If a child believed disclosing abuse could result in punishment, confidence in the child's statement may increase.
9. *Child's or adult's motive to fabricate.* Evidence that the child or an adult had a motive to fabricate allegations of abuse affects reliability.
10. *Medical evidence of abuse.* The child's statement may be corroborated by medical evidence (see Chapter 10).
11. *Changes in child's behavior.* When a child's behavior alters in a way that corroborates the child's description of abuse, it may be appropriate to place increased confidence in the child's statement (22).

None of the foregoing factors is a litmus test for reliability. Judges consider the totality of the circumstances to evaluate reliability, and professionals can assist the legal system by documenting anything that indicates the child was or was not telling the truth when describing abuse.

Importance of Documentation

Medical professionals are in an excellent position to document children's hearsay statements. Without careful documentation of exactly what questions are asked and exactly what children say, the professional will not likely remember months or years later, when the professional is called as a witness and asked to repeat what the child said. Documentation is needed not only to preserve the child's words, but also to preserve a record of the factors indicating that the child's hearsay statements meet the requirements of an exception to the hearsay rule.

Use of Suggestive or Leading Questions during Interviews of Children

There is no single "correct" way to interview children who may be abused or neglected (12,22,27). Increasingly, however, defense attorneys challenge the way professionals talk to children (21,22,24). Defense attorneys are particularly fond of criticizing leading questions. A leading question is a question that contains a suggestion of what the answer should be. Thus a leading question is a suggestive question—a question that tempts a child to give a particular answer.

When talking to a child who may be a victim of abuse, the professional should create an atmosphere in which the child feels comfortable. Initial questioning should be as nonsuggestive and nonleading as possible (12,22,27). The professional might begin with open-ended questions such as, "Can you tell me why you are here today?" If the child does not respond to open-ended questions, and many children do not, the professional then focuses the child's attention on a particular topic. When focused questions are used, the professional proceeds along a continuum, usually begin-

ning with questions that simply focus the child's attention on a particular subject, and then, when necessary, moving to more specific questions. Highly specific questions sometimes cross the line into leading questions.

Experienced professionals are skeptical of advice to begin interviews of young children with open-ended questions like, "Why are we here today?" Few young children understand, let alone disclose, abuse in response to such questions. Nevertheless, just as physicians are aware of the need for "defensive medicine" in other areas of practice, use of nonsuggestive, open-ended questions with children helps immunize professionals from legal challenge. A defense attorney has difficulty attacking a professional who begins an interview with open-ended questions, and who moves to more focused and, finally, mildly leading questions, only when open-ended questions prove unproductive. Thus the professional has little to lose and much to gain, forensically, by starting interviews with open-ended questions.

Although suggestive and leading questions should be avoided when possible, many occasions arise when suggestive and even mildly leading questions are necessary. The dynamics of abuse often work against disclosure (30,32). Many abused children are threatened into silence. Others are ambivalent about disclosure. In Lawson and Chaffin's (15) study of children with documented sexually transmitted disease, 57% of the children initially denied they had been abused.

The psychological dynamics of abuse are not the only barriers to disclosure. The developmental immaturity of young children further complicates the interview process. Young children are not so adept as older children and adolescents at responding to open-ended questions (10,22,24,27). It is not that young children have poor memories (6,28,29). Rather, young children often need cues to trigger their memories. In some cases, the necessary memory cue is a mildly leading question. When mildly leading questions are postponed until less suggestive methods prove unsuccessful, the professional is warranted in asking mildly leading questions (22,23).

CONFIDENTIAL RECORDS AND PRIVILEGED COMMUNICATIONS

Abused and neglected children interact with many professionals. Each professional who comes in contact with the child documents the interaction. Needless to say, much of this information is confidential and must be protected from inappropriate disclosure.

Sources of Confidentiality and Privilege

Confidentiality arises from three sources: (a) the broad ethical duty to protect confidential information, (b) laws that make certain records confidential, and (c) privileges that apply in legal proceedings.

Ethical Duty to Safeguard Confidential Information

The ethical principles of medicine, nursing, and other professions require professionals to safeguard confidential information revealed by patients. The principles of medical ethics of the American Medical Association require physicians to "safeguard patient confidences within the constraints of the law" (1). The Hippocratic oath states, "whatsoever I shall see or hear in the course of my profession . . . if it be what should not be published abroad, I will never divulge, holding such things to be holy secrets." The Code of Nurses of the American Nurses Association states that nurses safeguard the patient's right to privacy by carefully protecting information of a confidential nature (2).

Laws That Make Patient Records Confidential

Every state has laws that make certain records confidential. Some of the laws pertain to records compiled by government agencies, such as child-protective services, public hospitals, and the juvenile court. Other laws govern records created by professionals and institutions in the private sector, such as physicians, psychotherapists, and private hospitals.

Privileged Communications

The ethical duty to protect confidential information applies in all settings. In legal proceedings, however, certain professionals have an additional duty to protect confidential information. The law prohibits disclosure during legal proceedings of confidential communications between certain professionals and their patients. These laws are called privileges (20).

Unlike the across-the-board ethical obligation to protect confidential patient information, privileges apply only in legal proceedings. Privileges clearly apply when professionals testify in court and are asked to reveal privileged information. Privileges also apply during legal proceedings outside the courtroom. For example, in most civil cases, and in some criminal cases as well, attorneys take pretrial depositions of potential witnesses. If questions are asked during a deposition that call for privileged information, the professional or one of the attorneys should raise the privilege issue.

Communication between a patient and a professional is privileged when three requirements are fulfilled. First, the communication must be between a patient and a professional with whom privileged communication is possible. All states have some form of physician–patient privilege. Not all professions are covered by privilege statutes, however. For example, most states have a privilege for confidential communication between certain psychotherapists and their patients. If the patient communicates with a psychotherapist who is not covered by privilege law, however, no privilege applies. (A privilege may apply if the therapist not covered by a privilege is working under the supervision of a therapist who is covered by a privilege.) Of course, the fact that a privilege does not apply does nothing to undermine the therapist's ethical duty to protect confidential information.

In legal proceedings, the presence or absence of a privilege is important. In court, a professional may have to answer questions that require disclosure of information the professional is ethically bound to protect. By contrast, the professional generally does not have to answer questions that require disclosure of privileged information. Thus in legal proceedings, a privilege gives added protection to confidentiality, protection that is not available under the ethical duty to protect confidential information.

The second requirement for a privilege to apply is that the patient must seek professional services. The patient must consult the professional to obtain advice or therapy. If the patient enters therapy, the privilege applies to confidential communications leading up to and during therapy. If the patient does not formally enter therapy, the privilege may nevertheless apply to confidential communications between the patient and the professional. For example, a patient may consult a physician who refers the patient to a second professional. In most states, communication between the patient and the referring physician is privileged even though the patient does not receive treatment from the referring doctor.

The third requirement of privilege law is that only communications that the patient intends to be confidential are privileged. The privilege generally does not attach to communications that the patient intends to be released to other people.

The fact that a third person is present when a patient discloses information may or may not eliminate the confidentiality required for a privilege. The deciding factor usually is whether the third person is needed to assist the professional. For example, suppose a physician is conducting a physical examination and interview of a child. The presence of a nurse during the examination does not undermine the confidentiality of information revealed to the doctor. Furthermore, presence of the child's parents need not defeat confidentiality. Again, the important factor is whether the third person is needed to assist the professional. A privilege is not destroyed when colleagues consult about cases.

Privileged communications remain privileged when the relationship with the patient ends. In most situations, the patient's death does not end the privilege.

The privilege belongs to the patient, not the professional. In legal parlance, the patient is the "holder" of the privilege. As the privilege holder, the patient can prevent the professional from disclosing privileged information in legal proceedings. For example, suppose a treating physician is subpoenaed to testify about a patient. While the physician is on the witness stand, an attorney may ask a question that calls for privileged information. At that point, the patient's attorney should object. The patient's attorney asserts the privilege on behalf of the privilege holder—the patient. The judge then decides whether a privilege applies.

If the patient's attorney fails to object to a question calling for privileged information, or if the patient is not represented by an attorney, the professional may assert the privilege on behalf of the patient. Indeed, the professional may have an ethical duty to assert the privilege if no one else does. The professional might turn to the judge and say, "Your Honor, I would rather not answer that question because answering would require disclosure of information I believe is privileged." When the judge learns that a privilege may exist, the judge decides whether the question should be answered.

Disclosure of Confidential and Privileged Information

The following paragraphs concern disclosure of confidential and privileged information.

Patient Consent

Patient consent plays the central role in release of confidential or privileged information. As Gutheil and Appelbaum (11) observed, "With rare exceptions, identifiable data [about patients] can be transmitted to third parties only with the patient's explicit consent" (p. 5). A competent adult may consent to release of information to attorneys, courts, or anyone else. The patient's consent should be fully informed and voluntary. The professional should explain any disadvantages of disclosing confidential information. For example, the patient may be told that release to most third persons may waive privileges that would otherwise apply.

A professional who discloses confidential information without patient consent can be sued. With an eye toward such lawsuits, Gutheil and Appelbaum (11) wrote:

> [I]t is probably wise for therapists always to require the written consent of their patients before releasing information to third parties. Written consent is advisable for at least two reasons: (1) it makes clear to both parties involved that consent has, in fact, been given; (2) if the fact, nature or timing of the consent should ever be challenged, a documentary record exists. The consent should be made a part of the patient's permanent chart.

When the patient is a child, parents normally have authority to make decisions about confidential and privileged information. When a parent is accused of abusing or neglecting a child, however, it may be inappropriate for the parent to make decisions regarding the child's confidential information. In the event of a conflict between the interests of the child and the parents, the judge may appoint someone else, such as a guardian *ad litem,* to make decisions about confidential and privileged information.

Limitations on Privileges

Every privilege has limitations established by law. In most states, for example, the physician–patient privilege has numerous limitations. Mueller and Kirkpatrick (20) wrote "[m]ost states recognize numerous exceptions to the physician–patient privilege that significantly limit its scope. For example, the privilege is often made inapplicable in criminal cases . . . . (p. 466)."

Subpoenas

A subpoena is issued by a court at the request of an attorney. A subpoena is a court order, and it cannot be ignored. Disobedience of a subpoena can be punished as contempt of court.

The two types of subpoenas are (a) a subpoena requiring an individual to appear at a designated time and place to provide testimony, sometimes called a *subpoena ad testificandum,* and (b) a subpoena requiring a person to appear at a designated time and place, and to bring with them records or documents designated in the subpoena. A subpoena for records is sometimes called a *subpoena duces tecum.*

A subpoena does not override privileges such as the physician–patient and psychotherapist–patient privileges. The subpoena requires the professional to appear, but the subpoena does not mean the professional has to disclose privileged information. The judge decides whether a privilege applies and whether the professional has to answer questions or release records.

Before responding to a subpoena, the professional should contact the patient or, in the case of a child, a responsible adult. The patient may desire to release confidential or privileged information.

It is often useful, with the patient's permission, to communicate with the attorney issuing the subpoena. In some cases, the conversation lets the attorney know the professional has nothing that can assist the attorney, and the attorney withdraws the subpoena. Even if the attorney insists on compliance with the subpoena, the telephone conversation may clarify the limits of relevant information in the professional's possession. Naturally, care is taken during such conversations to avoid discussing confidential or privileged information.

If doubts exist concerning how to respond to a subpoena, consult an attorney. Needless to say, legal advice should not be obtained from the attorney who issued the subpoena.

Reviewing Client Records before or during Testimony

When a professional is asked to testify, portions of the child's medical record may be reviewed to refresh the professional's memory. In some cases, the professional leaves the record at the office, although sometimes the record is taken to court. In most cases, it is appropriate to review pertinent records before testifying. Indeed, such review is often essential for accurate and detailed testimony. Professionals should be aware, however, that reviewing records before or during testimony may compromise the confidentiality of the records.

Reviewing Records before *Testifying*

While the professional is on the witness stand, the attorney for the alleged perpetrator may ask whether the professional reviewed the child's record, and, if so, may request the judge to order the record produced for the attorney's inspection. In most states, the judge has authority to order the record produced. In favor of disclosure, the judge considers the attorney's right to cross-examine the professional, and the extent to which the record will assist cross-examination. Against disclosure, the judge evaluates the impact on the child of disclosing confidential information. The outcome turns on which of these factors predominates.

Referring to Records While *Testifying*

When records are reviewed *before* testifying, the judge is unlikely to order the record disclosed to the attorney for the alleged perpetrator. If the professional takes the record to court and refers to it *while* testifying, however, the judge is likely to order the record disclosed.

Protecting Records from Disclosure

Whether a professional reviews a child's record before or during testimony, a judge is more likely to require disclosure of nonprivileged records than of records that are protected by the physician–patient or psychotherapist–patient privileges. Unfortunately, in most states, the law is unsettled regarding the impact of record review on privileged communications. With the law unsettled, simple steps can be taken to reduce the likelihood that reviewing records will jeopardize confidentiality. Before implementing any of these recommendations, however, consult an attorney.

First, when reviewing a child's record before going to court, limit review to portions of the record that are needed to prepare for testifying. Document the parts of the record reviewed and not reviewed. In this way, if the

judge orders the record disclosed to the attorney for the alleged perpetrator, an argument can be made that disclosure should be limited to portions of the record actually used to prepare for testifying.

Second, recall that records containing privileged communications probably have greater protection from disclosure than do nonprivileged records. With this distinction in mind, professionals may wish to organize records so that privileged information is maintained separately from nonprivileged information. When a record organized in this manner is reviewed before testifying, it is sometimes possible to avoid review of privileged communications. This done, if a judge orders the record disclosed, the judge may be willing to limit disclosure to nonprivileged portions of the record. Although this approach entails the burden of separating records into privileged and nonprivileged sections, and may not persuade all judges, the technique is worth considering, especially for professionals who testify regularly.

Third, if it is necessary to take the record to court, consider taking only the portions of the record that will be useful during testimony and leaving the remainder at the office.

Fourth, if the record is taken to court, perhaps the record can remain in the briefcase rather than be taken to the witness stand. Make no mention of the record unless it becomes necessary to refer to it while testifying. Once the record is used during testimony, the attorney for the alleged perpetrator may have a right to inspect it.

Fifth, if the record is taken to court and to the witness stand, it may be possible to testify without referring to the record.

Again, legal advice should be obtained before implementing any of the foregoing suggestions. Some of the recommendations may not be permitted in some states.

Child Abuse Reporting Laws Override Confidentiality and Privilege

Child abuse reporting laws require professionals to report suspected child abuse and neglect to designated authorities (14). The reporting laws override the ethical duty to protect confidential client information. Moreover, the reporting requirement overrides privileges for confidential communications between professionals and their patients.

Although reporting laws abrogate privileges, abrogation usually is not complete. In many states, professionals may limit the information they report to the specific information required by law. Information that is not required to be reported remains privileged.

Psychotherapist's Duty to Warn Potential Victims about Dangerous Clients

In 1974, the California Supreme Court ruled in *Tarasoff v. Regents of the University of California* (33) that a psychotherapist has a legal duty to warn the potential victim of a psychiatric patient who threatens the victim. The duty to warn overcomes both the ethical duty to protect confidential information and the psychotherapist–patient privilege. If the therapist fails to take reasonable steps to warn the victim, and the patient carries out the threat, the therapist can be sued (22).

Since the *Tarasoff* case was decided, judges have grappled with the difficult question of when professionals have a legal duty to warn potential victims. Unfortunately, in most states, the law remains unsettled. Most judges agree that there is a legal duty to warn potential victims, but judges have not achieved consensus on when the duty applies. In 1985, California enacted a statute (4) on the subject, which limits the duty to warn to situations in which "the patient has communicated to the psychotherapist a serious threat of physical violence against a reasonably identifiable victim or victims." (Cal. Civil Code §43.92).

Emergencies

In emergencies, a professional may have little choice but to release confidential information without prior authorization from the patient. The law allows release of confidential information in genuine emergencies (11).

Court-Ordered Examinations

A judge may order an individual to submit to a medical examination or a psychological evaluation to help the judge decide the case. Because everyone knows from the outset that the professional's report will be shared with the judge and the attorneys, the obligation to protect confidential information is limited.

OBLIGATION TO REPORT SUSPECTED ABUSE AND NEGLECT

Professionals who work with children are required to report suspected abuse and neglect to designated authorities (14). The list of mandated reporters includes physicians, nurses, mental health professionals, social workers, and day-care providers. In most states, mandated reporters have no discretion whether to report. Reporting is mandatory, not optional.

The reporting requirement is triggered when a professional possesses a prescribed level of suspicion that a child is abused or neglected. The terms used to describe the triggering level of suspicion vary slightly from state to state, and include "cause to believe," "reasonable cause to believe," "known or suspected abuse," and "observation or examination which discloses evidence of abuse." Despite shades of difference, the basic meaning of the reporting laws is the same across the country. Reporting is required when a professional has evidence that would lead a reasonable professional to believe abuse or neglect is likely.

The duty to report does not require the professional to "know" that abuse or neglect occurred. All that is required is information that raises a reasonable suspicion of maltreatment. A mandated reporter who postpones reporting until all doubt is eliminated probably violates the reporting law.

A substantial number of reporting laws authorize designated professionals to photograph or radiograph children without parental consent.

EXPERT TESTIMONY IN CHILD ABUSE LITIGATION

Expert testimony plays a critical role in child abuse litigation (23). Such testimony is provided by physicians, nurses, psychologists, social workers, and other professionals.

Who Qualifies as an Expert Witness

Before a professional may testify as an expert witness, the judge must be convinced that the professional possesses sufficient knowledge, skill, experience, training, or education to qualify as an expert. Normally, the proposed expert takes the witness stand and answers questions about the professional's educational accomplishments, specialized training, and relevant experience.

Preparation for Expert Testimony

When a professional prepares to testify, it is important to meet with the attorney for whom the expert will testify. Nothing about pretrial conferences is ethically or legally improper. Chadwick (5) observed, "[f]ace-to-face conferences between . . . attorneys and [expert witnesses] are always desirable, and rarely impossible" (p. 936).

Form of Expert Testimony

Expert testimony usually takes one of three forms: (a) an opinion, (b) an answer to a hypothetical question, or (c) a lecture providing background information for the judge or jury. The most common form of expert testimony is an opinion, although in child sexual abuse cases, expert testimony often takes the form of a lecture designed to help jurors understand the psychological dynamics of sexual abuse.

Opinion Testimony

Expert witnesses are permitted to offer professional opinions. For example, in a physical abuse case, a physician could testify that, in the doctor's opinion, the child has battered child syndrome, and the child's injuries are not accidental. In a neglect case, an expert could offer an opinion that a child's failure to thrive is caused by parental behavior.

The expert must be reasonably confident of the opinion. Lawyers use the term "reasonable certainty" to describe the necessary degree of confidence. Unfortunately, reasonable certainty is not easily defined. How certain must the expert be to be reasonably certain? It is clear that expert witnesses may not speculate or guess. It is equally clear that experts do not have to be completely certain before offering opinions; thus the degree of certainty lies somewhere between guesswork and absolute certainty.

In the final analysis, the reasonable certainty standard provides little guidance. A more useful way to assess the strength of expert testimony looks beyond reasonable certainty, and asks questions that shed light on the factual and logical strength of the expert's opinion: In formulating the opinion, did the expert consider all relevant facts? Did the expert have adequate understanding of pertinent clinical and scientific principles? Did the expert use methods of assessment that are appropriate, reliable, and valid? Are the expert's assumptions and conclusions reasonable? Is the expert reasonably objective? In the end, the issue is whether the expert's reasoning is logical, consistent, and reasonably objective.

The Hypothetical Question

In some cases, expert testimony is elicited in response to a hypothetical question asked by the attorney who requested the expert's testimony. A hypothetical question contains facts that closely parallel the facts of the actual case on trial. In a physical abuse case, for example, the attorney might say, "Now doctor, let me ask you to assume that all of the following facts are true." The attorney then describes injuries suffered by a hypothetical child. After describing the hypothetical child, the attorney asks, "Doctor, based on these hypothetical facts, do you have an opinion, based on a reasonable degree of medical certainty, whether the hypothetical child's injuries were accidental or nonaccidental?" The doctor gives an opinion about the hypothetical child's injuries. The jury then applies the information supplied by the doctor regarding the hypothetical child to the injuries suffered by the actual child in the case on trial.

In bygone days, expert witnesses nearly always testified in response to a hypothetical question, yet the hypothetical question is a cumbersome device, and it gradually fell into disfavor. Today expert witnesses usually take the more direct approach of offering an opinion about the child in the case on trial, rather than an opinion about a hypothetical child. In modern trials, it is usually the cross-examining attorney who resorts to hypothetical questions. The cross-examiner seeks to undermine the expert's opinion by presenting a hypothetical set of facts that differs from the facts described by the expert. The cross-examiner then asks, "Now doctor, if the hypothetical facts I have suggested to you turn out to be true, would that change your opinion?" Chadwick (5) observed that it is "common to encounter hypothetical questions based on hypotheses that are extremely unlikely, and the [expert] witness may need to point out the unlikelihood" (p. 967).

A Background Lecture to Educate the Jury

Rather than offer an opinion, an expert may testify in the form of a lecture that provides the jury with background information on technical, clinical, or scientific issues. This form of expert testimony plays an important role in child sexual abuse litigation when the defense asserts that a child's delayed reporting or recantation means the child cannot be believed. When the defense attacks the child's credibility in this way, judges allow an expert witness to inform the jury that it is not uncommon for sexually abused children to delay reporting and to recant. Equipped with this background information, the jury is in a better position to evaluate the child's credibility (21).

Physical Abuse Cases

When physical abuse is alleged, the most common defense is that the child's injuries were accidental. Expert testimony plays a key role in proving nonaccidental injury. Judges routinely allow physicians to testify that a child has battered child syndrome. A physician may testify that a child's injuries are probably not accidental. In addition, judges allow physicians to describe the means used to inflict injury. For example, a physician may testify that a skull fracture was probably caused by a blow from a blunt instrument, such as a fist. Experts are permitted to estimate the amount of force required to inflict injury. Judges generally allow physicians to state whether a caretaker's explanation for injuries is reasonable. Judges allow expert witnesses to describe shaken baby syndrome, Munchausen syndrome by proxy, and other evidence of nonaccidental injury.

When physical abuse is suspected, the following information should be documented in the child's chart: (a) unexplained injury, (b) implausible explanation offered by caretaker, (c) caretakers with inconsistent explanations, (d) caretakers claim injuries inflicted by a sibling, and (e) delay in seeking medical care for serious or life-threatening conditions.

Sexual Abuse Litigation

Expert testimony regarding child sexual abuse can be divided into two categories: (a) expert testimony describing medical evidence of sexual abuse, and (b) expert testimony regarding the psychological effects of sexual abuse. Although these categories overlap, the distinction is important.

Medical and Laboratory Evidence

Uncertainty continues regarding some aspects of medical and laboratory evidence of sexual abuse (see Chapter 10). Nevertheless, when medical or laboratory evidence is available, judges permit medical professionals to describe such evidence. Moreover, judges allow physicians to describe the results of examinations aided by colposcopy. Judges permit physicians to use photographs and other visual aids to illustrate their testimony.

Psychological Effects of Sexual Abuse

Expert testimony regarding the psychological effects of sexual abuse is usefully divided into two categories. In the first category, the expert offers an opinion that a particular child was sexually abused, or that a child has a diagnosis of sexual abuse or symptoms consistent with sexual abuse. Expert testimony in this category focuses directly on the ultimate issue before the court: Was this child abused? Expert psychological testimony of this type is controversial (19,21,22).

The second category of expert testimony regarding the psychological effects of sexual abuse is less controversial than the first. In the second category, the expert does not offer an opinion that a particular child was sexually abused. Rather, the expert's testimony has the more limited purpose of explaining to the jury that certain behavior, such as delayed reporting and recantation, is relatively common in sexually abused children. As explained earlier, such expert testimony is permitted when the attorney for the alleged perpetrator attacks the child's credibility by attempting to persuade the jury to disbelieve the child because the child delayed reporting or recanted.

Expert Psychological Testimony That a Child Was Sexually Abused

When it comes to expert testimony from mental health professionals, commentators and judges disagree over whether such professionals should testify that particular children were sexually abused (19,21–23). Melton and Limber (18) wrote, "under no circumstances should a court admit the opinion of an expert about whether a particular child has been abused" (p. 1230). Contrary to this position, many professionals believe that, in some cases, properly qualified and experienced professionals can reach diagnostic decisions that help the courts decide whether children were sexually abused (21,22).

Expert Testimony to Rehabilitate Children's Credibility

One of the basic rules of the American legal system is that the credibility of a witness cannot be supported or bolstered until the witness's credibility is attacked. The process attorneys use to attack witnesses is called impeachment. In child sexual abuse litigation, two forms of impeachment are particularly common. First, the defense attorney may assert that a child's behavior is inconsistent with allegations of abuse. For example, defense counsel may argue that a child should not be believed because the child did not report abuse for a substantial period, or because the child recanted. Such impeachment is legitimate. When the defense concentrates on delay, recantation, and certain other behaviors, however, the prosecutor is generally allowed to respond with expert testimony to inform jurors that such behavior is relatively common in sexually abused children.

In the second form of impeachment, the defense attorney seeks to undermine the child's credibility by arguing that developmental differences between adults and children render children as a group less credible than adults. Defense counsel may assert that children are highly suggestible and have poor memories. In response to such impeachment, the prosecutor may offer expert testimony to inform jurors that children have adequate memories and are not as suggestible as many adults believe (12,16,21–24,28,29).

The following guidelines are suggested for professionals providing expert testimony to rehabilitate children's impeached credibility.

1. The prosecutor should tell the judge and the defense attorney which behavior(s) the expert will discuss. For example, if the defense attorney limits the attack on the child's credibility to delay in reporting, the prosecutor informs the judge and defense counsel that the expert's testimony will be limited to helping the jury understand delay. The expert who serves the limited function of rehabilitating a child's credibility should limit testimony to the behavior emphasized by the de-

.fense attorney, and should not offer a broad-ranging lecture on children's reactions to sexual abuse.

2. In many cases, expert rehabilitation testimony is limited to a description of behaviors seen in sexually abused children as a group, and the expert avoids mentioning the child in the present case.
3. If it is appropriate to refer to the child in the present case, avoid referring to the child as a "victim."
4. In most sexual abuse cases, avoid reference to syndromes such as child sexual abuse accommodation syndrome (CSAAS) (32). One does not need to use the word "syndrome" to help the jury understand that delay in reporting, recantation, and inconsistency are relatively common in sexually abused children.

Although experts are allowed to rehabilitate children's credibility by explaining behaviors such as delayed reporting and recantation, experts are not permitted to testify that particular children told the truth, or that sexually abused children as a group generally tell the truth about abuse.

Expert Testimony Regarding Syndromes

The legal system is comfortable with medical syndromes that are offered in court to prove physical abuse. Thus judges routinely allow expert testimony on battered child syndrome, shaken baby syndrome, and Munchausen syndrome by proxy. When it comes to sexual abuse, however, no syndrome—medical or psychological—detects or diagnoses sexual abuse. Although no psychological syndrome is pathognomonic of sexual abuse, several psychological syndromes play subsidiary roles in child sexual abuse litigation. Five psychological syndromes are briefly discussed.

Child Sexual Abuse Accommodation Syndrome

Summit (32) described CSAAS. CSAAS includes five characteristics commonly observed in sexually abused children: (a) se-

crecy; (b) helplessness; (c) entrapment and accommodation; (d) delayed, conflicted, and unconvincing disclosure; and (e) retraction. Summit's purpose in describing CSAAS was to provide a common language for professionals working to protect sexually abused children. Summit did not intend CSAAS as a diagnostic device. Summit observed, "[t]he accommodation syndrome is neither an illness nor a diagnosis, and it can't be used to measure whether or not a child has been sexually abused" (17). The accommodation syndrome does not detect sexual abuse. Rather, CSAAS assumes that abuse occurred, and explains the child's reaction to it.

The accommodation syndrome has a place in the courtroom, not as proof that a child was abused, but to help explain why many sexually abused children delay reporting their abuse, and why some children recant allegations of abuse. When the syndrome is confined to this explanatory purpose, the syndrome serves a useful forensic function.

Rape Trauma Syndrome

Rape trauma syndrome (RTS) was described by Burgess and Holmstrom in 1974 as

> . . . the acute phase and long-term reorganization process that occurs as a result of forcible rape or attempted forcible rape. This syndrome of behavioral, somatic, and psychological reactions is an acute stress reaction to a life-threatening situation (3).

Although expert testimony on RTS is used most frequently in litigation involving adult victims, RTS is sometimes useful in child sexual abuse litigation. Expert testimony on RTS has been offered by prosecutors for two purposes: (a) to prove lack of consent to sexual relations, and (b) to explain certain behaviors, such as delay in reporting rape, which jurors might misconstrue as evidence that rape did not occur.

Proving Lack of Consent

In rape cases involving adult victims, the evidence often focuses on whether the victim consented. Courts are divided on the admissibility of RTS to prove lack of consent. Some courts reject RTS to prove lack of consent. In *People v. Taylor* (26), for example, the New York Court of Appeals wrote, "evidence of rape trauma syndrome does not by itself prove that the complainant was raped" (p. 135). The court concluded, "evidence of rape trauma syndrome is inadmissible when it inescapably bears solely on proving that a rape occurred" (p. 138). The California Supreme Court reached a similar result in *People v. Bledsoe* (25), in which the Court ruled, "expert testimony that a complaining witness suffers from rape trauma syndrome is not admissible to prove that the witness was raped" (p. 301).

In contrast to the New York and California courts, several courts stated that RTS is admissible when the defendant asserts that the woman consented (21). In *State v. Marks* (31), for example, the Kansas Supreme Court wrote, "[w]hen consent is the defense in a prosecution for rape qualified expert psychiatric testimony regarding the existence of `rape trauma syndrome' is relevant and admissible" (p. 1294).

It should be remembered that when the victim is a child, consent is not generally an issue because children are legally incapable of consenting to sexual relations.

Rape Trauma Syndrome to Explain the Victim's Behavior after the Attack

Most courts allow expert testimony on RTS to rehabilitate a child or adult victim's credibility after the defense attorney attacks the victim's credibility by emphasizing delayed reporting and other behaviors that jurors might construe as evidence the rape did not occur. In *People v. Bledsoe* (25) for example, the California Supreme Court wrote, "expert testimony on rape trauma syndrome may play a particularly useful role by disabusing the jury of some widely held misconceptions about rape and rape victims, so that it may evaluate the evidence free of the constraints of, popular myths" (p. 457). In *People v.* Taylor (26), the New York Court of Appeals approved expert testimony explaining why a rape victim might not appear upset after the assault.

Courts that allow RTS to explain behaviors observed in rape victims place limits on such evidence. Thus several court decisions stated that the expert should describe behaviors observed in rape victims as a group, and should not refer to the victim in the case at hand (21).

Posttraumatic Stress Disorder

Judges generally permit qualified experts to testify that a patient has a diagnosis of posttraumatic stress disorder (21).

Parental Alienation Syndrome

Gardner (9) described parental alienation syndrome (PAS) as a psychiatric disorder that is observed in some parents fighting over custody of children in divorce court. One parent— the alienating parent—programs the child to revile the other parent. When one divorcing parent accuses the other of abusing their child, PAS is used to support an argument that the accusation is a lie. Of course, false accusations do arise in bitter custody disputes. Conversely, many accusations appear to be true. In still other cases, the accusation is unfounded, but the accusing parent makes the accusation in the good-faith belief that abuse happened. The important point here is that PAS does not help distinguish true from false accusations. PAS is not diagnostic. The syndrome does not detect false accusations or, for that matter, true accusations. Unfortunately, PAS is often used unfairly to attack the credibility of parents—usually mothers—who allege abuse. In the final analysis, everyone would be better off to discontinue use of the term PAS, and to evaluate accusations of abuse on their individual merits.

CROSS-EXAMINATION AND IMPEACHMENT OF EXPERT WITNESSES

Testifying begins with direct examination. During direct examination, the expert witness answers questions from the attorney who asked the expert to testify. After direct examination, the opposing attorney has the right to cross-examine. Cross-examination is sometimes followed by redirect examination. Redirect examination affords the attorney who asked the expert to testify an opportunity to clarify issues that were discussed during cross-examination.

Cross-examination causes anxiety. The following discussion is intended to demystify cross-examination by explaining six techniques commonly used by cross-examining attorneys.

Raise Doubts about the Expert's Testimony: Doubts That Will Be Emphasized during Closing Argument

At the end of the case, the attorneys present closing arguments. One goal of closing argument is to persuade the jury to disbelieve certain witnesses. With closing argument in mind, the attorney uses cross-examination to raise doubts about the expert's testimony. Closing argument is used to remind the jury of those doubts.

Leading Questions

The attorney conducting direct examination is generally not allowed to ask leading questions. By contrast, the cross-examiner is permitted to do so, and some attorneys ask only leading questions during cross-examination. The cross-examiner attempts to control the expert by using leading questions that require short, specific answers, answers the attorney wants the jury to hear. The cross-examiner keeps the witness hemmed in with leading questions, and seldom asks why or how something happened. How and why questions permit the witness to explain, and explanation is precisely what the cross-examiner does not want.

Limit the Expert's Ability to Explain

When an expert attempts to explain an answer, the cross-examining attorney may interrupt and say, "Please just answer yes or no." If the expert persists, the cross-examiner may ask the judge to admonish the expert to limit answers to the questions asked. Experts are understandably frustrated when an attorney thwarts efforts at clarification. It is sometimes proper to say, "Counsel, it is not possible for me to answer with a simple yes or no. May I explain myself?" Chadwick (5) advised, "[w]hen a question is posed in a strictly 'yes or no' fashion, but the correct answer is 'maybe,' the witness should find a way to express the true answer. A direct appeal to the judge may be helpful in some cases" (p. 967). Many judges permit witnesses to explain themselves during cross-examination if the jury needs more information to make sense of the witness's testimony.

Remember that after cross-examination comes redirect examination, during which the attorney who asked the expert to testify is allowed to ask further questions. During redirect examination, the expert has an opportunity to clarify matters that were left unclear during cross-examination.

Undermine the Expert's Assumptions

One of the most effective cross-examination techniques is to commit the expert witness to the facts and assumptions that support the expert's opinion, and then to dispute one or more of those facts or assumptions. Consider, for example, a case in which a physician testifies on direct examination that a child experienced vaginal penetration. The cross-examiner begins by committing the doctor to the facts and assumptions underlying the opinion. The attorney might say, "So doctor, your opinion is based exclusively on the history, the physical examination, and on what the child told you. Is that correct?" "And there is nothing else you relied on to form your opinion. Is that correct?" The cross-examiner commits the doctor to a specific set of facts and assumptions so that when the attorney disputes those facts or assumptions, the doctor's opinion cannot be justified on some other basis.

Once the cross-examiner pins down the basis of the doctor's opinion, the examiner attacks the opinion by disputing one or more of the facts or assumptions that support it. The attorney might ask whether the doctor's opinion would change if certain facts were different. The attorney might press the doctor to acknowledge alternative explanations for the doctor's conclusion. The attorney might ask the doctor whether experts could come to different conclusions based on the same facts. Finally, the cross-examiner might confront the doctor with a hypothetical question that favors the examiner's client.

Rather than attack the doctor's assumptions and conclusions during cross-examination, the attorney may limit cross-examination to pinning the doctor down to a limited set of facts and assumptions, and then, when the doctor has left the witness stand, offer another expert to contradict those facts and assumptions.

Impeach the Expert with a "Learned Treatise"

The judge may allow a cross-examining attorney to undermine an expert's testimony by confronting the expert with books or articles (called learned treatises) that contradict the expert. The rules on impeachment with learned treatises vary from state to state. There is agreement on one thing, however. When an expert is confronted with a sentence or a paragraph selected by an attorney from an article or chapter, the expert has the right to put the selected passage in context by reading surrounding material. The expert might say to the cross-examining attorney, "Counsel, I cannot comment on the sentence you have selected unless I first read the entire article. If you will permit me to read the article, I'll be happy to comment on the sentence that interests you."

Raise the Possibility of Bias

The cross-examiner may raise the possibility that the expert is biased in favor of one side of the litigation. For example, if the expert is part of a multidisciplinary child abuse team, the cross-examiner might proceed as follows:

Question 1: Now doctor, you are employed by Children's Hospital, isn't that correct?
Right.

Question 2: At the hospital, are you a member of the multidisciplinary team that investigates allegations of child abuse?
The team performs medical examinations and interviews. We do not investigate as the police investigate. But yes, I am a member of the hospital's multidisciplinary child abuse team.

Question 3: Your team regularly performs investigative examinations and interviews at the request of the prosecuting attorney's office, isn't that correct?
Yes.

Question 4: When you complete your investigation for the prosecutor, you prepare a report for the prosecutor, don't you?
A report and recommendation is prepared and placed in the child's medical record. On request, the team provides a copy of the report to the prosecutor and, I might add, to the defense.

Question 5: After your team prepares its report and provides a copy to the prosecutor, you often come to court to testify as an expert witness for the prosecution in child abuse cases, isn't that right, doctor?
Yes.

Question 6: Do you usually testify for the prosecution rather than the defense?
Correct.

Question 7: In fact, would I be correct in saying that you always testify for the prosecution and never for the defense?
I am willing to testify for the defense, but so far I have always testified for the prosecution.

Question 8: Thank you, doctor. I have no further questions.

Clearly, the cross-examiner is seeking to portray the doctor as biased in favor of the prosecution. Notice, however, that the cross-examiner is too cunning to ask, "Well then, doctor, isn't it a fact that because of your close working relationship with the prosecution, you are biased in favor of the prosecution?" The cross-examiner knows that the answer to that question is a truthful and indignant "No." So the cross-examiner refrains from asking directly about bias, and simply plants seeds of doubt in the jurors' minds. When it is time for the defense to give its closing argument, the defense attorney will remind the jury of the doctor's close working relationship with the prosecution, "A relationship, ladies and gentlemen of the jury, that is just a little too cozy." What is the antidote to this tactic? First, the doctor may find an opportunity to indicate lack of bias during cross-examination itself. Second, remember that cross-examination is followed by redirect examination. During redirect, the prosecutor may ask, "Doctor, in light of the defense attorney's questions about your job on the multidisciplinary team, are you biased in favor of the prosecution?" Now the doctor can set the record straight.

CONCLUSION

The professions of medicine and law sometimes seem like ships passing in the night, yet if children are to be protected, physicians and attorneys must put aside their differences and work together. Only genuine interdisciplinary cooperation holds realistic hope of reducing the tragic number of abused and neglected children.

REFERENCES

1. American Medical Association. *Principles of medical ethics.* Chicago: American Medical Association, 1989.
2. American Nurses Association. *Code for nurses.* Washington, DC: American Nurses Association, 1985.
3. Burgess A, Holmstrom L. Rape trauma syndrome. *Am J Psychiatry* 1974;131:981–986.
4. *California Civil Code.* St. Paul, MN. West Publishing, 1999.
5. Chadwick DL. Preparation for court testimony in child abuse cases. *Pediatr Clin North Am* 1990;37:955–970.
6. Fivush R. Developmental perspectives on autobiographical recall. In: Goodman GS, Bottoms BL, eds. *Child victims, child witnesses: understanding and improving children's testimony.* New York: Guilford Press, 1992:1–24.
7. Friedrich WN, Brambsch P, Broughton K, et al. Normative sexual behavior in children. *Pediatrics* 1991;88:456–464.
8. Friedrich WN, Brambsch P, Damon L, et al. Child Sexual Behavior Inventory: normative and clinical comparisons. *Psychol Assess* 1992;4:303–311.
9. Gardner RA. *The parental alienation syndrome: a guide for mental health and legal professionals.* Cresskil, NJ: Creative Therapeutics, 1992.
10. Goodman GS, Bottoms BL. *Child victims, child witnesses: understanding and improving testimony.* New York: Guilford, 1993.
11. Gutheil TG, Appelbaum PS. *Clinical handbook of psychiatry and the law.* New York: McGraw-Hill, 1982.
12. Hewitt SK. *Assessing allegations of sexual abuse in preschool children: understanding small voices.* Thousand Oaks, CA: Sage, 1998.
13. Jones DPH, McQuiston M. *Interviewing the sexually abused child.* Denver, CO: C. Henry Kempe National Center for the Prevention and Treatment of Child Abuse and Neglect, 1985.
14. Kalichman SC. *Mandated reporting of suspected child abuse: ethics, law, and policy.* Washington, DC: American Psychological Association, 1993.
15. Lawson L, Chaffin M. False negatives in sexual abuse disclosure interviews: incidence and influence of caretaker's belief in abuse cases of accidental abuse disclosure by diagnosis of STD. *J Interpersonal Violence* 1992;7:532–542.
16. Lyon TD. The new wave in children's suggestibility research: a critique. *Cornell Law J* 1999;84:1004–1086.
17. Meinig MB. Profile of Roland Summit. *Violence Update* 1991;1:6–7.
18. Melton GB, Limber S. Psychologists' involvement in cases of child maltreatment. *Am Psychol* 1989;44:1225–1233.
19. Melton GB, Petrila J, Poythress N, et al. *Psychological evaluations for the courts.* 2nd ed. New York: Guilford, 1997.
20. Mueller CB, Kirkpatrick LC. *Federal evidence.* 2nd ed. Rochester, NY: Lawyers Cooperative Publishing, 1994.
21. Myers JEB. *Evidence in child abuse and neglect cases.* 2nd ed. New York: Aspen Law & Business, 1997.
22. Myers JEB. *Legal issues in child abuse and neglect practice.* 2nd ed. Thousand Oaks, CA: Sage, 1998.
23. Myers JEB, Bays J, Becker JV, et al. Expert testimony in child sexual abuse litigation. *Nebr Law Rev* 1989;68:1–145.
24. Myers JEB, Saywitz KJ, Goodman GS. Psychological research on children as witnesses: practical implications for forensic interviews and courtroom testimony. *Pacific Law J* 1996;28:3–92.
25. *People v. Bledsoe,* 681 P.2d 291, California, 1984.
26. *People v. Taylor,* 552 N.E.2d 131, New York, 1990.
27. Poole DA, Lamb ME. *Investigative interviews of children.* Washington DC: American Psychological Association, 1998.
28. Quas JA, Goodman GS, Bidrose S, et al. Emotion and memory: children's long-term remembering, forgetting, and suggestibility. *J Exp Child Psychol* 1999;72:235–270.
29. Ricci CM, Beal CR. Child witnesses: effect of event knowledge on memory and suggestibility. *J Appl Dev Psychol* 1998;19:305–317.
30. Saywitz KJ, Goodman GS, Nicholas E, et al. Children's memories of a physical examination involving genital touch: implications for reports of child sexual abuse. *J Consult Clin Psychol* 1991;59:682–691.
31. *State v. Marks,* 647 P.2d 1292, Kansas, 1982.
32. Summit RC. The child sexual abuse accommodation syndrome. *Child Abuse Negl* 1983;7:177–193.
33. *Tarasoff v. Regents of the University of California,* 551 P.2d 334, California, 1976.

Subject Index

Page numbers followed by an f indicate figures; those followed by a t indicate tables.